Blood Group Serology

Useful Phenotype Frequencies (as approximate percentages) in the Western European Population

A_1	35	R_1R_1	18	Fy(a+b−)	18	Haptoglobin 1	16
A_2	10	R_1r	33	Fy(a+b+)	48	Haptoglobin 2–1	48
B	8	R_2R_2	3	Fy(a−b+)	34	Haptoglobin 2	36
O	44	R_2r	13				
A_1B	2.6	R_1R_2	14	Jk(a+b−)	26	Gc1	56
A_2B	0.6	R_0r	2	Jk(a+b+)	50	Gc2–1	38
		r′r	0.37	Jk(a−b+)	24	Gc 2	6
MS+	20	r″r	0.23				
MS−	10	rr	15	Lu(a+b−)	0.15		
NS+	6			Lu(a+b+)	7.5	Gm(1,−2)	36
NS−	15			Lu(a−b+)	92	Gm(1,2,)	23
MNS+	26	K+	9			Gm(−1−2)	42
MNS−	23	K−	91				
S+s−	11			Le(a+b−)	23		
S+s+	44	P_1	79	Le(a−b+)	71	Xg(a+) males	65.6
S−s+	45	P_2	21	Le(a−b−)	6	Xg(a+) females	88.7

Useful Gene Frequencies

A^1	0.21		Fy^a	0.43
A^2	0.07		Fy^b	0.56
B	0.06		Fy	0.01
O	0.66			
			Jk^a	0.51
MS	0.24		Jk^b	0.49
Ms	0.28			
NS	0.08		Lu^a	0.04
Ns	0.40		Lu^b	0.96
R^1 (CDe)	0.41		Le	0.82
R^2 (cDE)	0.14		le	0.18
R^0 (cDe)	0.03			
R^z (CDE)	0.002		Se	0.52
r′ (Cde)	0.01		se	0.48
r″ (cdE)	0.01			
r (cde)	0.39		Hp^1	0.42
			Hp^2	0.58
K	0.05			
k	0.95		Gc^1	0.73
			Gc^2	0.27
P^1	0.54		Xg^a	0.66
P^2	0.46		Xg	0.34

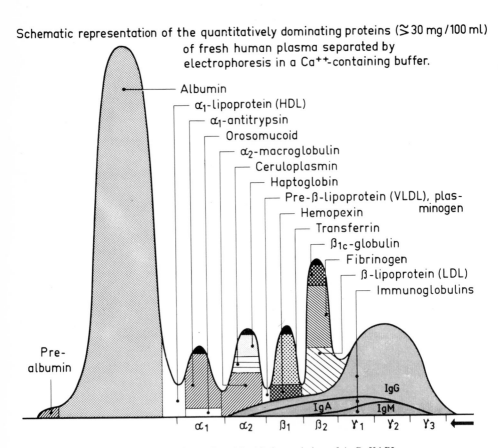

Schematic representation of the quantitatively dominating proteins ($\gtrsim 30$ mg/100 ml) of fresh human plasma separated by electrophoresis in a Ca^{++}-containing buffer.

Frontispiece.   Reproduced by kind permission of A. B. KABI

Blood Group Serology

THEORY, TECHNIQUES, PRACTICAL APPLICATIONS

Kathleen E. Boorman
M. I. Biol.
Formerly of South London Blood Transfusion Centre,
Tooting, London

Barbara E. Dodd
M.Sc. (Lond.), Ph.D. (Lond.), D.Sc. (Lond.)
Reader in Blood Group Serology
Departments of Forensic Medicine and Haematology
The London Hospital Medical College

P. J. Lincoln
B.Sc., Ph.D.
Senior Lecturer in Blood Group Serology,
Departments of Forensic Medicine and Haematology
The London Hospital Medical College

FIFTH EDITION

CHURCHILL LIVINGSTONE
EDINBURGH LONDON AND NEW YORK 1977

CHURCHILL LIVINGSTONE
Medical Division of Longman Group Limited

Distributed in the United States of America by
Longman Inc., 19 West 44th Street, New York, N.Y.
10036 and by associated companies, branches and
representatives throughout the world.

First Edition 1957
Second Edition 1961
Third Edition 1966
Fourth Edition 1970
  Reprinted 1973
Fifth edition 1977

ISBN 0 443 01475 2

Library of Congress Cataloging in Publication Data

Boorman, Kathleen E
  Blood group serology.

  First-4th ed. published under title: An introduction
to blood group serology.
  Includes bibliographies and index.
  1. Blood groups. 2. Blood–Examination. 3. Compatibility testing (Hematology). I. Dodd, Barbara E.,
joint author. II. Lincoln, Patrick J., joint author.
III. Title.
RB45.5 B66 1977   612′.11825   76-44375

Printed in Great Britain by T. & A. Constable Ltd., Edinburgh

Preface to the Fifth Edition

It will be apparent to readers familiar with our Fourth Edition that the book has now been considerably restyled. We have deleted the words 'An introduction to' from the book's title and have made Part I 'An introduction to blood group serology'. This is because much of Part II and Part III now contain more advanced and detailed accounts of various aspects of the subject than we have attempted in previous editions. There are a number of new chapters (nos. 15, 19, 21, 28, 30, 31, 32) and many of the old ones have been largely re-written.

We fully realise that some readers may find methods excluded which they would have liked to have seen described here, but it has always been our policy to restrict the number of techniques of which we have little personal experience to as few as possible.

We have maintained the practice of giving a short bibliography at the end of each section in Part I while in later chapters we include references which are intended to encourage further reading and we have included many papers which themselves have long lists of useful references. Thus, this new edition is directed towards a wider readership. While maintaining the simplicity of approach in Part I for the benefit of newcomers to this field of study, we hope that much of the remainder of the book will appeal to the more experienced, such as those who have elected to take haematology and blood transfusion as their subject for H.N.C. in medical laboratory sciences.

We also have in mind those who are studying for the Special Examination in Serology set by the Institute of Medical Laboratory Science, particularly people who are eligible for this examination through qualification in another specialty, but have limited experience in blood group serology. We hope that the extended chapters together with their appended references will form a useful addition to whatever course of lectures is being followed for this examination.

We also hope that pathologists taking M.R.C.Path. in Blood Transfusion will find chapters that cover some of their syllabus.

However, we remain chiefly interested in producing a book that will meet the requirements of the routine blood transfusion laboratories whether these are in Transfusion Centres or hospitals.

London, 1977

K.E.B.
B.E.D.
P.J.L.

Preface to the First Edition

Several books have been written relating to blood group serology. Each has had its own emphasis; in one, technical methods, in another, the clinical importance, in another, racial distribution, etc. In this book our aim has been to deal with all aspects of the subject in such a way as to give a general picture but concentrating on those which relate to the working of a serological laboratory. The approach, therefore, is threefold, firstly theory, secondly technique, and thirdly laboratory and bench organisation. It is intended as a reference book suitable for all engaged in routine blood group serology, whether in the large transfusion centres, in specialised or in general pathological laboratories. For the benefit of those who do not specialise in blood group serology a table of contents of a "shortened version" which will meet almost all their needs is included. Technicians will also, it is hoped, find that this book covers all the aspects of the subject needed for the final examination in blood transfusion techniques of the Institute of Medical Laboratory Technology. There are some deliberate omissions, mainly in highly specialised fields. In short, we are concerned not so much with the "peaks" dear to the heart of the research worker but with the "plains" of the safe and competent handling of the larger volume of routine work.

The ABO blood groups are studied first and in considerable detail because these, the first human blood groups to be discovered, are still the most important. Moreover, the techniques involved in their determination form the basis of almost all blood grouping methods, those used for other blood group systems being to a large extent modifications using different reagents, media and temperatures of reaction.

We are much indebted to Dr. R. A. Zeitlin, Director of the South London Blood Transfusion Centre, at which so much of the experience necessary for the writing of this book was gained. We are grateful also for his helpful criticism of many of the chapters and his permission to publish the method of preparation of dried Anti-A slides, including figure.

We should like to acknowledge the kindness of Professor F. E. Camps, Director of the Department of Forensic Medicine, The London Hospital Medical College, in granting facilities which have greatly expedited the writing of the book.

Dr. S. R. M. Bushby and Miss E. W. Ikin have patiently read much of the first draft of the text. We are most grateful for their many useful suggestions. We should like to thank Dr. M. E. Mackay for valuable help.

We have been fortunate in having help from Miss E. M. Brooks and Miss D. A. Eeles in various ways, not least in the tedious task of reading proofs. All the photographs, including the photo-micrographs, are the work of Mr. A. E. Densham, and the black-and-white figures were drawn by Mr. W. T. J. McRae. We much appreciate the endless pains that they have taken. We should like to thank those who typed and re-typed the manuscript, and particularly Mrs. L. Joiner for the tables and some of the more complicated parts of the text.

We are indebted to Drs. R. R. Race and A. E. Mourant and to Blackwell Scientific Publications for permission to quote figures for various gene and blood group frequencies from their books, and to Dr. J. V. Dacie for allowing us to reproduce his scheme for the serological investigation of auto-antibody types of haemolytic anaemia.

There are many others whose work has contributed either directly or indirectly to this book; we appreciate, although we cannot enumerate, all that they have done.

The literature on blood group serology is so extensive that we have not attempted a comprehensive bibliography. We have, in the main, concentrated upon those papers in which new discoveries are described and those which themselves contain extensive references which the interested reader can consult. At points in the text we have mentioned standard works which deal more fully with particular aspects of the subject; to these we continually refer, since they are not only excellent in themselves but contain extensive references to original work.

KATHLEEN E. BOORMAN

BARBARA E. DODD

Acknowledgements

It is first of all, with pleasure, that Boorman and Dodd welcome Lincoln as a co-author of the Fifth Edition of this book. He has shouldered the burden with great enthusiasm and has brought a fresh appraisal which has been of immense value for the task of revision.

Secondly, we all three join in thanking those who have helped us in various ways and in particular our gratitude goes to those members of the staff of the South London Blood Transfusion Centre who have contributed new chapters. Mr. F. Sherwood has contributed the chapter on the HLA system (Chapter 19) and in the writing of this has consulted Dr. J. A. Sachs of the Tissue Immunology Research Unit of the London Hospital Medical College. Mr. Sherwood has also given us material for Chapter 21. The Australia antigen chapter has been contributed by Miss Barbara Cant while Chapter 32 on Blood Products has been written by Dr. K. Ll. Rogers.

We are grateful to the late Dr. K. L. G. Goldsmith, Director of the Blood Group Reference Laboratory, for material included in the section on anti-human globulin preparation in Appendix II.

The authors have been much encouraged in their efforts by the kindness of Professor J. M. Cameron of the Department of Forensic Medicine at the London Hospital Medical College and Dr. K. Ll. Rogers, Director of the South London Transfusion Centre. We much appreciate their support.

Mr. F. Quinton has helped us greatly in collating material and in proof reading and we should like to record our thanks to him.

We should also like to thank our secretary Mrs. Barbara Vandersypen who, not for the first time, has patiently and expertly typed her way through our untidy and sometimes almost illegible manuscripts.

Contents

PART 1
AN INTRODUCTION TO BLOOD GROUP SEROLOGY

Section 1. General Introduction

"Let me introduce you . . . said the Red Queen, Alice—Mutton; Mutton—Alice."

Lewis Carroll, THROUGH THE LOOKING GLASS

Chapter 1. Human Blood Groups— What Are They?

Blood groups are inherited characters which give rise to antigen-antibody systems. A short résumé therefore of the relevant theory both of antigens and antibodies and of genetics, is a useful starting point for an introduction to human blood group serology. For those who are not beginners in the field, a more advanced account of present-day antigen-antibody theory with special reference to blood group antigens and antibodies is given in Chapter 15 of this volume. The modern concepts of blood group genetics are dealt with under the individual systems in Part II and there is also a short assessment of the contribution of the study of human blood groups to modern genetic theory.

BLOOD GROUPS AS ANTIGEN-ANTIBODY SYSTEMS

The classical definitions of antigen and antibody are as follows:

1. An antigen is any substance which, when introduced parenterally into an individual who himself lacks that substance, stimulates the production of an antibody, and, when mixed with the antibody, reacts specifically with it in some observable way.
2. An antibody is a substance which appears in the plasma or body fluids as a result of stimulation by an antigen and which reacts specifically with that antigen in some observable way.

Although these definitions are not perfect in that antigens and antibodies are found which do not (or do not appear to) conform strictly to them, they are still the most useful definitions and remain valuable criteria by which this class of substances may be recognised.

Antigens

Antigens are substances of large molecular size, usually protein, sometimes having a polysaccharide component which determines the specificity while the

3

amino-acid component determines the antigenicity (*i.e.* the ability to stimulate the production of antibodies). While this is broadly true, some polysaccharides of large molecular size are in themselves weakly antigenic.

Substances which possess specificity but little or no antigenicity are called haptens. The group specific blood group substances which are secreted in saliva are examples of haptens. However, the distinction between haptenic and antigenic blood group substances is not clear-cut and whereas purified substances (haptens) are not strongly antigenic in rabbits unless previously combined with a protein, they do cause considerable antibody production when injected into man. Blood group antigens, especially those of the ABO system, are probably present in all cells of the body but have been most carefully studied in the red cell. There is evidence that they are situated at varying depths in the cell envelope. Any individual red cell carries a large number and variety of blood group antigens.

Antibodies

Antibodies are immunoglobulins and form part of the serum globulin; they are also found in other body fluids, *e.g.* saliva and urine. The immunoglobulins are subdivided into three main classes IgG, IgA and IgM. These are clearly seen in the Frontispiece where they have been separated by electrophoresis. While some antibody activity is associated with IgA, most blood group antibodies are either IgG or IgM.

These three classes can be differentiated in a number of ways. IgG has a smaller molecule than IgM, mol. w. 150,000 as opposed to 900,000. IgM antibodies are usually agglutinins causing red cells which contain the corresponding antigen to agglutinate in saline while IgG antibodies are mainly the so-called 'incomplete' antibodies which become attached to red cells of the appropriate type but do not cause them to agglutinate when suspended in saline. IgA antibodies when they occur are either saline agglutinins or incomplete antibodies. IgG antibodies have the property of being able to cross the placenta freely from mother to infant, while it is most unusual for IgA or IgM antibodies to do so. This means that when we are considering the possible effect of a maternal antibody on the foetus *in utero* it is the presence and strength of the IgG antibodies that we must determine.

However, it is important to realise that some IgG antibodies cause agglutination of red cells suspended in saline and not all IgM antibodies are agglutinins, some only sensitise red cells suspended in saline. IgG agglutinins are not necessarily different, physico-chemically, from IgG-incomplete antibodies. They seem to occur principally in the ABO system, which suggests their agglutinating ability is probably a function of the antigen rather than the antibody as ABO sites are extremely plentiful and moreover protrude from the red-cell surface. IgG agglutinins are found in many immune group O sera and examples of IgM incomplete antibodies are not infrequently found in the Rh system.

The specificity of an antibody is not necessarily related to whether the antibody is IgG or IgM. In fact antibodies of most specificities can be either IgG or IgM or both. When we deal with the separate blood group systems we shall indicate whether the antibodies are likely to be IgG or IgM and where they are mixtures how to show this and to reveal the presence of IgG antibodies in a mixture of IgG and IgM.

Naturally Occurring Antibodies

Naturally occurring antibodies are those found in a serum for which no specific antigenic stimulus causing their production can be traced. These antibodies may belong to many blood group systems but their frequency is variable. However in the ABO system they are regularly present in the serum of individuals who lack the corresponding antigen and in whom they develop during infancy at about 4-8 months and in late childhood attain a level which is maintained with little variation throughout life, tending to decrease in old age. The evidence for these antibodies in reality being immune rather than naturally occurring is discussed in chapter 15. In the P system the antibody anti-P_1 is common in P_1 negative persons. Other naturally occurring antibodies are found in only a few persons who lack the corresponding antigen; for instance, nearly all persons are Wr^a negative and yet only one per cent of all sera contain anti-Wr^a.

Immune Antibodies

In contrast to naturally occurring antibodies, those that are formed in response to a traceable stimulation by the corresponding antigen are termed immune antibodies. The process of formation of immune antibodies is called immunisation. If the process is brought about by the introduction of an antigen from another member of the same species it is called allo-immunisation and the antibodies formed, allo-antibodies. This production and increase of antibody in a serum is known as an immune response. Usually the peak of an immune response occurs 10-20 days after the injection of the antigen. In the process of immunisation there is a wide spectrum of antibody production and antibodies are formed from the stimulation of a single antigen differing from one another in physical and chemical properties and even to a certain extent in specificity.

Immune antibodies can be IgM, IgA or most commonly IgG. Some of the blood group systems in which antibodies are naturally occurring, can also form immune antibodies of the same specificity if there is stimulation by the corresponding antigen. For instance, a serum may contain naturally occurring anti-A and immune anti-A, most of the former will be IgM while the latter will often be a mixture of IgM and IgG. In some systems, such as Rh in which naturally occurring antibodies are uncommon, the immune antibody produced often follows the usual pattern of antibody production, in which IgM is produced first, followed by IgG as the immunisation continues so that many anti-Rh sera eventually contain mostly IgG antibodies. In some sera, almost all the Rh antibody is IgM. It will be seen later that these can either be sera with a high titre of saline agglutinins or of the "enzyme-type" antibody only detected by enzyme techniques.

Identification of IgG and IgM Antibodies

On account of their difference in reaction and ability to cross the placenta and possibly damage the foetus *in utero*, it may sometimes be important to know whether a given antibody is IgG or IgM or even IgA. These immunoglobulins can now be distinguished in many ways. Precipitation in agar and immunoelectro-phoresis will both show if IgG, IgA and IgM are present in a serum. For our present purpose, however, these techniques are not particularly helpful (although modifications can be devised) as they will only show whether the serum contains the usual amounts of IgG, IgA and IgM and not in which immunoglobulin fraction the antibody in which we are interested occurs, as the total quantity of IgG, IgA or IgM is not significantly altered by antibody production.

Techniques which actually fractionate the sera separating IgG from IgM are useful because the fractions can be tested individually for their antibody content. Such techniques are fractionation by means of DEAE cellulose or Sephadex G200 or ultracentrifugation. These techniques are mainly confined to specialist and research laboratories and will not be described in detail, though a simple modification of the DEAE fractionation is given in the chapter on haemolytic disease of the foetus, as it is a quick and useful method by which the specific antibody content of the IgG constituent of any serum can be determined. The general theory of these three techniques is as follows. When serum is allowed to pass down a column of diethylamino-ethyl cellulose (DEAE) which has been equilibrated with a buffer of pH 8.0 and molarity 0.02 (pH and molarity can be slightly varied, Mollison recommends pH 7.6 and 0.01M) only the IgG passes down the column. The other immunoglobulins (and indeed other proteins) being adsorbed onto the column. These other immunoglobulins can be successively eluted by increasing the molarity and decreasing the pH. The fractions can be concentrated to the original volume of the serum and the antibody content of each estimated.

Sephadex acts as a molecular sieve and when serum is washed through a column of this material the larger molecules come through faster than the smaller ones. The IgM fraction is thus obtained first and the IgG later (together with the IgA). Fraction I from a DEAE column produces the purest IgG, while fraction I from Sephadex produces pure IgM. Ultracentrifugation separates the various immunoglobulin molecules according to their molecular weights. It is usually performed on sucrose density gradients in which layers of sucrose of decreasing concentration are placed one on top of the other in a tube with antibody containing serum making the final layer.

Ultracentrifugation also does not separate IgG satisfactorily from IgA; moreover, the IgM which is spun down to the bottom is not completely free of the other immunoglobulins.

IgM and IgG molecules may be differentiated by treatment of the serum with sulphydryl compounds, the usual one being 2-mercapto-ethanol, when the IgM molecules split and are no longer capable of agglutinating red cells although they are sometimes able to sensitise the cells as can be shown by performing an indirect anti-human globulin test. IgG molecules on the other hand are not inactivated by 2-mercaptoethenol. (*see* Chapter 15).

IgM molecules can also be inactivated by heat. One method is to heat the serum at 56°C for 3 hours. This inactivates some IgM molecules, *e.g.* anti-P_1, but is less satisfactory for anti-A or anti-B.

IMMUNISATION

This is the process by which an individual produces antibodies in response to an antigen which he himself lacks. When the process is brought about by the introduction of an antigen from another member of the same species, it is known as allo-immunisation and the antibodies formed are termed allo-antibodies.

The process of immunisation has been studied in great detail. We will confine ourselves to mentioning a few of the known facts which have a direct bearing on allo-immunisation to blood group antigens in man.

The ability of an antigen to stimulate antibody production depends both on the intrinsic antigenicity (*e.g.* B is a good antigen in all group O and A persons, while P_1 is a comparatively poor antigen in most persons who lack P_1) and partly on individual variation between individuals of the same blood type receiving the same dose of antigen (*e.g.* while some group A persons may have a fourfold increase in anti-B activity when stimulated by a small injection of group B cells, others will respond to the same small dose by a hundred-fold or greater increase). It is now known, particularly from animal experiments that the ability to respond to an antigenic stimulus is under genetic control. It is obvious that blood group antigens which are strongly antigenic and to which the majority of suitable individuals respond will be of greater clinical importance than those which are weakly antigenic.

The response to an antigen is also influenced by whether or not the individual concerned has previously had an injection of the antigen. The first "dose" of antigen is known as the primary or sensitising dose—the response to it is slow and usually very weak. The secondary dose, on the other hand, usually elicits a strong response, with large amounts of antibody being rapidly produced. This is of importance, both with regard to immunisation by transfusions—immune blood group antibodies will more often be found among persons who have already had previous transfusions and to immunisation by pregnancy, where antibodies are comparatively rarely produced during a first pregnancy. In some cases of course the primary stimulus may be a pregnancy and the secondary a blood transfusion, or vice versa. This means that obstetric history is important when considering transfusion and transfusion history important when dealing with pregnant women.

Antibodies once produced may remain in the circulation for many years. As a general rule IgM antibodies disappear more quickly than IgG. On the whole, individuals in which the antibodies persist are less at risk when a further transfusion is contemplated as these antibodies are detected at the time of the direct match and suitable compatible blood can be selected. When an antibody has almost or entirely disappeared, blood containing the same antigen may well appear compatible at direct match, but will act as a secondary stimulus, the antibody being restimulated and possibly destroying the transfused cells within a few days or even hours. If the former, the outcome may be merely a failure to obtain the expected haemoglobin level after transfusion—if the latter there may well be all the classical symptoms of a haemolytic transfusion reaction. A further discussion of blood group antigens and antibodies and the mechanisms of immunisation is found in Chapter 15.

ANTIGEN-ANTIBODY REACTION

Much has been written about the nature of antigen-antibody reaction, but it may be stated briefly as follows. Certain chemical groupings called "determinants" on the large molecule which is behaving like an antigen combine with certain other groupings on the molecule of globulin which is the corresponding antibody. These groupings are called receptors or combining sites. The combination is specific in that a given antigen will react only with its corresponding antibody and not with others. However, specificity is not always absolute as, particularly after prolonged stimulation, antibodies may be produced which will react, albeit not so strongly, with related antigens. The reason for this is probably that there are many different chemical groupings on the large antigenic macromolecule which vary individually both in their ability to stimulate antibody production and in the quality of the antibody which they cause to be produced. Some of these chemical groupings will be possessed in common by a number of related antigens. In blood grouping, cross reactions are occasionally encountered but the worker is more usually impressed by the high degree of specificity of reaction displayed.

The combination of antigen with antibody gives rise to the "observable ways" of reaction to which reference was made in the definition. In blood grouping three "observable ways" are relevant, namely precipitation, agglutination and haemolysis.

(a) *Precipitation*

When the antigen is soluble then mixture with its corresponding antibody often causes precipitation of the antigen-antibody complex provided certain conditions, in particular the correct proportion of antigen to antibody, are fulfilled. In blood grouping the precipitin reaction is not used routinely although valuable research work has been carried out in the ABO system using this technique with purified A and B substances.

(b) *Agglutination*

This is by far the most important and most widely observed phenomenon in blood grouping.

If the antigens are cellular, as in blood cells or bacteria, mixture with their corresponding antibodies may cause a clumping or agglutination of the cells containing the antigen. Hence the term agglutinogen for the antigen, and agglutinin for the antibody.

Thus in blood grouping, clumping or agglutination of red cells is the observable result of mixing cells containing a particular antigen (agglutinogen) with a serum containing the corresponding antibody (agglutinin)*.

The agglutination of red cells takes place in two stages. In the first stage the

---

*Even soluble blood group substances can be detected and measured using an agglutination method. The agglutinin is reduced in strength, or even completely neutralised by the corresponding soluble antigen. This is shown by its inability to agglutinate red cells to the same degree as before the addition of the antigen.

serum agglutinins become attached to agglutinogens on the red cell surface. A red cell which has thus taken up agglutinins is said to be sensitised. In the second stage the actual agglutination or clumping of the sensitised red cells takes place. The cells form aggregates which, if large enough, are visible to the naked eye (*see* Figs. 3.1 a,b). There are degrees of agglutination which cannot be seen without the aid of a microscope (*see* Figs. 3.1 c,d; 3.2 a,b). If the agglutinins are potent, the agglutinating stage of the process may, under certain conditions, follow the sensitisation of the red cells within a few seconds of mixing the red cells and the anti-serum together. As the potency of the agglutinins diminishes more time is required to develop the agglutination fully.

The red cells which form the clumps or aggregates are distorted in shape, and sometimes the red cell membranes break and liberate haemoglobin. However, unless the cells are haemolysed the reaction is in some measure a reversible one. Agglutinated cells can be partially and often completely dispersed and the attached agglutinin recovered from them by alteration of temperature. In most blood group systems a good deal of attached agglutinin can be recovered from agglutinated cells and collected in a small quantity of saline by raising the temperature of agglutinated cells to 56°C for a few minutes. This antibody solution is called an eluate.

Eluates are of value in proving that certain red cells have in fact taken up antibody. Moreover, information about the specificity of each component of a mixture of antibodies can often be obtained by an elution technique.

It might be considered that the mere agglutination of red cells is sufficient proof that they have become sensitised. This would indeed be true if it were not for the existence of factors which occasionally cause pseudo-agglutination; in appearance this is sometimes difficult to distinguish from true agglutination (*see*

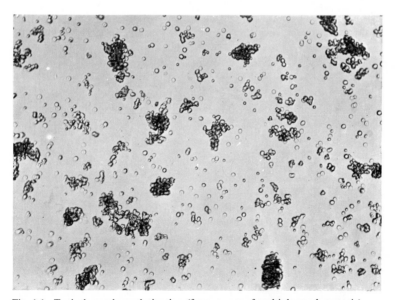

Fig. 1.1a Typical pseudo-agglutination (from a case of multiple myelomatosis).

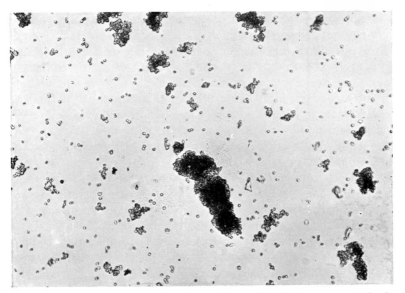

Fig. 1.1b Potent pseudo-agglutination almost indistinguishable from true agglutination.

Figs. 1.1 a,b). For example, an alteration in serum proteins (*e.g.* as occurs in multiple myelomatosis) will bring about a pseudo-agglutination of red cells which has no antigen-antibody basis. No eluate containing antibodies can be prepared from pseudo-agglutinated cells.

It is equally true that cells which are not agglutinated cannot *ipso facto* be considered to be unsensitised. There are three reasons for this. Firstly, the amount of antibody taken up by each red cell may not be sufficient to bring about actual agglutination of the cells. Secondly, the red cells may be subjected to such a temperature as will allow sensitisation of the cells but not their agglutination after sensitisation. Thirdly, the red cells may be sensitised by incomplete antibodies. These were first discovered in the Rh system but by now have been found for practically all the known blood group antigens. Much effort has been directed towards devising and improving the sensitivity of techniques which would induce incomplete antibodies to agglutinate red cells. At the present time three methods are used routinely, usually in parallel. (i) A substance of high molecular weight is introduced into the system. This is commonly bovine albumin and it has the effect of causing red cells sensitised with incomplete antibody to agglutinate. (ii) Another antibody is made by injecting human globulin into rabbits or other domestic animals. The globulin, as might be expected, considering its protein nature, stimulates the production of anti-human globulin antibodies. Treatment of red cells sensitised by antibody globulin, with anti-globulin, brings about agglutination. (iii) Various enzymes are used, notably trypsin, papain and ficin. Treatment of red cells with one of these enzymes renders them susceptible to agglutination by incomplete antibodies. Incomplete antibodies are sometimes capable of preventing the agglutination of cells by complete antibodies (agglutinins) because they occupy the same antigenic sites thus "blocking" agglutination by the complete antibodies.

The blocking nature of the incomplete antibody can be demonstrated by a simple experiment. A saline suspension of red cells of appropriate specificity is exposed to a serum containing incomplete antibodies. After the red cells have had time to become sensitised there is added to them agglutinins. of the same specificity as the incomplete antibodies. These would normally cause agglutination, but if the cells are already sensitised by incomplete antibodies they fail to do so. The agglutinogen of the red cells has been coated by the incomplete antibody and is, therefore, not available to react with an agglutinin of the same specificity.

The practice of employing a variety of techniques in parallel for the detection of incomplete antibodies has led to the finding of antibodies which will react better by one technique than another or which will even fail entirely to react by one method although detectable by another. These differences are not satisfactorily explained by variation in sensitivity of the methods used but almost certainly reflect differences in quality between antibodies which, however, are identical in specificity.

The name "incomplete" given to a class of antibodies merely reflects the fact that these antibodies sensitise red cells but do not cause them to agglutinate in a saline medium, it does not imply that these antibodies are defective.

Some incomplete antibodies only sensitise cells in the presence of fresh serum (provided either by using a freshly taken sample containing the antibodies or by adding fresh human serum of the same ABO group).

The factor in the fresh human serum is complement.

(c) *Haemolysis*

Sometimes, when cellular antigens are concerned, the corresponding antibody may cause a breaking up or lysis of the cells.

Some haemolysins are of blood group specificity. When these react with red cells containing the corresponding antigen haemolysis occurs, haemoglobin is liberated from the red cells and can readily be observed staining the supernatant fluid. The red cell envelopes remain undissolved but distorted in shape. The appearance of haemolysed red cells as viewed by means of the electron microscope suggests that a series of small round holes have been made all over the surface of the red cell. It has been found that haemolysins need complement before lysis can take place. Complement deteriorates upon storage. It is, therefore, essential to use fresh serum* as a source of complement for haemolysin tests. Complement is inactivated by heating the serum at 56°C for 30 minutes.

Experiment has shown that it is the complement rather than the specific haemolysin that actually lyses the red cell. The haemolysin sensitises the red cell and conditions it for the haemolytic action of complement. Red cells cannot be lysed by complement in the absence of the specific haemolysin, nor will their

---

*Fresh serum that has been frozen at –20°C or "freeze-dried" is a good source of complement provided it is used immediately upon reconstitution.

mixture with, followed by removal of, complement-containing serum permit subsequently added haemolysin to act. The sequential action of the various complement components is discussed briefly in Chapter 15.

The specificity of haemolysins is often the same as that of agglutinins and incomplete antibodies, which has suggested that the haemolysin may be the agglutinin or incomplete antibody producing a different effect under different conditions. This point is still controversial but all would agree that whatever the type of observable reaction between blood group antigen and its corresponding antibody *in vitro,* the evidence is in favour of a reaction which is largely haemolytic when it occurs intravenously.

BLOOD GROUPS AS INHERITED CHARACTERS

The following is an elementary discussion of the inheritance of blood group characters. In Part II, as the various blood groups are studied a more detailed concept of the genetic background will be obtained.

General Theory of Inheritance

The nucleus of each cell of the body contains thread-like structures called chromosomes. These chromosomes are divided along their length into more or less discrete regions each of which has distinct genetic properties. These regions are called genes and a large number of them are present on each chromosome. They are arranged in a characteristic order along its length so that each gene always occupies its own special position (or locus) on a particular chromosome. In man, it is now known that there are 46 chromosomes in 23 pairs. Each member of a pair contains the same number of genes and the gene loci are arranged in the same order. (The sex chromosomes are the only known exceptions to this rule.) The significance of the paired chromosomes can be seen in consideration of the gametes. In the sperm and ova there are only 23 chromosomes in each nucleus. This position is reached by special cell divisions (called meiosis) in which the homologous paired chromosomes part, one going into each of two gametes. Thus sex cells are produced which contain exactly half of the chromosome material of the body cells. When fusion of the male and female gametes occurs, the chromosome material doubles up again, each chromosome finding its homologue among chromosomes derived from the opposite sex, subsequent divisions giving rise to body cells containing 46 chromosomes in 23 pairs. Thus, every body cell (as opposed to sex cell) contains the same genes in its nucleus as every other body cell. Moreover, half of them have been derived from the male parent and half from the female.

A gene is usually extremely stable and its replication at cell division is complete. Occasionally, however, it may undergo a change, called a mutation, the new form of the gene being reproduced at each further cell division so that the mutant form persists. A number of alternative genes (possibly derived from a single gene by past mutations) occur at a particular locus. These are called alleles or.allelomorphic genes. It will be realised that the same locus will be represented twice in a fertilised ovum, once on each member of a pair of homologous chromosomes. Therefore, an individual possesses two and only two alleles for that locus, one from each parent. If the same allele is derived from each parent, the individual is said to be homozygous for the particular gene and if different, heterozygous. It follows, therefore, that if two alleles which can be designated L and l exist at a particular locus, three genetically different types of individual can occur, *LL, Ll* and *ll*. Sometimes it is possible to distinguish clearly each of these from the other but often only two classes can be recognised, one which may be called "L" comprising *LL* and *Ll* and the other "l" corresponding to the genotype *ll*. In such circumstances *L* is said to be dominant to *l* and *l* recessive to *L*. The class "L" is called the phenotype and contains the two genotypes *LL* and *Ll*.

With increased knowledge and improved techniques, geneticists are finding that truly recessive genes are becoming fewer or, in other words, in the heterozygote *Ll* characteristics differentiating *Ll* from *LL* and *ll* can be distinguished. In blood groups, with few exceptions, it is possible to distinguish the heterozygote from the homozygote, although a gene when present in single dose in the heterozygote may not express itself so strongly as when in double dose in the homozygote form. This dosage effect is sometimes so marked that it can be used to differentiate between the homo and heterozygote. If, for example, L and l were blood group antigens and anti-L was available but not anti-l, it might be possible on the results of titrations to say that titres over a certain figure indicated two doses of L (*i.e.* genotype *LL*) and titres below that figure one dose (*i.e.* genotype *Ll*).

Genes on the same chromosome are defined as syntenic, and linked if within measurable distance of each other. Sometimes linked genes become separated by crossing over at meiosis. Crossing over involves exchange of material between two homologous chromosomes. By and large, the further apart the linked genes are on the chromosome the more likely they are to be separated by crossing over and conversely, closely linked genes travel together through many generations before separation occurs.

Linkage and crossing over may be illustrated by supposing a gene *O* and its allele *o* carried on the same pair of chromosomes as the *Ll* genes discussed above. The possible gene arrangements are *L* with *O. L* with *o*, *l* with *O* and l with *o* and therefore, for example, people who are *Lo/lO* will hand on to their children *Lo* or *lO*; occasionally, however, due to crossing over they will hand on *LO* or *lo*.

When genes are more than a certain distance apart they cross over sufficiently often that they appear to segregate independently and it is not obvious that they are in fact in the same chromosome.

Linkage has been demonstrated between the Rh blood group systems and oval cells, also between ABO and nail-patella syndrome.

The Xg blood group system is sex-linked, being carried on the X chromosome. The study of this system has helped in the "mapping" of the X chromosome (*i.e.* in saying whereabouts in relation to each other some of the sex-linked genes are carried on the X chromosome).

A good deal of biochemical evidence has led geneticists to the conclusion that many genes control inherited characteristics by controlling the synthesis of specific enzymes. It is indeed suggested that in most cases genes bear a simple one-to-one relationship with enzymes. Moreover, any mutation that occurs in a gene may cause complete or partial failure in the synthesis of a particular enzyme, or alternatively a qualitatively different enzyme may be produced although its activity may not always be apparent. This subject of genes and enzymes will be briefly discussed again in relation to the most recent advances made in our knowledge of the ABO blood group system (*see* Chapter 16).

It is probable that instead of thinking of a single gene we should think of a section of chromosome with a large number of genes all acting and interacting to produce their effect. Such a section of chromosome is called a cistron—two genes belonging to one cistron would produce effects when on the same chromosome which might differ from those produced if they were one on each chromosome of a pair. Two genes on the same chromosome which belong to the same cistron are said to be in cis position, while two genes which are on opposite chromosomes are said to be in trans position.

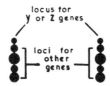

Fig. 1.2a Diagrammatic representation of a pair of chromosomes.

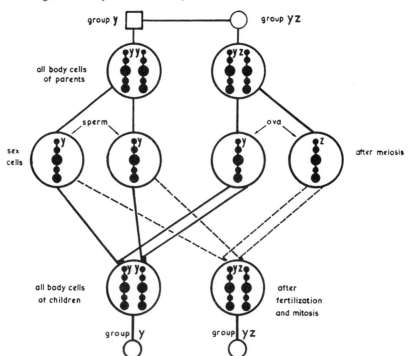

Fig. 1.2b The inheritance of the blood group system YZ, showing the segregation of the genes in the sperm and ova.

The Inheritance of Blood Groups

Every individual receives from each parent a gene or possibly, a linked combination of genes (*see* Rh factor) relating to each of the blood group systems. Figs. 1.2a and b show the inheritance of an imaginary blood group system YZ in which *Y* and *Z* are allelomorphic genes so that either *Y* or *Z* occupies the particular chromosomal locus for this system, never both.

It is customary to give the genes the same designation as the antigen whose development it controls. Gene *Y* gives rise to antigen Y, and gene *Z* to antigen Z. This is unfortunate in some respects as it tends to lead to confusion of thought and gives the erroneous impression that genes and antigens are identical. To help to clarify the situation it is now the practice to print genes and genotypes in italics as in this section.

In this hypothetical blood group system, three types of individual are possible, *YY*, *YZ* and *ZZ*. Fig.1.1b shows the mating of a group Y male with a group YZ female. It is clear the male of group Y must have received *Y* from each parent and so is of genotype *YY*, whereas the female has received *Y* from one parent and *Z* from the other and so is of genotype *YZ*.

In each body or somatic cell of the male each member of the relevant pair of chromosomes possess Y one of which has been derived from one parent and one from the other. The female has one chromosome of type *Y* inherited from one parent and one of type *Z* from the other. Her body cells, therefore contain chromosomes of two kinds with respect to the YZ system in question. After meiosis, the sperm cells are all alike and each possesses one chromosome having *Y*. Half the ova, however, have *Y* and half *Z* so that there are two kinds of ova. When fertilisation takes place the chromatin material is doubled and the body cells of the children from this mating (*see* Fig. 1.1) contain either two chromosomes each with *Y* or one with *Y* and one with *Z*. Children of the first type belong to group Y, children of the second type to group YZ.

All known blood group systems are inherited along similar lines to the hypothetical case described above, the chief differences being in the number of allelomorphs controlling a particular system and the way in which they are designated.

It should of course, be realised that in each body cell in the human species there are forty-six chromosomes in twenty-three pairs, and the different genes controlling the various blood group systems are not all situated on the same pair of chromosomes. In fact, many of them have been shown conclusively to be independent of each other and to occur on different chromosome pairs.

In this chapter we have simplified the actual position by assuming that the appearance of a blood group antigen, on for instance, a red cell is dependent on only one set of allelomorphic genes and for the general understanding of blood group genetics this simplification is justified. There are, however, other genes involved. Should these prevent the formation of an antigen which according to the individual's blood group genetic make-up he should possess, they are known as suppressor genes. Examples of such genes will be found in Chapter 17.

Section 2. The ABO Blood Group System

"..., now let us begin. When we have got to the end of the story we shall know more than we do at present...."

Hans Christian Andersen, THE SNOW QUEEN

Chapter 2. The ABO Blood Groups and Grouping Methods

Landsteiner discovered the phenomenon of allo-agglutination in 1900. In 1901 he published the results of experiments which made it possible to divide the population into three groups, which he called A, B, and O. A year later the existence of a fourth, less common group, AB, was established. This marked the beginning of the whole subject of blood group serology and made blood transfusion practicable.

The four groups are determined by the presence or absence in the red blood cells of the blood group antigens A and B, and, therefore, the blood group of the individual is either A, B, AB, or O (O denoting the absence of A and B).

In addition, it has been shown that corresponding to the antigens A and B there are antibodies anti-A (α) and anti-B (ß), which occur as agglutinins in the sera of individuals whose red cells lack the corresponding agglutinogen. The agglutinogen and agglutinin content of the red cells and serum of the four blood groups are shown in Table 2.1.

Table 2.1 Agglutinogen and agglutinin content of the red cells and serum of the four blood groups

Blood group	Agglutinogen in red cells	Agglutinin in serum	Frequency in English population
A	A	Anti-B	41.7
B	B	Anti-A	8.6
AB	A and B	Neither	3.0
O	Neither	Both Anti-A and Anti-B	46.7

Although all individuals of the same blood group have the same kind of agglutinogen in their red cells, the sensitivity of the cells to agglutination varies from individual to individual. Moreover, there are very wide variations in the amount of agglutinin in the serum of different individuals belonging to the same blood group.

16

Table 2.2 ABO grouping, using standard sera and standard red cells

Blood group	Reactions of red cells with standard sera		Reactions of sera with standard cells	
	Anti-A	Anti-B	A cells	B cells
A	C	–	–	C
B	–	C	C	–
AB	C	C	–	–
O	–	–	C	C

C = clumping (complete agglutination)
– = no reaction

It is by means of the agglutination reaction of red cells that the blood group of an individual is determined. This can be effected either by testing the individual's red cells with standard anti-A and anti-B sera (for selection and method of preparation of standard sera *see* Chapter 3) or by testing his serum with standard red cells of groups A and B. The most reliable grouping is achieved if both these methods are used, so that they form a check on each other. The pattern of reactions obtained for each blood group by these two methods is shown in Table 2.2.

It is very important to distinguish between true agglutination and rouleaux formation. This latter phenomenon is a running together of the red cells to form aggregates, like piles of coins (Figs. 2.1a and b). It is often well marked in the blood of patients suffering from acute infection, in conditions where the albumin-globulin serum protein balance is disturbed, and even in normal blood when

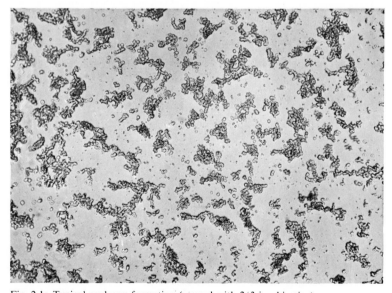

Fig. 2.1a Typical rouleaux formation (viewed with 2/3-in objective).

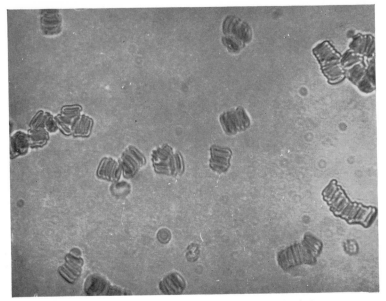

Fig. 2.1b Typical rouleaux formation (viewed with 1/6-in objective).

a smear is beginning to dry or when a too concentrated cell suspension is used. When rouleaux formation is very heavy it is sometimes difficult even for an experienced worker to distinguish it from true agglutination, as the piles form compact masses very similar to the appearance given by true agglutination (Fig. 1.2a). Usually, rouleaux formation can be dispersed readily by adding a drop of saline to the slide and gently rubbing. However, it should be borne in mind that this practice may be dangerous. The agglutination caused by the agglutinogen and agglutinins of the ABO system is tough and not easily broken down by the above treatment, but that caused by most other blood group systems is fragile, and, if present together with rouleaux, will also be dispersed and a false negative obtained.

TECHNIQUES

As has been mentioned, it is possible to determine the group of a specimen of blood either by testing the red cells with standard anti-A and anti-B sera (chosen for their good agglutinating power) or by testing the serum with standard group A and group B red cells (chosen for their sensitivity). It is more difficult to test unknown sera than unknown red cells because the strength of the agglutinins varies greatly in different sera. For reliable grouping both cells and serum should be examined and the tests repeated if there is any discrepancy. When using potent serum and red cells of good sensitivity agglutination takes place very rapidly. As the strength of the agglutinin or agglutinogen decreases. however, the speed of the reaction diminishes. Techniques which do not allow sufficient time for the reaction between the weakest agglutinogen and agglutinin can never be reliable.

To expedite the process the tests may be centrifuged after 15-20 minutes. If it is intended to spin the tests, the plastic 50-hole racks which fit the serological centrifuge should be used, so that each test is given the same treatment and the tubes do not have to be individually numbered.

The two methods described here are chosen for their reliability. In a grave emergency it may become necessary to risk a less reliable method; these are described and discussed in Chapter 24.

A description of a suggested bench lay-out and equipment including useful Pasteur pipettes etc. are to be found in Appendix I.

Technique No. 2.1 ABO grouping by the moist chamber slide technique

Apparatus

Moist chamber—this can vary from a Petri-dish lined with damp filter paper to a properly constructed cabinet to take many hundreds of tests—a useful one for the moderate sized laboratory is 22 cm × 32 cm and takes four 'long' slides each 22 cm × 8 cm allowing for 80 individual tests.

Cell-suspension tubes—round bottomed, 50 mm × 11 mm
Slides—Microscope slides or preferably glass (or perspex) slides with two rows of 10 divisions.
Microscope with 2/3 objective.

Reagents

Physiological saline (0.85 per cent solution of NaCl).

Standard anti-A and anti-B sera.
Standard Group O serum.
Control inert AB serum
Standard A_1, A_2, B and O red cells.

Method. This description is for the testing of seven blood samples with A_2, B and O controls; it can readily be adapted for any number.

Four slides are placed in the moist chamber giving 8 rows each of 10 divisions.

One drop of anti-A serum is added to each division of row one.

One drop of anti-B serum to each division of row two.

One drop of O serum to each division of row three.

One drop of control AB serum to each division of row four (see comment on use of this control).

The pipette is carefully rinsed between each row.

The samples to be tested are of clotted blood where the serum has separated (either by standing over-night or by centrifugation) sufficiently for clear serum to be pipetted from the top of the samples while free red cells can be obtained from the bottom of the tube.

The first unknown sample is held in the left hand, together with the first suspension tube, one drop of the unknown serum is placed in the first division of rows five, six, seven and eight; a 3–5 per cent cell suspension in saline is made in the cell suspension tube and one drop added to the first division of rows one, two, three and four. The pipette is then rinsed and the tubes exchanged for the second unknown sample and its suspension tube, serum and cells from the second sample being added in the same way to the second division in each row. The process is repeated for each of the seven samples. One drop of a 3–5 per cent suspension of standard group O cells is run into each division of row five and the last division of rows one, two, three and four; one drop of group A_1 cells is run into each division of row six; one drop of A_2 cells into each division of row seven and the eighth divisions of rows one, two, three and four; one drop of group B cells into each division of row eight and the ninth division of rows one to four. The lid is placed on the moist chamber and the whole gently rocked to ensure mixing of cells and serum in each division.

The tests are allowed to stand at room temperature for 25–30 minutes. The chamber is again gently rocked and the results recorded. The macroscopic readings are checked by removing the slides from the chamber and examining under the lower power (2/3) objective of the microscope. A typical protocol is given in Table 2.3).

Table 2.3 Protocol of ABO grouping moist chamber slide technique

Tested with	Samples							Controls		
	1	2	3	4	5	6	7	A_2	B	O
Anti-A	5+	–	5+	–	2+	–	4+	5+	–	–
Anti-B	–	–	–	5+	5+	–	5+	–	5+	–
O serum	5+	–	5+	5+	5+	–	5+	5+	5+	–
AB serum	–	–	–	–	–	–	–	–	–	–
O red cells	–	–	–	–	–	–	–			
A_1 red cells	–	5+	–	5+	2+	5+	–			
A_2 red cells	–	4+	–	3+	–	5+	–			
B red cells	5+	5+	5+	–	–	4+	–			
Group	A	O	A	B	for further tests	O	AB			

Comment

This slide technique allows adequate time for weak reactions to develop. Agreement should always be found between the results of testing the cells and serum (unless an atypical antibody is present in the serum (*see* section on anomalous results)). If the tests agree, this technique may be regarded as 100 per cent reliable, the main disadvantage being the dimension of the moist chamber required for the performance of a large number of grouping tests at one time. When a large number of normal samples are being tested, the AB serum control is sometimes omitted. This is probably quite safe but some prefer always to include this negative control. It should never be omitted in testing patients with auto-immune diseases or babies suffering from haemolytic disease of the new-born.

Technique No. 2.2 ABO grouping by tube technique—standard method

As this is the technique recommended for use whenever it is possible to leave the tests for at least 1½ hours, both the apparatus used and the technique are described in detail. Moreover, this is the basic typing technique for all blood group work.

Apparatus

Precipitin tubes, round bottomed glass tubes* size 50 mm × 5.5 mm internal diameter.
Cell-suspension tubes, round bottomed glass tubes* size 50 mm × 11 mm internal diameter.
Racks having 50 holes arranged in 5 rows of 10.
Capillary or Pasteur pipettes graduated to deliver one and two standard volumes. (The standard volume should be of the order of 0.03 ml)
Microscope slides.
Microscope with 2/3 objective.

Reagents

Physiological saline (0.85 per cent solution of NaCl).
Standard anti-A and anti-B sera and standard group O serum(*i.e.* anti-A + anti-B and control inert AB serum).
Standard group A_1, group A_2, group B, and group O red cells.

*Plastic disposable tubes of similar dimensions can be substituted if desired.

Testing of unknown cells. The method now described allows for the grouping of ten blood specimens, including controls of groups A_2, B, and O. Small precipitin tubes are placed in the first three rows of a 50-holed block or rack and the larger cell suspension tubes in the back row. In each tube of the front row are placed 1 volume of anti-A serum and 1 volume of saline, in each tube of the second row 1 volume of anti-B serum and 1 volume of saline and in the third row equal volumes of saline and group O serum using the graduated capillary pipette. The addition of saline minimises rouleaux formation. When large numbers of tests are being done the grouping serum may be diluted in bulk with an equal volume of saline and a double volume of this diluted serum placed in each tube. At the end of this stage the tubes are scrutinised carefully to make certain that each contains its allotted quantity of serum. Approximately 0.5 ml of saline is run into each of the cell suspension tubes in the back row. A 2–5 per cent cell suspension (judged by eye) of the first specimen of red cells to be tested is made with a Pasteur pipette in the corresponding cell suspension tube. Then, using the same Pasteur pipette and without rinsing, 1 volume of cell suspension is measured into the first tubes of all three rows. The pipette is then rinsed three times in normal saline, discarding each rinsing, and the process repeated along the row for each of the specimens to be grouped. Cell suspension tubes in positions 8, 9, and 10 on the rack will contain the standard red cells of groups A_2, B, and O, respectively, as controls. If several racks of grouping tests are set up at the same time, controls need only be placed in the final rack.

The tubes are then tapped to ensure good mixing of the cells and serum and the tests are allowed to stand at room temperature for at least 1½, preferably 2, hours. Each tube is then agitated by tapping with the finger. If the contents show agglutination which is obvious to the naked eye (*see* Figs. 3.1a,b) a positive result is recorded. The content of each tube not showing obvious agglutination is removed, spread evenly on a microscope slide and examined under the low power of the microscope. Control tubes should be read first, and only if these are satisfactory should the other tests be read.

Testing of unknown sera. These tests should be carried out independently of the tests for red cells and are therefore set up in a different rack. Four rows of precipitin tubes are placed in the front of the rack, as in the cell grouping test. One volume of serum from the first sample is placed in the first tube of all four rows, the pipette rinsed, and the process repeated along the row. One volume of a 2–5 per cent suspension of standard group A_1 red cells is placed in each tube of the front row and one volume of a similar suspension of standard A_2, B and O red cells in each tube of the second, third and fourth rows respectively. If the standard cells are run into the control tubes belonging to the cell tests at the same time these controls will serve for both tests otherwise controls must be set up for each test separately. The tubes are shaken and allowed to stand for 2 hours. The reading is the same as for the tests on the unknown cells.

Use of group O serum. Group O serum contains both anti-A and anti-B agglutinins. It can, therefore, be used to agglutinate all A, B, and AB bloods, leaving only group O bloods unagglutinated. This test should be read independently of the other two and then the results correlated. The anti-A in group O serum reacts more strongly than the anti-A in group B serum with some of the low sub-groups of A (A_3, A_x, A_m, etc.) and may prevent such bloods being wrongly diagnosed as group O.

Negative Control using inert AB serum. This can best be done as an additional test, the unknown cells being incubated with the AB serum and all results read

Table 2.4 Protocol of ABO grouping by tube technique*a*

Sample No.	Test on red cells				Tests on serum				Group
	Anti-A	Anti-B	Group 0 anti-A + anti-B	AB Serum	A_1 Cells	A_2 Cells	B Cells	O Cells	
1	C	-	C	-	-	-	C	-	A
2	-	-	-	-	C	V	C	-	O
3	C	-	C	-	-	-	C	-	A
4	-	C	C	-	C	V	-	-	B
5	++	C	C	-	+	-	-	-	Further tests
6	-	-	-	-	C	C	C	-	O
7	C	C	C	-	-	-	-	-	AB
Control A_2	C	-	C	-					
Control B	-	C	C	-					
Control O	-	-	-	-					

C = complete agglutination
V = visual agglutination
Other symbols see below under Anomalous results

microscopically. As in the covered slide test this control is sometimes omitted, the remarks made in discussing this procedure apply also to the tube technique.

Correlation of Results

The best method of reading and recording the results of a large number of tests is for two people to work together, one reading the macroscopic agglutination and preparing microscope slides from the tubes not showing obvious agglutination, while the other examines the prepared slides and records the results. Such a team with practice becomes extremely efficient. If only one worker is available, then he must record his results as they are read; it is permissible, however, to memorise consecutive identical results.

The recorded results are then correlated. Table 2.4 is a facsimile of results obtained on seven unknown red cell samples, together with controls. Sometimes (*e.g.* sample No. 5) the results are not typical. There are several reasons why this might be so; for convenience a list is given here. Some of the items will be better understood when the chapters on the sub-groups of A, Rh antibodies, etc., have been studied.

Anomalous Results

(1) *Weak Reactions.*

If agglutination is not clearly visible to the naked eye and has to be read microscopically the reaction is recorded according to the following table:

```
++ = very large clumps—few free cells.
 + = large clumps—more free cells.
(+) = an even distribution of clumps of about 8–16 cells.
 w = weak—an even distribution of clumps of about 3–10 cells.
 - = no agglutination.
```

(For a photograph of these degrees of agglutination *see* Figs. 3.1a-d; 3.2a-c)

The reaction ++ may be taken as denoting definite agglutination. Reactions of + or less mean that the tests must be repeated with further reagents.

(2) *Haemolysis*

The unknown sera may cause haemolysis of the standard red cells, If there is good agglutination also (*e.g.* C or ++ reaction), the haemolysis can be disregarded and the agglutination reaction recorded. If, however, the majority of the cells are haemolysed so that there is little or no agglutination, a further test is necessary. This is because although the haemolysis is probably due to the specific anti-A or anti-B haemolysins, it is not safe to assume that this is so. In these cases three or four serial dilutions of the unknown serum in saline (*see* titration technique No. 3.2) can be made and tested with red cells of the appropriate ABO group. The dilution giving little or no haemolysis will normally show agglutination. Alternatively the serum may be inactivated (*i.e.* heated at 56°C for 30 minutes) to destroy complement and the heated serum retested—by this means haemolysis is prevented while the agglutination reaction is unimpaired.

(3) *The Weak Agglutinogens of the Sub-groups of A*

Some cells may give consistently poor reactions with anti-A sera because they belong to one of the weaker sub-groups of A. Such blood should be tested with anti-A and group O sera which have been especially chosen for their good reactivity with weak A agglutinogens.

(4) *Reactions Due to the Cold Agglutinins of the Sub-groups of A*

Typical results given by samples which contain these agglutinins are shown below.

Table 2.5 Cold agglutinins of A sub-groups

Sample No.	Anti-A	Anti-B	O serum (anti-A + anti-B)	AB serum	A_1 cells	A_2 cells	B cells	O cells
I	C	-	C	-	+	-	C	-
II	+	C	C	-	(+)	-	-	-

If such reactions are obtained, the tests are repeated and, in addition, the red cells tested with anti-A_1 sera and the serum with two samples of A_1 and two samples of A_2 cells. (For a description of these reagents and the results which would be obtained *see* (Chapter 4).

(5) *Reactions Due to Other Atypical Agglutinins*

Among the most common atypical agglutinins whose presence in an unknown serum may give rise to anomalous results are the Rh antibodies. This difficulty may most easily be overcome by using Rh negative group A and group B standard cells. If there are still atypical reactions between the unknown sera and the standard cells these may be due to a variety of atypical antibodies. As a general rule, such cases are investigated by a specialist laboratory which has a large panel of standard cells available (*see also* Chapter 22).

(6) *Auto-agglutinins*

These are agglutinins which if present in the serum of an individual will cause agglutination of his own red cells. The phenomenon is usually observed at temperatures lower than 37°C. Thus if there is an auto-agglutinin in the unknown serum active at the temperature of the test, the red cells will be agglutinated before being tested. Washing the red cells at 37°C or, if necessary, 45°C, may disperse this agglutination and the red cells can be grouped in the usual way. If the results are still not clear cut, a fresh sample must be taken, the cells and serum separated, and the cells washed at 37°C without allowing the sample to cool, so that the agglutinin never becomes attached to the red cells (*see also* Chapter 14).

(7) *Grouping of Cord or Infants' Blood*

The ABO grouping of babies presents difficulty for two reasons. Firstly, the cell agglutinogens may not be fully developed at birth—this is particularly true of the sub-groups of A—and very weak reactions may be obtained. It is therefore recommended that the additional test, using group O sera, should always be used when typing infants' blood. Secondly, infants do not possess their own anti-A and anti-B agglutinins at birth; these usually start developing at about the third to the sixth month of life. Any antibodies found in the infants' sera at birth have been passively acquired from the maternal serum by passage across the placenta. This means that it is not possible to check the group of the child by means of the antibody content of its serum.

(8) *Grouping of cells sensitised with incomplete antibody*

It is unusual for cells sensitised with antibody *e.g.* cells from haemolytic anaemia patients to cause anomalies in ABO grouping as it is a saline agglutination technique. It is possible however that some may do so and these will be disclosed by the fact that a positive reaction is obtained in the AB serum control. The treatment in such cases is similar to that noted under section 6 where auto-agglutinins rather than sensitising antibodies are attached to the red cells. These sensitising auto antibodies may well be active at $37^\circ C$ and so washing at $45^\circ C$ or even $56^\circ C$ may be necessary. If this does not clear the false reaction, it is sometimes possible to type the cells with a strong agglutinating anti-serum diluted about 1 in 4 in saline.

Chapter 3. ABO Grouping Sera — Selection and Preparation

The standard sera for blood grouping have to be selected, for although all group A individuals have anti-B agglutinins, all group B individuals anti-A agglutinins, and all group O individuals both anti-A and anti-B agglutinins, only about 2 per cent have them in sufficient strength for the certain detection of the weakest agglutinogens.

CRITERIA FOR DETERMINING SERUM SUITABILITY

To determine the suitability of a given serum both the titre and the avidity of the agglutinins must be estimated. The determination of the titre involves making serial dilutions of serum in saline in a row of tubes and the addition to each tube of a volume of red cells of the appropriate group to cause agglutination. The reciprocal of the highest dilution of serum still causing agglutination (as viewed under the microscope) is the titre (or titration value) of a particular serum. Experience has shown that to be satisfactory for grouping a serum must have a titre of at least 512 against standard red cells of group A, or 256 against standard red cells of group B.

The avidity of a serum is its power to agglutinate red cells quickly and strongly, forming large clumps. It is possible to find a serum which satisfies the criterion for minimum titration value and yet agglutinates poorly at most dilutions. It is necessary, therefore, to select on the basis of a certain strength of agglutination at a given dilution as well as on the end point of the titre; an anti-A serum should show a V to ++ agglutination, and an anti-B serum a ++ to + agglutination at a dilution of 1 in 64. Sera should show "C" or "complete" agglutination in the four lowest dilutions.

The standard both for titre and avidity is higher for anti-A than for anti-B because there are weak sub-groups of A (see Chapter 4) and a more potent serum is needed for the detection of some of these. Anti-A sera should be titrated with A_2B and, if available, A_3B cells, and are only regarded as satisfactory if they give at least three macroscopic readings with A_2B or one macroscopic reading with A_3B cells.

When group O serum is used as an anti-A + anti-B ($\alpha\beta$) grouping serum it must satisfy the criteria for titre and avidity for both anti-A and anti-B. Fortunately, in most group O sera the anti-A titre is slightly higher than the anti-B, and if the serum satisifies the criteria for anti-B the anti-A is usually satisfactory also. The use of group O ($\alpha\beta$) sera is in the detection of cells belonging to the weaker sub-groups of A (A_3 and A_x). Whenever possible, therefore, sera giving titre of 16 or over with A_x cells should be selected. A description of sub-group A_x is given in Chapter 16.

It is also necessary before issuing ABO grouping sera as specific for agglutin-ogens A and B to test them against the cells of at least 30 group O individuals. This is a precautionary measure, as the sera may contain atypical agglutinins which would render them unsuitable for grouping purposes. Some of these agglutinins (*e.g.* anti-Lutheran) detect antigen of low frequency and could be missed if the panel of group O cells was too small. Alternatively, a much smaller panel of group O cells, specially selected for their ability to detect atypical antibodies belonging to any of the known blood group systems, can be used (*see also* Chapter 22).

Elimination of unsuitable sera

Large numbers of serum samples have to be tested in order to select grouping sera, as only about 2 per cent* of all individuals have anti-A or anti-B agglutinins of sufficient titre and avidity. It is convenient, therefore, to devise a screening method which avoids titrating fully the 98 per cent of sera which are unsuitable. The screening method which we recommend involves making a one in four dilution of each serum, adding red cells, and selecting for full and careful titration those sera causing complete (C) agglutination at the end of 1 hour. This method is a fairly accurate way of choosing good sera since only about one in ten thus selected have to be discarded upon further testing.

Use of immune sera

It is possible to prepare high titre grouping sera by the deliberate injection of A or B substances into human volunteers or animals (usually rabbits). Adequate supplies of grouping sera for routine purposes can be maintained without resorting to this procedure. The chief use of such immune sera is for research purposes (*see* particularly Chapter 16). Animal sera have to be absorbed before use to remove species specific or "anti-Man" agglutinins which agglutinate all human red cells.

Snail anti-A

An anti-A reagent can be prepared from snails. This is extremely powerful and reacts equally well with A_1 and A_2 blood, though not with A_3. The snail originally used was *Helix hortensis,* but other snails, in particular *Helix aspersa,* are equally good. A simple way of obtaining the reagent is to add the contents of snail's egg to 100 ml of saline—this reagent is often sufficiently potent to be diluted considerably, especially if tests are performed on enzyme treated red cells. It can be used very dilute in the AutoAnalyser. The reagent does however react with Group O and Group B cells as shown by the fact that active eluates can be prepared from them. This means that it must be suitably diluted so that the reaction is specific for A.

---

*This figure applies to random civilian donors in the south of England. A higher percentage of suitable sera is found in the north of the country. There is also an age-sex relationship, and if young males are tested, up to 20 per cent have antibody titres satisfying the grouping sera criteria.

The snail "anti-A" has been described as recognizing a "new" blood group receptor, A_{hel}.

Although this reagent seems attractive, we prefer human anti-A antisera (of which there is a quite adequate supply) mainly because this does detect the A_3 sub-group.

Principles of processing serum

When a serum has been selected for grouping purposes it is then prepared for use. After the serum has separated from the clot it is collected free of red cells either by gravity or centrifugation. The latter method is to be preferred since it is quicker and improves the yield. Speed is an advantage as the longer the serum is kept in an unfrozen state the greater is the risk of a reduction in titre. Nowadays it is usual to bleed 'serum' donors into ACD and to recalcify the plasma. This is a simple procedure and is described in technique No. 3.6.

In our experience the best way to sterilize a serum is by Seitz filtration, as this does not appreciably reduce the titre, whereas heating may easily do so. Moreover, Seitz filtration also clarifies serum. Whenever possible sera should be stored frozen solid at -10 to $-20°C$, but this is less essential for anti-A and anti-B sera than for anti-Rh sera. Grouping serum can also be "freeze-dried" without deterioration and it can then be stored at room temperature; this is useful when the serum is for transport, especially to places abroad. Grouping serum should never be kept in capillary tubes, in spite of the fact that it is more economical when only undertaking a few grouping tests on any one occasion. Serious mistakes leading to the death of patients have occurred through using sera stored in this way. For some reason, possibly related to the type of glass used for the making of capillaries, coupled with the greater surface area of serum exposed to it, serum stored in capillaries deteriorates very rapidly and also tends to give false positive reactions. It is possible for a pin-point hole in a capillary to remain undetected and thereby allow the serum to become infected. Moreover, as conditions vary from capillary to capillary no real control is possible

TECHNIQUES

Technique No. 3.1. Screening technique for ABO grouping sera

For anti-A and anti-B a one in four dilution of each of the unknown sera is made in saline with a Pasteur pipette graduated to deliver three unit volumes (*see* Appendix I). This quantity of saline is placed in a row of precipitin tubes equal in number to the sera to be tested. One unit volume of the first serum under test is added to the first tube and the contents thoroughly mixed. Three volumes of the mixture are then discarded, leaving one volume of a one in four dilution in the tube. The Pasteur pipette is carefully rinsed at least four times in saline and then once in the next serum to be tested; it is then ready to be used for making the second one in four dilution. When all the dilutions have been made one unit volume of a 2 per cent suspension of the appropriate standard cells is added and after the tests have stood for exactly 1 hour they are examined macroscopically for agglutination. Only those sera showing a "C" reaction are selected for full titration. About one in ten selected by this method prove unsuitable when titrated in full.

Screening for Group O ($\alpha\beta$) sera is best done by testing one volume of serum with one volume of A_x cells at room temperature for 1 hour. Sera giving visual agglutination will usually prove suitable on full titration.

Technique No. 3.2. Titration of agglutinins (anti-A and anti-B)

The method of performing and reading the titrations is a slight modification of that described by Taylor and Ikin (1939). The titrations are carried out in precipitin tubes, the diluent being normal saline. The standard red cells should be less than 24 hours old when used. With a Pasteur pipette graduated to deliver a constant unit volume (approximately 0.03 ml) twofold dilutions of serum are made in a row of tubes. To each of these serial dilutions 1 volume of the appropriate red cell suspension (4–5 per cent in terms of whole blood) in saline is added and the tubes shaken. The titrations are made in duplicate and are allowed to stand for 2 hours at room temperature. The cell deposit is then agitated by tapping the tube sharply, and the degree of agglutination read. No reaction is scored as negative until it has been examined microscopically, when an even distribution of clumps of three or more cells is accepted as evidence of agglutination. The titre of the serum is expressed as the reciprocal of the greatest dilution causing agglutination (the cell suspension volume is neglected in calculating the dilution)*. Some workers express the titre as the reciprocal of the highest dilution showing at least a (+) reaction, but in our experience this is a much more variable end-point and we do not recommend its adoption. In any case, when a titration value is quoted the method used and the end-point accepted should always be stated. A useful method of scoring reactions is given below.

Comment

The experimental error of this technique in the hands of an experienced worker rarely exceeds one dilution, in spite of the fact that the unit volume employed is small. The titration values are higher than those obtained when the serial dilutions are made with standard graduated pipettes, using a separate pipette for each dilution, because inevitably there is a slight carry-over from tube to tube when the same pipette is used for the whole titration. Furthermore, the method estimates only the amount of antibody bound to the red cells, not the total amount of antibody present in each dilution, and the proportion of bound antibody is influenced by the combining capacity of the antibody. It has been estimated that if two sera contain the same concentration of antibody, but one has a combining capacity ten times higher than the other, then the antibody with the higher combining capacity will have a titre approximately ten times greater than the other. This does not affect the validity of the results as only comparative values are required, and indeed no absolute standard of antibody strength exists. This means that the same titration method must be used throughout any series of estimations, and in stating any results or standards the method employed must be clearly indicated.

---

*Titres above 512 are usually approximated to the nearest thousand.

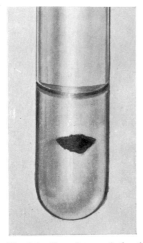

Fig: 3.1a Complete agglutination.

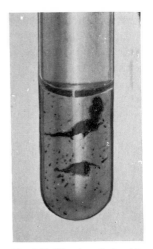

Fig. 3.1b Visual agglutinatión.

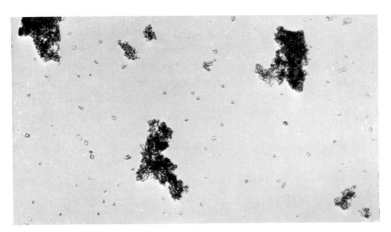

Fig. 3.1c ++ agglutination.

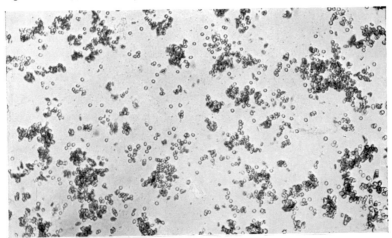

Fig. 3.1d + agglutination.

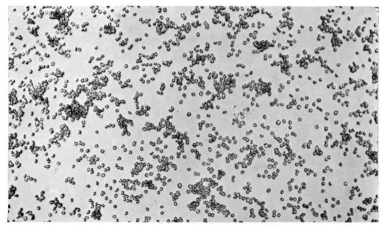

Fig. 3.2a (+) agglutination.

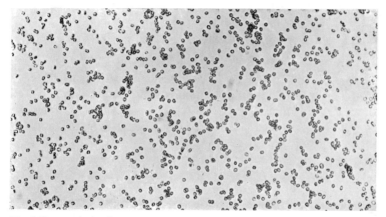

Fig. 3.2b w agglutination.

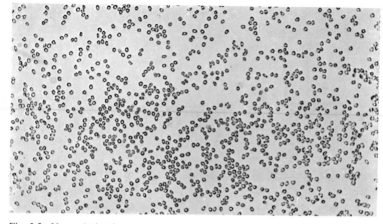

Fig. 3.2c No agglutination.

Sometimes a modification of the Pasteur pipette method is used, in which, instead of measured volumes, drops are used. This modification introduces a large source of error as the drops of saline, of serum and of cell suspension are not the same size. This objection is even more valid when, as we shall see later, it is sometimes necessary to perform titrations using a protein diluent. With practice it is almost, if not quite, as quick to use a graduated Pasteur pipette as to use a dropping pipette.

Macroscopic
   C = complete agglutination—large agglutinates surrounded by clear fluid (Fig. 3.1a).
   V = visual agglutination—while the agglutinates are still visible to the naked eye the surrounding fluid is pink (Fig. 3.1b).

Microscopic
   ++ = very large clumps—few free cells (Fig. 3.1c).
    + = large clumps—more free cells (Fig. 3.1d).
   (+) = an even distribution of clumps of about 8-16 cells (Fig. 3.2a).
   w = weak—an even distribution of clumps of about 3-10 cells (Fig. 3.2b).
   - = no agglutination (Fig. 3.2c).

Technique No. 3.3. Titration of agglutinins using standard graduated pipettes

Serial dilutions of not less than 0.5 ml of the serum are made in saline with standard graduated 1 ml "blow-out" pipettes, using a fresh pipette for each dilution. Then 0.1 ml of each dilution, beginning with the weakest, is placed (using a standard "run-out" pipette) in each of a row of precipitin tubes, and 0.1 ml of standard cells added to each. The tests are allowed to stand for 2 hours at room temperature and then read in the same way as for technique No. 3.2

The disadvantages of this method are that it requires larger volumes of serum and is more time-consuming.

Technique No. 3.4. Master titres

If it is required for any reason to titrate a serum against several different samples of red cells (*e.g.* when comparing the agglutinogen content of different cells of the same group, or when titrating more than one antibody in a serum containing a mixture) a "master" titre is made.

To be comparable with titrations made by technique No. 3.2 the master titre should be made with the master titre pipette shown in appendix, Fig. A1.1G*. On the other hand, to be comparable with results obtained by technique No. 3.3 the master dilutions are made using a fresh standard graduated pipette for each dilution.

After the dilutions have been made the one volume graduated Pasteur pipette (Fig. A1.1C) can be used to run out (commencing with the weakest dilution) as many rows of dilutions as there are different cells to be added. It is advisable that the "master" dilutions should be made in duplicate, as any error would affect all the titres involved.

*Appendix numbers will be preceded by "**A**" throughout the book.

Technique No. 3.5. Method of preparation of grouping serum

Serum is rendered sterile by Seitz filtration. For this purpose the serum is separated from the clot and made absolutely cell free. If this is done by centrifugation and the time between the opening of the blood bottle and the filtering of the serum is a matter of a few hours only, then no sterile precautions need be taken until after the serum is Seitz filtered. If the method of pouring off the serum and allowing it to stand for a day or two to settle is adopted, then aseptic precautions should be taken from the beginning of the manipulation. Cloudy or fatty serum should be clarified by passing it through a clarifying (grade 4) Seitz filter pad. For the actual sterilisation the Seitz pad HPEK must be used. The filtered serum is stored in sterile bottles in suitable quantities, e.g. 10ml for blood bank, 1ml for routine hospital use. It should be kept frozen preferably at or below –20°C.

Technique No. 3.6. Recalcification of human plasma for use as a typing reagent

The separated plasma is placed in a 37°C incubator for approximately 15 minutes. 2 ml calcium chloride (1M) are added for each 100 ml plasma, and the mixture is left for a further half an hour to allow the clot to form. The clot is then broken up by shaking and left in the incubator for 1½ hours. The fluid is stored at 4°C overnight and strained through muslin the following day, after which it is frozen at –20°C.

Chapter 4. The ABO sub-groups

There are a number of sub-groups of A but the main division is into A_1 and A_2 by means of anti-A_1 serum. Anti-A_1 which is specific for A_1 is a normal component of the anti-A found in group B and group O individuals. It can be isolated. This serum is usually prepared by absorbing an anti-A (group B) serum with group A_2 red cells, which remove anti-A and leave anti-A_1. Using anti-A_1 so prepared groups A and AB can be sub-divided into A_1 and A_2 A_1B and A_2B (Table 4.1)

Table 4.1 Reactions of various sub-groups of A with anti-A, anti-B, and anti-A_1. Key as in Table 2.2

Group	Reactions with:		
	Anti-A	Anti-B	Anti-A_1 (α_1)
A_1	C	–	C
A_2	C	–	–
A_1B	C	C	C
A_2B	C	C	–

Titration of a group B (*i.e.* an anti-A) serum against red cells of sub-groups A_1 and A_2, A_1B and A_2B shows that the strength of the A agglutinogen in each of the sub-groups is different. The titration values of the anti-A serum against red cells of each sub-group shows that these strengths are in the order $A_1 > A_1B > A_2 > A_2B$. The range of titre can be considerable. For example, in a particular case using an extremely potent anti-A serum, the titre with A_1 was 16,000, with A_1B 4000, with A_2, 1000 and A_2B 128. In another case in which the anti-A was of average standard for grouping, the times were A_1 256, A_1B 128 with A_2 64, A_2B 16. These figures show how necessary it is, when selecting anti-A grouping serum, to titrate against red cells of the weakly reacting sub-groups, especially A_2B.

If the titration method is used to differentiate between the sub-groups of A it soon becomes apparent that there are occasional examples of red cells encountered in which the A agglutinogen is even weaker than in the sub-group A_2B. Such red cells are called A_3 and A_3B. These give a characteristic appearance with anti-A sera, which consists of some quite large agglutinates with many free cells. It should be noted that typing with anti-A_1 serum will not allow a distinction to be made between A_2 and A_3 since the cells of both these sub-groups are negative with anti-A_1 serum. Further researches have revealed even weaker sub-groups of A which are all negative with anti-A_1 and differ from A_2 in other ways but chiefly

34

in the strength of the agglutinogen. In some, the antigen is so weak as not to be detectable with ordinary anti-A grouping serum and it is chiefly on account of these that group O serum is included in routine grouping tests.

Anti-A$_1$

Anti-A$_1$ (α_1) occurs as an atypical cold agglutinin in the sera of individuals who lack the corresponding antigen.

The frequency of occurrence varies with the sub-group. In A$_2$ it is about 2 per cent, in A$_2$B about 26 per cent and in the weaker sub-groups even higher to the extent of being almost a constant feature of some of them. The figures refer to the atypical anti-A$_1$ agglutinins sufficiently potent to be active at room temperature. If tests are done at 4°C many more will be found.

It must be emphasised that the anti-A$_1$ component of group B and group O sera is always present and is not a cold agglutinin. Its temperature range is similar to anti-A and anti-B, which, although slightly more active in the cold, show little change of titre with temperature and are always active at 37°C.

When active at room temperature the presence of an anti-A$_1$ agglutinin in the serum of persons of groups A$_2$ and A$_2$B often leads to anomalous blood grouping results. This has already been referred to in Chapter 2. The anomalous results, as might be expected from the percentage occurrence of anti-A$_1$ agglutinins, are most often associated with sub-group A$_2$B. For example, although the red cells of an individual of sub-group A$_2$B will give the normal reactions expected of those of AB, the serum, if it contains an anti-A$_1$ will give the reactions characteristic of group B (*see* Table 4.2). Such individuals cannot be said to belong to group AB until further tests have been carried out. These tests comprise typing the red cells with anti-A$_1$ serum to confirm that they do in fact belong to sub-group A$_2$B, and testing the serum with subgroup A$_2$ cells in addition to those of A$_1$ to show that the atypical agglutinin does not react with A$_2$ cells and is, therefore, anti-A$_1$. If anti-A$_1$ typing serum and cells of sub-group A$_2$ are not available the serum grouping test may be repeated at 37°C in which case the anti-A$_1$ being a cold agglutinin will be inactive and the results obtained will be those expected of group AB. However, this second test does not give so satisfactory a proof of the presence of anti-A$_1$ in a group A$_2$B sample as does the first.

The question naturally arises as to whether anomalous grouping results can be satisfactorily avoided by using sub-group A$_2$ cells for routine serum grouping tests rather than A$_1$. This procedure is not recommended for three main reasons. Firstly, A$_2$ cells do not react as crisply with the wide range of anti-A agglutinin strengths encountered in routine tests as do A$_1$ cells. Thus for the sake of avoiding a few anomalous results, the serum grouping tests would be rendered less reliable and more laborious to read as macroscopic agglutination would be less frequent. Secondly, the presence of atypical anti-A$_1$ agglutinins would go undetected which would mean that agglutinins potent enough for use as anti-A$_1$ typing sera could not be collected. In addition, and of greater importance, the occasional immune anti-A$_1$ which is active at 37°C and, therefore, may be of clinical significance, would be missed. Thirdly, A$_2$ cells will themselves be agglutinated by the anti-H and anti-HI types of atypical cold agglutinins (*see* below), and would thus give rise to a further set of anomalous results.

Table 4.2 Agglutination reactions of a sub-group A_2B, the serum of which contains an anti-A_1 active at room temperature

Sub-group A_2B	Anti-A serum	Anti-B serum	Anti-A_1 serum	Red cells		
				A_1	B	A_2
Reaction of red cells	+	C	−			
Reaction of serum				V	−	−

It is of great importance to realise it is just in the circumstance in which the presence of an atypical anti-A_1 may cause anomalous serum grouping results that the cell grouping test also may give an erroneous result. This takes the form of a false negative which may occur if the anti-A grouping serum being used is not of sufficient potency for the detection of the weak A agglutinogen which is characteristic of these low sub-groups of A. Herein lies the necessity for ensuring an adequate titre of anti-A grouping serum with cells of A_2B and for using group O serum as a check. The most usual mistake to occur if these precautions are omitted is the grouping as B of an A_2B with anti-A_1 in the serum. The use of A_2 cells as an extra serum check on all apparent group B samples will prevent such mistakes being made.

Sera reacting preferentially with group O cells

Atypical cold agglutinins also appear in the sera of individuals of sub-groups A_1 and A_1B (and rarely of group B). These agglutinins are distinguished by their ability to agglutinate all group O and A_2 cells, whereas cells of other groups are agglutinated only weakly or not at all. This preference for cells of groups O and A_2 resulted in these agglutinins being termed "anti-O" or "anti-A_2" (α_2) but they are now called anti-HI. Certain animal sera, particularly from oxen, occasionally contain an agglutinin which reacts preferentially with human O and A_2 red cells as also do certain plant extracts (*see* below). It was at first thought that all examples of such agglutinins whether of human or animal origin were of the same type and were detecting a product of the O gene, A_2 cells being agglutinated because they contained an O factor in addition to A. This is now known not to be the case and it is thought that the O gene is a 'silent' gene and does not produce a specific antigen.

The animal sera and seed extracts react with a substance called H. It is this substance on which the enzymes produced by the A and B genes act to produce A and B substances while in group O the H substance is unchanged. Apparently the production of A substance in A_2 uses less H than A_1 or B. We can see therefore why anti-H would react more strongly with O cells and with A_2 and less strongly with B and A_1. Some sera of human origin are also anti-H in specificity. H substance is secreted in saliva (*see* Chapter 6) and so anti-H sera are characterised by being inhibited by secretor saliva.

We are left with an assortment of human sera which react preferentially with group O cells. Some of these are detecting an antigen produced as a result of the interaction of the H and I genes (*see* Chapter 16) and they are called anti-HI.

Antibodies to the compound antigens IB and IA also occur, although they are very rare. Their presence is usually masked by the normal anti-B or anti-A of the serum in which they occur. They can be disclosed by absorbing the sera with cord cells of the appropriate ABO group as these cells are I negative and so do not react with anti-IB or anti-IA.

Those concerned mainly with the more practical aspects of these cold agglutinins should realise that these too can cause anomalous grouping results. When anomalous results are encountered the red cells of the individual should be typed with anti-A_1 and the serum shown to agglutinate O and A_2 cells either preferentially or exclusively.

Table 4.3 The ABO blood group system, showing the sub-groups of A, with particular reference to the antibody content of the serum

Group	Reactions with anti-A_1 (α_1)	Agglutinins always present (typical)[1]	Agglutinins sometimes present (atypical)[2]
A_1	+	Anti-B	AntiH and anti-HI
A_2 (and A_3, A_X, etc.)	-	Anti-B	Anti-A_1 (α_1)
A_1B	+	None	Anti-H and anti-HI
A_2B (and A_3B, A_XB, etc.)	-	None	Anti-A_1 (α_1)
B	-	Anti-A (α) and anti-A_1 (α_1)	Anti-H and anti-HI
O	-	Anti-A (α) and anti-A_1 (α_1) Anti-B	

[1] React strongly at 4°C, room temperature, and 37°C.
[2] React strongly at 4°C, less strongly or not at all at room temperature—very rarely active at 37°C.

The fact that the ABO system has both typical and atypical agglutinins is often found to be confusing, particularly as anti-A_1 occurs in both forms. Table 4.3 clearly differentiates between the two types of agglutinins and indicates the groups in which each antibody may be found.

Plant agglutinins (lectins)

It has long been known that extracts of certain seeds will agglutinate human red cells. Most of these extracts are of little importance in routine blood group serology as they do not clearly differentiate the blood groups.

Two extracts are, however, useful in testing for the sub-groups of A. *Dolichos biflorus* seeds are a rich source of an anti-A lectin which reacts very strongly with the sub-group A_1 much less strongly with A_2 and not at all with the other subgroups of A. By suitable dilution a specific anti-A_1 reagent can be prepared which is more potent and avid than most, if not all, the anti-A_1 reagents prepared from human serum.

Ulex europaeus on the other hand is a good source of anti-H, so that *Ulex* extract reacts much more strongly with A_2 and the weaker sub-groups of A than with A_1. It is possible to choose a dilution and technique by which these extracts used in parallel will react antithetically and distinguish the sub-groups A_1 and A_2.

Sub-groups of B

In group B there is no variation in antigen strength comparable to that of A nor is group B divisible into two main sub-groups as A is divided by anti-A_1. However, sub-groups of B do occur and may very rarely be the cause of anomalies in ABO grouping. An account of some of the recent work on the sub-groups of B is given in Chapter 16.

TECHNIQUES

Technique No. 4.1 Preparation of human anti-A₁ sera

To choose a suitable group B serum, a number of sera are titrated against A_1 and A_2 cells—a suitable serum has a titre of at least 512 with A_1 cells and shows a difference in titre between the A_1 and A_2 cells of several dilutions.

For the absorption the serum is mixed with half its own volume of packed washed group A_2 red cells (the cells are washed by shaking them in an excess of normal saline, centrifuging and removing the supernatant fluid. This process is repeated three times). The serum-cell mixture is allowed to stand in the ice chest at 3–5°C for 2 hours. The mixture is then centrifuged and the supernatant serum collected. If the absorption has been successful the serum will give no reaction with A_2 cells and a titre of 16 or greater with A_1 cells. If there is still a reaction with A_2 cells it may be necessary to reabsorb with half the quantity of cells but if there is only a slight reaction it is often better to dilute the serum to give a negative reaction with the A_2 cells rather than to reabsorb. Over absorption may result in the removal of some of the anti-A agglutinins.

Ideally the serum should give macroscopic agglutination with all A_1 and A_1B cells and be negative with A_2 and A_2B cells. In practice it will be found that some A_1 cells give much weaker reactions than others. Moreover, a serum that is negative with almost all A_2 and A_1B cells will occasionally give a weak reaction with cells from a few persons of these groups. It is for this reason that it is advisable to use at least two different anti-A_1 reagents for typing purposes.

Anti-A_1 also occurs in A_2 and A_2B as a cold agglutinin and when it is sufficiently strong (*i.e.* giving a titre of 16 or more at room temperature) such a serum can be used as an anti-A_1 typing serum. The main disadvantage is that being a cold agglutinin small changes in temperature may affect the titre and avidity of the serum very considerably. This difficulty is minimised if a cold water bath or incubator at 12–15°C is available.

The selected and absorbed sera are clarified if necessary and then Seitz-filtered. The sterile serum is stored at –20°C in 1 ml. quantities.

Technique No. 4.2 Sub-typing with human anti-A_1 sera

The technique is essentially the same as for ABO grouping. One unit volume of an anti-A_1 serum is mixed with one unit volume of a 2 per cent suspension of red cells in a precipitin tube. The mixture is allowed to stand at room temperature for 2 hours before reading. No reaction is scored as negative until it has been examined microscopically. It is important to include controls consisting of known A_1 and A_2 cells with each batch of tests. At least two anti-A_1 sera should be used.

Technique No. 4.3. Preparation of anti-A_1 from *Dolichos biflorus*

A 2-g packet of seeds is soaked overnight in approximately 25 ml of saline. The seeds are then ground, preferably in an electric grinder but a pepper mill may be used. The extract is poured off, a further 25 ml of saline added and the seeds reground. The process is repeated once more. The three amounts of fluid are pooled and stored at $-20°C$.

The ground seeds are again soaked overnight. The extraction procedure is repeated the next day until the seeds are thoroughly macerated and the volume of fluid has reached about 600 ml. The process can be completed on the third day or continued over several days.

The pooled extract is filtered through several layers of gauze to remove coarse particles and frozen overnight. After thawing, it is centrifuged hard after which the supernatant is collected, and frozen and thawed once more. It is examined for coarse particles which tend to come out when the extract is stored and if necessary it is refiltered and/or centrifuged to remove these. When the suspension is fine it is standardised by testing by both tile and tube techniques at various dilutions against A_1 and A_2 cells.

The *Dolichos* extract should be used at a dilution which gives strong agglutination with A_1 cells while being negative with A_2.

The extract can be freeze-dried, stored and reconstituted when required. This procedure is usually unnecessary, however, as it stores very well frozen at $-20°C$.

It is tested with a panel of known cells of sub-groups A_1 and A_2 as the extract may need dilution to give clear negatives with A_2 cells (*see* technique No. 4.5).

Technique No. 4.4. Preparation of anti-H from *Ulex europaeus*

The seeds are ground in a mill and to each gram of meal 10 ml of saline is added. The mixture is thoroughly agitated mechanically for at least 1 hour and then centrifuged at 3,000 r.p.m. for about five minutes and the sediment discarded. If the supernatant fluid is cloudy, the preparation may be re-centrifuged and/or filtered through a clarifying Seitz filter (grade 4). Alternatively a good product may be obtained by centrifugation in a high speed centrifuge at about 12,000 for 1 hour. It is sometimes possible to obtain a second active extract from the same ground seeds but the second extraction should be checked for activity before being pooled with the first one.

The resulting extract reacts with almost all human red cells, the reaction declining in strength in the direction $O \rightarrow A_2 \rightarrow B \rightarrow A_2B \rightarrow A_1 \rightarrow A_1B$. It is essential that the extract is used at a suitable dilution so that the A_1 and A_1B groups are negative and the A_2 and A_2B groups positive (*see* technique No. 4.5).

Technique 4.5. Sub-typing using *Dolichos* and *Ulex* extracts

When sub-typing using both *Ulex* and *Dolichos*, a slide-technique is very convenient. Both reagents are used diluted: a suitable dilution for *Dolichos* is 1:10 or 1:15 and *Ulex* 1:2 or undiluted.

One drop of a 5 per cent saline suspension of the unknown cells is mixed with one drop of *Dolichos* extract on a long slide, the controls being known A_1 and A_2 cells. At the same time one drop of the 5 per cent suspension is mixed with *Ulex* extract, the controls being O, A_2 and A_1 cells. A_1 cells are strongly agglutinated by the *Dolichos* and are negative with the *Ulex*. A_2 cells are positive with *Ulex* and negative with *Dolichos*. Occasionally a sample is encountered which gives weak positive reactions with both extracts; this belongs to a rare type known as A_{int} (*see also* Chapter 16). It is important that the tests are read as soon as the positive control is well developed and while the negative control is still completely unagglutinated. If the tests are read later, false positive results will certainly be obtained.

Sub-typing with *Dolichos* can be satisfactorily carried out by a tube-technique. This method is essentially the same as for testing with anti-A_1 serum (technique No. 6.2).

Practical Importance

Although of considerable academic interest the sub-groups of A are of limited practical importance. Anomalous grouping results due primarily to the occurrence of atypical anti-A_1 agglutinins will be encountered sooner or later and must be dealt with according to the methods described above. As a general rule cold agglutinins such as anti-A_1 and anti-H can be disregarded when selecting blood for transfusion. However, these antibodies are sometimes stimulated by transfusion or pregnancy, in which case, not only do they increase in titre but also become active at higher temperatures. It is only when they reach 37°C that blood of the same sub-group as the recipient must be selected for transfusion.

Chapter 5. The Inheritance of the ABO Groups

GENERAL CONSIDERATIONS

It is assumed that the reader will have an adequate knowledge of the principles underlying the Mendelian theory of inheritance. Its application to blood groups in general has been discussed briefly in Chapter 1. All the genetic terms used in this chapter are defined briefly in the Glossary to which reference should be made by any to whom the sense in which we have used them may not be quite clear.

The characters A, B, and O will be considered first; once the mode of inheritance of these is understood it is comparatively simple to expand the scheme to include the sub-groups of A.

Table 5.1 The ABO groups and their corresponding genotypes

Blood group or phenotype	Genotypes
A	AA
	AO
B	BB
	BO
O	OO
AB	AB

According to the generally accepted theory of Bernstein the characters A, B, and O are inherited by means of three allelomorphic genes, also called *A, B,* and *O*. Every individual has two chromosomes each carrying either *A, B,* or *O*, one chromosome from each parent. Thus the possible ABO genotypes are *AA, AO, BB, BO, AB,* and *OO*. ABO typing is normally only carried out using the two anti-sera, anti-A and anti-B detecting the characters A and B. This divides the population into the four blood groups, group A (phenotype A) comprising two genotypes *AA* (homozygous) and *AO* (heterozygous), group B (phenotype B) comprising two genotypes *BB* (homozygous) and *BO* (heterozygous), group O (phenotype O) genotype *OO* (homozygous) and group AB where the phenotype and the genotype are both *AB* (heterozygous) (Table 5.1).

To illustrate the mode of inheritance a particular type of mating, *e.g.* that in which a group A male mates with a group B female, can be considered. The group A male may be of genotype *AA* or *AO* and similarly the group B female may be of the genotype *BB* or *BO*, therefore within this one mating four possibilities exist, namely (*a*) *AA* with *BB*, (*b*) *AA* with *BO*, (*c*) *AO* with *BB* and (*d*) *AO* with *BO*. The outcome of the four matings is shown diagrammatically in Figs. 5.1a-d.

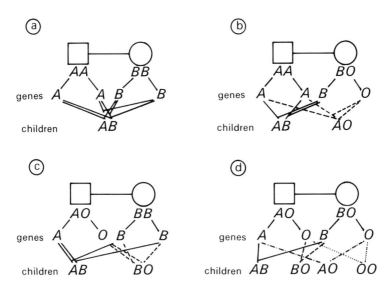

Fig. 5.1 a–d. The four genotype matings included in the phenotype mating A × B, and the children arising therefrom.

Table 5.2 The various ABO matings and the children which can arise from them

| Mating | | Children | |
Phenotypes	Genotypes	Genotypes	Phenotypes
A × A	(1) *AA × AA* (2) *AA × AO* (3) *AO × AO*	(1) *AA* (2) *AA* and *AO* (3) *AA, AO,* and *OO*	A and O
A × B	(1) *AA × BB* (2) *AA × BO* (3) *AO × BB* (4) *AO × BO*	(1) *AB* (2) *AB* and *AO* (3) *AB* and *BO* (4) *AB, AO, BO,* and *OO*	A, B, AB, and O
A × AB	(1) *AA × AB* (2) *AO × AB*	(1) *AA* and *AB* (2) *AA, AB, AO,* and *BO*	A, B, and AB
A × O	(1) *AA × OO* (2) *AO × OO*	(1) *AO* (2) *AO* and *OO*	A and O
B × B	(1) *BB × BB* (2) *BB × BO* (3) *BO × BO*	(1) *BB* (2) *BB* and *BO* (3) *BB, BO,* and *OO*	B and O
B × AB	(1) *BB × AB* (2) *BO × AB*	(1) *AB* and *BB* (2) *AB, BB, AO,* and *BO*	A, B, and AB
B × O	(1) *BB × OO* (2) *BO × OO*	(1) *BO* (2) *BO* and *OO*	B and O
AB × AB	(1) *AB × AB*	(1) *AA, AB,* and *BB*	A, B, and AB
AB × O	(1) *AB × OO*	(1) *AO* and *BO*	A and B
O × O	(1) *OO × OO*	(1) *OO*	O

It will be seen that this mating can result in children of all four blood groups or phenotypes, although it is only in mating d, AO with $BO,$ that children of all four blood groups can occur in the same family. This mating also shows that a determination of the groups of relatives will sometimes disclose the genotype of group A or group B individuals, *e.g.* the finding of a group O child in an A × B mating demonstrates the presence of the O gene in both parents, and it follows that any A or B children arising from this particular mating are heterozygous, *i.e.* AO or $BO.$ Table 5.2 shows all the possible ABO matings and the children which can arise from them. Naturally in considering a whole population all the possible genotype combinations will occur for each group of matings, but in considering a particular family only one genotype combination will represent the truth. For example, as we have seen there are four possible alternatives of the A × B mating and in the whole population each one of these four will be found; any particular family, however, can only belong to mating a, b, c, or d (Fig 5.1). Sometimes the particular genotype combination will be evident from the phenotypes found but often it will not be possible to determine the genotypes involved.

Table 5.3 ABO matings showing possible and impossible phenotypes of children

Mating	Possible phenotypes of children	Impossible phenotypes of children
A × A	A and O	B and AB
A × B	A, B, O, and AB	None
A × AB	A, B, and AB	O
A × O	A and O	B and AB
B × B	B and O	A and AB
B × AB	A, B, and AB	O
B × O	B and O	A and AB
AB × AB	A, B, and AB	O
AB × O	A and B	AB and O
O × O	O	A, B, and AB

This means that in Table 5.2 while the two genotype columns are important in enabling us to predict which phenotypes can occur among the offspring of any given mating, they can be omitted for most practical purposes. Table 5.3 is this simplified form of Table 5.2 with the addition of a column which gives the phenotypes which cannot occur among the children of each given mating. It is this column, of course, which is useful in the interpretation of paternity tests. It is obviously never possible to tell whether a man is the father of a given child as there will be many men of the same phenotype, but it is sometimes possible to say that he cannot be the father as, for instance, when he is group O and the child is group AB.

Extension to include sub-groups of A

The Bernstein theory of inheritance can now be extended to include the sub-groups of A by the simple expedient of replacing A by A_1 and A_2.

Table 5.4 shows the groups of phenotypes with their corresponding genotypes

Table 5.4 ABO blood group phenotypes and genotypes, including sub-groups of A

Blood group or phenotype	Genotypes
A_1	A^1A^1
	A^1O
	A^1A^2
A_2	A^2A^2
	A^2O
B	BB
	BO
O	OO
A_1B	A^1B
A_2B	A^2B

Table 5.5 ABO Matings, including the sub-groups of A

Mating	Possible phenotypes of children	Impossible phenotypes of children
$A_1 \times A_1$	A_1, O, A_2	B, A_1B, A_2B
$A_1 \times A_2$	A_1, A_2, O	B, A_1B, A_2B
$A_1 \times B$	A_1, A_2, B, O, A_1B, A_2B	None
$A_1 \times O$	A_1, A_2, O	B, A_1B, A_2B
$A_1 \times A_1B$	A_1, B, A_1B, A_2B	A_2, O
$A_1 \times A_2B$	A_1, A_2, B, A_1B, A_2B	O
$A_2 \times A_2$	A_2, O	A_1, B, A_1B, A_2B
$A_2 \times B$	A_2, B, O, A_2B	A_1, A_1B
$A_2 \times O$	A_2, O	A_1, B, A_1B, A_2B
$A_2 \times A_1B$	A_1, B, A_2B	A_2, O, A_1B
$A_2 \times A_2B$	A_2, B, A_2B	A_1, O, A_1B
$B \times B$	B, O	A_1, A_2, A_1B, A_2B
$B \times O$	B, O	A_1, A_2, A_1B, A_2B
$B \times A_1B$	A_1, A_1B, B	A_2, O, A_2B
$B \times A_2B$	A_2, B, A_2B	A_1, O, A_1B
$O \times O$	O	A_1, A_2, B, A_1B, A_2B
$O \times A_1B$	A_1, B	A_2, O, A_1B, A_2B
$O \times A_2B$	A_2, B	A_1, O, A_1B, A_2B
$A_1B \times A_1B$	A_1, B, A_1B	A_2, O, A_2B
$A_1B \times A_2B$	A_1, B, A_1B, A_2B	A_2, O
$A_2B \times A_2B$	A_2, B, A_2B	A_1, O, A_1B

Table 5.6 The mating $A_1 \times B$

Mating possible genotypes	Possible phenotypes of children	Impossible phenotypes of children
$A^1A^1 \times BB$	A_1B	A_1, B, A_2, A_2B, O
$A^1A^1 \times BO$	A_1B, A_1	B, A_2, A_2B, O
$A^1O \times BB$	A_1B, B	A_1, A_2, A_2B, O
$A^1O \times BO$	A_1, B, A_1B, O	A_2, A_2, B
$A^1A^2 \times BB$	A_1B, A_2B	A_1, B, A_2, O
$A^1A^2 \times BO$	A_1, A_2, A_1B, A_2B	B, O

and Table 5.5 the various matings and the groups which can and cannot arise from them. This table applies to the whole population. In considering any particular family, however, it must be remembered that although each parent may belong to any one of the genotypes of which has phenotype is comprised he cannot in fact belong to more than one. The six possible genotype matings included in the one phenotype mating $A_1 \times B$ are shown in Table 5.6 together with the phenotypes which can and cannot be found among the offspring of each mating. Sometimes by studying the phenotypes of the children it is possible to say to which genotype the parents belong. Moreover, it will be seen that for the mating $A_1 \times B$, A_2 and A_2B children never occur in the same family as B or O children so that—although, taking all $A_1 \times B$ matings together, all six phenotypes can occur—the finding of, for instance, a group O child in a family where other children are A_2 and A_2B would not be possible if they all had the same parents.

Chapter 6. The Group Specific Substances A, B and H in Tissues and Body Fluids

It has long been realised that the blood group substances A and B are not confined to the red cells but can be detected in tissue cells and particularly in body fluids. They have a wide distribution and have been found in serum, saliva, gastric juices, ovarian cyst fluid, semen, amniotic fluid, and in smaller quantity in sweat, urine, tears, bile and milk. One of the richest and most readily available sources of group specific substance is saliva, and so it is used extensively in detecting the presence of these substances in any given individual. In about 24 per cent of the population, however, ABO group specific substances are almost absent from the saliva and other body fluids. Those individuals whose saliva contains the appropriate ABO group specific substances are called secretors while those whose saliva is devoid of such substances are called non-secretors. Even in non-secretors a small amount of group specific substance is often detectable using sensitive techniques, *e.g.* elution, *see* Chapter 29.

It has been established that secretion of group specific substances is controlled by a pair of allelomorphic genes, *Se* and *se* with *Se* dominant over *se*. Thus individuals can be homozygous *SeSe,* heterozygous *Sese* or homozygous *sese*. The first two classes are secretors and the third class, non-secretors. There is evidence that there are two distinct forms of group specific substance, one a water soluble glycoprotein present in most body fluids and one alcohol soluble glycolipid present in red cells and almost all other tissues but absent from the secretions. The presence of the water soluble form is controlled by the secretor gene whereas the alcohol soluble form is not so controlled. In other words the tissue cells of every individual, whether secretor or non-secretor, contain a form of group specific substance which can be extracted with alcohol, but the secretor in addition to this possesses the water soluble form which appears in the body fluids. Group O persons are divided into secretors and non-secretors according to whether their saliva contains H. Secretors of A, B, and AB also have H in their saliva.

More precise knowledge of the distribution of ABH substances in the tissues has been acquired by the use of mixed agglutination and immunofluorescence techniques by means of which the substances may be traced to individual cells. For example, immunofluorescence staining has shown ABH substances in the cell membranes of all vascular endothelial cells and some epithelial cells. These membrane antigens are alcohol-soluble and occur in both secretors and non-secretors. ABH substances are secreted in a water-soluble form as glycoproteins in the mucous glands of many organs. These are controlled by the secretor gene. Strangely, the Brunner's glands situated more deeply in the mucosa of the pylorus and small intestine produce what appear to be water soluble glycoproteins in both secretors and non-secretors. However the ABH substances produced by the gastric parietal glands which are also found in both secretors and non-secretors are alcohol soluble and probably lipid in nature.

ABH substances appear in the milk of secretors but there is usually much more H than A and B. Small amounts are found in sweat and plasma but these are not controlled by the secretor gene and are largely alcohol-soluble glycolipids.

The fact that group specific substances are detectable in most tissues and body fluids, has led many workers to attempt their isolation with a view to studying their chemical nature. The richest sources of group specific substances in water soluble form are the body secretions, saliva, gastric juices and the fluid contained in pseudo-mucinous ovarian cysts. A similar non-human material which is rich in a substance showing A specificity is commercial hog pepsin. From these materials a purified form of group specific substance can be extracted. There are several methods but the phenol extraction method is, for practical purposes, the one used today.

When ovarian cyst fluids are used as the source of blood-group substance the crude freeze-dried cyst contents are extracted with cold 95 per cent phenol. The blood-group active material is then usually obtained as phenol-insoluble residue, whereas the contaminating protein goes into solution in phenol. The phenol-insoluble residue is then further purified by fractionation from aqueous solution with ethanol, high-speed centrifugation, etc. Sometimes some of the blood-group active material goes into solution in phenol and this can then be recovered from phenol solution by precipitation with 10 per cent ethanol. Higher concentrations of alcohol are needed to bring down the dissolved protein. If saliva or stomach mucosal linings are used as a source of blood-group substance these are usually digested with pepsin before they are freeze-dried and extracted with phenol. The pepsin treatment does not affect the serological properties of the substances but it alters the solubility in phenol in such a way that most of the material becomes soluble. The blood-group substance can again be recovered from the phenol solution by precipitation with 10 per cent ethanol.

The group specific substance thus prepared shows little or no antigenicity when injected into rabbits unless the substances are first combined with Shiga conjugated protein. In Man the response to the substances is quite marked without prior conjugation with protein. Extremely potent grouping sera can be obtained either in Man or animals by the injection of appropriately prepared substances.

In order to detect group specific substances in solution, advantage is taken of the fact that the soluble substance is capable of neutralising specifically its corresponding antibody. This neutralisation is reflected in a complete or partial inhibition of the agglutinin titre. This is the basis of the inhibition technique, which is of great importance in blood group serology as it can be adapted for many purposes. It can, for instance, be used for the detection of red cell agglutinogens in blood samples in which the red cells are too damaged to agglutinate properly and in forensic medicine it is used for the identification of antigens in blood stains. The tissue cells of the liver, spleen, kidney, etc., can be subjected to the inhibition test in order to find out whether or not they contain A or B substances, but in this case the difficulty of separating the tissue cells from blood cells must be overcome. This is most satisfactorily done by haemolysing the red cells in the well crushed tissue with distilled water and removing them as stromata after slow centrifugation. Because of the difficulty of ensuring complete removal of stromata, the inhibition technique is not now used for the detection of tissue antigens but is replaced by the mixed agglutination technique where this problem is overcome.

When detecting the presence of group specific substances it is advisable to test against both anti-A and anti-B agglutinins because except in the case of material from group AB individuals, one or other agglutinin forms a valuable negative control and so confirms the specificity of the group specific substance in question. If the available test material is small in quantity it can be tested against a mixture of anti-A and anti-B agglutinins rather than with each one separately. For this purpose a special mixture of anti-A and anti-B should be made. It is inadvisable to use group O sera as these may contain antibody molecules which cross react with both A and B.

The strength of the anti-A and anti-B agglutinins chosen for inhibition tests should be moderate, a titration value of 32 or 64 being convenient. If more potent sera are used the sensitivity of the test is decreased. When the group specific substance present in group O individuals is under investigation, anti-H must be used to measure the H content of the saliva. It is also important to include tests with anti-H in the identification of stains from body fluids (*e.g.* saliva, seminal fluid) in forensic work.

The group A cells used, particularly in testing saliva, should be of sub-group A_2 since the A group specific substance more readily neutralises the anti-A (α) component of the serum than the anti-A_1 (α_1). Consequently any inhibition which may occur will be more apparent if group A_2 cells, which only react with the anti-A (α) component, are used for the titration.

A modification of the method can be used in circumstances in which a more precise estimate of the strength of a particular group specific substance is required or when a comparison of the relative strengths of several fluids, *e.g.* salivas, is undertaken. This involves making serial dilutions of the saliva and testing each dilution against the standard anti-serum. By this method it is possible to obtain a titration value for the group specific substance itself.

TECHNIQUES

Technique No. 6.1. Preparation of saliva

Some saliva is collected in a suitable container. It is then transferred to a test-tube, diluted with an approximately equal quantity of saline, and placed in a boiling water bath for 10 minutes to destroy enzyme activity. The tube is then centifuged and the clear supernatant fluid is used in the following tests.

Technique No. 6.2. Determination of secretor status (screening test)

Suitable dilutions of anti-A, anti-B and anti-H reagents are made to give titres of 32 approximately. The saliva is tested 'neat' (*i.e.* diluted with one part of saline and inactivated as in technique No. 6.1) and at 1:10 to act as a confirmation. Each saliva preparation is tested against anti-A, anti-B and anti-H using equal volumes of saliva and antiserum. A control of one volume of saline in place of the saliva is included for each antiserum. The tests are allowed to stand for 30-60 minutes at room temperature. One volume of the appropriate A_2, B or O red cells is added to each tube. After 2 hours incubation at room temperature, the degree of agglutination is read. Secretor saliva will normally give complete inhibition of agglutination both 'neat' and at '1:10'.

Table 6.1 Determination of secretor status

	Saliva X Neat	1/10	Saline control
Anti-A	–	–	C
Anti-B	C	C	C
Anti-H	–	–	V

Conclusion

Saliva X is from a secretor of A and H substances.

Technique No. 6.3. Inhibition test using undiluted saliva

The crux of the test is the comparison of titration values of anti-A, anti-B and anti-H anti-sera before and after the addition of saliva from persons of groups A, B, or AB.

The anti-A and anti-B sera chosen should have titres of approximately 32. One unit volume of such an anti-A serum is mixed with one unit volume of saliva and similarly one unit volume of anti-B serum is mixed with one unit volume of saliva and for Anti-H equal volumes of *Ulex europeus* extract and saliva are mixed together. It is unlikely that this reagent will require dilution since its titre by saline technique is normally about 32. These mixtures are allowed to stand on the bench for 30 minutes and while waiting for them to absorb the dilutions for the original titres of the anti-A and anti-B sera can be carried out. The red cells of course should not be added at this stage. The procedure for making the dilutions is similar to the method already described for titration of anti-A and anti-B agglutinins (*see* technique No. 3.2) with the exception that a volume of saline is placed in all tubes of the row including the first and one volume only of the serum to be titrated is used and this is placed in the first tube of the row. Thus instead of having undiluted serum in the first tube it is diluted 1:2 with saline and is comparable with the serum which is diluted 1:2 with saliva. After 30 minutes the serum-saliva mixtures are titrated in exactly the same manner as the original anti-A and anti-B sera. Appropriate red cell suspensions are added to all the tubes and they are allowed to stand on the bench for 2 hours. They are then read and the results scored in the normal manner for titrations.

C

If the titration value of the anti-A serum is reduced after being mixed with the saliva, then the saliva contains the group specific substance A. Similarly, if the titration value of the anti-B is reduced the saliva contains group specific substance B. Saliva from secretors of all ABO groups will inhibit the anti-H but O and A_2 are most active for H, and A_1 and A_1B least active

Typical Result

$$\text{Original titre of anti-A serum} = 64$$
$$\text{Titre of anti-A serum} + \text{saliva} = 0$$
$$\text{Original titre of anti-B serum} = 32$$
$$\text{Titre of anti-B serum} + \text{saliva} = 32$$

Conclusion

Reduction in titre of anti-A from 64 to 0 indicates presence of group A substance in the saliva.

No reduction in titre of anti-B indicates absence of group B substance in the saliva.

Therefore saliva is from a secretor individual of group A.

This test can be made even more sensitive by adding one volume of saliva to each tube of the titre. This will detect the small amount of substance present in some non-secretor salivas. It can also be used for body fluids such as tears, plasma, etc. where the amount of group specific substance is much less than in saliva.

Technique No. 6.4. Inhibition technique using dilutions of saliva

When saliva from different secretors is being compared the technique given above is too sensitive in that the antibody will be neutralised completely using undiluted saliva from all secretors; thus it is necessary to dilute the saliva and then test against a standard quantity of antibody.

The standard serum should be of a titre of 32 or 64 giving two macroscopic reactions with standard cells and the saliva should be tested at dilutions ranging from 1:10 to 1:500. Suitable dilutions obtained by means of standard graduated pipettes are shown in the following table:

Table 6.2 Preparation of saliva dilutions

Saliva			Saline	Dilution
0.1 ml	neat saliva	+	0.9 ml	$\frac{1}{10}$
0.2 ml	$\frac{1}{10}$ "	+	0.8 ml	$\frac{1}{50}$
0.1 ml	$\frac{1}{10}$ "	+	0.9 ml	$\frac{1}{100}$
0.1 ml	$\frac{1}{50}$ "	+	0.2 ml	$\frac{1}{150}$
0.1 ml	$\frac{1}{100}$ "	+	0.1 ml	$\frac{1}{200}$
0.1 ml	$\frac{1}{50}$ "	+	0.4 ml	$\frac{1}{250}$
0.1 ml	$\frac{1}{100}$ "	+	0.2 ml	$\frac{1}{300}$
0.1 ml	$\frac{1}{50}$ "	+	0.6 ml	$\frac{1}{350}$
0.1 ml	$\frac{1}{100}$ "	+	0.3 ml	$\frac{1}{400}$
0.1 ml	$\frac{1}{100}$ "	+	0.4 ml	$\frac{1}{500}$

Using a Pasteur pipette and starting with the weakest dilution of saliva, one volume of each dilution is pipetted into a row of precipitin tubes, after which an equal volume of test serum is added to each tube, mixed with the saliva dilution and allowed to stand at room temperature for 30-60 minutes. Then one volume of cells of appropriate group added and the reaction read after a further 1½ to 2 hours at room temperature. In all cases a control of saline + serum is included. Most secretor salivas will give complete inhibition up to a point within the $\frac{1}{100}$ to $\frac{1}{1000}$ range. If pseudo mucinous cyst fluids are being tested a much wider range of dilutions should be tested as a screen—for instance $\frac{1}{10}, \frac{1}{250}, \frac{1}{500}, \frac{1}{1000}, \frac{1}{5000}, \frac{1}{10000}$, and then a further set of dilutions tested, closing in on the highest dilution which is giving complete inhibition.

Typical result

Dilutions of saliva	$\frac{1}{10}$	$\frac{1}{50}$	$\frac{1}{100}$	$\frac{1}{150}$	$\frac{1}{200}$	$\frac{1}{250}$	$\frac{1}{300}$	$\frac{1}{350}$	$\frac{1}{400}$	$\frac{1}{500}$	saline
Agglutination reaction											control
with standard cells	—	—	—	—	(+)	++	V	V	V	V	V

This shows that up to a dilution of $\frac{1}{150}$ there is enough group specific substance to neutralise completely a titre of 32 of the corresponding antibody and that at $\frac{1}{200}$ and $\frac{1}{250}$ there is partial inhibition. This shows that the saliva is from a secretor but not from one secreting large amounts of group specific substance.

General Bibliography for ABO Section
(*Arranged in chronological order)

Landsteiner, K. (1900) Zur Kenntnis der antifermentativen, lytischen und agglutinierenden Wirkungen des Blutserum und der Lymphe. *Zbl. Bakt.,* **27,** 357.

Landsteiner, K. (1901) Ueber Agglutination-serscheinungen normalen menschlichen Blutes. *Wien klin. Wschr.,* **14,** 1132.

Decastello, A. V. & Sturli, A. (1902) Ueber die Isoagglutinine im Serum gesunder und kranker Menschen. *Münch. med. Wschr.,* 1090.

Dungern, E. Von & Hirszfeld, L. (1910) Ueber Verebung gruppenspezifischer Strukturen des Blutes. *Z. Immun. Forsch,* **6,** 284.

Dungern, E. Von & Hirszfeld, L. (1911) Ueber gruppenspezifische Strukturen des Blutes III. *Z. Immun. Forsch.,* **8,** 526.

Bernstein, F. (1924) Ergebnisse einer biostatischen zusammenfassenden Betrachtung über die erblichen Blutstrukturen des Menschen. *Klin. Wschr.,* **3,** 1495.

Schiff, F. (1924) Ueber gruppenspezifische Serumprecipitine. *Klin. Woch.,* **1,** 679.

Schiff, F. & Adelsberger, L. (1924) Ueber blutgruppenspezifische Antikörper und Antigene. *Zbl. Bakt., I Orig.,* **93,** 172.

Bernstein, F. (1925)Zusammenfassende Betrachtungen über die erblichen Blutstrukturen des Menschen. *Z. indukt. Abstamm. U. Vererb. Lehre.* **37,** 237.

Landsteiner, K. & Van Der Scheer, J. (1925) On the antigens of red blood corpuscles. *J. exp. Med.,* **41,** 427.

Landsteiner, K. & Witt, D. (1926) Observation on the human blood groups. *J. Immunol.,* **11,** 221.

Friedenreich, V. (1936) Eine bisher unbekannte Blutgruppeneigenschaft (A_3). *Z. Immun, Forsch.,* **89,** 409.

Taylor, G. L. & Ikin, E. W. (1939) Observations on the performance of blood-group tests. *Brit. med. J.,* **i,** 1027.

Morgan, W. T. J. & King, H. K. (1943) Studies in immuno-chemistry. The isolation from hog gastric mucin of the polysaccharide-amino acid complex possessing blood group A specificity. *Biochem. J.,* **37,** 640.

Wiener, A. S. (1943) *Blood Groups and Transfusion.* Springfield, Ill: Charles C. Thomas.

Boorman, K. E., Dodd, B. E. & Mollison, P. L. (1945) Iso-immunisation to the Blood Group Factors A, B and Rh. *J. Path-Bact.,* **57,** 157.

Kabat, E. A. & Beser, A. E. (1945) Estimation of A and B iso-antibodies in human serum by the quantitative precipitin method. *J. exp. Med.,* **82,** 207.

Coombs, R. R. A., Bedford, D. & Rouillard, L. M. (1956) A and B blood group antigens on human epidermal cells demonstrated by mixed agglutination. *Lancet,* **i,** 461.

Kabat, E. A. (1956) *The Blood Group Substances.* New York: Academic Press.

*The full bibliography of the ABO blood groups would fill many pages; here we give a few papers mainly because of their historical interest.

Section 3. The Rh System

"And wouldst thou master Rhesus 'Fac',
The E that's 'two', the C that's 'one',
And learn the knack, how not to thwack
The fragile clumps, my son!"

With acknowledgments to E. H., Irish Medical
Journal, and to Lewis Carroll

Chapter 7. The Rh Blood Group System and Rh Typing methods

DISCOVERY AND IMPORTANCE

In 1940 Landsteiner and Wiener reported the discovery of a human blood factor which they called Rhesus or Rh. They immunised guinea pigs and rabbits with blood from the Macacus rhesus monkey and thereby obtained an anti-serum which, after suitable absorption, agglutinated not only the red cells of the rhesus monkey but also approximately 85 per cent of a panel of blood samples from the white population of New York. They realised that this serum was detecting a hitherto unknown human blood group antigen and they used it to type as Rh positive those whose red cells were agglutinated by the new antibody and as Rh negative those whose red cells were not so agglutinated. The antibody responsible they called anti-Rh. The distribution of the newly discovered Rh antigen was found to be the same in each ABO blood group, suggesting that the Rh and the ABO blood group systems were unrelated. Later family studies showed that, as expected, the Rh factor was segregating independently of A and B.

The real importance of the Rh factor was only realised when it was shown by Wiener and Peters (1940) that the sera of some people who had experienced hitherto unexplained incompatible transfusion reactions even when given blood of the correct ABO group, contained antibodies which gave parallel reactions to the animal anti-Rh sera. This meant that the Rh factor was antigenic in man and that the anti-Rh allo-agglutinins which were formed as a result of immunisation could destroy incompatible blood *in vivo*.

Levine and Stetson (1939) had described an atypical antibody which later was shown to be anti-Rh in specificity. This antibody occurred in the serum of a woman delivered of a stillborn foetus. Shortly after delivery she had required a blood transfusion and was given her husband's blood which caused a haemolytic transfusion reaction. Levine and Stetson postulated that the antibody had arisen as the result of immunisation of the mother by a foetal antigen which had been inherited from the father. This became the basis of their work reported in a series of papers in 1941 by Levine and his co-workers, which showed that not only

53

could an Rh negative mother become immunised to an Rh positive foetus *in utero* but also that the antibody could then traverse the placenta and give rise to erythroblastosis foetalis—or as it is now more generally called "haemolytic disease of the newborn".

Moreover, they showed that these antibodies were "warm" antibodies reacting more strongly at 37° C, *i.e.* body temperature, than in the cold or at room temperature.

The clinical significance of the Rh factor is, of course, the reason why the Rh system is second only to the ABO system in importance and why methods of Rh testing and antibody detection are so essential a part of the work of any laboratory which deals with blood group serology.

Later work has shown that the animal anti-serum used by Landsteiner and Wiener was not detecting the antigen which is detected by human anti-Rh serum but another antigen possessed by Rh positive and Rh negative persons but in much greater strength by Rh positives. It was suggested that this antigen should be re-christened LW after Landsteiner and Wiener who discovered it. Their work stimulated Wiener and Peters, and Levine and his co-workers to investigate the human Rh antibodies and was one of the most important discoveries in the history of blood grouping and transfusion.

PRINCIPLES OF Rh TYPING

Since its discovery the Rh system has been found to be composed of a series of antigens each with its corresponding antibody, so that it is much more complicated than was at first realised. However, the original Rh antigen (now called D or Rh_0) and its corresponding antibody, anti-Rh (anti-D or anti-Rh_0) account for over 90 per cent of all haemolytic reactions caused by the Rh blood groups. The techniques of testing are essentially the same for all the various Rh antigens and antibodies. In the interest of simplicity, therefore, tests using anti-D sera and tests for the detection of anti-D antibodies will be dealt with first. When the sub-groups of Rh, the Fisher nomenclature and theory of inheritance of the Rh factor (*see* Chapter 9) have been discussed, the modifications necessary to detect all the various antigens and antibodies will be described (*see* Chapters 10 and 11).

The original anti-Rh typing was done with animal sera but today human sera are almost universally used. Human anti-Rh sera can be obtained from Rh negative women who have recently been delivered of an Rh positive infant suffering from haemolytic disease of the newborn. Alternatively they can be obtained from human volunteers (usually Rh negative men) who have been deliberately immunised. The selection and preparation of the various types of anti-Rh sera will be dealt with in Chapter 12. For "D-typing" (*i.e.* dividing individuals into the two classes D positive and D negative) the human serum needs to be of the specificity anti-D, of high titre and avidity, and having had any anti-A or anti-B agglutinins removed so that it is suitable for testing blood of all ABO groups.

The standard sera belong to two distinct types called for convenience "saline anti-D" and "albumin anti-D". This is because human anti-D antibodies occur either as agglutinins (or "complete" antibodies), which can agglutinate cells containing the corresponding agglutinogen in a saline medium, or as "incomplete" antibodies, which sensitise the cells in saline but only cause them to agglutinate in a high protein medium. The protein medium usually employed in Rh testing is bovine albumin. This may be obtained from the manufacturers as a 30 per cent solution especially prepared for use in Rh testing. Thirty per cent bovine albumin can be diluted to give a 20 per cent solution using AB serum or normal saline as a diluent. This is preferred by some workers as it makes negative reactions easier to read; there is sometimes however a falling off in the strength of the positive reaction using a 20 per cent solution (*see* Appendix II).

There are two ways in which the bovine albumin may be introduced into the test if albumin anti-D sera are to be used for Rh typing.

(*a*) The test cells can be suspended in the albumin (making a 2 per cent suspension approximately). This, however, is timeconsuming, as red cell suspensions are not so quickly made in albumin as in saline—nor is the rinsing of the pipette so easy! In addition there is considerable wastage of expensive albumin as it is inevitable that more than the requisite amount of cell suspension will be made. This method has now been superseded by (*b*).

(*b*) The serum and saline suspended red cells are mixed and the test incubated so that the cells have time to become sensitised. The cells are then covered with a layer of bovine albumin without disturbing them. This can be done by removing the supernatant and replacing it with albumin, but it is preferable to run a drop of albumin down the inside of the tube without removing supernatant. Being heavier than the saline-serum mixture the albumin displaces it forming a layer immediately above the red cells. This method involves no undue wastage of albumin.

Controls

Whatever technique is used controls are necessary. For any anti-D testing three controls should be used: (1) known Rh positive cells with the standard anti-D serum, (2) known Rh negative cells with the standard anti-D serum, and (3) the unknown cells with a bland serum (group AB) with the addition of bovine albumin if the technique employed involves its use.

(1) *The positive control*

The cells chosen for this test should be standard Rh positive cells known to give the least strong reaction. Anti-D does not normally show "dosage" but as the D antigen in the R_1 phenotype is weaker than in the R_2, ideally cells belonging to group O R_1r should be used (*see* Chapter 12). Where the serum is known to react with all Rh sub-groups, R_1R_2 red cells may be used. This control should be set up under exactly the same conditions as the Rh(D) typing tests and unless it gives a satisfactory positive reaction all the tests should be repeated.

(2) *The negative control on the anti-serum*

This consists of known Rh negative cells incubated with the standard serum under exactly the same test conditions as the unknown cells. If the standard serum has had anti-A and/or anti-B agglutinins absorbed out of it, it is as well to check at least once with Rh negative cells of group AB as a negative reaction then shows that the anti-A and anti-B have been completely removed.

(3) *Negative control on the cells under test*

In this control the test is repeated replacing the standard serum with an AB serum. It is exceedingly important that it should be included in all slide and enzyme techniques, in tests on cord blood and on blood from patients whose protein balance may be disturbed. It may be omitted when the tube technique is used for testing normal blood samples, *i.e.* from blood donors, from routine ante-natal cases, husbands, etc. provided a saline anti-D is included in the typing.

If this control is positive no positive results obtained with standard antisera can be relied upon and the phenomenon should be fully investigated (*see* Chapter 14). It may be possible to type the cells successfully using suitably diluted saline antisera or alternatively it may be necessary first to elute an antibody from the cells; in the very rare case typing of the cells may be impossible.

Test sera

It is advisable in all typing to use two different sera of the same specificity. No blood group should be determined on the result of a single reaction. Any discrepancy between the two readings necessitates a further investigation.

TECHNIQUES

There are innumerable Rh typing methods, a few are so unreliable as to be best forgotten, most are reasonably accurate in the hands of an experienced worker and one or two are sufficiently proven to be used as the yardstick by which other methods are assessed. It is, perhaps, of interest to note in this connection that almost every worker if asked "What do you do in the event of this method giving you a doubtful result" replies "Oh, then I check it by the tube technique". The methods described in this chapter are those we consider to be the best. In Chapter 23 we describe others which are faster but, we feel, slightly less reliable. There are circumstances which make the adoption of such techniques essential but in our opinion they should be reserved for the case where the condition of the patient warrants the risk being taken. Sometimes the choice of method is dictated by the convenience of the laboratory (less washing-up!) rather than the safety of the patient. If one of the most reliable of the quick methods (*see* Chapter 24, Table 24.00) is selected and used in parallel to the tube technique for part at least of the day to day routine work, experience will be gained which will minimise the risk of errors when the method is used in an emergency.

Technique No. 7.1. Rh typing by the moist chamber slide technique

The apparatus used is the same as for the ABO moist chamber technique (technique No. 2.1). If a saline anti-D is used, one volume of serum is mixed on a slide with one volume of a 5 per cent suspension in saline of washed red cells. If an albumin anti-D is used, equal volumes of albumin, of serum and the red cell suspension are mixed together. The slide is gently rocked and placed in a moist chamber in the 37° C incubator for 30 minutes, controls of known D positive and

D negative cells being included. The control on rouleaux formation and pseudo-agglutination must be included also, it will consist of equal volumes of the suspension of unknown cells and group AB serum for the saline anti-D and for the albumin anti-D of equal volumes of cell suspension, of albumin and of group AB serum. The tests are read macroscopically and any negative reactions checked microscopically.

Comment. This method is a good one provided the sera are specially chosen and all the controls are satisfactory. It is important that the unknown cells under test should be thoroughly washed and that the control suspensions in group AB serum and in bovine albumin are included.

Occasionally weakly reacting D positive blood may appear to be D negative by this technique, but except in cases where the unknown cells are giving pseudo-agglutination with group AB serum alone or with group AB serum and bovine albumin, it is very unlikely that a false positive reaction will be obtained. If the cells are giving pseudo-agglutination, a more detailed investigation will have to be made.

Technique No. 7.2. Standard technique for Rh typing. One-stage method using saline anti-D

The apparatus for this technique is the same as for ABO grouping in tubes, with the addition of a 37°C incubator or water bath.

Ideally two different saline anti-D sera are used.

Precipitin tubes are placed in the first and second rows of a fifty-holed rack and larger cell suspension tubes in the back row.

One unit volume of the first anti-D serum is delivered into each tube of the frong row using the standard graduated Pasteur pipette. The second anti-D is run into the second row in the same way. The tubes are then examined to see that each does in fact contain one volume of anti-serum (This prevents those errors that can arise from serum going outside instead of inside the precipitin tubes, a mistake which can easily happen when dealing with such narrow tubes, or from serum leaking out of the tube through an almost invisible crack.) About 0.5 ml of saline is run into each of the cell suspension tubes. A 2 per cent cell suspension, judged by eye is then made in the first of these tubes from the first unknown sample—and one volume of this suspension added to the corresponding tubes in rows 1 and 2. The pipette is carefully rinsed at least three times in saline, discarding each rinsing, and the process repeated for each unknown sample to be tested. The known D positive and D negative cells must be included at the end of each batch of tests as controls. The serum-cell mixtures are then tapped to ensure good mixing and the tests incubated at 37°C for 2 hours.

The reading of the reactions is the most difficult part of the test; the clumps are quite easily dispersed by rough handling unless the anti-serum is unusually potent. The cell sediment should, therefore, be removed from the tube with a wider bore Pasteur pipette (*see* Fig. A1.1E) and very gently spread on to a microscope slide (for details of preparing film *see* Appendix I). The actual degree of agglutination should be recorded (*See* Fig. 1.1a for appropriate symbols.) It is advisable to check every test microscopically even when the agglutination can be seen with the naked eye, because occasionally macroscopic clumping may be observed which is not true agglutination.

Technique No. 7.3. Standard technique for Rh typing. Two-stage method (Albumin addition)

The tests are put up exactly as described above but the reagents used are anti-D sera containing incomplete antibodies, "albumin" sera and an AB serum as the negative control on the cells under test. The tests are incubated for 1 to 1½ hours at 37°C. Then one drop of bovine albumin is allowed to run down the side of each tube, taking care not to disturb the cell sediment. The albumin displaces the serum-saline mixture forming a layer immediately above the cell button. The tests are incubated for a further 30 minutes. It will be found that the agglutinates formed using this method are not easily broken down so that the tubes can be gently shaken, the positive reaction will almost invariably be macroscopic but all negatives are checked microscopically as weak positive reactions are occasionally encountered usually denoting the presence of the D^u antigen (*see* below).

Comment. This is a very convenient and reliable technique. The time factor is not critical, the first stage must be long enough to allow the cells to sediment, the second can be reduced to 15–20 minutes when the serum used is potent, on the other hand either stage can be left for 2–3 hours without detriment. This flexibility can be of considerable advantage in a busy laboratory. A certain amount of experience is needed in reading the negative reactions as there is sometimes a tendency for the cells to agglomerate; gentle rolling of the microscope slide will however disperse such clumps while having no such effect on the true agglutinates.

INTERPRETATION OF RESULTS

D-typing is always performed with two anti-D sera. A negative result with both sera will mean that the blood sample under test is probably D-negative— it should not, however, be regarded as completely Rh negative without further testing for the other Rh antigens (*see* Chapter 10). This further testing can be omitted in an emergency since a patient who is negative with two anti-D sera must always receive Rh negative blood. A positive result (V or ++) with both anti-D sera will mean that the sample is almost certainly Rh positive and for all practical purposes can be so considered. High grade D^u red cells (*see* Chapter 10) may also be positive with both anti-D sera, but such cells are treated as Rh positive for all practical purposes. Samples which give doubtful reactions [+, (+) or w] with one or both anti-sera should be re-tested, if possible, with a larger range of anti-D sera. If the blood sample is more than 48 hours old it is as well in these doubtful cases to wash the red cells with saline at 37°C as this will appreciably restore their diminished agglutinability. A negative result with one serum and a positive with the other is also an indication for testing against a number of anti-D sera. The reasons for these anomalous results (other than technical faults) are dealt with fully when the subject of D^u is considered in Chapters 9, 10 and 17).

Chapter 8. Methods of Detection of Anti-D Antibodies

Rh antibodies are with only one or two exceptions immune antibodies. Therefore the vast majority of D negative individuals will not have anti-D antibodies in their serum. When such antibodies have been formed as the result of immunisation they are of such clinical importance, especially in the aetiology of haemolytic disease of the newborn, that it is essential that their presence should be detected.

DETECTION METHODS

These fall into five main divisions.
(1) Saline agglutination tests.
(2) Tests in a high protein medium—especially bovine albumin.
(3) Tests using anti-human globulin ("Coombs tests").
(4) Tests using red cells partially digested with proteolytic enzymes.
(5) Blocking tests.

The general principles of the tests will be dealt with quite shortly, then will follow a full description of at least one method of each type. These methods while not exhaustive include sufficient techniques for the full investigation of any serum for the presence of Rh antibodies. Finally the correlation between the tests and the antibodies which they demonstrate will be considered.

(1) Saline Agglutination Tests

When anti-D is present in a serum as an agglutinin, mixture with a saline suspension of cells which have the D antigen results in agglutination. As mentioned in the previous chapter, the agglutination is often readily dispersed by rough handling of the agglutinates. This is particularly true when the anti-D is present in low titre as often will be the case when unknown sera are being tested for antibodies.

(2) Tests in High Protein Media

It has been found that there are antibodies which fail to agglutinate red cells in saline but do so in a high protein medium. One of the first used was the natural one, human serum—the resulting agglomeration of cells being called "conglutination". Various other media were tried; the most effective was found to be bovine albumin, fraction 5 of the Cohn separation. Incomplete anti-D antibodies will cause firm agglutination of D-positive red cells suspended in 20–30 per cent bovine albumin. No other protein medium has been found to be as effective as bovine albumin while giving negative reactions free from pseudo-agglutination.

(3) Tests Using Anti-human Globulin

Human globulin if injected into an animal of another species will act as an antigen and cause the animal to produce specific anti-human globulin antibodies. These antibodies are capable of reacting with all human globulin molecules including those which are antibodies. The reaction will still take place even if the antibodies (*e.g.* anti-D) are already specifically attached to red cells. In these circumstances the red cells will be clumped. Anti-human globulin (ahg or Coombs' reagent) is serum from animals, usually rabbits, immunised with either whole human serum or the precipitated globulin fraction. Unwanted antibodies are removed leaving a serum specific for human globulin. (For details of the preparation and standardisation of anti-human globulin *see* Appendix II) In the present chapter the method of using the anti-human globulin reaction to detect incomplete anti-D antibodies in human serum is described in great detail, for once the basic technique has been mastered it will be found easy to adapt it for other purposes.

(4) Tests Involving the Use of Proteolytic Enzymes

It has been stated that incomplete antibodies will not cause agglutination of red cells in a saline medium. This is true of untreated red cells but Pickles discovered in 1946 that cholera filtrate would modify red cells to make them agglutinable in saline by incomplete antibodies. This was considered to be due to a proteolytic action on the red cell surface and other enzymes known to have proteolytic activity were tested. Many of them were found to have the same effect and today four are in general use, namely papain, trypsin, ficin and bromelin. We shall describe techniques using all these enzymes although our personal preference is for papain. The mechanism by which these enzymes render cells capable of being agglutinated by incomplete antibodies is almost certainly partly a direct result of proteolytic action which removes polypeptides and thereby makes some antigen sites more accessible, making it easier for the small incomplete antibodies to combine with the cells. Enzymes also undoubtedly reduce the negative charge on the surface of red cells enabling them to approach one another more closely (*see also* Chapter 15). Most enzyme techniques are two-stage with the cells being first modified by the enzyme and then exposed to the antibody containing serum. It is however also possible to adjust the potency of enzyme preparation, usually by means of an activator, so that the cells are adequately digested even in the presence of serum, making a one-stage test possible. The advantages of the enzyme techniques are sensitivity, avidity and speed of reaction. The main disadvantage is that some sera contain auto-antibodies against enzyme-treated cells which normally react with all of the test cells used. These have to be removed before the serum can be tested for allo-antibodies.

(5) Blocking Tests

The blocking test is the test which was used originally to demonstrate the presence of "incomplete" antibodies. It cannot, however, be used to detect the presence of incomplete antibodies in a mixture of complete and incomplete unless the serum is first treated to remove the complete antibody. Moreover, not all types of incomplete antibody are capable of blocking red cell antigen sites.

The blocking antibodies will sensitise red cells in a saline diluent but will not cause them to agglutinate. In the presence of excess of incomplete anti-D all the D sites of the red cells will have this antibody attached to them and are said to be "blocked", that is incapable of taking up more antibody. When such blocked cells are mixed with serum containing saline anti-D agglutinins there are no free D sites with which the agglutinins can react, therefore no agglutination takes place. The absence of agglutination between cells containing the D antigen and serum containing anti-D agglutinins clearly demonstrates the presence of anti-D blocking incomplete antibodies attached to the D sites.

TECHNIQUES

In the following techniques standard cells from one D-positive and one D-negative individual are used. These will detect the presence of an antibody but for the complete establishment of the identity of the antibody further tests are necessary; these are discussed after the various Rh antibodies are described (Chapter 11).

Technique No. 8.1. Detection of Rh antibodies—saline

One unit volume of the serum under test is placed in each of two precipitin tubes. To one is added one unit volume of D positive and to the other one unit volume of D negative red cells (2 per cent suspensions in normal saline). The tests are incubated at 37° C for at least 2 hours. Whenever possible the tests are left for 3–4 hours as the agglutination becomes "tighter" and thus more easily read. The cell sediment is examined for agglutination under the low power of the microscope. It must be emphasised that the gentle handling of the sedimented cells in making the smear is even more important in all antibody detection tests than it is in the Rh typing of red cells because the antibodies are often very weak. Results are recorded as for Rh typing.

Any agglutination indicates that an agglutinin, not necessarily anti-D or indeed any of the Rh antibodies, is present and further tests in a saline medium with a panel of red cells should be done to establish specificity. The strength of the antibody should be found by titration technique or AutoAnalyser quantification.

Comment. The saline technique is the best for the detection of agglutinins and, therefore, should always be included in any antibody detection routine.

Technique No. 8.2. Detection of Rh antibodies—albumin, two-stage method

One volume of a 2 per cent suspension in saline of standard cells is mixed with one volume of unknown serum, each serum being tested with D positive and D negative cells. The mixtures are then incubated for 1½ hours at 37° C. Then one volume of 30 per cent bovine albumin is allowed to run down the side of each tube to form a layer over the red cell button, care being taken that the red cells are not disturbed. The tests are re-incubated for a further 30 minutes at 37° C, then read. Any antibody found should have its specificity determined and strength estimated by the albumin technique (as above).

Technique No. 8.3a. Indirect anti-human globulin (Coombs) test*

This test has three stages: (1) sensitisation of the red cells; (2) washing the cells free of all traces of serum; (3) mixing the washed red cells with the anti-human globulin serum (Coombs reagent).

There are an almost bewildering number of modifications of this technique but the following method has been selected as one giving very satisfactory results.

(1) *Sensitisation*

Two volumes (about 0.03 ml each) of test serum are mixed with two volumes of a 3 per cent cell suspension of D positive red cells and a similar test is set up using 3 per cent D negative red cells. The 50 × 11-mm tubes are convenient for these tests. The cells are washed three times prior to use as traces of plasma may result in small clots which interfere with the reading of the tests.

The same D positive and D negative red cells are mixed with a serum containing a weak incomplete anti-D to act as positive and negative controls. The tests are incubated at 37° C for a minimum period of 1 hour.

(2) *Washing*

The tubes are removed from the incubator without jolting so that the supernatant fluid may be discarded before the cells are washed; this is an important step and should not be omitted. The fluid may be sucked off carefully by hand or a vacuum pump. The cells are then washed three times. The same care is exercised in the removal of as much supernatant as possible between each wash. Thorough washing is essential as even minute traces of globulin left in solution may react with the anti-globulin afterwards applied, and so diminish its activity.

For each wash, therefore, the cells are completely re-suspended in at least 100 times their own volume of clean saline from a container set aside for this purpose.

It is the complete suspension of the cells, especially after centrifugation, which often presents difficulty. Fig. 8.1 shows both correct and incorrect washing of tests. An adequate method for washing is achieved by the addition of a small quantity of saline 8.1d in which the cells are evenly suspended either by a vigorous jarring of the rack or by lifting each tube and tapping with the finger. The tube is then filled to the top with saline and the result is an even suspension of cells in sufficient saline for adequate washing (8.1e). Of course if a jet of saline of sufficient force to cause even suspension of cells can be directed into each tube, then no further handling of the tubes is necessary, but in our experience this is difficult to achieve.

There are various machines designed for the automatic washing of red cells.

---

*When the indirect anti-human globulin is used as a typing technique and gives a positive result it is essential to include the direct anti-human globulin test on the unknown cells as a negative control.

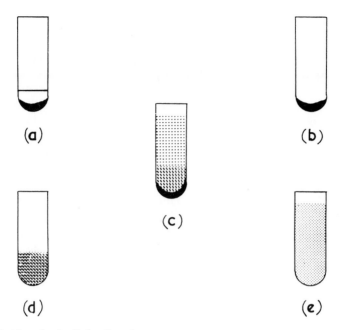

Fig. 8.1 Washing of red cells for Coombs tests.

(*a*) Red cell button and clear supernatant.
(*b*) Supernatant removed.
(*c*) Incorrect washing. Uneven suspension of cells can be corrected by mixing with a Pasteur pipette or tapping with the finger, inversion and vigorous shaking.
(*d*) Correct washing—Stage I. Resuspension of cells in a small quantity of saline (shake rack or tap tubes individually to ensure even suspension).
(*e*) Correct washing—Stage II. Tube filled with saline to give an even suspension throughout.

(3) *Mixture with anti-human globulin*

Directions for the dilution of the anti-globulin reagent are usually supplied with the reagent. The recommended dilution will probably be between 1:50 and 1:100. Some commercial reagents are pre-diluted and therefore should be used neat by the method recommended (usually a spin technique). Such reagents may be suitable for a slide technique but the worker will have first to standardise them for this method (*see* technique No. AII.13).

Great care must be exercised to ensure that all glassware used in making up and putting out anti-human globulin reagent is absolutely clean and free from traces of human serum which would inevitably react with some of the anti-human globulin in the reagent. If contamination of the diluted reagent is suspected, it should be centrifuged: the appearance of a white film on the bottom of the tube will confirm the suspicion of contamination with serum and the reagent should be discarded. Unused diluted reagent can be kept frozen at –20° C for about a week provided it is not thawed and re-frozen more than once a day and is always carefully checked by controls.

Slide technique. Before plating out, the washed packed cells in each tube are re-suspended in two drops of saline.

Mixture with anti-globulin is best performed on an opalescent tile. (The tile must be scrupulously cleaned with soap and water and rinsed thoroughly under running water, finally polishing with a clean cloth.) One drop of diluted reagent is then mixed with one drop of weakly sensitised D positive control cells to ensure the reagent is active. Then the requisite number of generous drops of anti-globulin reagent is delivered onto the tile after which a drop of the appropriate test red cells is mixed with each. A positive and negative control is set out with each batch of tests. Mixture can be conveniently done with a small plastic rod or with wooden applicator sticks. Glass mixing rods are not recommended since the presence of colloidal silica in the test fluid may cause false agglutination. The tile is then gently rocked, preferably on some kind of rotary machine since it is often necessary to rock the tests for at least 5 minutes; the time varies according to the kind of tests being performed. Just before reading the tests (Fig. 8.2) it is an advantage to allow the tile to remain motionless for about 10 seconds before picking it up and gently rolling while the tests are read. This pause often "crisps up" the agglutination.

Ideally after the tests are read one drop of strongly sensitised cells is added to each negative test to show that the reagent is active. This is not always carried out routinely but should at least be done if the tests show more negative results than are expected.

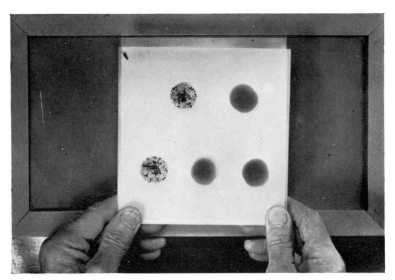

Fig. 8.2 Reading of the ahg test (from above).

Spin test. For this alternative method anti-human globulin is added to the washed cells in the tube in which they were washed adjusting the volume of cells to give a 2 per cent suspension to which an equal volume of anti-globulin is added. The mixture of cells and reagent are allowed to stand for about 2 minutes and then centrifuged lightly (*e.g.* 1000 r.p.m. for 2–3 minutes). The tubes are then gently rolled and examined for agglutination macroscopically either directly with the aid of a hand lens or by reflection in a concave mirror. Negative or doubtful reactions in our opinion should be checked microscopically after careful removal of the cells to a microscope slide.

Strongly sensitised cells may be added to each tube showing a negative reaction as mentioned above.

Comment. The anti-globulin test is a very delicate test, involving great care at every stage for reliable results. False positives are most likely to be obtained through dust particles in saline, colloidal silica or small plasma clots, false negatives through the reagent becoming inactive due to contamination with serum proteins. It cannot be recommended for large-scale routine work where time is not available for the unhurried performance of a complicated test. It is the best single test for almost all incomplete antibodies and should always be used in direct matching and special investigations. However as will be seen later some antibodies exist which are detectable only by enzyme technique.

The spin test is considered to be somewhat more sensitive than the tile test, but the tile test has the advantage that comparison may be more easily made and the speed at which reactions develop may be watched.

Technique No. 8.3b. Direct anti-human globulin (Coombs) test

The object of this test is to determine whether the red cells of certain patients (notably haemolytic anaemias and infants thought to be suffering from haemolytic disease of the newborn) have become sensitised by antibodies *in vivo*. The test is distinguished from that described above (8.3a) in that the first stage, *viz.* incubation of test serum with red cells in order to sensitise them, is omitted.

The red cells suspected to be sensitised *in vivo* are carefully washed at least three times in a large volume of saline. They are diluted with saline using a pipette which has never been in contact with serum, to give a 3 per cent suspension then mixed with anti-human globulin serum (Coombs reagent) on a tile or in a tube and read exactly in the manner described above. An extra control of the patient's washed red cells with a drop of saline to replace the anti-human globulin reagent is included. The development of agglutination in the anti-human globulin-red cell mixture shows that the red cells are sensitised by antibody. It should be noted that while this test reveals the presence of incomplete antibodies on the red cells it does not identify their specificity. This must be determined in other ways, one of which is to elute the antibody and to test the eluate with a panel of standard cells.

Technique No. 8.4. Trypsin technique

There are several preparations of trypsin which can be used partially to digest the test red cells (*See* Appendix II).

Preparation of trypsin treated cells. The standard D positive and D negative red cells are freshly bled, separated by centrifugation and washed three times with 0.85 per cent saline.

The washed packed cells then have the buffered trypsin solution added to them in the proportion of four parts of solution to each part of packed cells—both solution and cells should be at 37°C for ½ to ³/₄ hour, *i.e.* sufficient time to render the D positive cells agglutinable by an incomplete anti-D but not so long that they become pan-agglutin-able or even completely haemolysed.

The red cells are then washed twice with an excess of warm (37°C) saline and stored in bulk in the hot room or water bath until needed. Before adding the trypsin-treated cells to the test sera, a 4 per cent suspension of the cells is made in warm saline.

Antibody detection. One unit volume of each of the unknown sera is measured into each of two precipitin tubes and left at 37°C for 10 minutes before the addition of an equal volume of trypsin-treated red cells, D positive to one set of tubes and D negative to the other. They are then incubated for 1 hour. The tests are read by gently tapping the tubes and examining them macroscopically for agglutination, negatives are confirmed microscopically. A control serum known to contain a weak anti-D antibody is included in each batch of tests; only if this gives a macroscopic positive with the D positive and a clear negative with the D negative cells should the rest of the tests be read.

Comment. This is a very sensitive and useful technique. Occasionally sera are encountered which give pan-agglutination with trypsin treated red cells. The antibody responsible for the pan-agglutination can usually be quite easily removed by incubating the serum with an equal volume of the patient's own trypsin treated red cells. The absorbed serum can then be re-examined for the presence of specific antibodies with the standard trypsin treated cells.

Technique No. 8.5a. Papain technique for antibody detection—one stage

Equal volumes of the serum to be tested, papain (for preparation *see* appendix II) and a 2 per cent suspension of red cells are placed in a precipitin tube by a layering procedure, taking care to adhere strictly to the order: (*a*) serum, (*b*) papain, (*c*) red cells. It is also important that the serum/papain preparation should not be allowed to stand on the bench for more than about five minutes before the red cells are added. The effect of layering is to allow the red cells to to sink through both the papain and then the serum during the incubation period of the test. Therefore the contents of the tubes are not mixed up at the initial stage. The test is read after precisely one hour's incubation, controls of known D positive and D negative cells with a weak incomplete anti-D being included with each batch of tests. The time of incubation is critical since as papain is present, too long an incubation period results in destruction of the antibody by the enzyme.

Comment. This is a good and efficient technique and is excellent for the detection of Rh antibodies. In fact anti-D antibodies may be detectable by this technique when they are not apparent by any non-enzyme technique, even the anti-human globulin. It does, however, give positives when certain other antibodies are present such as anti-P₁ anti-Lewis, anti-H, etc., so that care must be taken in the establishment of the specificity of any antibody detected by this method. Auto-antibodies are also encountered and can be removed by absorption of the serum with an equal volume of the patient's own papain treated cells, after which the absorbed serum is retested.

Technique No. 8.5b. Papain technique—two stage

To treat cells with papain either a saturated solution of papain or the Löw's papain which contains cysteine as an activator (*see* Appendix II) can be used. The use of Löw's papain is preferable because it is a standard solution and the digestion time can be cut to 15 minutes.

For the preparation of papain treated cells, washed, packed cells are used as for the trypsin technique. One part of the Löw's papain is added to one part of 50 per cent of suspension of cells and incubated for 15 minutes. The red cells are then washed twice with an excess of saline; they should be used within 24 hours.

Antibody detection. One unit volume of each of the unknown sera is measured into a precipitin tube and left at 37° C for 10 minutes after which one volume of a pre-warmed 2 per cent suspension of papain treated cells is added. The test is incubated at 37° C for 1 hour—the sediment re-suspended by gentle tapping and the degree of agglutination read macroscopically and if necessary microscopically. The sensitivity can be increased by slow centrifugation before reading.

Comment. This technique is slightly more sensitive than the one stage papain test. It has the same disadvantages as the one stage technique, in that it detects some cold antibodies and auto-antibodies. The latter can be removed by absorption of the serum with the patient's own papain treated cells and the absorbed serum retested.

Technique No. 8.6. Detection of Rh antibodies using bromelin—one stage

A solution of bromelin is prepared as described in Appendix II or as directed on the manufacturer's leaflet.

The stock solution of bromelin is diluted 1 in 2 in saline, buffered with Sorensen's buffer ph 7.3 on the day of use. If kept, the diluted bromelin deteriorates rapidly.

Equal volumes of diluted bromelin solution, serum and red cells are placed in a precipitin tube and incubated at 37° C for 1 hour. The sediment is gently agitated and the tests read macroscopically for agglutination.

Comment. This technique is by no means as sensitive as papain for the detection of anti-D. The fact that fewer cold antibodies and auto-antibodies are detected by it does not compensate for its failure to detect some weak Rh antibodies. A further disadvantage is that batches of bromelin vary so that the sensitivity of the test varies also. Moreover the enzyme is less stable than papain or trypsin. For use 'on line' in the AutoAnalyser, however, bromelin is usually the enzyme of choice.

Technique No. 8.6b. Detection of Rh antibodies using bromelin—two stage

Bromelin-treated cells are prepared by adding one part of stock bromelin to one part of a 50 per cent suspension well washed cells, the mixture incubated at 37° C for 20 minutes, the cells washed three times with saline at 37° C and stored at 37° C—in this way they are ready for instant use; alternatively they may be stored at 4° C or room temperature but should be re-warmed to 37° C before use or unwanted reactions due to a cold antibodies may be encountered. Equal volumes of a 2 per cent suspension of the bromelin treated cells and test serum are incubated at 37°C for 15–20 minutes then centrifuged at 1000 r.p.m. for 1 minute and examined for macroscopic agglutination.

Technique No. 8.7. Detection of Rh antibodies using ficin

For the preparation of stock solution and Hendry's buffer *see* Appendix I.

Ficin treatment of cells. Ficin for use is made by adding 1 volume of stock solution to 39 volumes of Hendry's buffer. These 40 volumes are warmed to 37°C when one volume of packed washed cells is added and the mixture incubated for exactly 15 minutes at 37°C. The cells are then washed three times in saline and stored at 37°C until needed.

Antibody detection. One volume of test serum is measured into each of two precipitin tubes and left at 37°C for 10 minutes, after which one volume of ficin treated cells is added, D-positive cells to the first tube and D-negative to the second. They are incubated for 1 hour and then read macroscopically for agglutination.

Comment. This is a very sensitive technique. Its main disadvantages are firstly the care that must be taken with powdered ficin and secondly that the digestion time is very critical, a few moments over or under can result respectively in a false positive or a false negative reaction being obtained. Like the other enzyme techniques auto-antibodies are often detected which have to be removed by absorption with the patient's own treated cells before the test with standard cells can be performed.

Technique No. 8.8. Blocking test

This is not so sensitive a test for the presence of incomplete antibodies as either the albumin or the Coombs test but it is the only test that demonstrates their "blocking" nature and thus shows that complete and incomplete antibodies even when of the same specificity are not identical. It is an antibody-investiga-tion technique as opposed to a detection technique but is included here for completeness and to some extent as of historical interest, as it was the origi-nal technique by which the presence of incomplete antibodies was demonstrated.

One unit volume of unknown serum is mixed with one unit volume of a 2 per cent red cell suspension in saline of D-positive cells. The tests are incubated at 37° for 1 hour.

The controls on this test consist of (1) one unit volume of group AB serum, and (2) one unit volume of a serum known to contain incomplete anti-D, to each of which are added one volume of the 2 per cent suspension of D-positive cells. These are incubated for 1 hour at 37°C with the tests on the unknown sera. Then a unit volume of a saline agglutinating anti-D which has been diluted to give a ++ reaction is added to each tube. The tubes are well shaken and allowed to stand for a further 1½ hours after which they are examined for agglutination. Absence of agglutination or definitely diminished agglutination in the test as compared with control tube (1) together with no agglutination in control tube (2)

Table 8.1 Specimen results obtained by the blocking test

Serial No. of serum tested	Reaction after first stage	Reaction after second stage	Conclusion
1213	–	++	No antibody demonstrated
1306	–	(+)	Incomplete anti-D present
1175	–	–	Incomplete anti-D present
Control (1) AB serum	–	++	No antibody present
Control (2), incomplete anti-D	–	–	Incomplete anti-D present

indicates the presence of blocking antibody in the unknown serum. (*See* Table 8.1 for specimen results.)

It will be realised that this test for incomplete antibodies cannot be performed in the presence of saline agglutinins as the test cells would be agglutinated during the first stage. If for any reason it is important to show whether a serum does in fact contain incomplete as well as complete antibodies, it is necessary first to inactivate the latter. This may be done in several ways; probably the easiest is to dilute the serum with an equal part of saline (to minimise the risk of coagulation) and then heat at 70°C for approximately 10 minutes. The exact time needed to destroy all the agglutinins without appreciably increasing the viscosity of the serum varies and must be determined by trial and error.

Comment. This is not a sensitive technique and is only used when it is required to prove that a given antibody can specifically block red cell antigen sites.

TITRATION OF Rh ANTIBODIES

Technique No. 8.9. Saline.

Serial dilutions of the serum are made in saline as in technique No. 3.2 (or if desired techniques Nos. 3.3 or 3.4) and incubated at 37°C for 2 hours with standard D-positive red cells (2 per cent suspension) in saline. The tests are read taking the usual precautions against breaking down the agglutinates. The results are recorded as for ABO titres. *See* Figs. 3.1a–d and 3.2a–c.

Technique No. 8.10. Albumin two-stage method.

Tests are set up as for technique No. 8.9 but using AB serum as diluent. After 1½ hours' incubation bovine albumin is added without disturbing the cells. After a further 30 minutes' incubation the tests are read in the usual manner.

Technique No. 8.11. Indirect anti-human globulin (Coombs) technique.

Serial dilutions of the serum are made in saline using double unit volumes (0.06 ml) in the cell-suspension tubes. Two volumes of a 3 per cent suspension of D-positive red cells is added to each tube. From this point the procedure is exactly as in technique No. 8.3a.

Technique No. 8.12a. Two-stage Papain or Trypsin.

The serial dilutions of serum are made in saline and warmed to 37°C before the addition to each tube of an equal volume of papain treated or trypsin treated D-positive red cells. The tests are incubated for 1 hour, centrifuged and read by tapping the tubes and examining the contents macroscopically and if necessary microscopically for agglutination.

Technique No. 8.12b. One-stage Papain.

The serial dilutions are made as for technique No. 8.10 (it is important to use AB serum as diluent as if saline is used the enzyme will over papainise the cells and give false positive reactions), after which one volume of Löw's papain is added to each tube. This is followed immediately by an equal volume of a 2 per cent suspension in saline of D-positive red cells. Care is taken to layer the serum, papain and red cells, if they are mixed the titre will be substantially reduced. The tubes are incubated for exactly 1 hour and then read, first tapping the tube twice gently before examining the contents macroscopically and, if negative, microscopically.

Technique No. 8.13. Blocking Titre.

Serial dilutions of the serum containing blocking antibody are made and one volume of a 2 per cent suspension of D-positive red cells added to each tube. A control consisting of equal volumes of AB serum and the D-positive cells is set up at the same time. After 1 hour's incubation at 37°C a unit volume of a saline anti-D diluted to give a ++ reaction is added to each tube. The tubes are well shaken and incubated for a further $1\frac{1}{2}$ hours. The tests are read with the usual Rh precautions (for a specimen protocol *see* Table 8.2).

Table 8.2 Protocol of blocking titre

									Control of
Dilutions of serum containing incomplete antibody									AB serum
	Neat	$\frac{1}{2}$	$\frac{1}{4}$	$\frac{1}{8}$	$\frac{1}{32}$	$\frac{1}{32}$	$\frac{1}{64}$	$\frac{1}{128}$	
Reaction after adding saline anti-D	–	–	–	w	*(+)*	+	++	++	++

INTERPRETATION OF RESULTS

Sera are usually tested by at least two of the techniques, Nos. 8.1–5b in parallel; *e.g.* in the testing of Rh negative women ante-natally it is recommended that the saline (No. 8.1) albumin addition (No. 8.2) and one enzyme technique are used. Various patterns of reaction that may be obtained are shown in Table 8.3.

The finding of a positive reaction with D positive cells and a negative reaction with D negative cells with serum from an individual whose own cells are D negative means that there is a good probability that the antibody is in fact anti-D.

Table 8.3 Results that may be obtained in antibody tests

No.	Saline		Albumin		Papain		Conclusion and further investigation
	D+	D–	D+	D–	D+	D–	
1.	+	–	+	–	+	–	Probably Anti-D
2.	–	–	+	–	+	–	Probably Anti-D incomplete type
3.	–	–	–	–	+	–	Probably Anti-D incomplete type found either at beginning or end of immune process
4.	+	+	+	+	+	+	Not anti-D
5.	–	–	+	+	+	+	Not anti-D

Rows 1–3: Check with further D+ and D– cells and titrate
Row 4: Needs full antibody investigation
Row 5: "

Nevertheless, a confirmatory test with a slightly larger panel of known cells must be done. Three examples of D positive and two of D negative cells are adequate and should be used by the techniques by which the antibody is reacting best and it should only be reported as anti-D if clear-cut positives (ranging + to C) or negatives are obtained. If the positive reactions are inconclusive ((+) or w) the tests should be repeated and if still weak the presence of anti-D antibody should not be considered conclusive until confirmed in a later sample. It must be realised that a serum behaving like anti-D in the above tests may, in fact, be a mixture of Rh antibodies (*see* Chapter 11). Occasionally, as in examples 4 and 5, Table 8.3, the antibody belongs to one of the other blood group systems (*see* Section 4 in Chapter 26).

Classes of Rh antibody defined by their serological properties

As already stated Rh antibodies are either agglutinins capable of agglutinating Rh positive red cells in a saline suspension or incomplete antibodies capable of sensitising red cells in a saline medium but requiring albumin, anti-globulin or enzymes for the development of agglutination. Rh agglutinins are IgM immunoglobulins while the incomplete antibodies are usually IgG but may also be IgA or IgM.

Incomplete antibodies display a good deal of heterogeneity which is revealed when the various techniques for their detection are carried out in parallel.

The commonest kind of incomplete antibody is detectable by albumin, ahg and enzyme techniques and may or may not cause blocking. In fact, whether or not the incomplete antibody blocks the red cell determinant may be dependent upon its concentration in the serum rather than upon being a particular kind of incomplete antibody.

Other incomplete antibodies are characterised by being negative or at best weakly positive by anti-globulin technique. However they are consistently positive by enzyme techniques, particularly papain and may or may not be detected by albumin. Such antibodies are often precursor types; they occur in both IgM and IgG immunoglobulins.

Table 8.4 Types of Rh Antibodies and Techniques for their detection

Types	Reactions by various techniques					
	Saline	Albumin	ahg	Enzyme	Blocking	Ig class
Agglutinin	+	+	+	+	–	IgM
Incomplete antibodies						
(a)	–	+	+	+	Often +	IgG, some times with IgA.
(b)	–	+	Weak or –	+	–	Usually IgG
(c)	–	–	Weak or –	+	–	IgM or IgG

A summary of the various antibodies is found in Table 8.4. In any given serum the reactions are unlikely to be so clear cut because several types of antibody may occur together in varying amounts and the different kinds may mask each other. For example, (*see* Table 8.4) the Rh agglutinin (or indeed agglutinins of any other specificity gives a positive reaction by all techniques and therefore masks the presence of an incomplete antibody present in the same serum. The presence of the latter may be disclosed by titration or other methods. Similarly it is occasionally possible for incomplete antibodies to mask agglutinins (*see below*).

Interpretation of titres

In routine work titres are performed by saline and albumin techniques in parallel and in special cases by anti-human globulin and/or enzyme techniques as well. The finding of a negative or low titre in saline in association with a moderate or high titre in albumin establishes the presence of incomplete antibodies but it cannot be assumed that agglutinins are entirely absent since in the presence of incomplete antibodies capable of blocking the antigen sites, agglutinins may be prevented from reacting with the red cells. Evidence of this is sometimes obtained when sera are fractionated, for example, by column chromatography.

It should be noted that a titre of 1 or 2 with red cells suspended in saline is not good evidence of the presence of agglutinins since, at these low dilutions, there is often sufficient concentration of protein for agglutination of the cells to be caused by incomplete antibody.

A moderate or high titre by saline technique established unequivocably the presence of agglutinins but unless the titre in albumin is at least two dilutions higher, the assumption that incomplete antibodies are also present cannot be made without inactivating or removing the agglutinin; various methods which can be employed utilise heating diluted serum to 70°C for 5 to 10 minutes, treatment with 2-mercapto-ethanol or fractionation using DEAE or Sephadex.

Chapter 9. The Various Rh Antigens and Theory of Inheritance

It was not long before it was realised that important though the first described Rh antigen (now called D) and its corresponding antibody (anti-D) were, they were not by any means the whole of the Rh system.

In 1941 American workers noted that not all so called anti-Rh sera gave parallel results and it seemed, therefore, that more than one Rh antigen and its corresponding antibody might exist. Moreover the reactions obtained with some of the anti-sera suggested that they were in fact a mixture of two Rh antibodies. In addition another antibody was found which agglutinated all Rh negative red cells as well as many which were Rh positive. This antibody was called anti-Hr to show that its reactions were in some measure antithetical to those of anti-Rh. With these new antibodies it was found possible to subdivide the original Rh positive and Rh negative groups.

Concurrently with the American work three antibodies, which were obviously related to the Rh system, were being investigated in England.

One of these, which agglutinated the red cells of about 70 per cent of all individuals, was obviously related to anti-Rh in that almost all the red cells which were positive with this serum were also Rh positive. This antibody was called anti-Rh$_1$.

The second antibody was also related to anti-Rh in that almost all the cells with which it gave a positive reaction were Rh positive but differed strikingly in that it only agglutinated some 30 per cent of the samples with which it was tested. This antibody was called anti-Rh$_2$.

The third antibody agglutinated the cells of all Rh negative individuals and some Rh positives (including all those positive with anti-Rh$_2$) giving an overall frequency for the antigen it was detecting of approximately 80 per cent. It was called "St" after the woman in whom it was found, pending a nomenclature which would describe its place in the Rh system. This antibody was later found to be identical with the anti-Hr mentioned above.

These three sera enabled the English workers also to subdivide the Rh positive and Rh negative groups and it was very satisfying that the subdivisions made quite independently on both sides of the Atlantic were in all essentials the same.

This pattern of discovery, *i.e.* the finding of antibodies which are obviously reacting with antigens related to but not identical with the original antigen, is one which recurs in almost all blood group systems. A theory then has to be formulated to explain how the various sub-groups arise and are inherited. There are two main theories about the origin and inheritance of the Rh subtypes. We shall here describe in most detail that of Fisher because, in our opinion, it is the

73

clearest way to approach the subject and to gain a working knowledge of the main Rh subgroups and the antibodies with which they react. In Tables 9.1 and 9.2 the Wiener nomenclature is given in parallel to that of Fisher for the benefit of those readers who may wish to convert one to the other. A short paragraph explaining Wiener's theory appears below.

Table 9.1 The eight Rh gene complexes*

Fisher notation	Wiener notation	Frequency
CDe	R^1	0.421
cDE	R^2	0.141
cDe	R^0	0.026
CDE	R^z	0.002
Cde	r'	0.010
cdE	r''	0.012
CdE	r^y	Very low
cde	$\cdot r$	0.389

*All figures quoted in this table apply to the English population, being based on the figures quoted in *Blood Groups in Man*, Race & Sanger, 1975, p. 184, combining their frequencies for *CDe* and C'De.

Table 9.2 The eight Rh blood types and their reactions with the four most commonly used anti-sera

Wiener Agglutinogen	Blood Factors	Fisher Antigen Complex	Reactions with Serum			
			Anti-rh' Anti-C	Anti-rh" Anti-E	Anti-Rh$_0$ Anti-D	Anti-hr' Anti-c
Rh$_0$	Rh$_0$, hr' hr" and hr	cDe	–	–	+	+
Rh$_1$	Rh$_0$, rh' and hr"	CDe	+	–	+	–
Rh$_2$	Rh$_0$, rh" and hr'	cDE	–	+	+	+
Rh$_z$	Rh$_0$, rh' and rh"	CDE	+	+	+	–
rh	hr', hr" and hr	cde	–	–	–	+
rh'	rh' and hr"	Cde	+	–	–	–
rh"	rh" and hr'	cdE	–	+	–	+
rh$_y$	rh' and rh"	CdE	+	+	–	–

From a study of the results obtained Fisher noticed that the reactions of anti-Rh$_1$ and the serum St were antithetical and so he postulated that the genes responsible for the production of the antigens recognised by those two antibodies were allelomorphic. He chose to call them *C* and *c*. The two remaining antibodies, anti-Rh and anti-Rh$_2$ were not showing antithetical reactions. The antigen picked out by anti-Rh was called D and the antibody anti-D. Similarly the antigen picked out by anti-Rh$_2$ was called E and so anti-Rh$_2$ was called anti-E. It seemed likely that the genes for these antigens also would have allelomorphs which would fit into the system and be called *d* and *e*. Thus an Rh system

Table 9.3 The Rh genotypes arranged in phenotypes

C	D	E	c	e	Phenotypes	Per cent occurrence of phenotype	Genotypes	Per cent occurrence of genotype in total population	Percent occurrence of genotype in phenotype
−	−	−	+	(+)	ccddee (rr)	15.102	cde/cde (rr)	15.102	100.0
−	−	+	+	+	cddEe ($r''r$)	0.924	cdE/cde ($r''r$)	0.924	100.0
+	−	−	+	(+)	Ccddee ($r'r$)	0.764	Cde/cde ($r'r$)	0.764	100.0
+	−	+	+	(+)	CcddEe ($r'r''$)	0.023	Cde/cdE ($r'r''$)	0.023	100.0
							CdE/cde ($r^y r$)	0.000	0.0
−	−	+	+	(−)	cddEE ($r''r''$)	0.000	cdE/cdE ($r''r''$)	0.000	0.0
+	−	−	−	(+)	CCddee ($r'r'$)	0.014	Cde/Cde ($r'r'$)	0.014	100.0
+	−	+	−	+	CCddEe ($r'r^y$)	0.010	Cde/CdE ($r'r^y$)	0.010	100.0
+	−	+	−	(−)	CCddEE ($r^y r^y$)	0.000	CdE/CdE ($r^y r^y$)	0.000	100.0
+	−	+	+	(−)	CddEE ($r^y r''$)	0.000	CdE/cdE ($r^y r''$)	0.000	100.0
+	+	−	+	(+)	CcDee (R_1r)	34.890	CDe/cde (R_1r)	32.681	93.7
							CDe/cDe (R_1R_0)	2.159	6.2
							Cde/cDe ($r'R_0$)	0.050	0.1
+	+	−	−	+	CCDee (R_1R_1)	18.508	CDe/CDe (R_1R_1)	17.680	95.5
							CDe/Cde (R_1r')	0.828	4.5
+	+	+	+	+	CcDEe (R_1R_2)	13.342	CDe/cDE (R_1R_2)	11.865	88.9
							CDe/cdE (R_1r'')	0.999	7.5
							cDE/Cde (R_2r')	0.277	2.1
							cDe/CDE (R_0R_z)	0.189	1.4
							cDe/CdE (R_0r^y)	0.012	0.1
							CDE/cde (R_zr)	0.000	0.0
+	+	+	+	(−)	CcDEE (R_2R_z)	0.075	cDE/CDE (R_2R_z)	0.069	92.0
							cdE/CDE ($r''R_z$)	0.006	8.0
							CDE/CdE (R_zr^y)	0.000	0.0
−	+	+	+	+	ccDEe (R_2r)	11.751	cDE/cde (R_2r)	10.966	93.3
							cDE/cDe (R_2R_0)	0.724	6.2
							cDe/cdE (R_0r'')	0.061	0.5
−	+	+	+	−	ccDEE (R_2R_2)	2.326	cDE/cDE (R_2R_2)	1.991	85.6
							cDE/cdE (R_2r'')	0.335	14.4
−	+	−	+	(+)	ccDee (R_0r)	2.061	cDe/cde (R_0r)	1.995	96.8
							cDe/cDe (R_0R_0)	0.066	3.2
+	+	+	−	(+)	CCDEe (R_1R_z)	0.210	CDe/CDE (R_1R_z)	0.205	97.6
							CDE/Cde (R_zr')	0.005	2.4
							CDe/CdE (R_1r^y)	0.000	0.0
+	+	+	−	−	CCDEE (R_zR_z)	0.001	CDE/CDE (R_zR_z)	0.001	100.0
							CDE/CdE (R_zr^y)	0.000	0.0

controlled by three pairs of allelomorphic genes *Cc, Dd* and *Ee* had been formulated. Since many family studies with the four anti-sera had been made without a single example of a crossover being found it was assumed that the genes must be very closely linked.

Support for the theory was obtained through the discovery of an antibody which gave the exact reactions predicted for anti-e. Later the eighth gene combination r^y (*CdE*) was found.

However, an antibody with the predicted reactions for 'd' has not been discovered, despite several false alarms, and 'd' is now regarded as being 'silent'.

Table 9.2 shows the reactions between the antigens formed by the eight gene complexes and the four most commonly used antibodies. It is of course an over-simplification as it is not possible to test single antigen complexes with the anti-sera because every individual will have two of these gene combinations making up his genotype, one inherited from each parent.

In Table 9.3 the 36 Rh genotypes are arranged in groups according to their reactions with the four generally available anti-sera, and with anti-e. These groups are the Rh phenotypes into which individuals can be classified according to the pattern of reactions their blood gives with the various anti-sera. The number of phenotypes that can be distinguished depends of course on the number of different anti-sera with which red cells are tested; *e.g.* if anti-D alone is used only two phenotypes D-positive and D-negative can be distinguished. Table 9.4 presents the same information in terms of Wiener nomenclature.

From Table 9.3 it can be seen that testing with anti-D, anti-C, anti-E, anti-c and anti-e divides a population into eighteen phenotypes. In a few cases *e.g.* rr (ccddee) and r'r' (CCddee) the phenotype discloses the only possible genotype but some of the other phenotypes include a number of genotypes *e.g.* the phenotype R_1R_2 (CcDEe). The use of anti-e is usually confined to tests on red cells which are C negative, E positive since it is only in these circumstances that the additional information obtained justifies the use of an uncommon antiserum. In Table 9.3 reactions of anti-e with all other types is shown in brackets.

It will be appreciated that in only a few cases will tests, even with all the available anti-sera, disclose the actual genotype of an individual. At best a probable genotype may be deduced from the frequency with which each occurs within a particular phenotype, *e.g.* within the phenotype whose pattern of reaction is ++++ the genotype R^1R^2 (*CDe/cDE*) is 88.4 per cent of the phenotype. This means that the probable genotype, therefore, of an individual in this phenotype is R^1R^2 (*CDe/cDE*). This subject will be referred to again when discussing the interpretation of "genotyping" tests on husbands of women who have formed Rh antibodies. (*See* Chapter 30).

A more accurate assessment of genotype can sometimes be made with the aid of family studies.

The mode of inheritance of the Rh gene combinations is illustrated in the particular mating R^1R^2 (*CDe/cDE*) × R^1r (*CDe/cde*) (Fig. 9.1). The Rh gene combinations being composed of closely linked genes on adjacent loci on a single chromosome are inherited as a unit and behave in this connexion like simple Mendelian dominants. This means that for any given antigen combination (*e.g.*

Table 9.4 The Rh–Hr phenotypes and genotypes

Reactions with anti-sera					Name	Phenotypes Frequencies in whites (per cent)	Genotypes
Anti-Rh₀	Anti-rh'	Anti-rh"	Anti-hr'	Anti-hr"			
−	−	−	+	+	rh	14.4	rr
−	+	−	+	+	rh'rh	0.45	$r'r$
−	+	−	−	+	rh'rh'	0.0036	$r'r'$
−	−	+	+	+	rh"rh	0.38	$r''r$
−	−	+	+	−	rh"rh"	0.0025	$r''r''$
−	+	+	+	+	rh'rh"	0.006	$r'r''$ or $r^y r$
−	+	+	−	+	rhyrh'	0.001	$r^y r'$
−	+	+	+	−	rhyrh"	0.0001	$r^y r''$
−	+	+	−	−	rhyrhy	0.000001	$r^y r^y$
+	−	−	+	+	Rh₀	2.1	$R^0 R^0$ or $R^0 r$
+	+	−	+	+	Rh₁rh	33.4	$R^1 r$, $R^1 R^0$ or $R^0 r'$
+	+	−	−	+	Rh₁Rh₁	17.3	$R^1 R^1$ or $R^1 r'$
+	−	+	+	+	Rh₂rh	12.2	$R^2 r$, $R^2 R^0$ or $R^0 r''$
+	−	+	+	−	Rh₂Rh₂	2.4	$R^2 R^2$ or $R^2 r''$
+	+	+	+	+	Rh₁Rh₂	12.9	$R^1 R^2$, $R^1 r''$, $R^2 r'$, $R^z r$, $R^z R^0$, or $R^0 r^y$
+	+	+	−	+	Rh_zRh₁	0.2	$R^z R^1$, $R^1 r'$ or $R^1 r^y$
+	+	+	+	−	Rh_zRh₂	0.07	$R^z R^2$, $R^2 r''$ or $R^2 r^y$
+	+	+	−	−	Rh_zRh_z	0.0004	$R^z R^2$ or $R^z r^y$

Wiener uses the convention of italics for genes and genotypes, regular type for agglutinogens and phenotypes and bold face type for blood factors and corresponding antibodies.

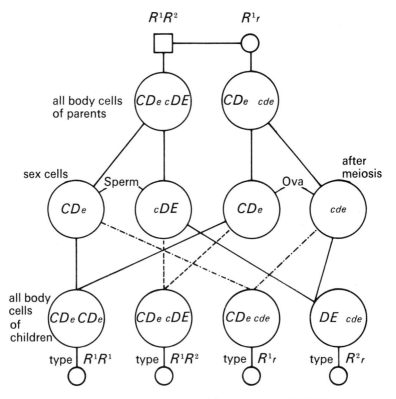

Fig. 9.1 The segregation of the Rh genes—illustrated by the mating $R^1R^2 \times R^1r$

CDe) to appear in the blood of a child it must be present in the blood of one or both parents.

Full tables giving all the possible matings to include every Rh sub-type and the sub-types of the children arising from such matings are too unwieldy to be given. Any required portion of such a table can readily be compiled when needed. For an example the mating R_1R_2 and R_1r can be taken. The phenotype R_1R_2 includes nine genotypes, namely, R^1R^2, $r'R^2$, R^1r'', R^0R^z, R^zr, r^yR^0, R^2R^z, $r''R^z$, $r''R^z$, r^yR^2, and the phenotype group R_1r includes the three genotypes R^1r, R^1R^0, and $r'R^0$. Within this one phenotype mating we have, therefore, twenty-seven possibilities for the genotype mating, each giving rise to different Rh sub-types among the offspring. Occasionally the phenotype of one or more children of a mating will throw light on the actual genotype of one or the other, or both, parents; in other cases, of course, the phenotype of the children is no help and may even be misleading, e.g. when a child whose genotype is really R^zr is thought of as R^1R^2 because this is the most common genotype in the phenotype to which R^zr belongs.

Some phenotype matings are much less complicated because there are fewer alternative genotypes in each phenotype and in a few cases e.g. rr and r'r there is only one genotype in the phenotype; thus the mating $r'r \times rr$ can be fully expressed in a one line table:

Phenotype mating	Genotypes of children	Phenotypes of children
r'r × rr	r'r and rr	r'r and rr

In this case of course it is possible to determine the actual genotype with the four anti-sera anti-C, anti-D, anti-E, and anti-c and family studies will merely confirm the findings.

The Theory of Wiener

Wiener favours the concept of one gene instead of three closely linked ones. However, to understand his theory fully, it is necessary to grasp his conception of agglutinogens and blood factors. He postulates that a gene gives rise to an agglutinogen on the red cell surface and that this in turn possesses a number of blood factors. For example, the gene R^1 (see Table 9.1) gives rise to the agglutinogen Rh_1 which possesses the three blood factors Rh_0, **rh'** and **hr"** (see Table 9.2). The blood factor **hr** appearing in Table 9.2 refers to the Fisher compound antigen ce (see Chapter 17).

It will be a relief to realise that the concept of one gene versus the concept of three closely linked genes has no significance in practical laboratory work beyond the unfortunate existence of a double nomenclature. However in our experience we have found that the subgroups of Rh are more comprehensible to students using the Fisher nomenclature than that of Wiener.

Rare Rh Genes

The Rh system is further complicated by such genes as C^W, C^x, c^v, C^u, G, V, etc., but it is not proposed to deal with these until Chapter 17. The antigen D^u however is discussed here because it is a common cause of anomalies in "D" typing.

D^u red cells

Red cells of the type D^u (Table 9.5) are recognised by the fact that they are agglutinated by some anti-D sera but not others. Specific anti-sera have not been

Table 9.5 Examples of the reactions given by D^u red cells

D^u red cells	Reactions with anti-D sera											
	In saline			In albumin				By ahg				
	1	2	3	4	5	6	7	8	9	10	11	12
(a) High grade	V	V	–	V	V	V	V	–	V	V	V	V
(b) Low grade	–	–	V	–	–	V	–	–	V	V	V	V
(c) Low grade	–	–	–	–	–	–	–	–	V	V	V	V
(d) Low grade	V	–	–	–	–	–	–	–	V	–	V	V
(e) High grade	w	(+)	w	(+)	w	+	(+)	w	V	V	V	V

found for them. D^u red cells have relatively few D-antigen sites compared with normal D red cells. With the same range of anti-D sera different examples of D^u cells behave differently and for convenience may be classified as high grade or low grade. A high grade D^u red cell is one that is agglutinated by the majority of anti-D sera by albumin technique. A type of high grade D^u is sometimes encountered which is agglutinated by all sera but only weakly. A low grade D^u red cell is one which is only agglutinated by albumin technique by one or two of a range of sera with which it is tested, although it is sensitised by most of them, as can be proved by testing with anti-human globulin (Coombs test) and it will normally react by papain two-stage technique. Sometimes the D^u is of such a low grade that the fact that it has reacted at all with anti-D can only be detected by the indirect anti-human globulin test, or by pre-treating the D^u cells with papain before testing with a powerful incomplete anti-D. In practice it is recommended that both these methods are used (*see* Chapter 10).

It is important to realise that pretreatment of a D^u cell with papain almost invariably renders it agglutinable by almost all anti-D sera.

It has been well established that D^u is inherited, *i.e.* a parent who is D^u can pass on to his child a D^u antigen which behaves towards anti-D sera as does the D^u antigen of the parent. The existence of D^u presents a problem when typing red cells using two anti-D sera; some red cells will be typed falsely as Rh negative when they are in fact D^u (*see* Chapter 10).

The D^u antigen if injected into individuals lacking D (*e.g. cde/cde* individuals) stimulates the production of normal anti-D antibodies which are in no way distinguishable from such antibodies which have been produced in response to a normal D but it is a less effective antigen.

The possible production of anti-D antibodies in a D^u individual has been widely considered and many D^u individuals, particularly of the low grade type, have had their serum examined for anti-D. It is unlikely that the true D^u is capable of being immunised by the D antigen therefore it is usual to regard them as Rh positive for all practical purposes (see also chapter 17). D positive people, who are found to have anti-D are most often those with a part of the D antigen missing who have formed an antibody against the missing fraction (*see* Chapter 17). These should be designated D variant and not D^u although they appear to be D^u on initial testing. Such people are usually discovered through having anti-D in their serum rather than showing anything unusual in their red cell reactions. Only a study of their cells with many unpooled anti-D typing sera reveals their particular antigenic structure. It is usual to regard all D^u individuals as Rh positive for all practical purposes. (*See also* Chapter 17).

Chapter 10. Rh Sub-Typing

The simple division of the Rh system into Rh positive (D positive) and Rh negative (D negative) using anti-D sera only, can now be extended by the use of the other Rh sera (anti-C, anti-E, etc.). These sera are not, however, in sufficiently good supply to allow of their routine use in Rh testing, nor indeed would the knowledge of the Rh sub-type be any real advantage for most purposes. This means that we have to consider how much testing is really necessary and the most economical way of using the available sera. The first step is always the division into D-positive and D-negative, therefore the further divisions and their appropriate techniques will be described under three headings: (1) subdivisions of D-negative; (2) subdivisions of D-positive ("genotyping"); (3) further investigation of anomalous results with anti-D.

SUBDIVISION OF D-NEGATIVE

The subdivisions of the D-negative individuals are: (1) *cde/cde* (*rr*); (2) *Cde/cde* (*r'r*); (3) *Cde/Cde* (*r'r'*); (4) *Cde/cdE* (*r'r"*); (5) *Cde/CdE* (*r'r*ʸ); (6) *cdE/cde* (*r"r*); (7) *cdE/cdE* (*r"r"*); (8) *cdE/CdE* (*r"r*ʸ); (9) *CdE/cde* (*r*ʸ*r*); (10) *CdE/CdE* (*r*ʸ*r*ʸ).

Most of the foregoing subdivisons are very rare and thus seldom encountered. The most important is, of course, No. (1) *cde/cde,* after which (2) *Cde/cde* and (6) *cdE/cde* are the most frequent. Individuals of these sub-groups are all capable of making anti-D if stimulated by the D antigen and should, if in need of a blood transfusion, receive blood which is either Rh negative (*cde/cde*) or of their own genotype. Since the latter alternative is impracticable all of these must be regarded as Rh negative recipients.

It can be seen that all but the true Rh negatives (*cde/cde*) have either C or E or both of these antigens and if they are used as Rh negative donors for transfusion they may stimulate the production of anti-C or anti-E in the recipient. This means that every donor who is negative to anti-D serum must be tested further with anti-C and anti-E. Whenever time allows it is advisable to test all D negative patients also with anti-C and anti-E.

In practice it is recommended that this testing is carried out, not with pure anti-C and anti-E sera but with mixtures which contain anti-D as well. As will be seen in Chapter 12 sera which contain anti-D and anti-C (called for convenience anti-C+ D or anti-CD sera) and those which contain anti-D and anti-E (called for convenience anti-D + E or anti-DE sera) are much more readily obtainable than the pure sera and are just as suitable, if not more so, for the testing of red cells which have already been shown to be D negative. A possible error which has

D

continually to be guarded against if Rh typing is to be done accurately is the designation rr, r′ or r″ to red cells which are in reality Rh positive but of the very low grade D^u type. It is not dangerous to mistake low grade D^u individuals for r′ or r″ since they will then be regarded as Rh positive if they are donors of blood and Rh negative if they themselves are recipients. It is very fortunate that in the white population D^u is usually associated with C or E, $cD^u e$ being very rare indeed. [However, with the increase in the number of non-white races in Britain now, it is becoming essential to test all anti-D negatives for D^u.] If several different anti-D sera are used to test any samples which appear to be D negative the chance of failure in detecting a D^u is reduced. Also, the further testing of D negatives with anti-CD and anti-DE mixtures is an advantage in this context. Another method for the detection of low grade D^u is the indirect anti-human globulin test, with a powerful incomplete anti-D.

If there is still any doubt, papain treated cells are tested with pure incomplete anti-D sera; almost all D^u cells give strong positive reactions by this technique. True D-variant cells will give negative reaction with some anti-sera even by this technique, because the anti-sera lack the fraction specific for the given variant (*see* Chapter 17).

The exact routine adopted for the confirmation of D negative blood samples is influenced by one or both of two main considerations: (*a*) whether the samples to be tested are from prospective donors or from patients who are, therefore, potential recipients; (*b*) the actual number of samples with which the laboratory has to deal. With regard to (*a*) it will by now have been appreciated that it is very important to diagnose accurately the "D" position of donors. If a patient's blood is found to be negative with two anti-D, one anti-CD and one anti-DE or even merely with two anti-D sera then it is called Rh(D) negative and the patient receives Rh negative blood. Donors, however, whose blood is negative with two anti-D sera have to be tested more extensively. At this point consideration (*b*) arises, for, on the whole, samples from prospective donors are dealt with in large numbers by the serological laboratories of the Transfusion Service so that the routine selected must of necessity be related to the problem of coping with large numbers of tests. We recommend that donors' samples be tested with four additional anti-D sera. This can be done either by using two anti-D, one anti-CD and one anti-DE or, rather than rely on one serum for C and one for E, with two anti-CD and two anti-DE sera (provided sufficient sera of these types are available). By this means adequate tests for D can be carried out simultaneously with tests for C and E. The indirect anti-human globulin test is too involved and time-consuming a technique for the detection of D^u in large-scale testing unless the staff position and time factor will allow for the careful and meticulous handling that is needed for this test. The papain technique is a slightly more convenient technique which will detect all but a very few low grade D^u samples. If only one ar.ti-CD and one anti-DE serum are used, further tests are necessary when a positive reaction is obtained with either the anti-CD or the anti-DE serum. This is for two reasons: (1) the presence of an antigen on the red cells should always be confirmed by testing with more than one anti-serum containing the corresponding antibody and (2) the possibility that the reaction is due to D^u. If two anti-CD and two anti-DE sera are used, providing the results are consistent, the first point is already covered but the second, the possibility of D^u, still remains.

It must be borne in mind that there are two antibodies operating in an anti-C + D or anti-D + E mixture so that any positive reaction obtained, in the one case might be due either to anti-C or anti-D and in the other to anti-D or anti-E. The cells being tested with such sera already will have been found negative with at least two anti-D sera so that any reaction obtained is more likely to be due to a C – anti-C or E – anti-E reaction than to D – anti-D. However, there is always the possibility that the blood sample in question may in fact be of a low grade D^u type which happens to react with the particular anti-D which is present in one of the mixtures. In view of this, therefore, it is advisable to confirm samples which appear to be r′ or r″ with at least one if not two further anti-C + D or anti-D + E mixtures where this has not already been done. Moreover, a large number of apparent r′ and r″ cells are in fact of the low grade D^u type which only reveals its D antigen by indirect anti-human globulin test. Any samples which give positive reactions with either the anti-CD or anti-DE mixtures should be tested against incomplete anti-D sera by the anti-human globulin and papain techniques. If pure anti-C, and anti-c sera are available r′ cells can be checked with these, similarly r″ cells with anti-E and anti-e. We do not describe the use of these sera in techniques 10.1–4 but reference can be made to technique No. 10.5.

Before describing details of techniques the choice of controls for anti-CD and anti-DE sera must be mentioned. (*See* Table 10.1.) These are selected to test the satisfactory working of each antibody *independently*. In effect this means that any red cell containing C and not D can be used as a positive control for the anti-C component of the anti-CD mixture and any red cell containing D and not C will be suitable as a positive control for the anti-D of the same mixture. The most readily available cells are r′r (Ccddee) and R_2r (ccDEe) respectively. Similarly for the proper control of the two components of the anti-DE mixture, red cells containing E and not D and others containing D and not E are suitable. The most easily obtained are r″r (ccddEe) and R_1r (CcDee). For both mixtures the negative control is rr (ccddee). (Table 10.1.)

Table 10.1 controls for Rh sub-typing

Anti-serum	Positive controls	Negative controls *
D	R_1r or R_1R_2	rr
CD	R_2r and r′r	rr
DE	R_1r and r″r	rr
C	R_1R_2	R_2r
C (from known D negative)	R_1R_2	R_2R_2
C (from known D positive)	R_1R_2	rr
E	R_1R_2	rr
c	R_1R_2	R_1R_1
e	R_1R_2	R_2R_2

* If group AB red cells of the required Rh sub-type are available, they form the best negative control, as they also control that the sera are adequately absorbed for anti-A and anti-B.

All the tests described in this chapter are done by the standard tube method, emergency techniques not being applicable to confirmatory tests. In the case of an urgent blood transfusion, a patient who is negative with one or two anti-D sera is given Rh negative blood.

TECHNIQUES

Technique No. 10.1. Testing of samples screened as D-negative

The tests are set up as described for Rh typing by tube technique (technique Nos. 7.2 or 7.3) except that four rows of tubes will be required in the fifty-holed rack so that the samples can be tested with either two anti-D, one anti-CD and one anti-DE 10. 1a or alternatively two anti-CD and two anti-DE mixtures(10. lb). The sera used will be either "saline" or "albumin" type according to availability; all the cell suspensions are made in saline, albumin being added to the appropriate tubes at the end of $1\frac{1}{2}$ hours' incubation. Positive and negative controls as described above are included with each batch of tests. The tubes are incubated at $37°$C for about 2 hours and read taking the usual precautions for dealing with delicate agglutination. For interpretation of results and indications for use of techniques Nos. 10.2–4 see Table 10.2. If tests have been done with two anti-CD and two anti-DE sera techniques Nos. 10.2 and 10.3 are omitted.

Technique No. 10.2. Further testing of samples found to be negative with anti-D but positive with anti-CD

Two rows of tubes are required for these tests. In each tube of the first row is placed one volume of an anti-CD serum while in each tube of the second row is placed one volume of a second anti-CD serum. The setting up of this test is completed as for Rh typing (techniques No. 7.2 or 7.3). Controls of Or'r, OR$_2$r and Orr cells are set up at the same time. The r'r and R$_2$r will control the two components of the anti-CD mixture independently. The tests are read in the usual way after 2 hours' incubation at $37°$C.

Technique No. 10.3. Further testing of samples found to be negative with anti-D but positive with anti-DE

The pattern of this test is exactly the same as that described immediately above, but instead of anti-CD sera, two anti-DE mixtures are used. Suitable controls are included (i.e. Or"r, OR$_1$r, and Orr) and the tests read after 2 hours' incubation.

Technique No. 10.4a. Detection of D^u in red cells apparently D-negative. Indirect anti-human globulin test

The technique is essentially the same as that described in Chapter 8 (technique No. 8.3a). The object of the test is, however, different. The test already outlined is for the detection of incomplete antibodies, using known standard cells. It is used in the present connexion conversely for the detection of the D^u antigen in unknown cells by means of known incomplete anti-D.

Table 10.2 Subdivision of D-negative cells. Interpretation of results

TECHNIQUE NO. 10.1a †

Samples tested	Anti-D	Anti-D	Anti-CD	Anti-DE	Further technique	Conclusion
F.G.	–	–	–	–	None*	rr
H.I.	–	⁓	+	–	10.2 and 4	
J.K.	–	–	–	+	10.3 and 4	
L.M.	+	–	+	–	10.2 and 4	
N.O.	–	+	–	+	10.3 and 4	
P.Q.	–	–	+	+	10.2, 3 and 4	
R.S.	–	–	+	–	10.2 and 4	

TECHNIQUE NO. 10.1b

Samples tested	Anti-CD	Anti-CD	Anti-DE	Anti-DE	Further technique	Conclusion
F.G.	–	–	–	–	None*	rr
H.I.	+	+	–	–		probably r′
J.K.	–	–	+	+		probably r″
L.M.	+	+	–	+	10.4	
N.O.	–	+	+	+		
P.Q.	+	+	+	+		probably r′r″
R.S.	+	+	–	–		probably r′

TECHNIQUE NO. 10.2 · TECHNIQUE NO. 10.4

Samples tested	Anti-CD	Anti-CD	Incomplete anti-D	Incomplete D anti-D	Conclusion
H.I.	+	+	–	–	r′
L.M.	+	+	+	+	D^u
P.Q.	+	+	–	–	See below
R.S.	+	+	+	+	Du

TECHNIQUE NO. 10.3

Samples tested	Anti-DE	Anti-DE			Conclusion
J.K.	+	+	–	–	r″
N.O.	+	+	+	+	D^u
P.Q.	+	+	see above		r′r″

†Depending upon availability of sera, technique 10.1 (a) or (b) will be used, not both.
*If negroid, technique 10.4 must be included.

The test is set up in the usual manner mixing two volumes of a potent incomplete anti-D with two volumes of 3 per cent cells from the sample to be tested. The anti-human globulin (Coombs reagent) must be used at the optimum dilution for the detection of IgG (*see* Appendix II). The controls and subsequent procedure are the same as in technique No. 8.3a.

Technique No. 10.4b. Detection of D^u in red cells apparently D-negative. Papain technique

The cells are papain treated by technique No. 8.5b. They are then washed and made up to a 2 per cent solution with saline. The cells are tested with two different pure anti-D sera and with AB serum as a negative control, one volume of cells is added to one volume of serum and the mixture incubated for 1 hour at 37° C.

The tests are read macro- and microscopically. Controls of Rh positive, Rh type D^u, r'r, r'' and rr cells are included in each batch of tests.

This test will detect almost all examples of D^u but the occasional cell will be encountered which is negative by this test but positive by the anti-human globulin technique (No. 10.4a).

Interpretation of Results

A summary of most of the various results which may be obtained from the above tests is shown in Table 10.2.

Although the testing of these D negative samples and the variety of possible results may seem confusing, it should be realised that in the majority of cases straightforward negative results will be obtained with anti-sera D, CD, and DE and the red cells will be designated Rh negative accordingly.

In a few cases a positive result may be obtained with either anti-CD or anti-DE which on confirmation will show the red cells to be r' or r'', or low grade D^u if the indirect anti-human globulin test is positive.

Very occasionally a D-variant type will be encountered. This may manifest itself by giving a positive reaction with one or more of the anti-D sera by all techniques used including indirect ahg and enzyme. (*See also* Table 9.5).

Very rarely indeed the r'r'' (which cannot be distinguished from the even more rare r^{y}r) may be found. This shows up as D negative but positive with both anti-CD and anti-DE mixtures. Its occurrence should be established carrying out a combination of techniques Nos. 10.2–4, wherein it will be found to be positive with all anti-CD and anti-DE sera but consistently negative with all examples of anti-D. Its distinction from r^y can only be made through family studies.

SUBDIVISION OF D-POSITIVE

It is only in special circumstances that a subdivision of D-positive red cells is required. This is fortunate because the sera necessary for such subdivision (commonly misnamed "genotyping") are in limited supply. There are situations, however, in which it is very useful to obtain as accurate an idea as possible of the actual Rh genotype of an individual. Cases in point are D positive persons suspected of having had a haemolytic transfusion reaction, infants suffering from haemolytic disease of the newborn, cases receiving multiple transfusions, persons whose sera contain atypical antibodies thought to belong to the Rh system, husbands of Rh negative women whose sera contain atypical antibodies, etc.

Before the actual technique of Rh sub-typing is described the choice of standard cells for controls on the anti-sera used must be discussed. (*See* Table 10.1.) The positive controls must be chosen bearing in mind that the strength of a positive reaction with anti-C, anti-E, anti-c, and anti-e is often considerably weaker with cells of a genotype containing only one "dose" of the corresponding antigen than with cells containing two "doses". This is particularly true of anti-c; cells containing a "double dose" of c through inheriting it from both parents (*e.g. cde/cde*) react more strongly with anti-c than do cells of genotype R^1r (*CDe/cde*) which contain only one c. A satisfactory positive control is one which corresponds to the weakest positive expected to be found in the tests. Accordingly, cells that are heterozygous for each antigen tested are used. R_1R_2 (CcDEe) cells are obviously the convenient choice for a positive control which satisfies the foregoing criterion for all anti-sera except anti-D for which R_1r (CcDee) cells are the best control. The negative control for each anti-serum has to be selected with the possible contaminants of that serum in mind. (*See* Chapter 12.).

Very strong anti-C, anti-E, and anti-c sera are rare and so weaker examples of them may have to be used for test sera than if the selection were wider. In spite of their rarity it is still recommended, therefore, that two examples of sera of each specificity be employed if available. In order to conserve stocks it is recommended that the unit volume for the test should be about 0.02 ml.

Technique No. 10.5. Further testing of samples found to be positive with anti-D—Rh phenotyping

The fifty-holed rack should be turned so that a row of seven precipitin tubes and one cell suspension tube can be placed in it for each sample to be tested.

Row 1 contains	anti-C	(1)
Row 2 "	"	(2)
Row 3 "	anti-E	(1)
Row 4 "	"	(2)
Row 5 "	anti-c	(1)
Row 6 "	"	(2)
Row 7 "	AB serum	

If the small unit volumes are used, they should be delivered very carefully to the bottom of the tubes using a Pasteur pipette specially graduated to deliver such small volumes (Fig. AI.1D). This avoids wetting the side of the tubes which may result in significant loss of fluid.

After the tubes have been checked for the presence of serum in each, an equal volume of a 2 per cent red cell suspension in saline is added to each one. This is also delivered to the bottom of the tube without touching the serum with the pipette; carrying out this manoeuvre with such a small volume necessitates lifting the tubes from the rack so that the contents can be seen. The tests are incubated for 2 hours and then read with even more care than usual owing to the small volume of fluid available for spreading on the slide. No reaction should be scored as definitely positive unless at least of "+" strength. Any discrepancy occurring between the results obtained with two sera of the same specificity necessitates repeating the test. If the anomalous results are confirmed the sample is tested with as large a panel of sera of the requisite specificity as is available. Typing sera containing incomplete antibodies should be used by albumin addition technique (No. 7.3) or Löw's papain technique (No. 8.5a or b) which ever is appropriate.

Interpretation of Results

Each possible pattern of reaction with the four anti-sera (including anti-D) will be discussed separately and in conjunction with Table 9.3. A step by step method of deducing the genotypes from first principles is given with the first set of reactions discussed. It should be pointed out that in Table 9.3 the frequency of each genotype is expressed as a percentage of the total population in Column 5 and as a percentage of the particular phenotype in Column 6.

Anti-D	Anti-C	Anti-E	Anti-c
+	+	-	-

This is the easiest pattern to interpret and therefore is dealt with first. Table 9.3 gives the two possible genotypes showing this pattern of reaction. The knack of working out the different alternatives without the aid of a table should be acquired.

A convenient line to adopt is given below.

Taking the result with anti-D first, the positive reaction obtained with this serum shows that at least one D occurs in the genotype. Whether the genotype is DD or Dd cannot be certainly determined because there is no antibody for the detection of "d."

So far then the genotype can be written:

$$D/D \text{ or } D/d$$

The result found with anti-C should be considered together with that for anti-c since these anti-sera are detecting antigens arising from allelomorphic genes. In this case the reaction with anti-C is positive and with anti-c is negative so the genotype must be CC which can now be included thus:

$$CD/CD \text{ or } CD/Cd$$

Lastly the anti-E result must be assessed. This is negative which indicates the absence of E so the genotype can be completed thus:

$$CDe/CDe \text{ or } CDe/Cde$$

i.e. the alternatives are R^1R^1 (*CDe/CDe*) or R^1r' (*CDe/Cde*).

From Table 9.3 it can be seen that the genotype $R'R'$ forms 95.5 per cent of the phenotype $R_1 R_1$.

It is, therefore, correct to conclude that the probable genotype of an individual whose cells give this pattern of agglutination reaction is R^1R^1. The fact that the "improbable" genotype R^1r' will occur in 4.5 per cent of the phenotype must not be overlooked!

Anti-D	Anti-C	Anti-E	Anti-c
+	+	-	+

Table 9.3 shows that there are three possible genotypes giving these reactions, but again the odds are overwhelmingly in favour of one; in this case R^1r. The probable genotype of such an individual is, therefore, R^1r.

Anti-D	Anti-C	Anti-E	Anti-c
+	+	+	+

A positive reaction with all four sera indicating the presence of all four antigens, D, C, E, and c gives rise to many more alternatives. From the table it can be seen that there are nine; R^1R^2 the probable genotype, comprising 88.4 per cent of the whole phenotype.

Anti-D	Anti-C	Anti-E	Anti-c
+	-	+	+

In the phenotype patterning as above there are five alternative genotypes of which the most common is R^2r (77.9 per cent) followed by R^2R^2 14.1 per cent.

It is often an advantage when it is realised that the blood under test falls into this category to use anti-e. If a positive reaction is obtained with this serum the probable genotype is R^2r (93.3 per cent) and if a negative reaction is obtained the probable genotype is R^2R^2 (85.6 per cent) (*see* Table 9.3). If no anti-e is available a titration with an anti-E known to show a marked dosage effect may be used instead although the results may not be so clear cut.

Anti-D	Anti-C	Anti-E	Anti-c
+	-	-	+

In this phenotype there are two alternative genotypes R^0r and R^0R^0. The probable genotype in this case R^0r (96.8 per cent):

Anti-D	Anti-C	Anti-E	Anti-c
+	+	+	-

Although this phenotype is rare, occurring in only 0.2 per cent of the total population, it comprises no less than five genotypes. The probable genotype is R^1R^z (97.1 per cent).

The circumstances in which it is of value to know the sub-group to which a D positive red cell belongs have already been listed and it will be seen that these differ widely. They must, therefore, be taken into account in the interpretation of results. For the identification of atypical antibodies which may be of the Rh system, a knowledge of the antigens lacking in the patient is more useful than assembling the results for the purpose of postulating a probable genotype. If, on the other hand, the blood of a husband whose wife's serum contains Rh antibodies is being considered, the important point is whether he is homozygous or heterozygous for the antigen corresponding to the antibody in her serum.

A knowledge of the husband's antigenic make-up may also be of help in confirming the identity of a maternal antibody. A more detailed discussion of the Rh genotypes of these husbands will be found in Chapter 17.

Chapter 11. Detection and Identification of Rh Antibodies, Including Mixtures

The emphasis of this chapter is on specificity, as it is important not only to detect but also to identify any of the Rh antibodies which may be present in a serum. Herein is also included the less straightforward identification of mixtures of Rh antibodies of different specificities occurring in one serum.

Choice of Standard Red Cells

The first step is the selection of suitable standard cells of known Rh sub-types for the routine testing of sera which may contain Rh antibodies. The object is to be able to detect any of the Rh antibodies with cells of a few readily available sub-types.

The trio R^1R^1 (CDe/CDe), R^2R^2 (cDE/cDE), and $rr(cde/cde)$ are the genotypes of choice. Table 11.1 shows not only that these detect any of the antibodies but also that they give a different pattern of reactions with each. A further advantage of using these genotypes is that they have two "doses" of those Rh antigens which show a "dosage" effect. R^1R^1 (CDe/CDe) has a double dose of C and e, R^2R^2 (cDE/cDE) has a double dose of c and E. These two also have a double dose of D but in R^1R^1 the D is partially suppressed by the C; R^2R^2 (cDE/cDE) is the best cell for the detection of anti-D. The third cell $rr(cde/cde)$ has a double dose of c and e. This means that if any of the antibodies anti-C, anti-E, anti-c, or anti-e are present they will be able to react to their maximum capacity with cells containing the double dose of antigen. Thus they are more readily detected. Indeed, when the antibody is weak the use of red cells containing only a single dose of the antibody would probably result in failure to detect the antibody.

Table 11.1 Identification of the five main Rh antibodies

Antibody	Standard cells			Mixtures giving same pattern of reaction
	R_1R_1	R_2R_2	rr	
(1) Anti-D	+	+	−	Anti-CD, anti-DE, anti-CDE, and anti-CE (v. rare)
(2) Anti-C	+	−	−	
(3) Anti-E	−	+	−	
(4) Anti-c	−	+	+	Anti-E+c
(5) Anti-e	+	−	+	Anti-C+e

In practice, as the actual genotypes of standard cells are not usually known, cells belonging to the corresponding phenotypes *i.e.* R_1R_1, R_2R_2 and rr are used. if R_1R_2 is unavailable it can be replaced by R_2r or even R_1R_2. If this is done, the antigen E will only be represented in single dose. Since E does not show dosage quite as markedly as c this is not too great a disadvantage, particularly if the technique of handling the cells sediments gently, while reading the tests, is strictly adhered to, so that weak agglutination is not missed.

Many laboratories favour the use of only R_1R_2 and rr red cells for Rh antibody detection tests, but these represent the absolute minimum. If these are used, the antigens C and E will be present in single dose. As anti-C and anti-E antibodies, in the main, occur as saline agglutinins, it is felt that R_1R_2 should not be substituted for R_1R_1 and R_2R_2 in the saline technique. Moreover, using R_1R_2 and rr cells the pattern of reaction given by anti-C, anti-D and anti-E will be identical, as will that given by anti-c and anti-e. Positive reactions with either or both of these red cells will require further investigation. However, even if a characteristic pattern is obtained with the ideal red cell combination R_1R_1, R_2R_2, and rr further tests are necessary with a larger panel of cells before the identity of the antibody can be established.

Choice of Techniques

Having selected the most satisfactory set of standard cells from those available it has to be decided which techniques to use. These, of course, must allow for the detection of antibodies occurring in either the complete or incomplete forms (or mixtures of both).

If only a few tests are being performed, saline (technique No. 8.1) indirect anti-human globulin (technique No. 8.3a), and papain (technique Nos. 8.5a or b) or one of the other enzyme techniques should be chosen. Where the number of sera to be examined for antibodies is very large the method using albumin (technique No. 8.2) can be substituted for the indirect anti-human globulin in spite of its slightly lower sensitivity. A rather different procedure is adopted when the AutoAnalyser is used (see chapter 21).

It may be asked whether a saline technique is necessary at all if albumin or indirect anti-human globulin tests are to be included. Will these not also detect agglutinins? Such agglutinins will often agglutinate red cells suspended in bovine albumin, but usually this agglutination is much weaker than when the red cells are suspended in saline. Occasionally, agglutination of cells by agglutinins is entirely inhibited by bovine albumin. Nor is the anti-human globulin test a satisfactory method of detecting agglutinins. If the latter are potent the cells are obviously agglutinated at the end of the incubation stage of the test and it is therefore unnecessary to add anti-human globulin reagent.

On the other hand, weak agglutination which has already taken place will often be enhanced by the addition of anti-human globulin. This is almost certainly because the red cells also have incomplete antibodies attached to them.

At this point it would seem appropriate to give a short account of the characteristics and method of identification of each Rh antibody separately, although a great deal about anti-D and a few facts about the others will have been dealt with in previous chapters.

Anti-D

Anti-D is not so frequent as it used to be due to the prophylactic treatment of Rh negative women with immunoglobulin. Anti-D has been discussed in Chapter 8.

It is produced by D-negative individuals in response to stimulation by the D antigen. The majority of people who form anti-D are rr, but persons of any sub-type lacking D are equally liable to produce it.

If an individual lacks antigen D and his serum gives the pattern of reaction (1) in Table 11.1, then the antibody present in the serum is probably anti-D. However, to confirm the specificity it is essential to test with a different set of known D positive and D negative cells by the techniques with which the antibody was detected. At least three examples of D positive cells and two of D negative must be used; if the serum is consistently positive with the D positive cells and negative with the D negative, then the serum certainly contains anti-D antibodies. Other antibodies may possibly be present but masked by the anti-D; for instance, anti-CD or anti-DE mixtures would give the same pattern of reaction as pure anti-D. Antibodies may also be present but undetected because no cell containing the corresponding antigen has been used in the test. The most common antibody which may be missed in this way is anti-Kell. It is recommended, therefore, that in addition to the test with D positive and D negative cells the serum should also be tested with r'r (*Cde/cde*), r"r (*cdE/cde*), and rr (*cde/cde*) Kell positive cells. A further fairly common antibody is anti-Wr^a rather less common but important contaminants are anti-Fy^a and anti-Jk^a.

Anti-D usually agglutinates equally well cells which are DD or Dd. It therefore does not normally show dosage. However, D is modified by its accompanying antigens (*see* Chapter 17) and the anti-D titre against D-positive cells of differing Rh genotypes will reflect this, the greatest titre being obtained with R^2R^2 (*cDE/cDE*) and the least with R^1r (*CDe/cde*) red cells.

Anti-C

Pure anti-C, *i.e.* unmixed with other Rh antibodies (No. 2 in Table 11.1) rarely occurs. Occasionally, however, it is formed by a D-positive, C-negative individual, *e.g.* R^2R^2 (*cDE/cDE*) or R^2r (*cDE/cde*) but not as often as might be expected from the number of opportunities for its production that arise. More often it occurs in a mixture with anti-D (*see* below). and has been found associated with anti-e (*see* below). If a serum gives the pattern of reaction characteristic of anti-C, the specificity should be checked by the use of three r'r, two R_2r and two rr samples of red cells. The patient's own cells are phenotyped, or at least tested and shown to be negative with anti-C.

Anti-C occurs in both complete and incomplete forms, but the complete form is more common.

The antibody sometimes shows a dosage effect, but not markedly.

There is a further discussion of various types of anti-C sera in Chapter 17. Before any serum is used as an anti-C typing serum it should be fully investigated along the lines suggested, by a laboratory having available cells of the various rare Rh sub-types necessary.

Anti-E

Pure anti-E occurs more frequently than pure anti-C, being found in general in the serum of R^1R^1 (CDe/CDe) or R^1r (CDe/cde) individuals.

The pattern of reaction it gives is No. 3 in Table 11.1. Confirmatory tests must be carried out to establish the specificity, using three r″r, two R_1R_1, and two rr samples of red cells; the individual's own cells are tested with anti-E. Anti-E sometimes displays a dosage effect, occasionally to such an extent that it is as reliable as anti-e in distinguishing between EE and Ee cells.

Anti-E is quite often present as an antibody detectable only by an enzyme technique, in which case it is probably naturally occurring. As such it has little clinical significance but may, upon stimulation, develop into a clinically significant antibody.

Anti-c

The pattern of agglutination reaction characteristic of anti-c is No. 4 in Table 11.1.

The antibody is almost always found in D positive persons, since D negatives lacking the antigen c are very rare indeed. The phenotype in which the antibody occurs is R_1R_1 which includes the genotype R^1r' (CDe/Cde). The antigen c, however, seems to be comparatively weak, and most people, even after a number of exposures to it, do not make anti-c.

It is important to confirm its specificity by testing against two rr, two R_1r and two R_1R_1 cell samples. It should also be tested with R_1R_z cells, if these are available as anti-c/anti-E mixtures are common (see below).

Anti-c is found in both complete and incomplete forms and almost always shows dosage to a high degree. Titres with cc (e.g. cde/cde cells) and Cc (e.g. CDe/cde) cells will help to confirm the identity of the antibody.

It is essential if it is proposed to use it for Rh typing purposes that it should give a satisfactory titration value with single dose c cells.

Anti-e

This is a rare antibody, partly because the e antigen seems to be a weak one, but mostly because there are very few individuals who lack it and are, therefore, capable of forming anti-e. The calculated total percentage of the population lacking e is 2.4 per cent, and of these the commonest genotype is R^2R^2 (cDE/cDE), which is 2.0 per cent. It is however now commercially available, as are other rare antibodies, the supply being increased by deliberate stimulation or re-stimulation and by plasmapheresis of the donor (*see* Chapter 30, technique No. 30.3).

The pattern of reaction of anti-e is number 5 in Table 11. It has been found in both complete and incomplete forms and usually displays marked dosage. When it occurs it is often detected preferentially or exclusively by enzyme technique. If a serum is suspected to contain anti-e, the red cells should be fully Rh typed, including testing with anti-e. Of the relatively common genotypes R^2R^2 (*cDE/cDE*) is the only one that will give a negative reaction with anti-e, and this will only occur once in fifty times among random samples. It is, therefore, a good plan to test the suspected anti-e against as many known R_2R_2 (ccDEE) red cells as can be procured. It should also be tested with R_2R_Z (CcDEE) for the possible presence of anti-C (*see* below). Dosage titrations can also be performed, using rr (ccddee) and R_2r (ccDEe) or R_1R_2 (CcDEe) cells as an added confirmation of the specificity.

Anti-CD, Anti-DE, and Anti-CDE Mixtures

These mixtures do not occur in all cases in which they are a theoretical possibility. Rather less than half the Rh antibodies found in Rh negative persons are mixtures of anti-D and anti-C, a much smaller number are anti-D + anti-E, and a very few are mixtures of all three antibodies. D is strongly antigenic and it is very rare indeed for anti-C or anti-E to be present and yet anti-D absent in D-negative individuals who are exposed to D as well as C or E.

Table 11.2 Differentiation of anti-D, anti-CD, anti-DE, anti-CDE and anti-CE

Antibody	r′r Ccddee	r″r ccddEe	R_0r ccDee
Anti-D	−	−	+
Anti-CD	+	−	+
Anti-DE	−	+	+
Anti-CDE	+	+	+
Anti-CE	+	+	−

As already stated above the panel of red cells recommended for routine antibody testing will not reveal the presence of anti-C and/or anti-E mixed with anti-D. These mixtures will give the same pattern as anti-D alone (Table 11.1). If anti-D is discovered in a serum, a further test is therefore necessary, using r′r (Ccddee) cells by saline, albumin and papain techniques, which will detect anti-C, and r″r (ccddEe) by the same techniques, which will detect anti-E (Table 11.2). In the apparent anti-CDE mixture the presence of anti-D must be confirmed with R_0r cells.

The quantities and forms of the antibodies in these mixtures vary considerably. Anti-D is normally present in higher titre than the others. Indeed, anti-C and anti-E are often only found in trace amounts. Sometimes both antibodies occur in the complete form, or one will be complete and the other incomplete. The anti-C and anti-E components are more often of the complete type and are occasionally accompanied by anti-D in the incomplete form only. This is useful, for such sera can be used as pure anti-C or anti-E if the saline technique is employed.

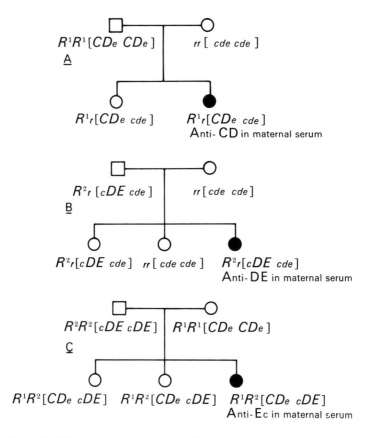

Fig. 11.1 A–C Families showing how mixtures of Rh antibodies may arise.

Examples of families in which these mixtures have occurred are shown in Fig. 11.1A and B. In Fig. 11.1A an Rh negative (*cde/cde*) woman married to an R^1R^1 (*CDe/CDe*) man was found to have anti-C and anti-D antibodies in her serum during her second pregnancy. Both children possessed the antigens C and D which the mother lacked, thus stimulating her to produce both anti-C and anti-D. In Fig. 11.1B where the mother was Rh negative (*cde/cde*) and the father R^2r (*cDE/cde*), the first and third children inherited the paternal D and E antigens, causing the formation of anti-D and anti-E in the mother.

Anti-CDE mixtures can occur in families where all three antigens are found among the children, *e.g.* if the mother is Rh negative (*cde/cde*), the father R^1R^2 (*CDe/cDE*), some of the children R^1r (*CDe/cde*) and others R^2r (*cDE/cde*).

Mixtures of antibodies also arise as a result of transfusions. Indeed, there is more opportunity for a mixture of two or more antibodies to be produced as a result of multiple transfusions than as a result of pregnancy.

Some anti-CD "mixtures" are in reality anti-G, an antibody reacting with part of the D and C antigens. Such "mixtures" are not separable into anti-D and anti-C components (*see also* Chapter 17).

Anti-E + anti-c Mixtures

Another not uncommon mixture of antibodies is anti-E + anti-c. Fig. 11.1C is an example of a family in which this mixture was found.

The identification of the components of mixtures discussed so far has been relatively simple because it has been possible to choose standard red cells specific for each separate component (*e.g.* the case of the anti-CD mixture, r'r (Ccddee) for the anti-C component and R_0r (ccDee) for the anti-D component). This is not always possible for an anti-Ec mixture, for although E-negative c-positive red cells (*e.g.* rr (ccddee)) are readily available, E-positive c-negative red cells are very rare indeed. Fortunately, the anti-E component is often present in higher titre than the anti-c, so that comparison of titration values against R_1r (CcDee), rr (ccddee), R_2r (ccDEe), and R_2R_2 (ccDEE) will clearly reveal the presence of both antibodies. Where a serum appears to contain anti-c and is known to have arisen as the result of stimulation by cells containing E as well as c, then it is essential to test for the possible presence of anti-E with cells of one of the rare E-positive c-negative genotypes, *e.g.* R_1R_z (CCDEe). If necessary, the serum must be sent to a reference laboratory for this purpose.

Anti-C and anti-e Mixtures

Another mixture which has been found on several occasions is that of anti-C + anti-e. The anti-e in such a mixture can be readily identified by the use of rr ccddee and R_2R_2 (ccDEE) without interference from the anti-C. The presence of anti-C can be revealed by a comparison of titration values against R_1r (CcDee), R_1R_1 (CCDee), R_2r (ccDEe), and rr (ccddee) red cells if the titre of anti-C is greater than that of anti-e. Otherwise, the only alternative is the testing with red cells of the very rare genotype R^2R^z (*cDE/CDE*) which is C-positive but e-negative.

The identification of the components in anti-E + anti-c, anti-C + anti-e mixtures may sometimes be facilitated by absorption and elution experiments. Absorption of both these mixtures with ccddee cells may leave behind identifiable anti-E or anti-C components. Anti-c can be recovered from the ccddee cells if desired (*see* technique 26.3) and identified.

Sometimes the individual antibodies may be tested for separately by the use of two different antibody detection techniques, *e.g.* anti-E or anti-C by saline and anti-c and anti-e by anti-globulin methods.

If the above treatment is unsuccessful it will be necessary to locate cells of the rare genotypes mentioned above.

Antibodies to Compound Antigens

Rh antibodies can also be made to compound antigens, *e.g.* cE, and they will only react with cells that have cE on the same chromosome, *i.e.* in the cis position. In normal tests such antibodies can be mistaken for mixtures of antibodies. They are discussed further in Chapter 17.

TECHNIQUES

There are no new techniques mentioned in this chapter, but there are a few points which should be mentioned about the adaptation of already described methods.

Saline, Albumin or Anti-human Globulin and Enzyme Techniques in Parallel

The test serum required for all three techniques should be run out in one operation. This reduces handling to a minimum and saves many rinses of the pipette. The standard cells can be run out in rows after checking that each tube contains serum.

The reading of a rack full of saline or albumin antibody tests takes some time, since the contents of every tube have to be examined microscopically. It is therefore inadvisable to remove from the incubator more than one rack at a time.

Titration of Mixtures

The technique for titration of mixtures of antibodies is the same as those described in Chapter 8 for the titration of complete and incomplete anti-D. The standard cells used, however, must be selected with the purpose of estimating the strength of each antibody in the mixture independently. Thus for an anti-CD mixture r'r (Ccddee) cells must be used to estimate the anti-C content, and R_0r (ccDee) or R_2r (ccDEe) cells the content of anti-D.

Chapter 12. Selection and Preparation of Rh Typing Sera

There are two main essentials for a satisfactory Rh typing serum:
 (1) It must be of sufficient strength to detect the corresponding antigen even when this is weak.
 (2) It must be specific for its corresponding antigen.

SELECTION

A serum is earmarked as useful for typing purposes because its titration value reaches or exceeds a required minimum and because it is sufficiently avid. Either saline agglutinins or incomplete antibodies or a mixture of both can be used equally well.

The various Rh antisera each present individual problems when being selected for typing purposes; they are, therefore, considered separately from this point of view although subsequently they are dealt with together.

Anti-D

Anti-D is the most frequently encountered of the Rh antibodies but the original plentiful supply of this antibody has been reduced by about two-thirds owing to the present prophylactic treatment for haemolytic disease of the newborn which consists of giving mothers at risk one or more doses of Rh immunoglobulin after the birth of an Rh positive infant. The main source of supply is therefore changing from being a mother at ten days post-partum to being re-stimulated women beyond child bearing age and males often stimulated *de novo*. The practice of plasmaphoresis (*see* below and Chapter 30) increases the quantity of antibody that may be safely collected from such donors.

To determine suitability for use as a typing reagent, samples of sera should first be titrated according to the methods given in Chapter 8 (technique Nos. 8.9 and 8.10). No anti-D with a titre of less than 64 with R_1r red cells should be selected. In addition there should be macroscopic readings at least to a dilution of 1 in 8. These criteria are the minimum required for typing by tube methods. For other techniques, Slide, Chown, etc., the titrations must be carried out by the particular technique for which it is proposed to use the serum and give satisfactory results at a dilution of at least 1:16.

The antibody is suitable whether in the complete or incomplete form or a mixture of both, except for those techniques for which a particular type of serum has been specified. In practice it will be found that potent incomplete anti-D sera are fairly easily obtainable, titres of 512 or over being by no means uncommon. Such a serum of high titre can be used very economically since it will withstand considerable dilution. It is recommended that AB serum (for preparation of suitable AB serum *see* Appendix II) should be used as the diluting fluid.

The importance of checking the specificity of the selected anti-D cannot be over-emphasised. It has already been seen that anti-D is often mixed with anti-C or anti-E or even with both. If serum containing these antibodies is inadvertently used as an anti-D typing serum patients who are C positive or E positive but D negative will be incorrectly typed as D positive. This can have dangerous consequences.

To check the purity of the anti-D, saline and albumin tests against *r'r* (*Cde/cde*) and *r″r* (*cdE/cde*) are made with at least five examples of each kind of red cell. This will ensure that any anti-C or anti-E which would give positive reactions with such D negative cells will not go undetected. If the serum is to be used for any but the standard techniques, in particular for the very sensitive Löw's papain technique, it must be examined for anti-C and anti-E by the appropriate method.

Anti-CD and Anti-DE Mixtures

The suitability of mixtures for Rh typing purposes depends on the strength of each antibody in the mixture reaching a required minimum standard. While it is not difficult to find sera in which the anti-D reaches the minimum requirements laid down above, it is not so easy to find anti-C or anti-E antibodies that do so. The standard, therefore, unavoidably, has to be lowered by one or two dilutions for the anti-C or anti-E component. Nevertheless if titres of sixteen are accepted care must be taken that the serum chosen is avid and gives macroscopic readings to at least a dilution of 1 in 4. It is obvious that the foregoing remarks with regard to choice of serum for a particular method apply also to anti-CD and anti-DE mixtures.

Anti-C

The pure anti-C which is produced by an Rh positive individual, e.g of genotype *R²r*, providing the titre is at least sixteen against r'r cells with two or more macroscopic readings, is the most satisfactory source of this reagent. Unfortunately anti-C is only rarely so produced and even when it is the titre is often inadequate. Anti-C sera are, therefore, usually prepared from specially selected anti-CD mixtures. Suitable mixtures are either those in which the anti-C titre greatly exceeds the anti-D or those in which the anti-C antibodies are complete and the anti-D mainly incomplete. In either case it is usually possible to choose a dilution of the serum at which it will behave as pure anti-C. The alternative course of preparing pure anti-C by removing the anti-D with D positive C negative red cells is seldom successful (*see* below). Such an absorbed serum, however, gives more consistent and reliable results since absorption, in contrast to dilution, actually removes the anti-D component from the serum.

It should be noted that anti-C/anti-e mixtures are not usually satisfactory for the preparation of anti-C but they are valuable for the e typing of C negative individuals.

Anti-C sera prepared by dilution or absorption may still contain anti-C^w and/or anti-C^we components but their presence does not make the anti-C unsatisfactory for typing purposes. Sera being used as anti-C should be tested with R_1^wr (C^wcDee) cells so that the strength of any anti-C^w component can be determined. It must be appreciated that C^wc cells will be typed as Cc if the anti-C typing serum contains strongly reacting anti-C^w. In this case only a specific anti-C^w will disclose C^wc red cells.

Anti-E

As anti-E is fairly readily available it is often possible to choose sera with minimum titration values of 64 with R_2r red cells. Even if this standard cannot be maintained it should at least reach that required for anti-C, namely a titration value of 16 with macroscopic readings at least as far as the 1 in 4 dilution.

The best source of anti-E is the serum of an R_1r individual where it occurs unmixed with other Rh antibodies. The other source of anti-E is from an individual of genotype R^1R^1, in which case it is usually mixed with anti-c. Such a mixture has been discussed in the previous chapter. Since the anti-E is usually considerably more potent than the anti-c the latter is often diluted out, or removed from the serum by absorption with Rh negative red cells. The absorption, however, will almost certainly reduce the titre of the anti-E as well as removing the anti-c because some of the antibody is likely to be anti-cE so that only those sera having titres which will allow for a reduction are suitable for this treatment.

Anti-c

Anti-c to be suitable for typing purposes must have a minimum titration value of 16 with R_1r red cells with macroscopic readings at least as far as a dilution of 1 in 4.

As mentioned above (*see also* Fig. 11.1C) anti-c may occur in the same serum as anti-E (see above), but usually such a serum is used as an anti-E rather than anti-c since the anti-E is almost always present in far greater titre.

Anti-e

Owing to the comparative rarity of this antibody, almost all examples of it, unless very weak, are used for typing purposes, even if this necessitates the use of an enzyme technique.

As mentioned above, when an anti-C/anti-e mixture is found it is usually used as anti-e for typing red cells which are C negative.

PREPARATION

Collection and Separation of Serum

A donor found to have suitable antibodies for the preparation of an Rh typing serum will donate from 100 to 480 ml. of blood according to his or her clinical condition. The blood is taken into a dry bottle and allowed to clot. Although clot retraction is slower in the cold the antibody may deteriorate slightly if the blood is allowed to clot at 37°C; it is preferable, therefore, to leave the bottle at 4°C for 24 hours by which time the serum will be well separated. After this as much serum as possible is collected, cell free, taking aseptic precautions. A further yield can almost certainly be obtained by centrifuging the clot. The separated serum is stored in bulk at −20°C until it is processed.

Sometimes donors are bled by the process of plasmapheresis which consists of withdrawing blood from a donor, retaining the plasma containing the wanted antibody and returning the red cells. In this way a larger volume of plasma can be obtained either at one donation or the usual amount of blood (500 ml) may be withdrawn at weekly intervals. Both methods enable a larger amount of a valuable antibody to be obtained. The plasma is recalcified [technique No. 3.6] and subsequently processed as for serum.

Pooling of Sera

With anti-D, anti-CD and anti-DE sera it is often an advantage to make a pool of sera from four or five donors. A serum which is just below the minimum standards can be included in a pool with stronger sera, and thus increase the total amount of reliable serum available. Moreover such pools are more likely to detect the D^u antigen than a serum from a single donor. Another advantage of a pool is that one standard serum can be used for several weeks or even months thus giving results which are strictly comparable.

It is not recommended, however, that the rarer sera should be pooled. A laboratory will only have a limited number of anti-C, anti-E, anti-c, etc., sera available and more reliable results are obtained by using them in parallel rather than mixed in a pool.

When it is decided to make a pool it should be done before the absorption and sterilisation stage. If the sera are of differing ABO groups this is an advantage as the pool will then be easier to absorb for anti-A and anti-B. If possible at least one very good serum (titre 512 or over) should be included in each pool. The pooled serum should be tested to see that it fulfils the criteria; if the constituents have been well chosen it will usually have a titre considerably above the minimum in spite of the inclusion of one weaker serum. On the other hand the final titre is occasionally disappointingly low and the pool will need the addition of a further very potent serum.

Pooled serum is processed as for single sera except that for the absorption of anti-A and anti-B agglutinins the quantity of red cells can be reduced by half if the pool is made from sera of differing ABO blood groups as the A and B substances in the sera will neutralise some of the anti-A and anti-B agglutinins.

Removal of Unwanted Antibodies

Unwanted antibodies fall into three classes; (a) other Rh antibodies; (b) anti-A and anti-B agglutinins; (c) antibodies of other blood group systems.

a) *Removal of other Rh antibodies.*

It has already been seen that Rh antibodies often occur as mixtures so that a serum chosen for typing purposes may have a component which it is desirable to remove.

A trace of unwanted antibody can be diluted out if by so doing the titre of the required antibody is not reduced below the minimum. A satisfactory dilution is one which goes well beyond the range of activity of the antibody which is being diluted out. For example, if the titre of an unwanted anti-C in an anti-CD mixture is two, then the serum must be diluted at least to 1 in 10 before it can be used with safety as pure anti-D; this means that the initial anti-D titre would have to be at least 2,000. The best diluting fluid to use is specially prepared AB serum (for preparation *see* Appendix II).

The alternative method of ridding the serum of unwanted Rh antibodies is that of absorption. The serum is mixed with cells which will specifically combine with the unwanted antibodies. After a suitable time interval the serum-cell mixture is centrifuged and the supernatant serum collected while the cells are discarded and with them the unwanted antibodies. This is the method of choice for the removal of anti-A and anti-B agglutinins (*see* below) but a complication often arises if it is used for the removal of one Rh antibody from another which it is desired to retain in the serum. It would seem that in many instances when antibodies of different specificites yet of the same blood group system co-exist in a serum, some of the antibody molecules have double specificity. For example, if R_2R_2 or R_2r cells are used to remove anti-D from an anti-CD mixture in an attempt to make the serum a pure anti-C some of the anti-C also will be removed from the serum. This is mainly due to the presence of anti-G, an antibody which reacts with C and D and which is removed by absorption with D positive C negative cells (*see also* Chapter 17). Absorption is not, therefore, advisable unless the titre of the required antibody is sufficiently great to withstand a certain reduction without rendering it unfit for use. The titre of the component that is to remain in the serum should well exceed the titre of the antibody that is to be removed. Before the absorption of the main bulk of serum is undertaken pilot tests, using small quantities of cells and serum, should be carried out. These will show whether it is possible to prepare a pure reagent from the selected mixture and also the optimum proportion of cells to serum for the bulk absorption.

It is sometimes useful to absorb with papain-treated red cells by technique No. 12.2 to remove traces of unwanted antibody. Here again pilot absorptions will give an indication as to whether it is possible to prepare a pure reagent.

When the titres of the separate antibodies making up a given mixture approximate each other it is almost always impossible to prepare a pure reagent from the serum.

b) *Removal of agglutinins belonging to the ABO blood group system.*

In any serum selected as a suitable typing reagent there are almost always unwanted ABO agglutinins present. It is a very worth while procedure to remove these from the serum which otherwise can only be used for the typing of cells of compatible ABO group.

Anti-A (including anti-A_1) and anti-B agglutinins are removed by absorption with red cells of the appropriate group. The most useful red cells to use are those of group A_1B. These will remove anti-A, anti-A_1 and anti-B agglutinins if present. If A_2B cells are used, the anti-A_1 fraction will remain in the serum. It is, of course, possible to use group B cells to absorb anti-B from a group A serum or group A_1 cells to absorb anti-A from a group B serum. However, if these are used they require an extra wash as they contain anti-A or anti-B agglutinins which it is obviously undesirable to add to the serum being absorbed.

The Rh sub-type of the cells chosen will of course depend upon the specificity of the anti-serum being prepared. Anti-D, anti-CD, and anti-DE mixtures will be absorbed by A_1B rr (ccddee) cells; these are often the cells of choice for the absorption of anti-C and anti-E sera also, unless considerations dealt with in section (a) indicate the use of cells of a different Rh sub-type. Absorption of anti-c requires cells of A_1B R_1R_1 (CCDee) and anti-e of A_1B R_2R_2 (ccDEE).

The red cells used for absorption can have been stored up to fourteen days provided they have been preserved in the standard acid-citrate-dextrose anti-coagulant solution (ACD see Appendix I). They must be washed free of their own plasma, for this would on mixture with the serum to be absorbed, form a plasma clot which could make the subsequent handling of the mixture extremely difficult.

The quantity of red cells required for the removal of anti-A and anti-B agglutinins will naturally vary according to the potency of these agglutinins. It is advisable to aim at excess. It will usually be found that a volume of packed washed cells equal to the volume of serum to be absorbed is satisfactory. If the agglutinins are immune and of exceptionally high titre a larger quantitiy of cells may be needed. If the serum is freshly bled it is advisable to inactivate it by heating at 56°C for 30 minutes to prevent haemolysis of the absorbing red cells by any anti-A or anti-B haemolysins which may be present. The serum-cell mixture is left at 4°C for at least 2 hours or preferably overnight.

In order to confirm that the anti-A and anti-B agglutinins have been removed from the serum, tests should be made against red cells from a number of group A and/or group B individuals. Red cells from different individuals vary in their reactivity to traces of antibody remaining in a serum and it is not uncommon to find that small quantities of antibody are detected by some cells but not by others. If even small quantities of anti-A or anti-B agglutinins remain in the serum after absorption it is advisable to reabsorb unless it is proposed to use the serum considerably diluted. If, for any reason, absorption of the serum with red cells is impracticable, the unwanted agglutinins can be "neutralised" by the addition of A or B group specific substances either in saliva or purified. This method of suppressing their activity is not recommended since the agglutinins are not actually removed from the serum. Neutralised sera should not be stored.

The use of enzyme techniques is so widespread that it is advisable that sera should have a final absorption with one-quarter volume of papain-treated red cells to remove the last traces of anti-A and anti-B (technique No. 12.2).

c) *Removal of antibodies of other blood group systems.*

Antibodies belonging to other blood group systems may occur in a serum chosen for Rh typing. The range and characteristics of these are described in Chapter 13. If present it is advisable to remove them with appropriate red cells containing their corresponding antigen. This can usually be combined with the absorption of anti-A and anti-B agglutinins, *e.g* if the serum also contains an unwanted anti-P_1 agglutinin A_1B cells of suitable Rh genotype which are also P_1 positive can be selected.

Of course the other antibody (*e.g.* anti-S) may be more valuable as a typing reagent than the anti-D in which case the latter is removed using D positive red cells. The separation of two or more antibodies by absorption followed by elution is attractive in theory but is seldom satisfactory and only attempted when the antibodies are rare.

The use of fortified antisera

Some commercial antisera of the incomplete type are "fortified" by the addition of albumin or other macromolecular substances so that the incomplete antibodies behave as agglutinins thus allowing the antisera to be used with saline suspended red cells. Such sera are satisfactory provided it is remembered that they are in reality incomplete antibodies in a high protein medium and are therefore likely to give false positives if used to type red cells already sensitised by antibodies *in vivo, e.g.* the red cells of infants with haemolytic disease or of patients with anti-immune haemolytic anaemia. However the AB serum/albumin control which is normally negative will be positive with these sensitised red cells so testing must then be repeated using an anti-serum reacting with cells in saline. Fortified antisera should be supplied with directions for the use of such a control and a warning of the unsuitability of the fortified reagent for any red cell which is positive in the ahg test. Ideally the medium in which the antibody is supplied shall be available for use in addition to the AB/albumin control. In cases of suspected haemolytic disease due to any allo-antibody, including anti-A or anti-B, fortified antisera should not be used regardless of whether the infant's cells appear to be negative or positive with anti-globulin.

Standardisation

Having selected and absorbed a serum, it must be standardised. At this stage the two main essentials for a satisfactory anti-serum mentioned at the outset, namely potency and specificity, should more than ever be borne in mind.

The serum must first be re-titrated although normally the titration value will not have altered appreciably during the absorption process. If the titre is well above the minimum with red cells containing a single dose of the corresponding antigen, the serum can be tried out at several different dilutions.

The serum, both undiluted and suitably diluted if strong enough, must then be tested against at least thirty random red cell samples in parallel with a known typing serum of the same specificity. In addition it should be tested against a number of specially selected samples of appropriate ABO groups and known Rh genotype to find out whether or not all unwanted antibodies have been successfully removed. In fact the final tests must be so designed to ensure that the typing serum will detect the presence of the corresponding antigen, however weak, and that it will be specific for it.

Panels of cells containing rare antigens Wr^a, By^a, Vw, etc. should be available for the final checking of all standard sera as although the antigens are rare the corresponding antibodies are more common.

Sterilisation and storage

It is strongly recommended that Rh typing sera should be stored in a sterile condition. This is particularly important if such sera are ever distributed by post.

The titres of Rh antibodies are not often reduced by Seitz filtration of the serum, therefore this method of sterilisation can be adopted. It should be remembered that at least 5 ml of serum will be lost in the Seitz filtration process. For very small quantities (up to 4 ml) the Hemmings filter can be used. This is a small filter which uses a Ford sterimat of 1.375 sq. cm in area, i.e. of $^{11}/_{16}''$ diameter—the loss of serum will not be more than 0.4 ml. Alternatively it is suggested that small amounts of a rare serum are apportioned out in such small quantities that sterility will not be so important. The method of sterilisation by heating at 56°C for 30 minutes on three successive days while the serum stands at room temperature between the applications of heat is definitely detrimental to Rh antibodies. A small knife-point of sodium azide can be added after the individual containers have been opened and taken into use. Rh typing sera should be stored at approximately –20°C. At higher temperatures than this, although the serum is completely frozen, the potency of the antibody may decrease quite rapidly. If kept under satisfactory conditions the sera will usually remain efficient for several years. However, some sera do not maintain their properties as well as others, so that if sera are kept for a long time they should be restandardised at regular intervals.

TECHNIQUES
Technique No. 12.1. Absorption of ABO agglutinins from an Rh typing serum

Rh negative cells are used for anti-D, for other antibodies the appropriate cells have to be selected e.g. A$_1$B R$_1$R$_1$ for anti-c.

If the serum has been frozen it is thawed out gradually at room temperature or 37°C but not more rapidly than this. It is then inactivated by heating at 56°C for 30 minutes. While the serum is being thawed and inactivated, the red cells for the absorption can be washed, twice if they are of group AB or three times if of groups A or B. The proportional volume of saline to cells for washing should be at least 4 to 1. It is convenient to use an MSE Mistral centrifuge specially designed for MRC transfusion bottles and plastic packs or the washing can be carried out in universal containers or large test-tubes. Sterile precautions are not essential. The red cells used should be well sedimented so that most of the supernatant plasma can be sucked off before the first aliquot of saline is added. If the plasma is not removed, one extra washing of the cells must be included.

The serum to be absorbed and an equal volume of well packed, washed cells are mixed and left at 4°C for 2 hours or preferably overnight.

The serum-cell mixture is centifuged and the supernatant absorbed serum collected. This is then standardised and if found satisfactory, Seitz-filtered. If, however, more than trace amounts of ABO agglutinins remain after absorption, the serum must be re-absorbed. For a re-absorption, an amount of red cells equal to a quarter of the volume of serum to be absorbed should be sufficient. Alternatively an absorption using a quarter volume of papain treated cells may be more efficient. The sera should be bottled in quantities which are related to the normal turnover. Large laboratories will find 10 ml amounts of anti-D sera convenient. On the other hand rare sera which are used slowly should be stored in quantities not greater than 0.25 ml to avoid continual alternate freezing and thawing which is detrimental to the serum.

Technique No. 12.2 The use of papain-treated red cells for absorption of sera

Some forms of antibody, including even anti-A and anti-B require enzyme treatment of the cells for absorption before they can be taken up by the red cells.

A_1B Rh negative cells are papain-treated either by mixing two parts of Löw's papain solution or alternatively two parts of a 1 per cent solution of papain (without activator) to one part of packed washed red cells and the mixture incubated for 15″ at 37°C. The red cells are then washed twice in a large volume of saline and packed. The serum to be absorbed is mixed with one-quarter of its volume of papain-treated cells and incubated for 15″ at 37°C, spun and separated. The process is repeated until there is no agglutination of the papain-treated cells. The separated serum is then tested for complete absorption with a panel of A and B Rh negative cells.

Technique No. 12.3. Standardisation of an Rh typing serum

Tests to Show that the Serum is free from ABO Agglutinins.

The serum is tested by saline tube technique against ten red cell samples of each appropriate ABO group and Rh type at 4°C, RT and 37°C. In addition the serum is tested against the same red cell samples by albumin technique and also by any method by which it is proposed to use the serum. If any appreciable reaction is obtained the residual antibody should be titrated; according to the titre it is decided whether to re-absorb or rely upon diluting out the antibody.

Tests to Show that the Serum is Free from Other Contaminants.

The serum is tested by saline, albumin and any other appropriate techniques at room temperature and 37°C against at least five red cell samples which are chosen because they contain the antigen corresponding to the contaminating antibody. It is particularly important that if possible some of them should contain the appropriate antigen in "double dose". Any residual contaminant is titrated and if present in appreciable amount removed by reabsorption.

Selection of Dilution for Use.

The following tests will be done by the method by which it is proposed to use the serum, usually saline or albumin but occasionally others, *e.g.* indirect anti-human globulin for a serum which is to be used to detect D^u.

Table 12.1 Red cell samples required for the standardisation of the various Rh anti- sera

Anti-serum	Red cell samples needed					
	Random	r'r	r"r	R_2r	Arr	Brr
Anti-D	30	5	5		10	10
Anti-CD	30	8	5	10	10	10
Anti-DE	30	5	8		10	10
Anti-C	30	8	5	10	10	10
Anti-E	30	5	8	10	10	10
					AR_1R_1	BR_1R_1
Anti-c	30				10	10
Anti-e	This presents a particular problem, but as many R_2R_2 and R_2r samples as possible must be included.					

Each component of the serum is investigated separately. The serum is tested at one or more dilutions, each of which must fulfil the criteria for the antibody or antibodies concerned. Table 12.1 shows the number and type of red cell samples with which each typing serum should be tested. The neat serum, or a dilution, is regarded as being satisfactory for use when all the positive reactions are V or ++ and there is no reaction whatever in the negative controls.

BIBLIOGRAPHY FOR Rh SECTION*

Levine, P., & Stetson, R.E. (1939) An unusual case of intragroup agglutination. *J. Amer. med. Ass.*, **113,** 126.

Wiener, A.S., & Peters, H.R. (1940) Hemolytic reactions following transfusions of blood of the homologous group, with three cases in which the same agglutinogen was responsible. *Ann. int. Med.*, 13, 2306.

Landsteiner, K., & Wiener, A.S. (1940) An agglutinable factor in human blood recognised by immune sera for Rhesus blood. *Proc. Soc. exp. Biol. N.Y.*, **43,** 223.

Landsteiner, K. & Wiener, A.S. (1941) Studies on an agglutinogen (Rh) in human blood reacting with anti-rhesus sera and with human iso-antibodies. *J. exp. Med.*, **74,** 309.

Levine, P., Katzin, E.M. & Burnham, L. (1941) Iso-immunisation in pregnancy, its possible bearing on the etiology of erythroblastosis fetalis. *J. Amer. med. Ass.*, **116,** 825.

Levine, P., Vogel, P., Katzin, E.M. & Burnham, L. (1941) Pathogenesis of erythroblastosis fetalis: statistical evidence. *Science,* **94,** 371.

Levine, P., Burnham, L., Katzin, E.M. & Vogel, P. (1941) The role of iso-immunisation in the pathogenesis of erythroblastosis fetalis. *Amer. J. Obstet. Gynec.*, **42,** 925.

Race, R.R. & Taylor, G.L. (1943) A serum that discloses the genotype of some Rh positive people. *Nature (Lond.),* **152,** 300.

Race, R.R., Taylor, G.L., Boorman, Kathleen E., & Dodd, Barbara E. (1943) Recognition of Rh genotypes in man. *Nature (Lond.),* **152, 563.**

Race, R.R. (1944) An 'incomplete' antibody in human serum.' *Nature (Lond.),* **153,** 771.

Race, R.R., Taylor, G.L., Cappell, D.F. & McFarlane, Marjory N. (1944) Recognition of a further common Rh genotype in man. *Nature (Lond.),* **153,** 52.

Coombs, R.R.A., Mourant, A.E., & Race, R.R. (1945) A new test for the detection of weak and 'incomplete' Rh agglutinins. *Brit. J. exp. Path.*, **26,** 255.

Mourant, A.E. (1945) A new rhesus antibody. *Nature (Lond.),* **155,** 542.

Wiener, A.S. (1945) Conglutination test for Rh sensitization. *J. Lab. clin. Med.*, **30,** 662.

Hill, J.M., Haberman, S. & Jones, Frances (1946) Hemolytic Rh immune globulins: evidence for a possible third order of antibodies incapable of agglutination or blocking. *Blood, Special Issue,* No. 2, 80.

Pickles, Margaret M. (1946) Effects of cholera filtrate on red cells as demonstrated by incomplete Rh antibodies. *Nature (Lond.),* **158,** 880.

Stratton, F. (1946) A new Rh allelomorph. *Nature (Lond.),* **158,** 25.

Morton, J.A., and Pickles, M.M. (1947) Use of trypsin in the detection of incomplete anti-Rh antibodies. *Nature,* **159,** 779.

Race, R.R., Sanger, Ruth, and Lawler, Sylvia D. (1948) Allelomorphs of the Rh gene C. *Heredity,* 2, 237.

Löw, B. (1955) A practical method using papain and incomplete Rh antibodies in routine Rh blood grouping *Vox Sang.*, **5,** 94.

Levine, P., Celano, M.J., Wallace, J. & Sanger, R. (1963) A human D-like antibody. *Nature (Lond.),* **198.**

*These are mostly papers of historical interest. They are arranged in date order. See also references Chapters 17 and 26.

Section 4. Other Systems and red cell agglutination phenomena

*"And thick and fast they came at last,
And more, and more, and more—"*

Lewis Carroll, THROUGH THE LOOKING GLASS

Chapter 13. General Introduction to Other Blood Group Systems

We now approach the other major blood group systems. These are of great interest and importance but their practical aspects are by no means as far reaching as those of the ABO and Rh groups. This does not mean that they are without clinical significance, indeed any antibody active at 37°C has to be taken into consideration when selecting blood for transfusion and if it is an IgG antibody it may cause haemolytic disease of the foetus. Fortunately the occurrence of these antibodies is comparatively rare and therefore routine antibody detection tests are not undertaken for each system individually. The identification of any atypical antibody that may be detected during routine ABO and Rh testing, and the full investigation of any serum suspected to contain atypical antibodies is described in Chapter 22.

INTRODUCTION

First we discuss what constitutes a blood group system and then describe the common antigens and antibodies of the MNSs, Kell, Duffy, Kidd, Lutheran, Lewis, P and I systems. A more detailed study of these together with the sex-linked blood group system Xg will be found in Part II as well as a consideration of the less important systems *e.g.* Diego, Yt, etc.

The discovery of a blood group system is made through the finding of an antibody either accidentally or through the deliberate immunisation of animals, carried out in the hope that hitherto unknown antibodies will be produced as a result. The MN system is, like Rh, an example of one which was disclosed by animal antibodies, although other antigens connected with the system were revealed later by antibodies of human origin.

Occasionally the discovery of a new system follows on the heels of the discovery of a new antibody detection technique. For example, the Kell groups were discovered within a few weeks of the development of the anti-human globulin technique. Not every new antibody heralds a new system. Some are found to detect antigens belonging to systems already described. Nor is it always at first easy to see the connexion between new antibodies and their antigens and old systems. Very often relationships only fall into place after thousands of tests have been performed or after inspection and correlation of the results of several teams of workers. Family studies also provide valuable evidence as to whether or not a "new" antigen belongs to one of the known blood group systems. These are undertaken both to see whether a newly-found antigen is travelling with a known antigen of one of the established systems (in which case the genes are said to segregate together) and also to determine whether the antigen detected could be the product of a gene allelomorphic to one already known.

The MN system, as we shall see was extended in both ways, a gene *S* was found to segregate with the *M* or *N* gene, *MS* being more common than *NS*; later an antiserum was found which reacted with s, a product of a gene allelomorphic to *S*.

New antigens are thus divided into three categories, those that belong to previously discovered systems; those that can be shown to be segregating independently of all previous known systems and therefore comprise new systems; and a large category where their precise position has not been determined.

Family studies are obviously difficult where the antigen is either very frequent or very rare and it is no wonder that there are many blood group antigens which are not yet accorded system status as it has not been possible to show their complete independence of all known systems.

In the P system, the antigen Luke falls into a new category in that it is a genetically independent part of the system—this is discussed in more detail in Chapter 18.

H, in the ABO system and LW in the Rh system are other examples of antigens that are genetically independent; that is, their production is controlled from a locus other than that controlling the main allelic antigens (*see also* Part II). Such genes are included in a particular system because, in spite of being inherited independently, they have some influence at the phenotypic level *e.g.* H is the necessary precursor for the formation of A and B substances.

The frequencies of the blood group antigens vary from being so infrequent that they seem to be confined to the members of one family (private antigens) to being so common that they seem to be "non specific" and require long, patient testing before a pattern of reaction for them can be worked out. Of the first category the antigen Di^a is an example, being found in four members of one family while 2600 random bloods were negative and of the second anti-k of the Kell system where in the original tests of 2500 blood specimens only five were negative with the new antibody.

Racial variations in antigen frequency very often occur; these may be striking and result in interesting findings. A comparison between the bloods of negroid and white races yields many instances of differences in antigenic frequencies, *e.g.* in the Duffy system Fy(a–b–) is almost unknown in whites but common in negroes. These racial distinctions occasionally account for the finding of apparent "private" antigens when mixed marriages occur.

The Di^a antigen mentioned above is a case in point. Admixture of white with native Indian blood accounted for the appearance in the family of what seemed to be a rare antigen. Subsequent studies of North and South American Indians, Chinese and Japanese bloods showed an incidence of Di^a ranging from 3 to 45 per cent. There are other examples of this.

Mixed marriages and the transfusion of blood from members of one race to another is a rich field for the study of new antigens and antibodies.

The progress of all blood group systems, following their discovery, seems to be through a period of clarity into the fog of increased complications as new alleles are discovered and afterwards, emergence, still in many cases partial, into a new understanding of the ramifications of the system in question. And how is all this related to routine work? As stated earlier, the antibodies of the blood groups to be described below have limited practical importance owing either to their infrequent occurrence, their low potency, or low temperature of reaction.

As expected, it is the warm antibodies that cause haemolytic disease or transfusion reactions. However, potent cold antibodies may react at 37°C either as agglutinins or as incomplete antibodies requiring complement, e.g. anti-P, anti-Le^a, or even if reactive below 37°C, may be stimulated to become active at 37°C by the corresponding antigen. This means that for transfusion purposes it is better not to use blood containing antigens corresponding to antibodies strongly reactive at room temperature.

The practical importance of a blood group system is not only related to the efficiency of its antigens in the production of warm antibodies, but also upon their opportunity for stimulating antibody formation; this is related to their frequency. For example, the k antigen is so common that only 1 in 500 people lack it, so inevitably, however good an antigen k may be, the antibody will always be comparatively rare.

At the other end of the scale are very rare antigens, e.g. Mg, V^w, Wr^a, etc., for which the antibodies are comparatively common. These antibodies are usually of the "cold" type and occur in the sera of people who apparently have not been stimulated to produce them by the corresponding antigen. A serum, which is found to agglutinate only one red cell sample when tested with many, thus merits special investigation. The possibility of standard sera containing such antibodies and therefore giving a false positive with blood containing the rare antigen is an extra reason why two sera of the same specificity should be used for all testing. Wherever possible, of course, the laboratory preparing the serum will have checked it against cells containing the known rare antigens but they may not possess a "full set" and new rare antigens with common antibodies will probably continue to be found for many years to come.

Most blood group antigens show dosage so that wherever possible the double dose cell (e.g. KK, Fy^a Fy^a) should be used for antibody detection techniques. The distinction between the homo- and heterozygote is not usually sufficiently clear cut however for genotyping to be done on dosage alone.

We now turn to the individual blood group systems of most importance. In each section we deal with the most common phenotypes, discuss the clinical and theoretical importance and the techniques most commonly used for their determination.

THE MNSs SYSTEM

The MN groups were discovered by Landsteiner and Levine (1927a and b, 1928) when experimenting with rabbit sera after the animals had received injections of human red cells. Two antibodies, called anti-M and anti-N, were identified and these were found to divide the human population into three groups:

(1) Persons whose red cells were agglutinated only by anti-M—group M.
(2) Persons whose red cells were agglutinated only by anti-N—group N.
(3) Persons whose red cells were agglutinated by both anti-M and anti-N— group MN.

No persons were found whose cells did not agglutinate with either of the two anti-sera.

The frequency of the three groups in the English population has been found to be:

<blockquote>
Group M   About 28 per cent
Group N   About 22 per cent
Group MN   About 50 per cent
</blockquote>

The two antigens have been shown to be derived from a single pair of genes which are allelomorphic and co-dominant. Chromosomes, therefore, can only be of two kinds M or N with three ways of pairing:

(a) M can pair with M giving rise to genotype *MM*—phenotype or group M.
(b) N can pair with N giving rise to genotype *NN*—phenotype or group N.
(c) M can pair with N giving rise to genotype *MN*—phenotype or group MN.

Thus it can be seen that given suitable anti-M and anti-N anti-sera three phenotypes can be differentiated.

The possible matings and the children that may arise from them are shown in Table 13.1. The last column in the table sets out the MN groupings that cannot arise from each given mating.

The clinical significance of MN groups is slight. One or two cases of

Table 13.1 Matings within the MN system

MN group of parents	Possible MN groups of children			Impossible MN groups of children	
M × M	M			N	MN
M × N		MN	M	N	
M × MN	M		MN	N	
N × N		N		M	MN
N × MN		N	MN	M	
MN × MN	M	N	MN		

E

transfusion reaction and haemolytic disease of the newborn incriminating anti-M have been reported.

The system is helpful in cases of disputed paternity since the genotypes are easily determined and for the most part unequivocal. In addition the MN groups are often used when it is desired to trace the survival *in vivo* of transfused red cells. The antigens are so weakly antigenic in Man that it is perfectly safe, for example, to transfuse type N blood to type M patient.

The production of good anti-sera for MN typing purposes is by no means easy. Anti-M and anti-N antibodies are of comparatively rare occurrence in human sera. They are neither regularly present in individuals lacking the antigen as in the ABO system nor are they fairly readily produced in response to stimulation by the appropriate antigen as in the Rh system. When they are found anti-N are almost invariably rather weak naturally occurring cold antibodies; anti-M antibodies tend to be stronger and can often be used for MN typing by technique No. 13.1.

Anti-sera for MN typing are most satisfactorily made in rabbits in similar fashion to those of the original experiments which disclosed the existence of the system.

The main problem with regard to the production of good anti-sera is that of satisfactory absorption. The production of a potent specific anti-serum from the raw material is by no means easy and not comparable with the simple process of absorption which is adequate for most Rh sera. The serum of any rabbit normally contains various agglutinins for human red cells, in particular one which reacts preferentially with human group A red cells; these agglutinins are collectively known as "anti-Man". When human red cells of type M or type N are injected for the purpose of producing anti-M or anti-N agglutinins, the "anti-Man" antibodies rise in titre as might be expected. Moreover, unless group O red cells are used immune anti-A and/or anti-B agglutinins may be produced in the rabbit, and these also must be removed. The amount of red cells required for absorption is very critical—too few red cells leave a serum which is not specific and gives false positive reactions—too many red cells cause a "non-specific" absorption of the anti-M or anti-N agglutinins which may make the serum too weak for typing purposes. In this respect anti-N agglutinins are more readily non-specifically absorbed by type M cells than are anti-M agglutinins by type N cells (*see* below).

The seeds of the plant *Vicia graminea* on extraction with saline in a similar manner to technique No. 4.4 yield a potent anti-N reagent although this may require some adjustment of dilution to give a specific reaction. This reagent is suitable for use by either technique Nos. 13.1 or 13.2.

For the accurate MN typing of red cells at least two examples of both anti-M and anti-N sera should be used. An extract of *Vicia graminea* can be substituted for one of the anti-N sera. The anti-sera usually show quite marked dosage effect giving stronger results with genotypes *MM* or *NN* than with *MN;* no typing therefore should be done without a control of MN cells. Rare forms of M and N have been described which are agglutinated by some anti-sera but not others. These together with rare alleles at the MN locus are considered in Chapter 18.

The Ss System and its Association with MN

In 1947 a new antibody was discovered which defined an antigen in human red cells associated with the MN groups (Walsh and Montgomery, 1947; Sanger and Race, 1947). The newly discovered antigen and its corresponding antibody were termed S and anti-S. In the English population the proportion of blood samples agglutinated by anti-S is approximately 55 per cent. However, this proportion varies if the three groups M, N, and MN are considered separately. Of M samples about 73 per cent are agglutinated by anti-S, of N samples 32 per cent are agglutinated and of MN samples 54 per cent are agglutinated. These figures show that S occurs in association with M rather than with N which suggests that there is some relationship between the MN system and S. This relationship can be confirmed using statistical methods.

In 1951 (Levine *et al.*, 1951) another antibody was found which was shown to detect the product of a gene allelomorphic to *S*. This antibody, therefore, was designated anti-s and the antigen detected by it, s. The discovery of this second antibody makes the existence of a pair of genes, separate from *M* and *N* but closely associated, the most likely explanation of the connexion between *MN* and *Ss*.

Individuals can be of genotype *SS, Ss,* or *ss*. The frequencies of these are as follows:

Genotype *SS*	About 11 per cent
Genotype *Ss*	About 44 per cent
Genotype *ss*	About 45 per cent

Anti-S and anti-s, therefore, agglutinate the red cells of about 55 per cent and 89 per cent of the population respectively. Unlike anti-M and anti-N, these antibodies are usually active at 37°C. Anti-S has been shown to be responsible for both haemolytic disease of the newborn and haemolytic transfusion reactions and so has the rarer anti-s. In routine work anti-S may be available, although it is rare, but not anti-s. Typing of red cells with anti-S is carried out by saline or

Table 13.2 The MNSs phenotypes as defined by anti-M, anti-N, and anti-S, and the corresponding genotypes

	Reactions with		Phenotype	Genotype
Anti-M	Anti-N	Anti-S		
+	−	+	MS	*MSMS*
				MSMs
+	−	−	Ms	*MsMs*
+	+	+	MNS	*MSNS*
				MSNs
				MsNS
+	+	−	MNs	*MsNs*
−	+	+	NS	*NSNS*
				NSNs
−	+	−	Ns	*NsNs*

albumin tube technique, usually at 37°C, or the indirect anti-human globulin test may have to be used. The method chosen will depend on the optimum for each individual anti-serum.

The various phenotypes and genotypes are shown in Table 13.2. Results of large numbers of family studies have shown that each M or N gene has S or s closely related to it, so closely in fact that no crossovers have been discovered and they segregate as though they were one gene. This means, as can be seen in Table 13.2, there are 10 ways in which the four genes can be arranged. The phenotypes given in this table are those defined by the anti-sera M, N, and S.

In spite of the association between the MN and Ss genes, which has led to their being regarded as belonging to the same blood group system, for most practical purposes they can be considered quite separately. Indeed their antibodies have widely diverse characteristics. Anti-M and anti-N are cold agglutinins which rarely become active at 37°C and are of little clinical significance. Anti-S and anti-s are immune antibodies active at 37°C appearing in both complete and incomplete forms and have been responsible for both haemolytic disease of the newborn and haemolytic transfusion reactions.

Cross Reactions between M and N

There is often marked cross-reactivity between anti-N and M cells. In fact continual absorption of rabbit anti-N with human M cells may result in almost complete uptake of the anti-N although there is little or no uptake of anti-M by N cells. Cross reactions between M and anti-N are increased by lowering the temperature. The plant anti-N from Vicia graminea also cross reacts. The cross reactions are thought to be due to an N-like receptor on M red cells, or alternatively that N is a basic substance acted on by M and m genes so that all cells would be likely to have some N specificity, most in mm and least in MM (*See also* Chapter 18).

In practice, the tendency for cross reactivity means that care has to be taken in the absorption of sera when preparing anti-M and anti-N grouping reagents and in the carrying out of the M and N typing tests.

The Effect of Enzymes

Papain, trypsin, ficin and bromelin inhibit MNSs reactions, though the cross reaction of anti-N with M cells is enhanced by trypsin.

TECHNIQUES

Technique No. 13.1. Typing of red cells for M and N—tube technique

At least two anti-M and anti-N typing sera are used at the recommended dilution in saline (*see* technique No. 13.5). One unit volume (approximately 0.03 ml) of each serum is delivered into the required number of precipitin tubes including three tubes for each serum with control cells of types M, N, and MN.

To each tube is added an equal volume of the red cells to be tested made up to a

2 per cent suspension in saline (judged by eye). The tests are left at 20°C (room temperature) for two hours.

The tests are then read as for ABO grouping, including gentle tapping of the tube as false positive results may be obtained if the cell sediment is not agitated.

The controls must be read first. The results obtained with an antiserum which is giving more than a weak (w) reaction with the negative control must be discarded.

Technique No. 13.2. Typing of red cells for M and N—tile technique

Two examples of each anti-serum are used at a dilution suitable for tile grouping (*see* technique No. 13.5).

The test is performed on a white opalescent glass tile appropriately marked out in squares. One drop of antiserum is placed in each square of a row of the required length, allowing for controls of M, N, and MN cells. One drop of a 5 per cent suspension of the red cells to be tested (previously washed in saline) is added to each drop of antiserum. The serum and cells are mixed thoroughly with the corner of a microscope slide or with a glass rod. After standing for two or three minutes, the tile is gently rocked. When the MN control is giving a good reaction and while the negative controls are still completely clear, the results are read.

Technique No. 13.3. Typing of red cells with anti-S

The method of testing will depend upon the nature of the antibody.

If the anti-S is an agglutinin the saline tube technique as for Rh typing is employed (technique No. 7.2) incubating either at 37°C or room temperature according to the reactivity of the particular antibody. The reading is also done in the manner recommended for Rh tests. An incomplete anti-S is best used by anti-human globulin technique (technique No. 8.3a) although bovine albumin methods (technique No. 7.3) may occasionally be found satisfactory.

With each batch of tests known S positive and S negative red cells are included as controls.

Technique No. 13.4. Preparation of anti-M and anti-N typing sera

The following account is based on the methods used by Dr. E. W. Ikin of the Medical Research Council Blood Group Reference Laboratory.

Injection of Rabbits.

To obtain several satisfactory sera, at least six rabbits should be used to produce anti-M sera, and at least six to produce anti-N sera. Cells of the type OM are given to the "anti-M" rabbits, and ON cells to the "anti-N" rabbits. The best antisera are usually produced by rabbits bred selectively from good producers. A course consists of injecting 0.5 ml washed packed cells from an OM (or ON) person into each rabbit, intraperitoneally on the first day and intravenously on the five successive days. The intra-peritoneal dose is given on the first day to prevent anaphylactic shock. The vein most easily used is the posterior peripheral auricular vein. On the ninth or tenth day after the last injections the rabbits are bled about 30–40 ml from the peripheral auricular vein.

Absorption of Anti-M Sera.

Rabbits sometimes possess a naturally occurring anti-A and thus it is best to use group A_1 rather than group O blood for absorption. Very rarely they possess a naturally occurring anti-B which may necessitate a special absorption with group BN red cells. Alternatively if available, group A_1BN cells can be used routinely for these absorptions. The sera are always absorbed after dilution with saline, and trial 2 ml. absorptions will show whether $\frac{1}{10}$, $\frac{1}{20}$, $\frac{1}{30}$, $\frac{1}{40}$, or even even $\frac{1}{80}$ is the optimum dilution, (Table 13.3).

Table 13.3 Preliminary trial absorption (unknown rabbit serum)

Formula	Amount of blood for absorption (washed packed cells) (ml)	Amount of saline (ml)	Amount of serum (ml)
2 ml dil. $(\frac{1}{10}) \times A_1 N \frac{1}{4}$	0.5	1.8	0.2
" " $(\frac{1}{10}) \times A_1 N \frac{1}{2}$	1	1.8	0.2
" " $(\frac{1}{20}) \times A_1 N \frac{1}{4}$	0.5	1.9	0.1
" " $(\frac{1}{20}) \times A_1 N \frac{1}{2}$	1	1.9	0.1
" " $(\frac{1}{40}) \times A_1 N \frac{1}{4}$	0.5	1.95	0.05
" " $(\frac{1}{40}) \times A_1 N \frac{1}{2}$	1	1.95	0.05
" " $(\frac{1}{40}) \times A_1 N \ 1$	2	1.95	0.05

The absorptions are carried out at room temperature for 1 hour.

The absorbed sera are then titrated with M, MN, and N cells. An absorption will be regarded as satisfactory if the titre against M cells is at least thirty-two, against MN cells sixteen and there is no reaction at 1 in 2 with N cells.

If none of the absorptions give entirely satisfactory results further trial absorptions can be attempted according to the titrations on the first trial sera. For example, in the above case, supposing that the most satisfactory trial serum was $(\frac{1}{20}) \times A_1 N \frac{1}{2}$ and the titration with the three standard cells (M, MN, and N) was as in Table 13.4.

Table 13.4 Titration after first trial absorption

Type of red cell	Dilutions of serum						
	1	$\frac{1}{2}$	$\frac{1}{4}$	$\frac{1}{8}$	$\frac{1}{16}$	$\frac{1}{32}$	$\frac{1}{64}$
M	C	C	V	V	++	+	w
MN	C	C	V	++	+	w	–
N	+	w	–	–	–	–	–

Then a satisfactory serum could probably be prepared with the following formula—$(\frac{1}{20}) \times A_1 N \frac{5}{8}$; and this might have the titration shown in Table 13.5. It is advisable not to over-absorb sera as this tends to remove some of the

Table 13.5 Titration after second trial absorption

Type of red cell	Dilutions of serum						
	1	$\frac{1}{2}$	$\frac{1}{4}$	$\frac{1}{8}$	$\frac{1}{16}$	$\frac{1}{32}$	$\frac{1}{64}$
M	C	C	V	++	+	(+)	w
MN	C	V	V	++	(+)	w	–
N	w	–	–	–	–	–	–

required anti-M. Moreover, a second absorption following an insufficient first absorption is often most unsatisfactory, much of the anti-M also being removed. It has been found worth while to experiment until a good formula has been obtained and then to do a large absorption (say 50 ml) with this formula.

Successive bleedings after a further course of injections of the same rabbit will usually yield sera to which the same or a very similar formula can be applied. For example, a further bleeding from the rabbit above whose optimum formula was $(\frac{1}{20}) \times A_1N\frac{5}{8}$ might work best at the formula $(\frac{1}{20}) \times A_1N\frac{3}{4}$. As a rule, later bleedings from the same rabbit require slightly more absorption.

Absorption of Anti-N Sera.

These are carried out exactly as for the anti-M sera except that the sera from rabbits which have been injected with ON cells are absorbed with cells from an A_1M person. As mentioned above, there is a greater tendency for the titre of the anti-N to be reduced by absorption with the heterologous (M) cells.

Technique No. 13.5. Standardisation of anti-M and anti-N typing sera

After absorbing the main portion of serum, it must be retitrated with appropriate red cells since the values obtained at this stage may not be quite the same as those for the serum absorbed in the pilot experiment. It will usually be found that, however successful the absorption, small amounts of "anti-Man" antibodies will remain in the serum and cause agglutination of the heterologous red cells. It is more satisfactory to dilute these out than to embark upon a reabsorption, providing the specific titre after the necessary dilution still reaches the required minimum. As seen above (technique No. 13.1) trace amounts of anti-Man antibodies can be dispersed when handling the tests at the reading stage since the specific agglutination is usually so firm that it is not appreciably broken down, whereas the agglutination caused by residual anti-Man antibodies is eliminated. When using the tile method (technique No. 13.2) the careful timing of the tests will avoid any slight reaction caused by traces of anti-Man antibodies.

The next step is to run the serum in parallel with known sera against at least thirty random red cell samples and in addition to include red cells of types AM, AN, BM, and BN. With these additional samples it is possible to detect any residual antibody in the rabbit specific for A and B red cells. If this antibody is too potent to be diluted out a further absorption with red cells of the appropriate ABO and MN type may be necessary, but this should be avoided if possible. This system is further discussed in Chapter 18.

THE KELL SYSTEM

This system was first described by Coombs *et al.,* 1946; the antibody being found in the serum of a mother whose infant suffered from haemolytic disease of the newborn. The antigen K was found to occur in 10 per cent of the British population and it was postulated that the system was governed by a pair of allelomorphic genes called K and k which controlled the production of the corresponding antigens K and k. The groups, therefore, are as follows:

Phenotype as defined by anti-K	Genotype
Kell positive	*KK* about 0.2 per cent
	Kk " 10 per cent
Kell negative	*kk* " 90 per cent

There is evidence supporting the view that K is rather strongly antigenic and indeed anti-K, although the antigen occurs in only 1 in 10 of the population, is the next most common immune antibody after anti-D and anti-C. Anti-K is almost invariably active at 37°C and often associated with a haemolytic transfusion reaction or haemolytic disease of the newborn. If the ABO and Rh systems cannot be incriminated in such clinical conditions it is well worth considering the possibility of Kell being the cause of the haemolysis. Anti-K is quite often found in persons who have made anti-D and occasionally it is the anti-K and not the anti-D which is incriminated. Anti-K is most readily detected by the indirect antiglobulin test. Some anti-K antibodies are detectable only by antiglobulin technique while some are detectable by other techniques even occasionally in saline. However, the indirect anti-globulin test is the most reliable way of detecting the presence of the antibody and of Kell typing unknown red cells.

Anti-k originally called anti-Cellano (Levine *et al.,* 1949) has been found but owing to the rarity of *KK* (the only genotype in which it can occur), anti-k will always be one of the less common antibodies.

This once simple system is now known to be highly complex (see chapter 18).

TECHNIQUE

Technique No. 13.6. Typing of red cells with anti-K.

It will be found that anti-K sera are individual in their behaviour and, therefore, the optimum working conditions for any given anti-serum must be found by trial and error. Some react by saline technique. The reactions of such Kell agglutinins may be enhanced by centrifuging the tests before reading them. Most sera react best by anti-globulin technique and this is undoubtedly the method of choice for typing.

The following is an anti-human globulin technique which usually works satisfactorily. Two anti-K sera should be used. Two volumes of each anti-K are mixed with an equal volume of a 2–3 per cent cell suspension and incubated at 37°C for 1–2 hours. It is important to include known K positive and known K negative controls. After incubation, the supernatant is removed and the cells are washed carefully at least three times in a large volume of saline, and then mixed with an anti-human globulin serum on an opalescent tile in exactly the same manner as described for indirect anti-human globulin technique. (Technique No. 8.3a.) When the agglutination of the known K positive cells has developed fully the tests are read.

THE DUFFY SYSTEM

The Duffy blood group system was discovered by Cutbush and Chanarin, (1950). The new antibody was found in the serum of a man suffering from haemophilia who had had a number of blood transfusions. The antigen which the new antibody detected was found in the red cells of about 65 per cent of the English population. It was called Fy^a, and the antibody anti-Fy^a, in accordance with the plan adopted for some other blood group systems. The phenotypes and genotypes of the system as defined by anti-Fy^a are as follows:

Phenotype as defined by anti-Fy^a	Genotype	Occurrence
Fy(a+)	Fy^aFy^a	About 17 per cent
	Fy^aFy^b	About 49 per cent
Fy(a−)	Fy^bFy^b	About 34 per cent

The anti-Fy^a antibody has been shown to cause haemolytic transfusion reactions, one of which was fatal, and haemolytic disease. The first anti-Fy^a antibodies discovered were only detectable by the indirect anti-human globulin technique but later ones were found which reacted by saline and albumin techniques. The antibody does not react in papain; indeed, even when an anti-Fy^a is capable of causing agglutination by saline technique, the agglutination can be dispersed by addition of papain. The indirect anti-human globulin method is by far the most reliable way of detecting and using this antibody. Occasionally anti-Fy^a fixes complement in which case an antiglobulin for the detection of complement may give improved results. Some eighteen months after the discovery of Fy^a and anti-Fy^a the expected allelomorph Fy^b was found when a "new" antibody proved to be anti-Fy^b (Ikin et al., 1951). This antibody was found in the serum of a woman who had had three children and no history of blood transfusion. None of the children had suffered from haemolytic disease.

The phenotype Fy (a− b−) has been found in a high proportion of negroes. For discussion of the Fy(a− b−) phenotype and recent work on the subtypes of Fy, see Chapter 18.

TECHNIQUE

Technique No. 13.7. Typing of red cells with anti-Fy^a.

Anti-Fy^a may not be in sufficiently good supply to allow the use of two anti-sera in parallel. In this case, unless the anti-Fy^a is particularly strongly reacting and reliable, it is recommended that negative reactions are checked with a second anti-Fy^a. It is usually found most satisfactory to use an indirect anti-human globulin method (technique No. 8.3a), even though the particular antibody selected for typing purposes may react by other methods. Two volumes of anti-Fy^a serum are mixed with an equal volume of a 2-3 per cent cell suspension and incubated at 37°C for 1-2 hours. Known Fy^a positive and Fy$^{a\cdot}$negative controls are included.

THE KIDD BLOOD GROUP SYSTEM

The Kidd blood group system was discovered by Allen *et al.* (1951), the antibody being found in the serum of a woman whose sixth child suffered from haemolytic disease of the newborn. The role of the new antibody in connexion with this disease could not be assessed because the maternal serum also contained anti-Kell. Since this time a few cases have been reported where the Kidd antibody has been stimulated either by transfusion, or pregnancy or both. In most instances this antibody has been accompanied by other blood group antibodies; a case in which it caused kernicterus has been reported.

The antibody was called anti-Jk^a and phenotypes and genotypes were postulated as follows:

Phenotype as defined by anti-Jk^a	Genotype	Occurrence
Jk(a+)	Jk^aJk^a	About 25 per cent
	Jk^aJk^b	About 50 per cent
Jk(a−)	Jk^bJk^b	About 25 per cent

Later anti-Jk^b was discovered (Plaut *et al.*, 1953). This antibody was found in association with anti- Fy^a and seemed to have been stimulated by transfusion. Many other examples of anti- Jk^b have since been found.

Later still the phenotype Jk(a− b−) was found through detection of an antibody following a transfusion reaction (Pinkerton *et al.*, 1959). The antibody reacted with all cells tested except the patient's own and was found to contain anti- Jk^a and anti- Jk^b which consisted of separable anti-Jk^b and inseparable anti-Jk^{a}Jk^b (anti-Jk^3). The phenotype was found in a Filipina with Spanish and Chinese ancestry. It has not yet been detected in negroes or whites.

The original anti- Jk^a serum worked at first as a saline agglutinin but later it became necessary to use the anti-human globulin test. Most Kidd anti-sera seem to give the best reactions by anti-human globulin technique, particularly if this is performed on enzyme treated red cells or in the presence of complement. The sera at the present time are too rare for routine use.

Unlike most other blood group systems, Kidd has not yet expanded to reveal further complexities so nothing further about this system will be found in Chapter 18.

TECHNIQUES

Technique No. 13.8. Typing of red cells with anti-Jk^a by indirect anti-human globulin on enzyme-treated cells.

This is a method involving the performance of an indirect anti-human globulin test on enzyme-treated red cells. The unknown cells together with known Jk^a positive and negative controls are enzyme-treated and then incubated with anti-Jk^a serum for 30–45 minutes in the proportion of two volumes of serum to two volumes of 2–3 per cent treated red cells. The subsequent procedure is identical with the indirect anti-human globulin technique (No. 8.3a) from the washing stage onwards.

Technique No. 13.9.* Typing of red cells with anti-Jk^a by anti-human globulin with the addition of complement. EDTA two-stage method for complement-binding antibodies and the anti-human globulin test.

(a) *Inactivation of complement and complementoid with EDTA (diaminoethanetetra-acetic acid)*
A neutral solution of EDTA is prepared:

$$\left.\begin{array}{l} \text{14.8 g EDTA (dipotassium salt)} \\ \text{1.1 g NaOH} \\ \text{333.3 ml water} \end{array}\right\} \text{pH 7.0-7.4}$$

This solution is placed in tubes in proportionate amounts and allowed to evaporate at 37°C; *e.g.* 0.1 ml of EDTA solution for 1.0 ml of serum.

It has been estimated that 4 mg of EDTA should be added to 1 ml of serum to inactivate it completely. Inactivation is immediate and permanent, and no dilution of antibody in the serum takes place since the serum is added to a dry tube.

(b) *Two-stage technique with fresh human complement and anti-human globulin*
   (i) The serum to be tested is transferred to the dry EDTA tube for inactivation.
   (ii) Two volumes of this serum (i) are incubated with 1 volume of washed packed red cells for 1½ hours at 37°C.
   (iii) The cells are washed four times with a large excess of saline to remove all traces of anti-complementary EDTA.
   (iv) The washed cells (iii) are packed and incubated with 2 volumes of fresh human complement at 37°C in a *water bath* for 15–20 minutes.
   (v) The cells (iv) are again washed four times.
   (vi) The washed cells (v) are tested as a 50 per cent suspension with an ahg diluted optimally for anti-ß$_1$ (principally anti-C3 and anti-C4).

---

*For a description of this technique we are indebted to Miss Caroline Giles of the Blood Group Reference Laboratory.

Notes

    (i) Fresh human complement will retain its activity for two weeks when stored at –20°C. Storage at –50°C or lower is advisable for longer periods.

    (ii) The anti-human globulin (ahg) reagent must contain anti-β_1; a broad spectrum reagent is recommended. It should have been standardised by this technique and found satisfactory. The dilutions used would probably be in the range of 1 in 8 to 1 in 60.

    (iii) This technique is ideal for incomplete Lewis antisera, good for many Kidd antisera and possibly helpful with some Kell and Duffy antisera that will bind complement.

    (iv) Haemolysis may occur with very potent antibodies on addition of complement to the sensitised cells. This can be overcome by dilution of the antiserum.

LUTHERAN

This system was first defined in 1946 when a hitherto unknown antibody appeared in the blood of a patient who had received many blood transfusions. (Callender and Race, 1946.) The antibody was immune, the stimulating antigen being present in one of the donors whose name was Lutheran; thus the antibody was called anti-Lu^a and the phenotypes Lu(a+) and Lu(a–).

Experiment has shown that anti-Lu^a can be produced as a result of transfusion of Lu(a+) blood into Lu(a–) persons; Mainwaring and Pickles (1948) found antibodies in two out of eight Lu(a–) patients who had received Lu(a+) blood.

Anti-Lu^a has not been incriminated in haemolytic disease of the newborn and has not so far produced a haemolytic transfusion reaction of any degree of severity. The anti-Lu^a antibodies are characteristically saline agglutinins and are usually more reactive at room temperature than at 37°C, although some examples have been found which have given stronger agglutination reactions at 37°C. The optimum temperature of reactivity has been shown in some cases to vary with the Lu(a+) cells used.

Later, anti-Lu^b was found in an individual who proved to be of the very rare genotype $Lu^a Lu^a$ Cutbush and Chanarin (1956). The antibody was a saline agglutinin. Only a few anti-Lu^b antibodies have been discovered since. None of them have had great clinical significance.

The phenotypes and genotypes can be summarised as follows:

Phenotypes defined by anti-Lu^a	Genotypes	Occurrence
Lu(a+)	$Lu^a Lu^b$	About 8 per cent
	$Lu^a Lu^a$	About 0.2 per cent
Lu(a–)	$Lu^b Lu^b$	About 92 per cent

This apparently simple system has been shown to be of great complexity. Not only was the phenotype Lu(a–b–) discovered but was found to arise in two distinct ways, one dominant and the other recessive in character. In Chapter 18 we shall see how this was merely the introduction to a fascinating blood-group study.

TECHNIQUE

Technique No. 13.10. Lutheran typing of red cells.

One unit volume of anti-Lu^a serum is mixed with one unit volume of a 2 per cent suspension of test cells. It is advisable to use small volumes of about 0.02 ml since the anti-serum is rare. A positive and a negative control consisting of known Lu(a+) and Lu(a−) red cells must be included with each batch of tests. After 2 hours' incubation at the optimum temperature for the anti-Lu^a serum being used (usually 15°C) the contents of each tube are pipetted gently on to a microscope slide and read for presence or absence of agglutination.

Lutheran agglutination is characteristic, being composed of loose clumps (morulae) in a field of free cells.

THE LEWIS BLOOD GROUP SYSTEM

A hitherto unknown antibody, believed to be naturally occurring, was found by Mourant in samples of blood from two different persons (Mourant, 1946). This antibody recognised an antigen present in about 22 per cent of the English population. The system was called Lewis after one of the two individuals in which it was first found. In accordance with the adopted convention the antigen is now designated Le^a and the antibody anti-Le^a.

Le^a typing of red cells can be carried out quite satisfactorily by tube technique in saline or papain at room temperature or 15°C. Occasionally an anti-Le^a antibody is found which reacts well by indirect anti-globulin technique especially in the presence of complement.

Anti-Le^a sera will sometimes haemolyse Le^a positive cells in the presence of complement. Haemolysis is a regular feature if ficin enzyme technique is used; this is a helpful fact in the identification of these antibodies. Haemolysis also occurs using papain treated Le^a positive cells with many but not all anti-Lewis antibodies.

Le^a has been found to be unique among blood groups in several respects. Firstly, there is a connexion between Le^a and the secretion of A, B, and H substances. All Le^a positives are nonsecretors of the blood group substances A, B, and H, but secretors of Le^a substance, *see* Chapter 16. The associations between Le^a positives and non-secretors of A, B, H substances is caused by an interaction at the phenotypic level. The Lewis and secretor genes are inherited quite independently of each other (*see* Fig. 16.5).

The frequency of Le^a positives in infants up to eighteen months is higher than in adults. Le^a appears to develop more rapidly than Le^b and there is plenty of Le^a substance in infants' plasma which is then taken up on the red cells.

Antibodies have been found, indeed they are not uncommon, whose reactions with red cells are to a great extent antithetical to those of anti-Le^a. These antibodies, therefore, have been designated anti-Le^b and the corresponding antigen Le^t. It is now known that the Le^b antigen does not arise from a separate gene *Le^b* but is a product of interaction between the *Le^a* and *H* genes (*see* Chapter 16). Four to six per cent individuals are both Le^a negative and Le^b negative. Moreover, most anti-Le^b sera do not give the same number of positive reactions in all ABO groups, in particular in groups A$_1$ and A$_1$B which contain a far higher proportion of Le^b negatives than groups O, A$_2$, B, and A$_2$B.

Work by Sneath and Sneath (1955) showed that the system is primarily composed of soluble antigens existing in the serum and body fluids and is not an erythrocyte blood group system at all. Thus, the most reliable way of determining the Lewis status of an individual is by testing the saliva by inhibition technique against appropriate antisera. The presence of the antigen on the red cells depends on there being a sufficient quantity in the serum for it to be taken up by the cells.

The great importance of the Lewis system in the understanding of the development of the ABO blood group antigens is discussed in Chapter 16.

Most anti-Le^a sera originate from people of the phenotype Le(a− b−) and very often contain weak anti-Le^b. Anti-Le^b sera are also usually made by people of phenotype Le(a−b−) but they are the non-secretors of ABH, Le^a and Le^b substances. Anti-Le^b sera often contain anti-H. It is obvious therefore that these sera need to be carefully controlled if used for typing.

TECHNIQUE

Technique No. 13.11. Typing of red cells with anti-Le^a and anti-Le^b

Equal volumes of serum and a 2 per cent suspension of the red cells to be typed are mixed in precipitin tubes and left for 2 hours at room temperature or preferably at 15°C in a water bath. Known Le^a and Le^b positive and negative red cells are included as controls. These should all be of group O.

The tests are read microscopically. The negative reactions are not always clear cut but if the sera used are selected to give good macroscopic readings with the true positives the distinction between the true positives and negatives is not difficult to make.

THE BLOOD GROUP SYSTEM P

This was one of the earlier known blood group systems, being discovered during the same experimental immunisation of rabbits with human red cells which led to the finding of M and N (Landsteiner and Levine, 1927).

The serum of one rabbit after absorption with certain human red cells was found to contain an antibody which did not appear to belong to the ABO or MN systems, the only two known at the time. The human red cells which were positive with the rabbit anti-P, now called anti-P$_1$ (Chapter 18), were designated P positive and those which were negative with it, P negative. Anti-P$_1$ frequently occurs in the serum of P$_1$ negative individuals as a naturally occurring cold agglutinin and also in the serum of some animals, in particular horses, rabbits, pigs and cattle. Unfortunately these anti-P$_1$ sera are usually of low titre.

The estimation of the frequency of P_1 is difficult owing both to the rarity of potent anti-sera and to the existence of individuals whose red cells only react weakly even with the best available anti-sera. Among the P_1 positives, three classes can be distinguished according to their strength of reaction with anti-P_1 sera: (1) P_1 strong; (2) P_1 medium; (3) P_1 weak. There is no evidence, to date, that there is any qualitative difference between them. In fact the result of absorption tests with P_1 weak cells and anti-P_1 sera show that these cells are as efficient in removal of anti-P_1 from a serum as are cells which are P_1 strong. Much of the variation in agglutinability of P_1 positive red cells seems to depend upon their genotype.

Anti-P_1 is rarely of importance from the clinical viewpoint. A few cases of haemolytic disease and one or two transfusion reactions have been attributed to it. The absence of clinical significance is undoubtedly due to the fact that anti-P_1 is characteristically a cold agglutinin of the agglutinating type. Nevertheless, a few anti-P_1 antibodies have been found active at $37°C$ and such antibodies are potential causes of haemolytic reactions. Moreover, some anti-P_1 sera in which the antibody is not active at $37°C$ by a saline technique can be shown to react at this temperature if the indirect anti-human globulin plus complement method is used. (Technique No. 22.6.) However, it is as a cold agglutinin that anti-P_1 will be encountered by those who do routine blood grouping tests.

Henningsen (1949) by the use of delicate techniques has demonstrated the presence of anti-P_1 active at $4°C$ in a high proportion of P_1 negative individuals. Anti-P_1 reacting at room temperature is comparatively rare but when it does occur it often produces anomalous results in ABO serum grouping tests. These anomalous results due to anti-P_1 can only be avoided if P_1 negative A and B red cells are chosen as standard cells. This choice is not usually convenient. When the occasion arises it is advisable to carry out tests which will establish the cause of the anomalous results. (*See* Chapter 22.) In the event of an anti-P_1 agglutinin being identified it should be secured as an anti-P_1 typing serum if sufficiently potent since those that can be relied upon to detect all P_1 weak cells are rare. Accurate P_1 typing of red cells is not easily accomplished and should always be performed with at least two, preferably more, anti-P_1 sera. P_1 weak cells should always be included among the positive controls.

For further antigens of the P system, Chapter 18 should be consulted.

TECHNIQUE

Technique No. 13.12. Typing of red cells with anti-P_1.

The standard tube technique is used. Equal volumes of a suitable anti-P_1 anti-serum and a 2 per cent suspension of red cells to be tested are mixed and left for 2 hours. Known P strong, P weak and P negative cells are included with each batch of tests. Each sample is tested with two anti-P_1 anti-sera whenever possible. The temperature at which the tests are incubated will depend upon the particular anti-sera used. It is preferable to choose anti-sera which will work well at a cool room temperature, *e.g.* $15°C$. At $4°C$ other cold agglutinins may interfere with the results although with well tried and well controlled anti-sera this temperature may be found to be satisfactory.

The tests are read in the same manner as for Rh typing since the agglutinated clumps are often fragile.

THE I BLOOD GROUP SYSTEM

This system is complicated and is of practical importance because the blood group serologist is unlikely to be able to avoid encountering anti-I antibodies.

In 1956 Wiener *et al.* gave the name anti-I to an antibody found in the serum of a patient suffering from haemolytic anaemia of the "cold" antibody type. Of 22,000 donors tested, only five were negative and therefore designated i.

In 1960 Jenkins *et al.* described a blood donor whose cells were i and whose serum contained anti-I. With the cells of this donor it was possible to show that a number of cases of acquired haemolytic anaemia of the cold type have anti-I and in addition many so-called non-specific antibodies in normal sera are anti-I. This work led to the recognition of two types of anti-I, one called "natural" which occurs regularly in the serum of i individuals and one called "auto anti-I", as found associated with haemolytic anaemia.

The differences between I and i are not completely clear-cut in that using certain techniques (*e.g.* ficin) it can be shown that i cells react with anti-I, although to a lesser degree than the cells from I individuals. Moreover, there is a great range of I activity in I positive people. Cord cells give relatively very weak reactions with potent anti-I and fail to react at all with most anti-I sera, but they are strongly i-positive. The I antigen reaches adult strength approximately 18 months from birth and at the same time the amount of i falls.

The Identification of Anti-I in Practice

Anti-I is usually detected as a saline cold agglutinin. Its activity is often enhanced by such enzymes as ficin, papain or bromelin, in fact it is sometimes only detectable by enzyme techniques. It is characterised by reacting strongly with adult cells (usually including the patient's own cells) but being negative or at most very weak with cord cells. It is differentiated from other antibodies which are weak or negative with cord cells, *e.g.* anti-H, anti-P$_1$ and anti-Le^a plus anti-Le^b mixtures, by the fact that it is usually an auto-antibody and also that it is uninhibited by human saliva. If the anti-I is not an auto-antibody the patient's cells will be strongly positive for i. The other similar antibody from which anti-I needs to be differentiated is anti-HI, an antibody which reacts preferentially with O cells (like anti-H) but is not inhibited by human saliva (like anti-I). Many workers believe that this antibody is detecting a compound antigen and so the designation anti-HI is appropriate. It has also been called anti-OI, as it is the antibody which used to be called anti-O. We feel that this is not a good name as it is not detecting a product of the *O* gene. If the rare i-adult cells are available for testing, anti-I will be weak or negative with these (as will be anti-H or anti-HI). All i-adult cells so far found are both I and H negative or only weakly positive.

REFERENCES

Allen, F.H., Diamond, L.K. & Niedziela, B. (1951) A new blood group antigen. *Nature (Lond.)* 167, 482.

Callender, S.T. & Race, R.R. (1946) A serological and genetical study of multiple antibodies formed in response to blood transfusion by a patient with *lupus erythematosus diffusus. Ann. Eugen. (Lond.),* 13, 102.

Coombs, R.R.A., Mourant, A.E., & Race, R.R. (1946) *In vivo* iso-sensitisation of red cells in babies with haemolytic disease. *Lancet,* i, 264.

Cutbush, M. & Chanarin, I. (1950) The Duffy blood group. *Heredity,* 4, 383.

Cutbush, M. & Chanarin, I. (1956) The expected blood group antibody anti-Lu^b. *Nature (Lond.),* 178, 855.

Henningsen, K. (1949). Investigations on the blood factor P. *Acta path. microbiol. scand.,* 26, 769.

Ikin, E.W., Mourant, A.E., Pettenkofer, H.J. & Bluementhal, G. (1951) Discovery of the expected haemagglutinin, anti-Fy^b. *Nature (Lond.),* 168, 1077.

Jenkins, W.J., Marsh, W.L., Noades, J., Tippett, P., Sanger, R. & Race, R.R. (1960) The I antigen and antibody. *Vox Sang,* 5, 97.

Landsteiner, K. & Levine, P. (1927) Further observations on individual differences of human blood. *Proc. Soc. exp. Biol. N.Y.,* 24, 941.

Landsteiner, K. & Levine, P. (1927) A new agglutinable factor differentiating individual human bloods. *Proc. Soc. exp. Biol. N.Y.* 24, 600.

Landsteiner, K. and Levine, P. (1928) On individual differences in human blood. *J. exp. Med.* 47, 757.

Levine, P., Wigod, M., Backer, A.M., & Ponder, R. (1949) A new human hereditary blood group property (Cellano) present in 99.8 per cent of all bloods. *Science,* 109, 474.

Levine, P., Kuhmichel, A.B., Wigod, M. & Koch, E. (1951) A new blood factor, s allelic to S. *Proc. Soc. exp. Biol. N.Y.* 78, 218.

Mainwaring, V.R. & Pickles, M.M. (1948) A further case of anti-Lutheran immunisation with some studies on its capacity for human sensitisation. *J. clin. Path.* 1, 292.

Mourant, A.E. (1946) A 'new' human blood group antigen of frequent occurrence. *Nature (Lond.),* 158, 237.

Pinkerton, F.J., Mermod, L.E., Liles, B.A., Jack, J.A. Jr. & Noades, J. (1959) The phenotype Jk(a–b–) in the Kidd blood group system. *Vox. Sang.* 4, 155.

Plaut, G., Ikin, E.W., Mourant, A.E. Sanger, R. & Race, R.R. (1953) A new blood group antibody. anti-Jk^b. *Nature, (Lond.),* 171, 431.

Sanger, R. & Race, R.R. (1947) Subdivisions of the MN blood groups in man. *Nature (Lond.),* 160, 505.

Sneath, J.S. & Sneath, P.H.A. (1955) Transformation of the Lewis groups of human red cells. *Nature (Lond.),* 176, 172.

Walsh, R.J. & Montgomery, C. (1947) A new human isoagglutinin subdividing the MN blood groups. *Nature (Lond.),* 160, 504.

Wiener, A.S., Unger, L.J., Cohen, L. & Feldman, J. (1956). Type specific cold auto-antibodies as a cause of acquired hemolytic anaemia and hemolytic transfusion reactions; biologic test with bovine red cells. *Ann intern. Med,* 44, 221.

Chapter 14. Various Red Cell Agglutination Phenomena

This chapter is concerned with auto-agglutination and bacteriogenic agglutination because both of these phenomena may interfere with routine tests. The agglutination is not always produced by antibodies belonging to easily recognisable blood group systems.

Auto-agglutination

This type of agglutination is caused by auto-antibodies the essential characteristic of which is that they react upon the red cells of the individual in whose serum they occur. Some of them seem to detect an antigen common to all, or almost all, human red cells since they give a positive reaction with the cells of all individuals irrespective of any known blood group system. Both complete and incomplete auto-antibodies are found.

In some cases the auto-antibody can be identified. For instance anti-H and anti-I both occur as cold auto-antibodies; among warm auto-antibodies anti-e is the most common although warm auto-antibodies of the other Rh specificities have been described. These auto-Rh antibodies are associated with auto-immune haemolytic anaemias (*See* Chapter 27).

Atypical auto-antibodies in virus pneumonia are usually anti-I, possibly because mycoplasma are also associated with this disease, and are believed to destroy the I antigen.

In patients with cold auto-agglutinins most of the antibody appears to be in the serum while in the patients with warm auto-antibodies most of the antibody is on the cells.

Complete Auto-antibodies

These are agglutinins and are normally active only in the cold. They occur in the sera of very many healthy individuals as can be readily ascertained by testing 2 per cent suspensions of red cells against an equal volume of serum from the same individuals at 4°C. Very occasionally auto-agglutinins may become active to the extent of having appreciable titres at room temperature or even at temperatures approaching 37°C. These more potent cold auto-agglutinins can also occur in healthy individuals but are often associated with pathological states, *e.g.* haemolytic anaemia. Auto-agglutinins having titres at 4°C of 1000 or over are often associated with virus pneumonia and are of value in differential diagnosis.

Auto-agglutination that confines its activity to low temperatures does not interfere with blood grouping tests but that which takes place at laboratory or higher temperatures must be dealt with before blood grouping is attempted. When auto-agglutination is sufficiently strong to interfere with tests it is usually obvious to the naked eye and will be seen during the handling of the sample of the patient's blood. Less strong auto-agglutination may be missed at this stage in which case it may cause anomalous results. Warm washing the red cells in saline at 37°C will usually free them of auto-agglutinins. Occasionally it may be necessary to wash at a temperature higher than 37°C or even allow the cells to remain at a higher temperature for 5–10 minutes in order to break down the auto-agglutination. (Technique No. 14.1.)

Incomplete Auto-antibodies

Incomplete auto-antibodies can be of both "cold" and "warm" types. If clotted or defibrinated normal blood is allowed to stand at 0°–2°C and thereafter an anti-human globulin test carried out on the red cells, the reaction is often positive due to absorption of incomplete cold auto-antibodies from the serum. These normal incomplete antibodies have anti-H specificity and react far more strongly with O than with A_1B cells. The reaction can be inhibited by the saliva of secretors but not by that of non-secretors. Blood samples containing anti-coagulant, *e.g.* sequestrine, heparin, citrate, etc., do not give this reaction. This phenomenon does not interfere with most blood grouping tests, but accounts for some anomalous positive anti-human globulin tests, if red cells stored overnight in the refrigerator as clotted samples are used. It is, however, possible to overcome this difficulty by the choice of a suitably diluted anti-human globulin reagent or especially prepared anti-IgG anti-human globulin that does not react with these antibodies of the cold type. (*See* Appendix II.)

The presence of "warm" incomplete auto-antibodies is usually associated with pathological states especially haemolytic anaemias. For a discussion of these and other auto-antibodies, including the Donath-Landsteiner antibody, which are concerned in the aetiology of haemolytic anaemia, *see* Chapter 27.

Bacteriogenic Agglutination

This agglutination is unlike any discussed so far in that it is bacteriogenic. It can occur in one of two ways. Either red cells are acted upon by certain bacteria and viruses in such a way that they become agglutinated by all human sera and are, therefore, said to be pan-agglutinable, or a sample of serum may become infected with certain organisms rendering it capable of agglutinating all samples of red cells; in this case the serum is said to be pan-agglutinating. In practice, the agglutination is variable according to the degree of bacterial infection, and the cells are usually poly- rather than pan-agglutinable.

Poly-agglutinable cells

Certain bacteria have the power of modifying red cells *in vitro* by causing the exposure of receptors for which there is a corresponding antibody in normal human sera. This is the basis of "T" agglutination. A latent receptor "T" on the human red cell acts as an agglutinogen when exposed by the action of certain bacteria, *e.g. Cl. Welchii, Vibrio cholerae* and also *staphylocci.* A corresponding antibody, anti-T, is present in all human sera (with the exception of the sera of newborn infants) so that cells which have been modified by the bacteria are agglutinated by all sera. Anti-T can be specifically removed from serum samples with such modified cells. The enzyme which activates the T antigen on red cells is now known to be neuraminidase. An anti-T lectin can be extracted from peanuts.

A few individuals have been described whose red cells are agglutinated by a proportion of normal human sera which are compatible from the point of view of all known blood groups. This agglutination may also be of bacterial origin but no proof of this exists. Sterile samples taken from the patient are poly-agglutinable and incapable of passing on their agglutinability to normal cells. This is quite different from the *in vitro* pan-agglutination where an inoculum of infected cells will within 24–48 hours infect normal cells causing them to become pan-agglutinable. On the other hand poly-agglutinability is not a constant characteristic of the cells of the individual, persisting for several weeks only in most of the cases described. From a practical point of view cells from such an individual would appear to be group AB while the serum would give the reactions typical of his true ABO group. Tests with AB sera would reveal that the red cells were agglutinated by the majority of these sera. The ABO group of the patient can be determined on serum reactions.

The cell typing for ABO, Rh type, etc., can be done in one of two ways.

(*a*) A standard anti-serum can be used to prepare a saline eluate of the required antibody (technique No. 22.3). Such an eluate will not contain the poly-agglutinating antibody whose presence in almost all sera makes their use for typing poly-agglutinable cells impossible.

(*b*) Poly-agglutinable red cells can be typed by inhibition technique, a modification of technique No. 6.3 being used. Briefly an anti-serum (titre approximately 32) is titrated both before and after absorption with an equal quantity of the red cells. A definite reduction in titration value of the anti-serum indicates that the corresponding antigen is present in the unknown poly-agglutinable red cells.

Pan-agglutinating Serum

Davidsohn and Toharsky showed that when serum became infected with a strain of *corynebacterium* which they called H, it agglutinated all samples of human red cells. This agglutination was caused by the organism acting upon adult and infant serum *in vitro* to produce "anti-h" agglutinins for which there is a corresponding agglutinogen H in all red cells. The H–anti-h agglutination has been shown to be distinct from T–anti-T. It should not be confused with H–anti-H which has already been described in connexion with the ABO blood group system. One of the chief dangers associated with pan-agglutinating serum is an error of blood group caused by a grouping serum becoming infected and thus pan-agglutinating. Such a possibility, however, presents no problem to those who consistently include adequate controls as the phenomenon would be detected in the negative control and the tests repeated with fresh serum.

Pseudo-agglutination

Pseudo-agglutination is the clumping of red cells by other means than antigen-antibody reaction. It is chiefly associated with a protein shift in the serum, *e.g.* in case of multiple myelomatosis or with the addition of certain substances which alter the serum viscosity, *e.g.* dextran (*see* Figs. 1.2a and b).

It is mentioned again here because it may easily be confused in practice with auto-agglutination, pan-agglutination, etc. The method by which it may most easily be distinguished from true agglutination is the indirect anti-human globulin technique.

TECHNIQUES

Technique No. 14.1. The washing of red cells to free them from auto-agglutinins

Any required quantity of red cells showing auto-agglutination are suspended in saline and allowed to reach a temperature of 37°C, either in an incubator or water bath, and left for 5–10 minutes. They are then centrifuged in warm centrifuge cups and the supernatant saline is quickly removed. The cells are washed twice more in warm saline and allowed to cool to room temperature. If examination under the microscope reveals that they are completely unagglutinated they may be used for grouping purposes. If on the other hand, they still show agglutination the process should be repeated raising the temperature to 45°C or even 56°C if necessary. In cases where a temperature above 37°C is needed it is preferable wherever possible to obtain washed cells from a sample which is not allowed to cool below 37°C from the moment of withdrawal from the patient to the completion of the washing process.

Technique No. 14.2. Titration of a serum containing auto-agglutinins

Serial dilutions of the serum are made in saline in the usual manner, technique No. 3.2 or by master titre technique No. 3.4. The number of rows prepared should allow for titrations using the patient's own cells prepared by technique No. 14.1 and two standards, one of group O and the other of the same ABO group as the patient, at 4°, 18°, 32°, and 37°C. The serial dilutions and the appropriate cells must be warmed to 32°C and 37°C respectively before they are mixed together. This ensures that agglutination does not begin to take place at a lower temperature. The titrations are left for 2 hours at the various temperatures before being read.

PART II

A MORE ADVANCED ACCOUNT OF SOME ASPECTS OF BLOOD GROUPS

Section 1. General Immunology

"It stimulated the phagocytes; and the phagocytes did the rest."

G.B. Shaw, THE DOCTOR'S DILEMMA

Chapter 15. General properties of antigens and antibodies

As long ago as 1939 Tiselius and Kabat showed that plasma proteins could be separated on the basis of their mobilities in an electric field into four main components, albumin, alpha (α), beta (ß) and gamma (γ) globulins. It was observed that antibodies occurred mainly in the gamma or occasionally the beta globulins. An example of such a separation can be seen in the plate which forms the frontispiece to this book.

In 1964 it was decided by international agreement to designate the antibody—containing proteins, immunoglobulins, based on their common properties; for example, they are all secreted by special cells of the lymphocyte-plasma series (immunologically competent cells) and all immunoglobulin molecules have basically a similar molecular structure.

However despite family resemblances within themselves the great feature of immunoglobulins is their heterogeneity. Thus, they can be divided into five different subclasses on the basis of physico-chemical, immuno-chemical and biological behaviour. These classes are internationally known as IgG, IgA, IgM, IgD and IgE. As already mentioned in Chapter 1, blood groups antibodies are found almost exclusively in the first three classes and in practice the most important division is into IgG and IgM. However Burkart *et al.* (1974) have described a potent example of anti-Tj[a] which occurred in all five immunoglobulin classes.

The division into subclasses can be achieved by ion-exchange chromatography on diethylaminoethyl (DEAE) cellulose or by Sephadex G 200. The first method depends on differences in net charge on the molecules and the second on molecular size since Sephadex acts as a molecular sieve. Pure IgG can be eluted from the DEAE column as fraction I, early in the elution process, while pure IgM can be collected as fraction I from Sephadex G 200. Immunoglobulins may also be separated by means of sedimentation rates when subjected to ultra centrifugation, the heavier molecules being deposited more rapidly than the lighter. The rate of sedimentation is calculated in Svedberg (S) units and a convenient technique is by ultra centrifugation on a sucrose-density gradient. It is found that

137

IgG molecules have a value of 7S approximately while the larger IgM molecules are 19S. IgA has a wider range, the average value being 6.5S.

Distinctions may also be made by the preparation in animals, usually rabbits, of antibodies which are specific for the various immunoglobulin classes. As well as taking part in precipitin tests these antibodies can be used either as antiglobulin reagents in a straight-forward anti-human globulin test or by the antiglobulin-consumption technique, although the latter test works most effectively for the identification of the immunoglobulin class of eluted antibodies. This is because eluates have a low protein concentration which is almost entirely antibody active in contrast to whole serum in which the globulin concentration is too high for satisfactory inhibition of antibody activity to be effected by the appropriate anti-Ig reagent.

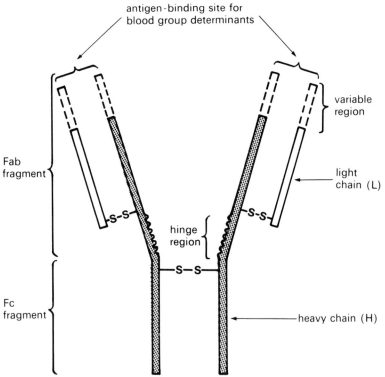

Fig. 15.1 Structure of the immunoglobulin molecule.

The structure of the immunoglobulin molecule

The basic immunoglobulin molecule is a bilaterally symmetrical four chain structure (see Fig. 15.1). At the centre and parallel to each other are two identical heavy polypeptide chains (H) bound together by disulphide bonds. Attached to each H-chain, also by disulphide bonds, are small polypeptide chains, the light chains (L). There are two antigenically different types of L-chain called Kappa (K) and Lambda (L) although the two L-chains of any given molecule are identical being either *K* or *L*. About two-thirds of the molecules of any immunoglobulin class (IgG, IgM, etc.) have Kappa L-chains and about one-third have Lambda L-chains. The H-chains of an immunoglobulin molecule which are structurally different for each class are given the Greek letter corresponding to the class letter. Thus the H-chain of IgA is alpha (α), IgG—gamma (γ), IgD—delta (δ), IgE—epsilon (Σ) and IgM—mu (μ). It is the fact that the H-chains are characteristic for each class of immunoglobulin which has permitted the preparation of class specific anti-sera *e.g.* anti-IgG, anti-IgA and anti-IgM.

The hinge region of the molecule which creates its flexibility is susceptible to attack by enzymes. Papain, in the presence of cysteine, cleaves the molecule at a point near the hinge region and just beyond the last sulphide bond between the heavy chains. This produces three fragments, two identical ones called Fab fragments which include the antigen-binding region and are therefore capable of binding antigen, and a third Fc fragment which can be crystallised and is made up of the constant portion of the H-chains. This latter portion has the complement binding site if the antibody binds complement and is also the site of the Gm allotypes. The primary structure of each chain is composed of two parts, a constant and a variable portion. The first 108 amino acids of the L-chain and the first 114 amino acids of the H-chain constitute the variable portions. In this region there is a great variety of amino acid sequence which influences the way the chain is folded because each different sequence produces its own characteristic folding. This in turn causes different groups to be exposed on the surface and

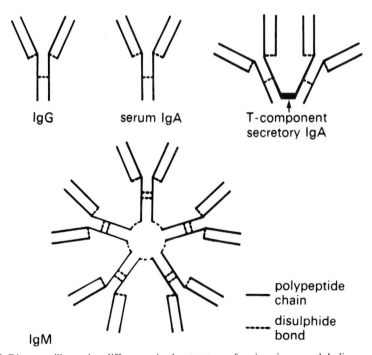

Fig. 15.2 Diagrams illustrating differences in the structure of various immunoglobulins.

in part accounts for the heterogeneity of the immunoglobulins. The structure of the immunoglobulin molecule is therefore designed to give it flexibility and thus it is able to adapt itself to fit an antigenic determinant. If the fit is good there is high complementarity between the antigen and antibody but if the fit is poor, the complementarity is low. Goodness of fit between antigen and antibody influences the combining constant (K) of the antibody. This is further discussed later in this chapter.

An IgG molecule is composed of one structural unit (a monomer) but the IgM molecule consists of five units (a polymer, *see* Fig. 15.2). It is this configuration no doubt that confers the ability of most IgM molecules to agglutinate red cells suspended in a saline medium. A small amount of IgM may occur in monomeric form in serum (IgMs). Mild treatment of IgM molecules with 0.1M 2-mercaptoethanol dissociates the IgM pentamer into the monomer form by splitting the intermonomer disulphide bonds. These units have no agglutinating power but in some cases e.g. anti-D, retain the ability to combine with the antigen and their presence on red cells can often be shown by an anti-globulin test Holborn et al (1971). It has been shown that IgM anti-Le^a after treatment with 2-ME does not retain the ability to sensitize red cells (Holborn 1973).

IgA in serum is usually composed of one unit but in external secretions it seems to occur as a dimer of two individual molecules joined by a secretory piece (*see* Fig. 15.2). IgA is the chief immunoglobulin of saliva and colostrum so blood group antibodies found in these fluids are likely to be IgA.

IgG Subclasses

Through work on myeloma proteins, IgG immunoglobulins have been divided into subclasses. Myeloma proteins are informative since they are derived as a clone from a single cell and all synthesise the same immunoglobulin. Thus, although individual myelomas may differ from each other, those of a particular patient have IgG molecules all identical in structure. Injection of myeloma proteins from different patients into suitable animals has resulted in the production of four different anti-IgG antibodies recognising four distinct IgG subclasses (IgG 1-4) each with different characteristics. From the limited amount of work yet carried out on the identification of the subclasses to which blood group IgG antibodies belong, those of the Rh system have been shown distributed among all four subclasses although they are mainly composed of IgG$_1$ and IgG$_3$.

A summary of some of the characteristics of immunoglobulins is given in Table 15.1.

Serological behaviour of IgM and IgG Antibodies

IgM antibodies are characteristically agglutinins (*i.e.* capable of agglutinating red cells in saline suspension) presumably because their molecules are large and because they have more combining sites than IgG molecules. However IgG anti-A and anti-B antibodies found in sera after immunisation with A or B antigens, are sometimes capable of agglutinating saline suspended cells. It is thought that it

Table 15.1 Summary of some characteristics of immunoglobulin classes in which blood group antibodies may be found.

Characteristic	WHO nomenclature		
	IgG (γ^G)	IgM (γ^M)	IgA (γ^A)
Approx. molecular weight	160,000	900,000	180,000
Sedimentation coefficient	7S	19S	6.5S
Plasma conc. (mg/100 ml (approx.)	1100	100	140
Usual red-cell antibody behaviour	Incomplete antibody	Agglutinin	Incomplete antibody
No. of combining sites per molecule	2	10	2
Treatment with 2-mercapto-ethanol	Unaffected	Reduced to subunits	Partially reduced
Serological activity after heating at 56°C	Unaffected	Heat labile	Unaffected
Complement fixation	Yes	Yes	No
Passage across placenta	Yes	No	No

is the density of A and B antigen sites on the red cell which enables IgG anti-A and anti-B to behave as agglutinins. Group A_1 cells have been shown to have 800,000-1,000,000 sites while group B cells boast 750,000 B sites (Economidou *et al.*, 1967). This view is supported by the fact that, whereas IgG anti-D fails to agglutinate ordinary D-positive cells in saline suspension where the maximum number of sites are in the region of 35,000, selected examples of IgG anti-D are capable of behaving as agglutinins with -D- cells, the sites upon which, range from 110,000-202,000 (Hughes-Jones *et al.* (1971)). The position of the antigen sites as well as their number is likely to be important. There is evidence that group A antigen sites protrude from the cell surface whereas at least some Rh antigen sites are in crypts.

However, IgG antibodies are highly effective agglutinators provided steps are taken to reduce the distance between individual cells. Normally red cells have a negative charge on their surface which keeps them apart and they are also surrounded by a cloud of charged particles. The capacity of the medium therefore to dissipate electric charge, *i.e.* its dielectric constant is thought to play a part in allowing the cells to aggregate to the point where agglutination of the cells by incomplete IgG antibodies can take place. Various colloids, among which bovine albumin is the most commonly used, are effective in increasing the dielectric constant of the medium thus reducing the electric repulsion between the cells (Pollack, 1965).

Enzymes are believed to be effective because they lower the negative surface charge and thus the zeta potential on the red cell by removing sialic acid. They may also remove certain structures (*e.g.* polypeptides) from the red-cell surface so that the accessibility of antigen sites is improved although others are removed *e.g.* Fy^a, M and N.

Recent work, however, has shown that these generally accepted views of the role of albumin and enzymes in promoting agglutination of cells by IgG incomplete antibodies may require modification. For example, although the enzyme neuraminidase is as efficient in reducing the net surface charge on red cells, as is papain, titres of incomplete Rh antibodies with neuraminidase-treated cells are far less than those with papain-treated cells (Stratton *et al.*, 1973). The fact that papain, being a protease, removes polypeptides as well as sialic acid groups from the red-cell surface may be of significance particularly if some blood group antigen sites are situated some distance below the surface of the red cell. Voak *et al.* (1974) have shown by means of electron microscope studies with D and anti-D that enzymes bring about clustering of the D-antigen sites which they consider is important in providing conditions for more antibody bridging than would take place with a non-clustered distribution of sites. In the same studies, these workers found that albumin does not increase site density but has the effect of increasing areas of cell-to-cell contact, which may be caused by adsorption between adjacent cells rather than by any reduction in zeta potential.

The antigen-antibody reaction

Before an antigen-antibody reaction occurs a bond must be formed between the antibody combining site and its corresponding antigenic determinant after which the reaction may become visible, *e.g.* as agglutination of cells.

Whether an antigen and its corresponding antibody meet is a chance affair but can be assisted in various ways. Agitation of the reacting mixture or centrifugation increases the likelihood of antigen and antibody coming into contact and obviously the process will be affected by the concentration of the reactants. Also, an antibody molecule when faced with an antigenic determinant must enter into a suitable spatial relationship with it before bonding can occur. Also, the complementarity or goodness of fit between antigen and antibody is important because antigens and antibodies do not form covalent bonds and the forces holding an antigen-antibody complex together are short range and relatively weak. This means that the antigen and corresponding antibody must be capable of achieving close proximity for the successful operation of such short range forces.

The antigen-antibody reaction is reversible and antigens and corresponding antibodies maintain a state of dynamic equilibrium in which random bonding is constantly made and broken. However at equilibrium, the relative concentration of reactants and products remain constant.

The whole process can be expressed in terms of a reversible reaction according to the following equation (Hughes-Jones, 1963):-

$$Ag + Ab \underset{k_2}{\overset{k_1}{\rightleftharpoons}} AgAb$$

where Ag = antigen, Ab = antibody, AgAb = antigen-antibody complex, k_1 = association constant, k_2 = dissociation constant.

By applying the law of mass action, the following equation is obtained:-

$$\frac{(AbAg)}{(Ab) \times (Ag)} = \frac{k_1}{k_2} = K$$

where (Ab), (Ag) and (AbAg) represent the concentrations of reactants and products and K is the equilibrium or combining constant.
Therefore at equilibrium:-

$$\frac{(AbAg)eq}{(Ab)eq} = K\,(Ag)eq$$

In blood grouping terms this means that the amount of antigen, *i.e.* the red cell concentration including the number of antigen sites per cell and the concentration of antibody will affect the uptake of antibody by the cells, which in turn will influence the degree of agglutination.

Thus, the equation may be used as a guide for finding the optimum conditions for particular purposes. For the maximum uptake of antibody, antigen excess is required *i.e.* an excess of red cells over antibody. These conditions are ideal for the inhibition test or when it is desired to remove unwanted antibodies from a serum. However, if a high degree of sensitivity is required in terms of agglutination, excess red cells are undesirable because too few antibody molecules combine with each cell. In this case antibody excess is the goal and this is achieved by altering the ratio of serum to cells. Maximum sensitivity is probably acquired by using 5 ml antibody to 5 μl of red cells but this is rarely practical. Increase in sensitivity may be attained by using very weak red cell suspension (*see* Chapter 29 in which is described a micro-elution technique for the detection of eluted antibodies).

The equilibrium constant (K) may be regarded as a measure of the goodness of fit between antigen and antibody and when this is high the bonds between the two will be difficult to break. Very different equilibrium constants are found for various examples of antibodies even of the same specificity and such differences are reflected in the variation in avidity displayed by antibodies. Clinically, it is the high K antibodies that are the most important as these do most damage to red cells *in vivo*.

Most sera are heterogeneous with regard to the combining constant of the antibodies they contain and any measurement of K is an average for a whole spectrum of antibodies with differing combining capacities.

The effect of ionic strength on antigen-antibody reaction
Lowering the ionic strength of the medium is remarkably effective in speeding up the rate of association between antibody and antigen and increasing the value of K. Normally when agglutination reactions are carried out in isotonic saline, the sodium ions accumulate around the negatively charged antigen while the negatively charged chloride ions form a cloud round the positively charged antibody thus partially neutralising the two opposing charges on the antigen and antibody. Removal of some of these ions exposes the charges on the antigen and antibody and they combine more effectively. For example, for anti-D the rate of association between antigen and antibody is almost 1000 times greater at 0.03 M than at 0.17 M concentration of NaCl. In practice, care has to be exercised when using a medium of low ionic strength that non-specific uptake of antibody onto red cells does not occur. However Löw and Messeter (1974) recommend a low

ionic strength of NaCl with glycine of molarity 0.03 which appears to be successful and specific.

The effect of temperature on agglutination of red cells

The effect of temperature upon agglutination cannot be discussed without reference to the type of antibody which is taking part in any particular agglutination reaction. In this context antibodies fall into two broad categories, "cold" and "warm" according to whether their optimum temperature of reactivity is at 4°C or at 37°C. The so-called naturally occurring antibodies are usually of the "cold" type while those traceable to production by an antigenic stimulus are "warm". The main difference between them is that while temperature has little or no effect upon the equilibrium constant of warm antibodies, it has considerable effect upon the equilibrium constant of cold antibodies.

Naturally occurring anti-A and anti-B react most strongly in the cold and their titre at 0°C may be about 8 times higher than at 37°C. After stimulation by the corresponding antigen "immune" anti-A and anti-B antibodies are formed. These are mainly IgG but may include IgM. Voak *et al.* (1973) present evidence that immune IgG anti-A shows equal activity at 4°C and 37°C.

In the case of those "warm" antibodies which have been studied in detail *e.g.* anti-D and anti-c, the effect of temperature seems to be mainly upon the rate of the reaction rather than upon the equilibrium constant (K) even though the antigen-antibody reaction is an exothermic one. For example, lowering the temperature from 37°C to 4°C while scarcely increasing the equilibrium constant, slows by approximately twenty-fold the rate at which the antigen and antibody combine and reach equilibrium (Hughes-Jones *et al.,* 1964). Therefore in laboratory practice Rh antibodies are tested at 37°C while tests with anti-A and anti-B are left at laboratory temperature. In general, incubation at 4°C is avoided since at this temperature unwanted "cold" reactions may occur.

Many naturally occurring "cold" antibodies fail to agglutinate red cells at all above 20-25°C, often their threshold is lower than this. This means that unlike the "warm" antibodies discussed above, temperature has a marked effect upon their equilibrium constants since an increase in temperature favours dissociation (k_2) between antigen and antibody to a point on the temperature scale when K is zero and no antigen-antibody complexes are formed. Anti-M, anti--N, anti-P_1 are typical examples of such "cold" antibodies.

Certain sera containing cold antibodies, although incapable of agglutinating red cells above 25°C to 30°C, have an antibody population which is able to sensitise cells at 37°C as can be shown by performing an anti-globulin test. Anti-P_1 if potent, and most anti-$Le^{a'}$ antibodies have this ability.

Cold antibodies of blood group specificity have little or no clinical effect with the exception of those described above which are capable of sensitising red cells at 37°C. These antibodies are discussed again later in connection with blood transfusion.

Haemolysis

Antibodies with haemolytic properties are common within the ABO, Lewis, P and Ii systems. Occasionally, anti-Jk^a (of the Kidd system) will haemolyse cells although with enzyme-treated cells (see below) it will regularly do so. The haemolytic phenomenon requires complement but not in every case when complement is bound to the red cell does haemolysis occur. This is particularly true if the antibody is not very potent.

When enzyme-treated cells are used, the haemolytic properties of such antibodies which have them, are considerably increased. In fact, many examples of such antibodies may produce no haemolysis of untreated cells but will readily haemolyse enzyme-treated cells.

Antibodies producing rapid haemolysis *in vitro* have considerable clinical significance because they usually produce rapid intravascular lysis *in vivo*. In the ABO system, probably all examples of anti-A and anti-B can be induced to produce some degree of haemolysis of the appropriate cells if the optimum proportion of serum to cells is found: a ratio as high as 80 parts of serum to one of packed cells may be necessary. The clinically significant anti-A and anti-B haemolysins however are those which are found in individuals who have been immunised by A or B antigens. Their titres however are never as high as the corresponding agglutinin titres of the same sera, and are of the order of 2-32; usually they can be detected using equal amounts of serum and a 2-5 per cent cell suspension.

In investigating a suspected incompatible transfusion, haemolysis by the patient's serum of A and/or B red cells is a pointer to an incompatibility within the ABO system. In circumstances (which should be few!) in which group O blood has to be used for transfusion to patients of other ABO groups, a screening test for haemolytic anti-A and anti-B in the donor is often used for the detection of dangerous universal donors although there are alternative methods such as the use of subgroup A$_x$ cells.

A haemolysin test is also invaluable in establishing whether or not an infant is suffering from ABO haemolytic disease. Absence of haemolysis between the mother's serum and infant's red cells almost certainly excludes this diagnosis.

Antibodies do not have to exhibit haemolytic properties in vitro in order to qualify as clinically important. Anti-D for the Rh system used to account for 95 per cent of the cases of haemolytic disease of the newborn yet only one anti-D has been described which showed haemolysis *in vitro*! As a general rule (although there are exceptions) an antibody which gives haemolysis *in vitro* will cause intra-vascular haemolysis *in vivo,* while with one which does not, *e.g.* Rh, the haemolysis will be mainly extravascular.

Complement

The term complement refers to a complex system of factors (some of them enzymes), present in normal serum which interacts with antibodies and other factors to play an important part in immune reactions.

Complement was first recognised as a heat-labile serum factor which was essential for the lysis of antibodies of red cells and some bacteria. It was found that heating a serum to 56°C for 30 minutes destroyed complement activity and

F

although the lytic antibodies were still capable of sensitising the cells no lysis occurred.

It soon became apparent that complement was more than a single substance as several fractions of serum were required for the haemolytic activity of complement to be effective. Complement is now considered to be composed of 11 proteins labelled C1-9 of which C1 has three components, C1q, C1r and C1s (for a review *see* Mayer, 1973).

The function of complement is the destruction of foreign cells but it is normally unable to attack such cells until they have become sensitised by the appropriate antibody and thus labelled as foreign.

When complement is activated by antibody it threatens the destruction not only of invading micro-organisms but of the hosts own cells. It is perhaps for the purpose of regulating complement activity that the complicated stepwise activation of complement operates. Complement activity is also limited by spontaneous decay and by inhibitor enzymes.

It is possible that the change in shape of the antibody molecule when it combines with the antigen may trigger off the complement sequence or the siting of two antibody molecules on adjacent antigenic determinants. Thereafter, the complement components act sequentially except that C4 reacts between C1 and C2 (after a component is activated it is usual to represent the number with a bar above it). $\overline{C14}$ in the presence of Mg^{++} activates C2 and the complex $\overline{C42}$ acts upon C3 after which the C3 molecule is split into two fragments (not shown in Fig. 15.3) C3a and C3b. C3b by a series of processes becomes converted to C3c and C3d. $\overline{C423}$ activates the complex $\overline{C567}$ which becomes attached to the cell surface and binds C8. C8 is capable of causing slow haemolysis but the reaction is enhanced by C9.

If the antigen taking part is situated on a red cell (*e.g.* blood group antigen A with anti-A haemolysin attached) the bonding of the last two components in the sequence produces holes in the cell membrane and haemolysis occurs. In effect therefore it is the complement rather than the sensitising antibody which finally causes haemolysis of the cells.

The reaction of the complement sequence is not equimolecular. One molecule of activated C1 is able to convert many C4 molecules and similarly one activated C42 complex can bind more than 100 C3 molecules. This amplification explains the greater sensitivity of the anti-globulin reaction when complement-binding antibodies are being detected by an anti-complement globulin.

Many of the complement components have now been isolated and characterised beginning with the identification of C3 as β_{1C} globulin (Müller-Eberhard and Nilsson, 1960). Others have been characterised as follows:- $C4 = \beta_{1E}$ $C3c = \beta_{1A}$ and $C3d = \alpha_{2D}$.

When red cells are treated *in vitro* with a complement-binding antibody such as anti-Le^a both β_{1A}, β_{1E} and α_{2D} can be demonstrated on the cell surface but on the cells of patients with auto-immune haemolytic anaemia of the cold type, (sometimes called cold agglutinin disease), only α_{2D} can be demonstrated. It is important therefore that the anti-globulin reagent used in such cases should contain an anti-α_{2D} component.

Table 15.2 Reactions of red cells coated with complement and complement components and various antibodies in the antiglobulin test

Anti-globulin sera	Test cells[a]						
	EC	EHC	EC4 (Anti-I)	EC3	CAHA	ELe^{a}C	EKC
Anti-complement	+++++	+++++	+++++	+++	+++++	+++++	+++++
Anti-C4 (anti-β_{1E})	+++++	+++++	+++	-	-	+++++	+++++
Anti-C3c (anti-β_{1A})	+++++	+	-	+++++	-	+++++	+++
Anti-C3D (anti-α_{2D})	+++	++	-	-	+++++	+++++	+++
Anti-C5	-	-	-	-	+	+++	+
Anti-IgM	-	-	-	-	-	-	-
Anti-IgA	-	-	-	-	-	-	-
Anti-IgG	-	-	-	-	-	-	+++++

aTest cells coated with:-EC complement; EHC incomplete anti-H; EC4 anti-I; EC3 third complement component; CAHA antibody from cold acquired haemolytic anaemia; ELe^{a}C Anti-Le^a; EKC anti-Kell.

Table 15.2 adapted from Stratton and Rawlinson (1974) shows the reaction of test cells coated with complement and various complement components in anti-globulin tests. Also shown are the reactions of variously coated cells with anti-IgM—IgA—IgG reagents.

The preparation of cells coated with the appropriate complement components and antibodies is described in Chapter 27.

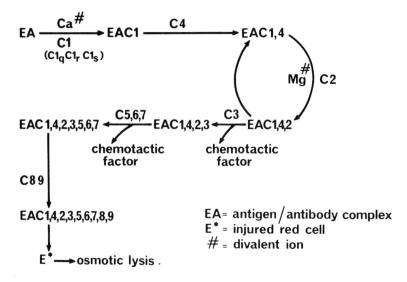

Fig. 15.3 The sequential activity of complement.

Figure 15.3 summarises what has come to be called the classical pathway for the activation of complement, but more recent work has shown that there exists an alternative pathway. This process does not involve C1, C4 or C2 and requires only Mg^{++} and not Ca^{++}. Nor does it apparently require an antigen-antibody complex to trigger off the mechanism. Zymosan and inulin have been found to be activating agents and aggregates of various classes of immunoglobulin (*e.g.* complexes of IgA) which fail to activate the classical pathway do activate the alternative pathway.

The alternative pathway has little relevance for blood group serology. A detailed account may be found in Lachmann (1975).

The reasons why some blood group antibodies activate complement while others do not is not fully understood, nor why, some antibody-complement complexes are more efficient in causing haemolysis than others.

There are some strong clues. For example, there is evidence that while a single IgM molecule attached to a red cell can activate complement, it requires two *adjacent* molecules of IgG. It has been calculated that if there are 600,000 sites of a particular antigen on the surface of the cell, 1000 IgG molecules must be attached to provide an even chance that somewhere on the surface there will be two molecules occupying adjacent sites (Humphrey and Dourmashkin, 1965). Thus it appears that the number of antigen sites on the red cell for a particular antigen and the distance between them must have considerable influence on complement activation.

Scarcity of antigen sites may explain the failure of D antibodies to activate complement. This may also explain the failure of even IgM anti-D to bind complement since it would seem that although a single IgM molecule is capable of activating complement it has to combine with more than one antigen site in order to do this (Ishizaka, *et al.,* 1968).

Additional evidence that the number of antigen sites may play a part in complement fixation is obtained from the experiments of Rosse (1968), who treated red cells with IgG Rh antibodies of three different specificities *e.g.* anti-c, anti-D and anti-e simultaneously and found complement ($C\overline{1}$) was thereby fixed.

The number and distribution of antigen sites do not wholly determine complement activation since there is variation in behaviour of the antibodies themselves. One example of IgG anti-Kell, for instance, will fix complement whereas with the same sample of red cells another anti-Kell may fail to do so.

Although in blood group reactions complement is incapable of becoming attached to the red cell without the intermediary of a complement-fixing antibody, it is often found that the antibody can be eluted from the cell while the complement remains attached.

Red cells sensitised *in vivo* by complement-fixing antibodies whether destroyed intravascularly or extravascularly are cleared by the liver whereas red cells sensitised *in vivo* by non-complement fixing antibodies are removed predominantly by the spleen.

Inactivation of complement

Complement activity is reduced on storage. Polley and Mollison (1961) found that serum stored at $4°C$ for 24 hours or 2 months at $-50°C$ was as effective as fresh serum. Storage at $-20°C$ for one month did not reduce the activity appreciably but after longer periods at $4°C$ and at $-20°C$ complement deteriorates and may have to be supplied from other sources if it is to be effective in causing haemolysis.

As well as being inactivated by heating serum at $56°C$ for 30 minutes, complement activity is prevented by the presence of ethylene-diamino tetra-acetic acid (EDTA) or indeed any other chelator of Ca^{++} and Mg^{++} which are required for the activation of the C1 and C2 complement components (Fig. 15.3).

Heparin is also anti-complementary but is required in large amounts to be completely effective.

Zymosan and inulin inactivate components required for the later stages of complement activation and are sometimes used for sensitising cells with a powerful haemolytic antibody, while preventing actual haemolysis.

In stored sera, C1 molecules become denatured and although complement binding antibodies can bind the denatured C1, the attachment of C4 is prevented and thus subsequent complexes, $C\overline{142}$ or $C\overline{1423}$ cannot be formed. This has an effect upon the strength of reaction obtained when blood group antibodies which bind complement are being detected by means of an anti-complement ahg reagent. It is in this situation that EDTA is useful because it can be used to prevent the uptake of altered C1. Thus in tests using anti-complement globulin for the detection of blood group antibodies a two-stage test may be performed in which complement is first inactivated with EDTA and then fresh complement is added before proceeding with the anti-globulin test (*see* technique No. 13.9).

The Immune Response

In this section a general account of the immune process is given beginning with its cellular aspects. Since our interest is in the production of blood group antibodies our illustrations are drawn mainly from blood group antigen-antibody phenomena.

The classical "instructive theory" of the way animals (including Man) synthesise antibodies has given way to the "selective theory". The older idea postulated that the antigen acted instructively as a template around which a γ-globulin chain could be shaped to make it complementary to the antigen. On separation from the template the molecule would have a specific combining site for the antigen.

This old idea that the antigen acts as a template for antibody formation is not substantiated by experimental findings. For example, it has been shown using auto-radiography and immunofluorescence that cells containing intracellular antibody do not have demonstrable antigen molecules. Amino acid analysis of a variety of purified myeloma proteins which represent individual immunoglobulin molecules has shown that within an immunoglobulin class the N-terminal portion of both heavy and light chains shows considerable variation while the remaining parts of the chains are relatively constant in structure. Within these variable regions on both heavy and light chains there are areas of hyper-variability (Kabat and Wu, 1972) and these areas are believed to form the antigen binding site their amino acid heterogeneity making them particularly able to cope with a variety of antigenic determinants.

Thus, present theory favours the view that the information required for the synthesis of different antibodies is already present in the antibody-producing cells and is under genetic control.

Genetic studies in mice have shown that animals of one strain may respond well to one particular antigen but poorly to another showing that the ability of a given strain to give a good or poor response is not a general one but varies from antigen to antigen.

There are two types of immune response to an antigen. 1. The synthesis and release of antibody into the blood stream. 2. Cell-mediated immunity resulting in graft rejection and delayed hyper-sensitivity.

In studying what happens in individuals stimulated by blood group antigens we are concerned with the type-1 effect.

The cellular aspects of the immune response

Small lymphocytes are of major importance in initiating antibody production and there are two populations of lymphocytes concerned. Both are derived from bone-marrow stem cells but one population, the T lymphocytes are processed through the thymus while the other "Bursa processed" or B lymphocytes are probably developed through gut lymphoid tissue and/or haemopoietic tissue.

Both populations proliferate when stimulated by antigen and show morphological changes. The B lymphocytes develop into the plasma cell series which synthesise and secrete antibodies. However they often seem to require the co-operation of T lymphocytes which do not themselves synthesise antibodies but function as antigen carriers presenting the antigenic determinant to the B lymphocyte, particularly when the antigen is small.

The modern view, the clonal selection model, is that each B lymphocyte is genetically geared to make one particular antibody and molecules of this antibody are built into the cell surface as receptors. Different lymphocytes have different antibodies, so between the many body lymphocytes there exists a large potential for the production of a wide spectrum of specificities. An antigen will combine with those lymphocytes which have the best-fitting antibody. This provides the stimulus for cell division and the formation of clones of daughter cells each producing the same antibody as the parent cell.

The response to the first encounter with an antigen is termed the primary response and usually only gives rise to a small amount of circulating antibody after considerable delay. Indeed it is not uncommon for the process to halt at the point of clone production. Cells which have formed clones but have not finally matured are known as "primed" cells. This type of immune response is seen in Rh-immunisation.

When a second dose of antigen is given there is a secondary response which manifests itself in high levels of antibody in the serum which reaches a peak a few weeks after the secondary stimulus (see Fig. 15.4). The nature of the antibody population changes. The first antibodies initiated by the primary response are predominantly IgM while after the secondary response IgG takes over and the combining constant (K) increases through greater complementarity between antigen and antibody.

The ease with which a second dose of antigen evokes a brisk response is partly due to the fact that after the primary stimulus some plasma cells revert to small lymphocytes and act as memory cells. These memory cells take part in the secondary response and together with primed cells initiate rapid antibody production.

Cross reactivity

Antibodies stimulated by a given antigen can sometimes cross react with a related antigen which possesses one or more identical or similar determinants. The avidity of the antibody for the related antigen is usually less than it is for the antigen affording the primary stimulus. It binds less strongly because it fits less well. Cross reactivity is more likely to occur when the immunisation process has been continuing for some time because this gives maximum opportunity for weaker antigenic determinants shared by related antigens to bring about an antibody response.

The most studied among blood group antibodies of those which cross react are found in group O sera (see Chapter 16). Such sera, particularly after an immune response to the A or B antigens has taken place contain antibodies cross reacting with both A and B antigens.

Other cross reacting antibodies are seen in the Rh system in the sera of individuals of genotype –D–. These people often make antibodies cross reacting with both C and c antigen and also E and e.

Suppression of the immune response

Antibody production is almost certainly controlled by a feed back mechanism *i.e.* the amount of antibody produced moderates the production rate. The control is probably effected by competition for the available antigen between circulating antibody and the antigen receptor sites on the antibody producing plasma cells, the latter obtaining a progressively smaller share of the antigen.

There is considerable evidence that T-lymphocytes may as well as co-operating in antibody formation, play a part in suppressing B cell activity (Allison, 1973). By passive administration of sufficient antibody at the same time as the primary dose of antigen, suppression of the primary response may be achieved, but giving small amounts of antibody may enhance the response. The prevention of Rh sensitisation by giving anti-D to mothers at risk (*see* Chapter 26) is a good example of suppression. Presumably the anti-D removes D positive cells from the maternal circulation before they have time to activate antigen sensitive cells.

A natural suppression of the immune response occurs during foetal life and enables the organism to recognise cells which might otherwise be antigenic as 'self'. It is thought that the lymphoid cells while in an immunologically immature stage are prevented by the individual's own potential antigens from ever producing auto-antibodies. Chimera twins are excellent examples of tolerance acquired before birth. This phenomenon was first described by Owen in 1945 when investigating the vascular anastomoses which are common between dissimilar bovine twin embryos. Primitive cells of one twin take root in the other, and continue to produce red cells of the genotype of the original donor, which are tolerated by the host as readily as the host's own cells.

Dunsford *et al.* (1953) found a similar state of affairs in human twin embryos. For example a twin who was genetically of group O was found to have grafted A cells and moreover lacked anti-A presumably through exposure to the A antigen during foetal life (see also chapter 28).

Tolerance can also be induced in adults under certain circumstances particularly when very large doses of antigen are given.

The Immune Response to Blood Group Antigens

The most important antigens to be considered are those of the ABO and Rh systems since these have most clinical significance. Rh makes a better starting point since the existence of so-called naturally occurring anti-A and anti-B makes the immune response due to the A and B antigens a rather special case.

Rh immunisation by transfusion or injection of red cells

The above description of the immune process applies in general to Rh immunisation. The initial challenge by the antigen in the form of a large single unit (500 ml) of Rh positive blood is likely to induce antibody formation in at least 50 per cent of cases at varying periods between 2 and 6 months. For example Pollack *et al.* (1971) gave 22 Rh-negative volunteers 500 ml of Rh positive blood;

18 responded with the formation of antibodies although in several recipients they took 3 to 5 months to develop.

Even if Rh antibodies fail to appear following a first dose of antigen, the individual can be shown to be primed. This is sometimes seen when Rh negative women inadvertently transfused with Rh positive blood do not show detectable antibodies following the transfusion and yet have a first Rh positive child affected with haemolytic disease.

The amount of antigen injected influences the response, and also probably the Rh phenotype of the red cells providing the antigenic stimulus. Experience based on many deliberate immunisation experiments of Rh negative volunteers suggests that it is not necessarily the large doses of antigen that illicit the best responses.

Sometimes when *in vitro* tests fail to reveal the presence of antibodies evidence of immunisation can be obtained *in vivo* by observing the rapid elimination from the circulation of suitably labelled Rh positive cells. This is usually followed at a later date by the formation of antibodies.

Non-responders. It would appear that some people are naturally "non-responders". About one-third of Rh negative individuals appear to be incapable of forming Rh antibodies.

Fletcher *et al.* (1971) report a series of 124 Rh negative male volunteers who were given an initial dose of 5-10 ml of R_2r blood followed by 1-5 ml doses at 5 weekly intervals until Rh antibodies appeared. After periods of time varying between about 10 weeks (one subject) and 18 months, 63.4 per cent of the volunteers formed detectable antibodies. Two more individuals first developed detectable antibodies at 2-2½ years. A further series of 86 subjects given a larger initial dose of 40 ml of R_2r blood followed by 5-ml doses every 3 months achieved detectable antibodies by 18 months in 72.8 per cent of cases.

A point of interest is that if radio-active labelled red cells are injected it can be shown that all those individuals who will subsequently form detectable antibodies show diminished red cell survival after the second injection of Rh positive cells while those whose second injection of Rh positive cells survives normally, never do so (Woodrow *et al.,* 1969).

Not all responders are equally ready responders. A few are 'poor responders' who require more than the usual number of doses of antigen before their response becomes apparent.

Whether or not an individual is capable of antibody formation is almost certainly at least partially under genetic control.

Rh immunisation due to pregnancy

This is a natural method of immunisation in contrast to deliberate injection of red cells or inadvertent incompatible transfusion. In the majority of cases in which Rh immunisation has taken place the mother is D negative and the antibody is anti-D, the stimulus being a foetus with the D antigen inherited from the father.

The primary challenge which does not usually illicit an antibody response may be provided by small bleeds from foetus to mother during the first pregnancy in which the foetus is D positive. It would seem however that these small bleeds are insufficient for antibody production since Rh antibodies are seen in the maternal circulation in only about 2 per cent of cases at the end of a first pregnancy with an ABO compatible Rh positive foetus.

The transplacental haemorrhage which contributes most to the formation of antibodies is that which occurs during normal delivery at which time the amount of foetal blood entering the maternal circulation varies between a trace to 10 ml or more. Amniocentesis, Caesarean section and manual removal of the placenta increase the risk of appreciable leakage of foetal cells into the maternal circulation, as do stillbirth, spontaneous miscarriage and 'D and C.'

Within 6 months after delivery about 7 per cent of those Rh negative women have detectable antibodies there being a relationship between the number of foetal red cells in the mother's circulation at delivery and the chance of the appearance of an antibody.

When pregnancy with a second Rh positive infant happens, provided the infant is ABO compatible with the mother (*see below*) about 17 per cent of women form antibodies by the end of this pregnancy, the antibodies often being detectable by the fifth month (Woodrow and Donohoe, 1968). Figure 15.4 illustrates some of these points.

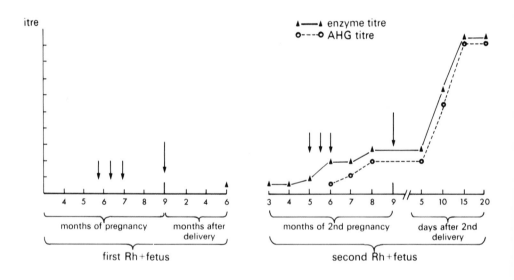

Fig. 15.4 Immune response to the first and second Rh-positive foetus.

During the months preceding delivery of a first Rh positive foetus there may be small bleeds of foetal cells into the maternal circulation (indicated by short arrows in Fig. 15.4). These are evidently sub-minimal doses of antigen since they fail to illicit a detectable immune response. The main primary stimulus (indicated by long arrows) is the trans-placental haemorrhage occuring at delivery of the Rh-positive infant. The case illustrated is one of those where a small amount of antibody is detectable by an enzyme technique at about 6 months after delivery.

During the second pregnancy, also with an Rh positive foetus, small bleeds of foetal cells into the mother occur but this time, since they are secondary doses of antigen they are able to initiate the production of antibodies in the maternal serum.

These antibodies are shown increasing in concentration towards the end of pregnancy and becoming detectable by anti-globulin as well as enzyme technique. The peak of the immune response is shown occurring 10-15 days following delivery.

The influence of ABO incompatibility on Rh immunisation

If Rh positive cells of incompatbile ABO group are given to Rh negative individuals, formation of Rh antibodies is less likely to occur than when the Rh positive cells are ABO compatible. The reason for this at the moment seems to be obscure, although several explanations have been suggested. The fact that ABO antibody forming cells are already well-established and able to take up the A antigen whereas the Rh must start *de novo* may be the key to the partial protection affected by ABO incompatibility. Also anti-A and anti-B lysins may play a part.

Similarly, immunisation due to Rh through pregnancy is less common when the foetus is ABO incompatible with the mother. Although once the mother does become immunised to the Rh antigen further ABO incompatible infants in the family are not protected. The protection is greater where group O women have either A or B children than where for example group A women have group B children and most protection is afforded by the combination O mother with A child. It may be relevant to note (*see below*) that group O individuals are capable of becoming more highly immune to incompatible ABO antigens than those of groups A or B.

The pattern of Rh immune response and the immunoglobulin types produced

A manual enzyme technique, particularly papain or an Auto Analyser system, will often reveal the presence of Rh antibodies at an earlier time following stimulation than any other method, even anti-globulin. This is not only because the technique has greater sensitivity, but because there are low affinity Rh antibodies which exist in both IgM and IgG classes, which when present even in appreciable concentration fail to be detected by anti-human globulin (although a few of them are detectable by albumin) but are detectable by enzyme techniques.

As the immune response develops these antibodies are followed by others which are commonly IgG of the incomplete type. Much less often IgM antibodies of the complete type *i.e.* capable of agglutinating red cells suspended in saline, are found. Occasionally Rh antibodies appear in the IgA fraction.

The development of Rh antibodies during pregnancy in a particular case between 18 and 38 weeks is shown in Table 15.3. At 18 weeks the precursor antibody predominates. At 31 weeks the antibody is detectable by all techniques and by the end of pregnancy agglutinins are established, and there has been a steady rise in titre of incomplete antibodies.

Increase in the immune response in general leads to greater potency of incomplete IgG antibodies with increase in antibody binding constant (K)

Table 15.3 Development in an Rh negative woman of an immune response to an Rh positive fetus

Titration technique	Weeks of pregnancy					
	18	31	33	35	37	38
Papain	128	512	2000	64,000	64,000	128,000
Trypsin	1	64	128	128	256	256
Albumin	2	16	128	128	256	256
Anti-human globulin	0	128	256	2000	1000	1000
Saline	0	4	0	64	64	64

resulting in antibodies which are clinically more damaging. After delivery, the titre of incomplete antibodies often continues to increase (*see* Fig. 15.4) before a levelling off after which the titres may be maintained at a high level for many months or even years.

Indeed Rh antibodies can be found persisting in the serum for a long time even many years after the last known stimulus. Again such antibodies are usually more readily detectable by an enzyme technique; it is unusual, although not entirely unknown, for Rh agglutinins to persist for long periods.

Immune responses to Rh antigens other than D and to antigens of other systems

Antibodies to Rh antigens other than D are less common but when they do occur they may have considerable clinical significance.

Deliberate intravenous injections or transfusions of blood containing the appropriate antigen have not been conspicuously successful. Thus, among 74 C negative, D negative patients transfused with one or more units of C positive, D negative blood, only 2 developed anti-C. Moreover, not one of 66 C negative D positive patients in the same series formed anti-C (Schorr *et al.*, 1971). The response to c appears to be slightly more readily invoked. Jones *et al.* (1954) produced anti-c in two out of 9 volunteers given repeated injections of c positive blood throughout a period of 10 months. The same workers attempted to produce anti-e in a volunteer lacking antigen e and after 6 years anti-e was found for the first time! However (*see* Chapter 27) anti-e is an antibody not infrequently found as an auto-antibody in patients with auto-immune disease who are themselves e positive.

The frequency with which an antigen occurs in the population will of course influence the frequency of finding the corresponding antibody. When the antigen is common, there are fewer opportunities for the antibody to be produced except as an auto-antibody.

A valuable survey by Giblett (1964) reveals the relative frequency of occurrence of various antibodies when the stimulating antigen was provided by a foetus *in utero*.

Anti-D has been shown to be outstandingly the most commonly produced antibody. In Giblett's series of 2024 cases in which incomplete antibodies were identified, 94.7 per cent of the antibodies were anti-D or anti-CD. Other Rh antibodies were anti-c 1.3 per cent anti-E 2.0 per cent and anti-Ce 0.2 per cent. Antibodies belonging to their blood group systems were found in 1.8 per cent of cases which included 1.4 per cent of cases of anti-Kell. It follows that other immune antibodies active at 37°C are but rarely encountered; however, when they are, they are every whit as important clinically as anti-D, since many of them have caused haemolytic disease of the newborn and all of them are potential causes of incompatible transfusions.

Immunisation to the A and B antigens

In the ABO system in contrast to Rh, the antibodies anti-A and anti-B are regularly present in the serum of individuals lacking the corresponding antigen so their mere presence does not prove that an immune response has occurred.

A popular view is that natural anti-A and anti-B antibodies are in fact immune since A, B and H blood group substances are widely distributed in nature and so frequently present in bacteria, diet, gut flora, dust particles, etc. that all individuals are likely to be exposed to these antigens from birth onwards and could therefore become immunised in this way. Support for this theory comes from the fact that most infants do not synthesise their own anti-A and anti-B until 3-6 months after birth. Moreover Springer *et al.* (1959) have shown that chicks which regularly form anti-blood group B antibodies, do not do so if kept in a germ-free condition. Feeding group B antigens in the form of B-active *Escherichia coli* 086 produced high titres of anti-B in the germ free chicks. Springer and Horton (1969) went further and fed blood group active *E.coli* to babies between the ages of 2 weeks and 9 months and showed the development of anti-B and to a lesser extent of anti-A by this experiment.

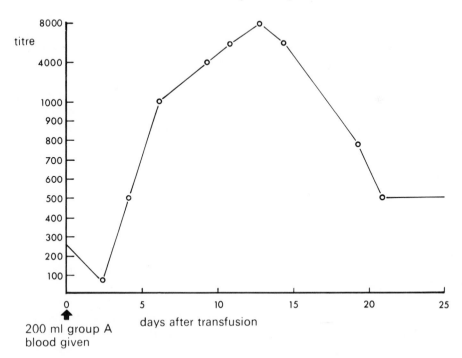

Fig. 15.5 Changes in titre following incompatible transfusion of group A blood to group O recipient

Nevertheless even if so-called naturally occurring anti-A and anti-B antibodies are produced after a challenge by commonly distributed A and B antigens, there is no doubt that a brisk immune response takes place if the individual receives a well-defined stimulus afforded either by the injection of red cells, a foetus *in utero* or particularly by giving purified soluble A or B substances. Some of the characteristics of such an immune response are shown in Fig. 15.5. This followed the inadvertant transfusion of one unit of incompatible blood. It is interesting to note that there was sufficient antigen circulating to absorb the antibody and cause a negative phase before the immune response started, the incompatible anti-A agglutinin titre actually showing a fall compared with the pre-stimulation level. Titration of agglutinins at intervals following the stimulus shows a steady increase to a peak after a period of 10-14 days followed by a slow decline.

Such immune responses result in a proliferation of IgG incomplete antibodies which are not always easy to demonstrate by titration since their presence is liable to be masked by the agglutinins. Also some IgG anti-A or anti-B themselves behave as agglutinins and add to the value of the agglutinin titre. However titration values as measured by anti-globulin or enzyme techniques are frequently several dilutions higher than the agglutinin titres and thus measure the concentration of incomplete antibodies. Nevertheless, differences in titration value do not have to be relied upon to detect IgG incomplete anti-A or anti-B since there are several other ways of disclosing their presence when masked by agglutinins. These methods, which include the "Witebsky" Test, DEAE separation by a batch method or treatment of the serum with 2-mercapto-ethanol are described in Chapter 26, in connection with haemolytic disease of the newborn.

IgM anti-A and anti-B in common with most IgM antibodies are more susceptible to heat than IgG antibodies and treatment at 56°C for 3 hours or a shorter period at higher temperatures markedly diminishes or may abolish completely any IgM activity.

Haemolysins are readily demonstrable in anti-A and anti-B immune sera. Both IgG and IgM anti-A have been shown to have haemolytic properties and to bind complement. IgA anti-A, on the other hand, although produced in response to stimulation fails to haemolyse group-A cells.

The appearance of haemolysins is indicative of a recent stimulation by the corresponding antigen since although non-immune sera may contain weak haemolysins, their presence is usually only demonstrable by very sensitive techniques. A useful distinction between immune and so called naturally occurring anti-A can be made with the red cells of pigs, some of which have A-like antigen, Ap. Ap cells are agglutinated by haemolytic IgM anti-A but not by the IgM anti-A which is naturally occurring. They are also sensitised but not agglutinated by IgG anti-A, and can therefore be agglutinated by anti-globulin reagents (Winstanley et al. 1957, Konugres and Coombs 1958).

It is commonly observed that group O subjects are much more readily immunised to A or B antigens than are subjects of other groups. This may be related to the fact that in group O there is a lack of both A and B antigens, whereas the similarity between the two antigens may act as a restraining influence on immune antibody production when one or other antigen is present.

In immune anti-A and anti-B sera from subjects of groups B and A respectively IgM antibody predominates. The titration values achieved are not so high, suggesting that the immune process does not proceed so far.

An additional account of anti-A and anti-B antibodies, including the antibodies found in group O sera which cross react with A and B red cells and in which immune group O sera are particularly rich, is found in Chapter 16 which takes a further look at the ABO system.

REFERENCES

Allison, A.C. (1973) Interacting of thymus-dependent and bone marrow derived lymphocytes in immunological tolerance. *Proc. Roy. Soc. Med.* **66**, 463.

Burkart, P., Rosenfield, R.E., Hsu, T.C.S., Wong, K.Y., Nusbacher, J., Shaikh, S.H. & Kochwa, S. (1974) Instrumental PVP—Augmented antiglobulin tests. *Vox. Sang.* **26**, 289.

Dunsford, I., Bowley, C.C., Hutchinson, A.M., Thomson, J.S., Sanger, R. & Race, R.R. (1953) A human blood chimaera. *Brit. med. J.,* **ii**, 81.

Economidou, J., Hughes-Jones, N.C. & Gardner, B. (1967) Quantitative measurement concerning A and B antigen sites. *Vox Sang. (Basel),* **12**, 321.

Fletcher, G., Cooke, B.R. & McDowall, J. (1971) Attempts to immunise Rh (D) negative volunteers against the D antigen. *Proc. 2nd Meet. Asian & Pac. Divn. Int. Soc. Haemat.,* Melbourne, p. 69.

Giblett, E.R. (1964) Blood group antibodies causing haemolytic disease of the newborn. *Clin. Obstet. Gynec.* 7, 1044.

Holburn A.M., Cartron J.P., Economidou J., Gardner B., & Hughes-Jones W.C. (1971) Observations on the reactions between D-positive red cells and ^{125}I IgM anti-D molecules and subunits. Immunology **21**, 499.

Holburn A.M. (1973 Quantitative Studies with ^{125}I IgM anti-Le^{a} Immunology **24**, 1019.

Hughes-Jones, N.C., (1963) Nature of the reaction between antigen and antibody. *Brit. med. Bull.* **19**, 171.

Hughes-Jones, N.C., Gardner, B. & Lincoln, P.J. (1971) Observations of the number of available c, D and E antigen sites on red cells. *Vox Sang. (Basel),* **21**, 210.

Hughes-Jones, N.C., Polley, M.J., Telford, R., Gardner, B. & Kleinschmidt, G. (1964) Optimal conditions for detection of blood group antibodies by the antiglobulin test. *Vox Sang. (Basel),* **9**, 385.

Humphrey, J.H. & Dourmashkin, R.R. (1965) Electron microscope studies of immune cell lysis in Ciba Foundation Symposium Complement. London: J. & A. Churchill.

Ishizaka, T., Tada, T. & Ishizaka, K. (1968) Fixation of C' and C'1a by rabbit γG and γM antibodies with particular and soluble antigens. *J. Immunol.,* **100**, 1145.

Jones, A.R., Diamond, L.K. & Allen, F.H. Jr. (1954) A decade of progress in the Rh blood group system. *New Engl. J. Med.,* **250**, 283 & 324.

Kabat, E.A. & Wu, T.T. (1972) Construction of a 3-dimensional model of the polypeptide backbone of the variable region of the Kappa immunoglobulin light chains. *Proc. Nat. Acad. Sci.* **69**, 960.

Konugres A.A. & Coombs R.R.A. (1958) Studies on human anti-A sera with special reference to so called immune anti-A. Brit. J. Haemat **4**, 261.

Lachmann, P.J. (1975) Complement. In *Clinical Aspects of Immunology.* 3rd edn., Ch. 14 Oxford: Blackwell.

Löw, B. & Messeter, L. (1974) Antiglobulin test in low-ionic strength salt solution for rapid antibody screening and cross-matching. *Vox Sang.,* **26**, 53.

Mayer M.M. (1973) The Complement System Sci. Amer. Nov. p.54.

Müller-Eberhard, H.J. & Nilsson, U. (1960) Relation of a ß$_1$ glycoprotein of human serum to the complement system. *J. exp. Med.* **iii**, 217.

Owen, R.D. (1945) Immunogenetic consequences of vascular anastomoses between bovine twins. *Science,* **102**, 400.

Pollack, W., Ascari, W.Q., Crispen, J.F., O'Connor, R.R. & Ho, T.Y., (1971) Studies on Rh prophylaxis 11. Rh immune prophylaxis after transfusion with Rh positive blood. *Transfusion (Philad.),* **11**, 333.

Pollack, W. (1965) Some physico-chemical aspects of haemagglutination. *Ann. N.Y. Acad. Sci.,* **127,** 892.

Polley, M.J. & Mollison, P.L. (1961) The role of complement in the detection of blood group antibodies. Special reference to the antiglobulin test. *Transfusion (Philad.),* **1,** 9.

Rosse, W.F. (1968) Fixation of the first component of complement (C'a) by human antibodies. *J. clin. Invest.,* **47,** 2430.

Schorr, J.B., Schorr, P.T., Francis, R., Spierer, G. & Dugan, E. (1971) The antigenicity of C and E antigen when transfused into Rh negative and Rh positive recipients. Cited in Mollison P.L. (1972). *Blood Transfusion in Clinical Medicine.* 5th edn., p. 294. Oxford: Blackwell.

Springer, G.F., & Horton, R.E. (1969) Blood group isoantibody stimulation in man by feeding blood group active bacteria. *J. clin. Invest.,* **48,** 1280.

Springer, G.F., Horton, R.E. & Forbes, M. (1959) Origin of anti-human blood group B agglutinins in white leghorn chicks. *J. exp. Med.,* **110,** 221.

Stratton, F. & Rawlinson, V.I. (1974) Preparation of test cells for the antiglobulin test. *J. clin. Path.,* **27,** 359.

Stratton, F., Rawlinson, V.I., Gunson, H.H. & Phillips, P.K. (1973) The role of zeta-potential in Rh agglutination. *Vox Sang. (Basel),* **24,** 273.

Tiselius, A. & Kabat, E.A. (1939) An electrophoretic study of immune sera and purified antibody preparations. *J. exp. Med.,* **69,** 119.

Voak, D., Abu-Sin, A.Y. & Downie, D.M. (1973) Observations on the thermal optimum, saline agglutinating activity and partial neutralisation characteristics of IgG anti-A antibodies. *Vox Sang. (Basel),* **24,** 246.

Voak, D., Cawley, J.C., Emmines, J.P. & Barker, C.R., (1974) The role of enzymes and albumen in haemagglutination reactions. A serological and ultrastructural study with ferritin-labelled anti-D. *Vox Sang. (Basel),* **27,** 156.

Winstanley D.P., Konugres A.A. & Coombs R.R.A. (1957) Studies on human anti-A sera with special reference to so called "immune" anti-A 1 the A^P antigen and the specificity of the haemolysin in anti-A sera. Brit. J. Haemat. **3,** 341.

Woodrow, J.C. & Donohoe, W.T.A. (1968) Rh-immunisation by pregnancy results of a survey and their relevance to prophylactic therapy. *Brit. med. J.,* **iv,** 139.

Woodrow, J.C., Finn, R., & Koevans, J.R. (1969) Rapid clearance of Rh positive blood during experimental Rh immunisation. *Vox Sang.,* **17,** 349.

Section 2.   An expanded account of individual blood group systems

"Curiouser and curiouser."

Lewis Carroll, THROUGH THE LOOKING GLASS

Chapter 16. A further look at the ABO and Lewis systems

This chapter looks at some of the complexities of a system the investigation of which in the routine laboratory is essentially simple and absolutely basic for clinical work. It is with the ABO system that every beginner starts, yet it is the system which at a deeper level has contributed most to an understanding of the fundamental principles upon which all blood group systems appear to be constructed.

The first section deals with ABO variants, which are mostly quite rare and this is followed by an account of the biochemistry of the ABH blood group substances, which, it is hoped is sufficiently detailed to form a basis for further study of this aspect of the system by those interested in pursuing it.

There follows an account of the antibodies of the ABO system with particular reference to those found in group O sera which cross react with both A and B antigens.

ABO VARIANTS

As early as 1935, ABO variants were beginning to be described and the number found has steadily increased, particularly in the past few years when constant searches through large numbers of blood samples have been rewarded.

The rare variants can be divided on genetic grounds into four categories:

(1) Those resulting from rare alleles occurring at the ABO locus.
(2) Those caused by rare genes modifying in some respect the expression of the common A and B genes.
(3) Cis AB.
(4) ABO variants due to disease.

(1) Rare Alleles

Rare alleles which show an A_3-like agglutination appearance.

A_3. Blood of sub-type A_3 can be recognised by its characteristic appearance

161

after agglutination by anti-A serum (Friedenreich, 1936). An even distribution of small clumps is seen accompanied by large numbers of unagglutinated red cells. One is reminded of the "mixed blood" picture which occurs when, for example, a mixture of group A and group O red cells is treated with anti-A serum. In fact, the suggestion that A_3 blood is in reality a moasaic of A_2 and O has been made; however, the free cells have been shown to take up anti-A and also certain group O (anti-A plus anti-B) sera, exist which can agglutinate all the cells of A_3 people. Moreover, if the free cells are separated from the agglutinated cells and mixed with a further volume of the original anti-A serum, a proportion of them are agglutinated, a "mixed blood" picture almost identical with the original being obtained.

Secretors belonging to sub-group A_3 have A substance in their saliva. A_3 does not usually have anti-A_1. On the other hand, A_3B persons often have anti-A_1 occasionally active at $37°C$ and may have anti-A also, at low temperatures. The conclusion that A_3 is an allele at the ABO locus is in accordance with the results of family studies.

A_{end}. (Weiner et al, 1959; Sturgeon et al., 1964). This very weak A was found in two generations of a family and behaved like a weak A_3. Unlike A_3 the saliva contained H but no A. Several similar families have since been described.

A_{finn}. (Mohn et al., 1973). This weak form of A appears to be distinguished from A_{end} mainly by its weak agglutination reaction being enhanced by enzymes and anti-globulin, particularly when selected potent anti-A sera from both O and B sources are used. However, even though the size of the agglutinates is increased the "mixed cell" appearance of clumps of cells among many free cells, is maintained. This antigen is commoner in Finland than has so far been found elsewhere. An interesting and intensive population study has been recorded by Nevanlinna and Pirkola (1973). A subgroup A_{RV} (Chaves et al. 1975) is now considered by the authors to be an English example of A_{finn}. A comparison with A_{finn} using the same selected high titre antisera shows enhancement of agglutination by enzymes and anti-globulin while maintaining the characteristic "mixed cell" appearance. In spite of the occurrence of many free cells, various experiments have demonstrated that the cells of both A_{finn} and A_{RV} all appear to possess at least some A antigen. The salivas of secretors of both A_{finn} and A_{RV} have H but no A.

A_{bantu} (Brain, 1966). This kind of A occurring in 4 per cent of Bantu A samples, gives an agglutination pattern like A_3, but the saliva of secretors contains H but no A and anti-A_1 is commonly present in the serum.

A_{el}. A rare type of A detectable only by elution.
Reed and Moore (1964) recognised this phenotype in an Italian Canadian donor who presented as apparently group O with a missing anti-A. Her sister was of the same unusual type. The inheritance of this type was demonstrated in three generations of an American family (Solomon and Sturgeon, 1964).

The red cells are not agglutinated by "natural" or "immune" anti-A, anti-A+B, anti-A_1 or anti-B with or without enzyme pretreatment of the cells. Anti-A of group O or B sera is absorbed and may be eluted from the cells. Secretors of H have no detectable A substances.

A_x. *A family of variants whose cells are not usually agglutinated by anti-A typing sera but are consistently agglutinated by selected group O sera.*

This variant is by no means as strictly defined as A_3 and, since the discovery of the first example by Fischer and Hahn in 1935, other examples have been variously named A_4, A_5, A_z and A_o. Broadly, the cells can be distinguished by the fact that they give negative or weak reactions with anti-A from group B, but positive reactions with specially chosen group O sera (anti-A + anti-B). The percentage of group O sera with which they react varies from example to example, some being agglutinated by almost all, others by as little as 10-20 per cent of sera. Fortunately it is possible to select O sera which will detect all A_x samples; sera where the anti-A component is immune are particularly effective. The anti-A of most examples which give negative reactions with A_x cells whether these be from group B or group O sera, can be recovered from A_x cells by elution, thus showing that, although they do not cause direct agglutination, they do at least sensitise the A_x cells.

There is little or no A group specific substance in A_x saliva. The serum usually contains anti-A_1 agglutinins and may also contain anti-A reacting in the cold.

The variation, especially in antigen strength of the red cells from individual to individual which occurs even in members of one family, raises a doubt as to whether A_x is a rare allele at the ABO locus or whether it is the result of modifying genes and should be more properly included in the section below. It would appear that some examples of the A_x phenotype are due to an allele at the ABO locus and others to the action of suppressor genes. Families in which A_x children have occurred when the parents were both group O and one in which an A_2B man transmitted an A_x gene may well belong to the latter category (Van Loghem and Van der Hart, 1954; Cahan *et al.*, 1957).

A_m. *A weak form with abundant A substance in the saliva of secretors.*

This phenotype is extremely rare and is usually found when an apparent group O individual lacks anti-A. It gives negative reactions with anti-A sera (from group B) and is distinguished from A_x by giving negative reactions with all but a few group O sera. However, the cells do absorb anti-A from both kinds of sera and anti-A may be recovered from them by elution. A further distinction from A_x is in the amount of A substance in the saliva which is often equivalent to the amount found in group A_2.

One example at least, of A_m, first described in 1957 by Dodd and Gilbey (known as Mrs R) was quite strongly agglutinated by group O sera where the anti-A was immune and particularly when an enzyme technique was used (Lincoln and Dodd, 1969).

A number of authors have shown quite unequivocally that an allele at the ABO locus can produce A_m (Salmon *et al.*, 1958; Hrubîsko *et al.*, 1966). However as seen in the next section it can also be produced by modifying genes at another locus.

A_{int}. *This is a type of A acquiring the name "intermediate" from its weak reaction with anti-A_1*

(Landsteiner and Levine, 1930). It is commoner in Negroes than in Whites.

Although the variant might be thought to be intermediate between A_1 and A_2 on account of its behaviour with anti-A_1, it has been found to have more H than has A_2 and therefore does not fit into such an intermediate position.

Variants at the B locus are even more rare than those at the A locus. They can however be placed in categories.

The B_v type.

This subgroup is characterised by having anti-B in the serum and weak B in the saliva. It was originally discovered by Mäkelä and Mäkelä (1955) and later studied in another family by Boorman and Zeitlin (1958) where it was apparently a dominant character found in two generations of an English family. The reactions with anti-B serum are weak compared with normal group B cells. The subgroup is similar to A_x, in that it reacts more strongly with O sera than with the anti-B of group A sera. It is not, however, reacting with the same antibody component as the A_x. The cells do not react with anti-B serum prepared in a rabbit, and there is no reaction between B_v cells and human anti-B sera completely absorbed with rabbit cells. The serum contains anti-B agglutinins reacting with all normal group B cells, though not with B_v, and agglutinates $A_{\bar{x}}$ cells, in this respect behaving like a group O rather than a group B serum. B substance is found in the saliva but usually can be demonstrated only when the individual's own B_v cells are used as indicator cells. Thus it appears that the saliva contains only a fraction of the normal B antigens.

The B_m type.

All examples of this subgroup have no anti-B in the serum and normal amounts of B in the saliva. Many B variants which qualify for this section with properties analogous to A_m have been described by various authors but they are not all called B_m. Yokoyama et al. (1957) described a dominant character which they called B_x. (A variant which is more properly designated B_x is mentioned later.) The cells of this subgroup behave as O, being unagglutinated by anti-B or by group O sera. The saliva contained a normal quantity of B substance and so did the serum. The B_w of Levine et al. (1958) has similar characteristics but the red cells apparently gave the mixed field appearance with anti-B and with group O serum. Later studies of B_m types have been made by Ikemoto et al. (1964) and Kogure and Iseki (1970). In the latter case the B_m seemed to be caused by a modifying gene.

The B_3 type.

This variant has no anti-B in the serum, and H but usually no B in the saliva. Moullec et al. (1955) have described an allele at the B locus which they called B_3, characterized by a weaker reaction with anti-B serum together with free cells similar to that given by A_3 with anti-A serum. Unlike A_3, where secretors have plenty of A substance, two B_3 secretors had no B substance in their saliva. The serum did not contain any anti-B. Some families classified as B_3 whose saliva contained B are described by Bhatia et al. (1965). Studies of similar variants have been made by Sussman, et al. (1960) and others.

B_x corresponding to A_x

The first example of a rare B variant corresponding to A_x has been found by Yamaguchi *et al.* 1970) in the course of a large survey. The propositus was A_1B_x, his father B_x and a sib B_x. The cells of the B_x individuals were not agglutinated by anti-B but by most group O sera. Anti-B could be recovered from the cells after pretreatment with anti-B serum. There was H but not B in the saliva and weak anti-B in the serum.

* * * * * *

The differences in behaviour towards the corresponding antibody displayed by the rare subgroups of A and B compared with the behaviour of their common A and B relatives is probably largely attributable to the number and arrangement of the specific antigenic determinants on the red-cell surface and also the depth at which they are situated. The number of antigenic determinants on A and B cells has been estimated by Economidou *et al.* (1967) and also by Cartron *et al.* (1974) who included counts on most of the better known variants of A (*see* Table 16.1). These latter workers also made a comparison between agglutinability and antigen site density using a Coulter counter and a standard anti-A, Salmon *et al.* (1977). A study of weak B variants has been made by Salmon and Reviron (1964).

Table 16.1 Antigen site counts of various subgroups of A (from Cartron *et al.*, 1974)

Subgroup	No. of sites per red cell
A_1	800,000 — 900,000
A_2	160,000 — 440,000
A_3	70,000 — 100,000
A_x	1400 — 10,300
A_{end}	1100 — 4400
A_m	200 — 1090
A_{el}	100 — 1400

It is worth summarising here a few immunological properties that the rare subgroups of A (and also of B) tend to have in common and which are of practical value when investigating these variants in the laboratory.

(1) Their agglutinability is often improved if selected highly immune anti-A or anti-B (whichever is appropriate) sera are used. The sera of group O individuals immunised against purified A or B glycoproteins are particularly effective. Almost certainly cross reacting antibodies play a part here.

(2) Pre-treatment of the red cells with an enzyme (*e.g.* papain) is often an advantage.

(3) Although their agglutinability may be weak, their absorptive power may be appreciable *e.g.* A_x, A_m and B_v.

(4) As a consequence of (3) very active eluates may be prepared particularly if A_1 (or B) cells are used for detection of the eluted antibody. This is not only

because these cells are the most sensitive for the detection of the eluted antibody but because there is evidence that the cells of weak variants bind the corresponding antibody less strongly than A_1 or B cells and therefore the antibody is more readily recovered in the eluate (Lincoln and Dodd, 1969; Dodd and Lincoln 1974).

Some of the difficulty encountered in assigning a rare variant to a particular category may be due to variation in the reagents used by different laboratories.

(2) Genes modifying the expression of the A and B genes

To explain some of the ABO variants it is necessary to postulate the existence of modifying genes at independent loci which vary the expression of the ABO genes.

Bombay bloods

The most striking example of such genes is found in the "Strange case of the Bombay Bloods", first described by Bhende *et al.* (1952). Levine *et al.* (1955) described a family (shown in Fig. 16.1) which illustrates the way in which this rare phenotype arises. The parents of the propositus are first cousins. The propositus has handed on her mother's B gene to her own daughter but lacks expression of the gene in her own red cells or her saliva. In fact with anti-A and anti-B grouping sera, the propositus behaves as group O, but the agglutination expected of normal group O cells with anti-H serum is missing and a powerful anti-H is present in her serum. With "immune" anti-B from O serum there is weak agglutination. A further significant feature is that the mating of two

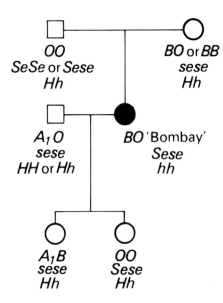

Fig. 16.1 Family study showing gene interaction resulting in suppression of B (modified from Levine *et al.*, 1955).

apparent non-secretors (Le^a positive) has given rise to a daughter who is a secretor and has Le^b. In fact, of course the propositus is not a true non-secretor. She possesses the *Se* gene but fails to secrete A, B or H because her *hh* genes do not allow the formation of these substances.

Levine and his associates believed that the best explanation for all the unusual findings in this family was given by postulating a rare gene *x* which in homozygous state suppresses both the ABO pheno-type and the ABO secretion. If this was so, it followed that there probably existed a common gene *X* possessed by almost all people which in either single or double dose played a part in the synthesis of A and B substances.

In the light of later biochemical work Watkins and Morgan (1955) suggested that the H antigen was the result of a genetically independent blood group system H-h. The Bombay type of blood would therefore be homozygous *hh*. The *h* gene has to be very rare and therefore most normal individuals are homozygous *HH*.

This view is now generally accepted, with some reservations (Race and Sanger, 1975a-c). Recent work on enzymes by Watkins and others has shown that the α-2-L-fucosyl-transferase which is the *H* gene product responsible for the production of H antigen, is absent from Bombay cells (Schenkel-Brunner *et al.*, 1972). However the appropriate A and B transferases are present but are unable to bring about the production of A and B because of the lack of H. In family studies such as that described by Levine *et al.* shown in Figure 16.1, the A and B transferases (in Levine's case B transferase) can be traced passing through to the next generation where if the *A* and *B* genes pair with a normal *H* gene, A and B antigens can be expressed on the red cell.

However in many Bombay (O_h) phenotypes the suppressed A or B antigens can be identified by means of elution tests. Lanset *et al.* (1966) first demonstrated this property when testing a family with four sibs, three of whom shown to be O_h^B· and one Oh_h^{AB}. It will be remembered that in Levine's original family the suppressed B could be detected weakly with a potent immune anti-B.

Para Bombay types

From the number of Bombay families already investigated it seems clear that the amount of suppression of A, B and H antigens is variable and ranges from suppression in which the antigens can be detected only by elution to some (called para Bombay phenotypes) where H is absent from the red cells but where A and B can be detected weakly in straight agglutination tests. The biochemical view of these types is that h does not necessarily represent absolute absence of α-2-L-fucosyltransferase but several alleles of h giving rise to varying amounts of the enzyme too small to be detected in present day enzyme assays may exist; the subsequently formed trace of H is seized upon by the A or B transferases which are present in normal amounts and fully converted into A and B substances although in a few instances a weak agglutination is obtained with anti-H.

The anti-A and anti-B in the sera of para Bombay types are often weaker or occasionally may be absent when the corresponding antigen is detected on the red cell and/or the secretions. These anti-A and anti-B antibodies do not agglutinate the individuals own red cells thus suggesting that the antigens detectable on the red cells are only partially expressed.

There is a further collection of curious Bombay like families which have to be accounted for; these have red cells which can be agglutinated directly but weakly by certain anti-A and anti-B sera; some of them have trace amounts of H on the red cell but their *Se* gene allows normal amounts of the appropriate A, B and H substances to appear in their saliva. To account for these a different locus sometimes called *Zz* is suggested. Some workers (Yamaguchi *et al.*, 1972) consider that there is a regulator gene controlling the expression of the H gene at the sites of biosynthesis of the secreted glycoproteins. This gene if it exists is opposite in its effects to the secretor (*Se*) gene.

The various categories (1-3) of Bombay phenotypes are briefly summarised as follows:-

(1) O_h, O_h^A, O_h^B and O_h^{AB}

These may be described as the true Bombay types in which A, B and occasionally H is detectable by elution tests. Anti-H, anti-A and anti-B is present in the serum. They have no A, B or H in their saliva.

(2) A_h and B_h (Levine *et al.*, 1961; Beranová *et al.*, 1969). The red cells of these types are negative or very weak with anti-H but agglutinate directly albeit weakly with anti-A and anti-B. Anti-H is present in the serum. There is again no A, B or H in the saliva.

(3) O_{Hm}, O_{Hm}^A, O_{Hm}^{AB} Hrubisko *et al.* (1970). Fawcett *et al.* (1970).

These types are distinguished from (2) mainly by being normal secretors of A, B or H substances. The weak anti-H in their serum is probably anti-HI.

A recent paper by Moores *et al.* (1975) offers evidence of an O_h phenotype in which the suppression is so complete that A and B substances are not detectable on the red cells even by elution tests with selected sera and subsequent testing of the eluates by enzyme and ahg techniques.

A_m types which require modifying genes (Yy) to explain them

Weiner *et al.* (1957) suggested the existence of modifying genes called for convenience *Yy* to explain the findings in two A_m families.

The groups of the family of a blood donor of phenotype A_m showed that his genotype was in fact A_1O.

In the second family, the A_m was paired with B giving an A_mB phenotype. However the family groups showed the propositus to be A_1B. A further case described by Darnborough *et al.* (1973) is a good example of A_m produced by a modifying gene as shown below (Fig. 16.2).

A similar case providing evidence for the existence of a modifying gene is reported by Ducos *et al.* (1975). Family studies showed the parents of the A_m propositus to be A_1O and A_2O.

It is postulated that a very common gene Y is necessary for the development of the A antigen on red cells and its absence in the genotype yy inhibits the production of A on red cells but not in saliva. The suggested Yy position of the family of Darnborough *et al.* (1973) is shown below.

Family studies (Weiner *et al.*, 1957) showed that the modifying gene did not

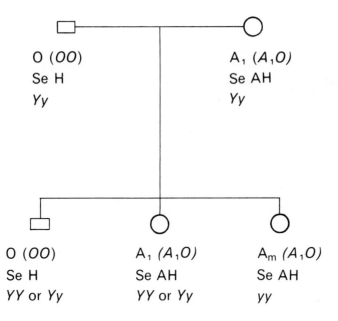

O *(OO)*
Se H
Yy

A₁ *(A₁O)*
Se AH
Yy

O *(OO)*
Se H
YY or *Yy*

A₁ *(A₁O)*
Se AH
YY or *Yy*

A_m *(A₁O)*
Se AH
yy

Fig. 16.2 The Yy suppressor genes.

affect the development of B or H. There are however a few families showing recessive inhibition of B (*e.g.* Gundolf and Andersen, 1970). The propositus in this case had *BO* parents with normal B antigens.

(3) Cis AB

Several families have been found in which some members who are AB appear to have inherited both the *A* and *B* genes from one parent. The first family in which this occurred was one described by Seyfried *et al.* (1964). An A₂B daughter with a group O mother was married to a group O husband and had two A₂B children. The B antigen was weaker than normal and the serum contained some form of anti-B. Her saliva contained a normal amount of a A but little B.

A similar family, again involving A₂B was reported by Yamaguchi, *et al.* (1965). At least twelve such families are now on record; it would seem that the condition is less rare in Japan than in Europe.

The first example of cis A₁B (as distinct from A₂B) was reported by Reviron *et al.* (1968). These workers showed that the B antigen associated with the A₁ was but a part of the normal B antigen. The two A₁B/O members of the family secreted in the saliva the same partial B found on their red cells. The anti-B present in the serum did not agglutinate their own cells but was directed against the remaining part of the B antigen.

Race and Sanger (1975b) remarked "although recombination with a complex locus is the most attractive and by analogy with the MNSs, Rh and Kell systems the most likely explanation of the families, it can be argued that a rare allele is responsible, one which results in an antigen with some of the properties of A and of B . . . But, anyhow a new ABO group has certainly emerged."

(4) ABO variants due to disease

The effect of leukaemia and other diseases on blood group antigens.

An early observation made by Van Loghem (1957) was the finding of a weak A in a patient with myeloblastic leukaemia who a year previously had grouped as a normal A. Stratton *et al.* (1958) observed a similar phenomenon in a patient suffering from hypoplastic anaemia. From previous grouping the patient was group A_1 but his cells lost the power to be agglutinated by anti-A although they were still able to absorb anti-A. For other examples of modified A see Gold (1964). A case in which the group A reaction improved during a remission of the disease and became weak again just before the death of the patient was recorded by Gold *et al.* (1959).

Salmon *et al.* (1961) had the idea of injecting A_1 cells into 3 patients with an A antigen modified by disease and found that the antigen of the foreign cells was not weakened like the patient's own.

Other diseases than leukaemia, for example, Hodgkin's disease and cases of refractory anaemia have been shown to have their H and Ii antigens modified.

Acquired B

Man cannot claim to be the sole species possessing A, B and H substances since they are found distributed throughout the natural world and are even found in numerous micro-organisms. Some of these gain the opportunity, usually through disease processes, of imposing antigens similar in specificity to ABO antigens, on human red cells.

Springer has shown that from Gram-negative bacteria, particularly *E.coli,* substances can be isolated which are similar to the A, B and H substances of human origin (for a review, *see* Springer, 1970).

Earlier, Cameron *et al.* (1959) described a B-like antigen in seven patients who otherwise appeared to be group A_1. Four of them had group O children and therefore were presumably of genotype A_1O. Their sera contained anti-B. Those who were secretors contained A and H but not B in their saliva. Other examples of acquired B have been discovered and it has become clear that the phenomenon is seen particularly in sufferers from diseases of the gut.

Race and Sanger (1975) reported over forty examples of acquired B, thirty-nine of which were A_1, two were A_2 and one was an inhibited A. The shortage of A_2 is significant and so is the fact that none of the patients were group O although, curiously, it is possible to produce a bacterially acquired B on group O cells *in vitro*.

In spite of the almost conclusive evidence that acquired B is of bacterial origin, most attempts to isolate organisms from the actual blood stream of the host, failed. However Garratty *et al.* (1971) have achieved success in isolating *Proteus vulgaris* from the blood of a patient with acquired B.

The problem of acquired B is ever present in forensic serology since post mortem tissue from human organs and muscle particularly if they have been in contact with water readily produce blood group specificity of B and sometimes A. This problem is discussed by Jenkins *et al.* (1972).

A summary of all ABO variables mentioned in this chapter is given in Table 16.2

Table 16.2 Summary of ABO variants

Cause	Major Distinguishing Features	Cell type
Rare alleles		
A variants		
(a)	"Mixed blood" appearance	A_3
		A_{end}
		A_{finn}
		A_{RV}
		A_{bantu}
(b)	Detectable only by elution	A_{el}
(c)	Weak or negative reactions with group B sera but positive with selected group O sera	A_x type (A_4, A_5, A_r and A_0)
(d)	Negative with group B and group O sera but can absorb anti-A from both. Normal amounts of A and H in saliva	A_m type (see also below)
B variants		
(e)	Weak reactions with group A serum. Stronger with O serum. Anti-B in serum. Weak B in saliva.	B_v type
(f)	No anti-B in serum. Normal B in saliva, but variable	B_m type
(g)	No anti-B in serum, H but no B in saliva	Variously named B_3, B
Cis AB		
(h)	A and B antigens both inherited from one parent	Cis AB
Produced by modifying genes		
(i)	A_m reactions same as (d). Distinguished only by family studies	A_m
(j)	A, B and H only detected by elution anti-H, anti-A, anti-B present in serum. No A, B, or H in saliva	True Bombays O_h, O_h^A, O_h^B and O_{hm}^{AB}
(k)	Cells weakly agglutinated by anti-A and anti-B. No A, B or H in saliva	A_h and B_h
(l)	Different from (b) mainly by being normal secretors of A, B and H	O_{Hm}, O_{Hm}^A, O_{Hm}^{AB}
Modification due to disease		
(m)	Loss of A activity	Weakened A antigen
(n)	Predominantly A_1 patients acquiring B-like antigen which is negative with patient's own anti-B	Acquired B

THE BIOCHEMISTRY OF THE ABO SYSTEM

Our present level of understanding of the genetics of the ABO system has been reached in large part through the brilliant work of the biochemists. We give here a short summary of the results of a tremendous volume of biochemical work followed by a discussion of its genetic implications. Readers who would like a more complete account are referred to the review articles of Morgan and Watkins (1969), Marcus (1969) and Watkins (1974).

The pioneer work on the isolation and purification of A, B, H, Le^a, Le^b substances has used body secretions as a source of raw material because of the difficulty of obtaining adequate quantities of active material from red cells. In recent years with more sophisticated techniques becoming available more attention has been devoted to chemical study of red cell substances. Even so, large volumes of blood are required to obtain a few milligrams of purified material.

The following is first of all an account of ABH blood group substances isolated from body fluids, after which we consider briefly some of the characteristics of red cell substances.

As already described (*see* Chapter 6) A, B, H and Lewis blood group substances occur as glycoproteins in a water-soluble form in the body secretions of people with at least one *Se* gene.

To study the chemical composition of such substances it has been necessary to purify them. The best source of raw material for this purpose is the fluid obtained from ovarian cysts which contain active substances in considerable amounts.

The purified glycoproteins obtained are macro-molecules composed of 80-90 per cent carbohydrate and the remainder of the molecule is made up of amino acids. Irrespective of specificity within the ABO and Lewis system, each macro-molecule contains the sugars L-fucose, D-galactose, N-acetyl- D-glucosamine, N-acetyl-galactosamine and N-acetylneuraminic acid. The average molecular weights range from 3×10^5 to 1×10^6. A single secretion contains a family of molecules of varying sizes all closely related in structure and composition. Each molecule consists of a peptide backbone to which many relatively short carbohydrate chains are attached. The peptide backbone does not influence the serological specificity of the molecule but holds the carbohydrate chains whose terminal groupings are responsible for specificity, in a particular spatial relationship to each other and the rest of the molecule. The actual specificity of the molecule is determined by the sugar occurring as a non-reducing group at the end of the chain. N-acetyl- D-galactosamine is the terminal sugar responsible for A specificity, while D-galactose in a similar position determines B specificity and L-fucose is the sugar associated with H (and also with Le^a see below).

Diagrams of the terminal sugars responsible for A and B specificity are shown in Fig. 16.3. Their striking similarity should be noted. In fact the difference between the A and B specific structures is determined solely by the substituent at

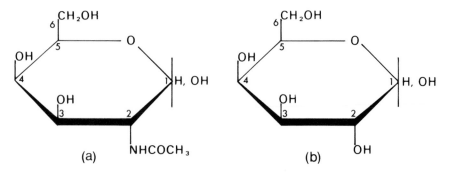

Fig. 16.3 The terminal sugars responsible for A and B specificities. (a), N-acetylgalactosamine (A-specific); (b), D-galactose (B-specific).

the carbon 2 position; an $NHCOCH_3$ group being characteristic of A which when replaced by OH determines B specificity.

The sequence of the sugar units was largely determined by the use of enzymes which released single sugars from the whole specific substance. The A and B substances were converted to give H specificity through release of N-acetylgalactosamine and galactose respectively. The H substance was then changed to Le^a by the liberation of L-fucose. Finally the Le^a substance through the action of a further enzyme lost its Le^a specificity and a structure remained which reacted strongly with Type XIV pneumococcal anti-serum. This stepwise degradation process thus throws light on how the final group specific substances are synthesised. The molecule which reacts with the Type XIV pneumococcal anti-serum is the precursor molecule to which the various sugar units are added. The sugar units responsible for A and B specificity can only be added to chains on which fucose has already been added. This explains why, when H is absent, as in *sese* individuals, no A and B can appear in the body fluids. A simple diagram illustrating the formation of A, B and H specificities is shown in Fig. 16.4. Only

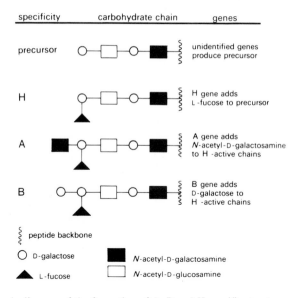

Fig. 16.4 A simple diagram of the formation of A, B and H specific structures.

one carbohydrate chain is shown and the relationship of the *Le* gene to the formation of the various specificities is omitted. This diagram should be studied as a preliminary to the study of Table 16.3.

Here, it can be seen that the precursor structure comprises two different carbohydrate chains. The type 1 chain has the terminal β-galactosyl unit linked in the 1-3 position while the type 2 chain has the terminal β-galactosyl unit linked in the 1-4 position. The *H* gene is able to control the addition of H at the terminal position to both types of chain by adding L-fucose. The Lewis (*Le*) gene also adds L-fucose, but to a subterminal position, to produce Le^a specificity. It is only able

Table 16.3 The formation of blood-group-specific A, B, H, Le^a and Le^b structures

Gene	Enzymic product of gene	Precursor type	Structure of terminal sugars	Serological specificity
Unknown	Unknown	Type 1	β-Gal-(1→3)-GNAc-	Unknown
Unknown	Unknown	Type 2	β-Gal-(1→4)-GNAc-	Type XIV
H	α-L-Fucosyltransferase	Type 1	β-Gal-(1→3)-GNAc- ↑1,2 α-Fuc	H
		Type 2	β-Gal-(1→4)-GNAc- ↑1,2 α-Fuc	H
Le	α-L-Fucosyltransferase	Type 1	β-Gal-(1→3)-GNAc- ↑1,4 α-Fuc	Le^a
H and Le	α-L-Fucosyltransferase	Type 2, Type 1	β-Gal-(1→4)-GNAc-, β-Gal-(1→3)-GNAc- ↑1,2 ↑1,4 α-Fuc α-Fuc	Type XIV, Le^b
		Type 2	β-Gal-(1→4)-GNAc- ↑1,2 α-Fuc	H
H and A	α-L-Fucosyltransferase and α-N-acetylgalactosaminyltransferase	Type 1	α-GalNAc-(1→3)-β-Gal-(1→3)-GNAc- ↑1,2 α-Fuc	A
		Type 2	α-GalNAc-(1→3)-β-Gal-(1→4)-GNAc- ↑1,2 α-Fuc	A
H and B	α-L-Fucosyltransferase and α-D-galactosyltransferase	Type 1	α-Gal-(1→3)-β-Gal-(1→3)-GNAc- ↑1,2 α-Fuc	B
		Type 2	α-Gal-(1→3)-β-Gal-(1→4)-GNAc- ↑1,2 α-Fuc	B

to add L-fucose to a type 1 chain. When both the *H* and *Le* genes are present therefore, substitutions with L-fucose occur at two positions on a type 1 chain. This gives rise to a structure with Le^b specificity. The Le^b structure is thus an interaction product of the *H* and *Le* genes and it is unnecessary to postulate the existence of an ·Le^b gene to account for this specificity.

The primary products of the *A, B* and *H* genes are specific transferase enzymes which catalyse the addition of the appropriate sugar units to give the various A, B and H specificities.

It is important to realise that the various transferases do not always effect conversion of all available chains and there is also competition for the various essential substrates. It can be seen from Table 16.2, for example, that the *H* and Le genes are in competition for type-1 chain precursor substance. When H is absent as in non-secretors considerable amounts of Le^a substance are present in the secretions, but in secretors H and Le^b predominate and only a small amount of Le^a substance is present.

H and Le^b co-exist because only the type-1 chain can be converted into Le^b.

Le^a specific structures are not converted into A or B structures nor is the Le^b structure once formed an acceptor for A or B transferases. However evidence exists for the formation of Le^b structures underlying A and B which is accomplished by the transfer of fucose to the C-4 position of N-acetylglucosamine by the Le transferase *after* the A or B transferases have effected the conversion to A and B specificities.

When both H and A transferases are present many of the precursor chains are converted first to H active structures and then to A active structures and a similar conversion to B is effected by H and B transferases. The N-acetylgalactosamine and galactose endings to the chains mask the H specificity of the structure to which they are added.

Since, as mentioned above, the conversions are never complete, a person who has, for example, the genes *A, H, Se* and Le will have the antigens A, H, Le^a and Le^b in the saliva although Le^a will be present in but small amounts and the quantity of H is of course less than in a group-O person in whose fluids H remain unconverted on all type II chains although many of type 1 will be converted to Le^b.

More than one blood group specificity may be carried on a single macro-molecule. In fact all five specificities *i.e.* A, B, H, Le^a and Le^b, if present, may occupy one macro-molecule. Evidence for this was shown in precipitation experiments in which a mono-specific antiserum was found to carry down in the precipitate all the specificities although they were readily separable by this means in artificial mixtures.

Table 16.4 taken from Morgan and Watkins (1969) is useful for serologists. It must be emphasised that although the *ABO, Hh, Sese* and *Lele* genes profoundly influence one another they are genetically independent and occupy separate loci.

The proposed genetic pathways showing the various gene interactions can be seen in Fig. 16.5. The genes *Le, H, Se, A* and *B* are transforming genes which control certain stages in the conversion of the precursor substance to the specific products secreted. The genes *le, h, se* and *O* can in this connexion be thought of as

Table 16.4 Gene combinations giving rise to A, B, H, Le^a and Le^b activities on the red cell and in secretions

Gene combinations	Antigens on red cells					Substances in secretions				
	A	B	H	Le^a	Le^b	A	B	H	Le^a	Le^b
ABO, H, Se, Le	+	+	+	−	+	+	+	+	+	+
ABO, H, sese, Le	+	+	+	+	−	−	−	−	+	−
ABO, H, Se, lele	+	+	+	−	−	+	+	+	−	−
ABO, H, sese, lele	+	+	+	−	−	−	−	−	−	−
*ABO, hh, Se or sese, Le**	−	−	−	+	−	−	−	−	+	−
*ABO, hh, Se or sese, lele**	−	−	−	−	−	−	−	−	−	−

*Bombay genotype

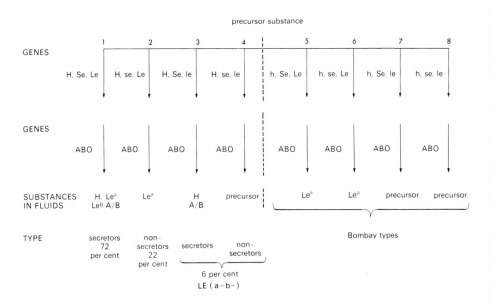

Fig. 16.5 The proposed biosynthetic pathways for the production of group-specific substances in body fluids.

inactive genes or amorphs as they play no part in the conversion of the precursor substance (they may, however, have other functions).

A and B substances cannot appear in saliva or ovarian cyst fluids without the prior conversion of precursor substance into H. This conversion is blocked in the absence of the *Se* gene and, of course, in the rare absence of the *H* gene as in Bombay individuals. The activity of the *Le* gene is not dependent upon the *H* or *Se* genes, therefore Le^a substance is produced whether or not these genes are present. However in secretors (having *Se*) when *H* and *Le* genes are both present they tend to compete for the precursor substances.

It is interesting to note (*see* Fig. 16.5) that although the gene combinations 2, 5 and 6 are different they all result in a fluid in which Le^{a}substance only is present. Similarly, the gene combinations found in numbers 4, 7 and 8 for different reasons allow no A, B, H, Le^a or Le^b substances through into the body fluids.

Much work has now been done on the isolation and identification of the various enzymes (transferases) necessary for the synthesis of the various group specific substances. Such enzymes have been demonstrated in an insoluble form in human stomach mucosal tissue, submaxillary glands and ovarian cyst linings (Ziderman *et al.*, 1967; Hearn *et al.*, 1972) and as soluble enzymes in human milk and in plasma or serum (Kobata and Ginsburg, 1970; Sawicka, 1971).

Group O red cells have been converted into A-active and B-active cells by means of enzyme preparations containing N-acetyl-galactosaminyl and α-galactosyl transferases respectively. The acceptors for the transferred sugars are almost certainly the H determinants on the group O red cell surface.

The work on enzymes is among the later developments of the subject and has beautifully confirmed the serological and biochemical findings that have preceded it. For example α-2- L-fucosyltransferase responsible for H activity is present in both secretions and serum of ABH secretors, while in non-secretors it is absent from secretion but present in serum. The enzyme is absent in individuals of the Bombay *hh* type.

Although A and B transferases are unable to confer A or B specificity in the absence of a fucosyltransferase they are nevertheless present in appropriate individuals. Thus fluids, *e.g.* milk and submaxillary homogenates from both secretors and non-secretors contain A and B transferases indicating that failure to secrete A or B substance depends on the absence of the requisite H structure and not on the absence of the products of the A and B genes. This latter fact is strikingly confirmed when the blood group transferases of Bombay O$_h$ individuals are investigated. The serum of nine such individuals was tested by Race and Watkins (1972) for the presence of α-N-acetylgalactosaminyl and α- D-galactosyl transferases. Whenever possible the findings were correlated with the serological family data which enabled the probable genotype of the O$_h$ individuals to be deduced. The results showed that the enzymes are readily detectable and that their assay supplied information as to whether or not the *A* and *B* genes are present in people of the *hh* genotype.

By providing the right preconditions and ingredients it is apparently possible to transform Bombay (O$_h$) cells into H active cells and finally into cells having A specificity. The transformation requires prior incubation of the Bombay cells with neuraminidase followed by treatment with GDP-fucose and $\alpha(1-2)$ fucosyl transferase. Once H specificity is achieved, A specified transferases can be induced to transfer α-N-acetylgalactosamine residues to the terminal sugar structures (Schenkel-Brunner *et al.*, 1975). Conversion to B has so far not been reported.

G

Substances on red cells

The A, B and H substances on the red cell are predominantly glycolipids and may be extracted from stromata with ethanol. The extracted material is a crude glycosphingolipid fraction which is further purified by various processes and then tested for homogeneity which is not an easy procedure. It is of interest that in contrast to blood group active glycoproteins in secretions, N-acetylgalactosamine is not an essential component of the glycolipids and is found regularly only in those with blood group A activity (Hakomori and Strycharz, 1968). The isolated blood group active sugars whether A, B or H are of varying complexity from simple to branched structures with chains of varying lengths. The composition of the fatty moieties of the active glycolipids are very similar irrespective of blood group specificity.

The yields of blood group active material are very low. For example, from 30 litres of blood, Hakomori and Strycharz (1968) isolated only a few milligrams of purified A and B active glycolipids. These active materials are water soluble and can be tested for serological activity. Their activity is enhanced if the purified materials are complexed with inactive carrier lipid which possibly produces its effect through the provision of a suitable surface configuration for optimum combination with the corresponding antibody.

Although the A, B and H antigens on the red cell appear to be predominantly glycolipids there is evidence that they are partly glycoprotein. There would seem to be a relationship with secretor status as it is only in the red cell stromata of secretors that blood group substances in the glycoprotein form are found. (Gardas and Koscielak, 1971.)

The genetic pathway envisaged for the production of A, B and H substances on the red cells is shown in Figure 16.6.

The Lewis antigens Le^a and Le^b do not appear here since they are not controlled by the genes responsible for the production of red cell substances but are passively acquired from the plasma (see section below on Lewis groups). Presumably Le^a and Le^b structures cannot become incorporated in red cell glycosphingolipids because they can be built only on type 1 chain endings (*see* Table 16.2) and type-1 chains appear to be absent from red cells. For some years it was assumed that the Lewis substances taken up from the plasma were the secreted glycoprotein Le^a and Le^b substances. However red cells suspended in saliva containing Le^a and Le^b substances failed to become coated. Subsequently, Marcus and Cass (1969) produced evidence that the Lewis substances in plasma are glycosphingolipids.

The A_1, A_2 controversy

Although there is a good deal of persuasive serological and indeed clinical evidence for a qualitative distinction between the antigens A_1 and A_2, it is not supported by any but rather controversial biochemical data which tends with equal persuasiveness in the opposite direction *i.e.* that the difference between A_1 and A_2 is a quantitative rather than a qualitative one.

On the basis of certain immuno chemical findings Moreno *et al.* (1971) suggested that the difference between A_1 and A_2 was explicable on the grounds that the A_1 gene-specified-transferase conveyed N-acetylgalactosamine to both

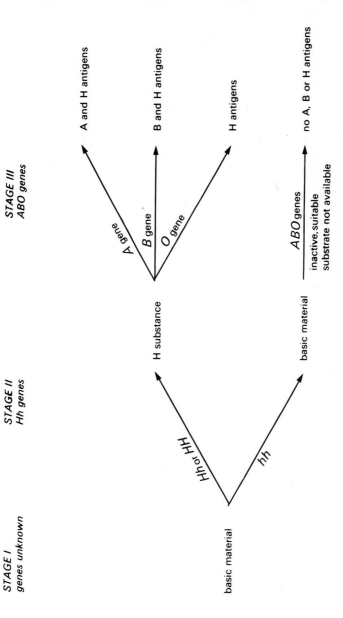

Fig. 16.6 Stages in the production of the blood-group determinants of red cells.

type 1 and type 2 chain endings in the glycoprotein molecule whereas the corresponding A_2 transferase conveyed this sugar only to type 2 chain endings.

However Hearn and Watkins (cited Watkins, 1974) experimenting with A_1 and A_2-gene-specified-transferases isolated from submaxillary glands and stomach mucosal tissue and low-molecular-weight oligosaccharides containing type-1 and type-2 chains as acceptors have failed to find any differences in specificity between A_1 and A_2 transferases in that the A_2-gene-associated enzyme was able to convey N-acetylgalactosamine to *both* type-1 and type-2 chain endings. However kinetic studies on N-acetylgalactosamyl-transferases in human serum made by Schachter *et al.* (1973) revealed a lower activity of the transferase in the serum from A_2 donors than in that from A_1 donors and also pH optima and other factors were different thus the view of Watkins (1974) is that the A_2 gene produces an enzyme which performs the same function as the A_1-gene-specified transferase but does so less efficiently so that fewer of the precursor H structures are changed into A active determinants.

Furthermore, when A-active glycoproteins from either A_1 or A_2 individuals are enzyme treated to remove terminal N-acetylgalactosamine residues there is a rise in Le^b activity and since Le^b can be built only on type-1 chains, the development of Le^b activity in the glycoproteins of A_2 individuals is not in accord with the idea of Moreno *et al.* (1971) that only type-2 chains are transformed by the A_2 transferase.

The distinction which is perceived between A_1 and A_2 by anti-A_1 antibodies is attributed to there being a population of anti-A antibodies for which A site density is critical. These anti-A_1 antibodies may have receptor site requirements which allow optimum reactivity with the A_1 antigen although there must be some reaction with A_2 to account for the well-known observation that repeated absorption of anti-A_1 by A_2 red cells gradually removes anti-A_1 from the serum.

There is no doubt that the occasional group A_2 patient acquires an anti-A_1 which is reactive at 37°C and recognises a transfusion of A_1 cells as foreign (Boorman *et al.*, 1946; Lundberg and McGinnis, 1975).

Another approach to the problem has been explored by Mohn *et al.* (1975). Sonicated human erythrocyte stromata were tested in agar gel against immune anti-A. Immuno-diffusion studies on A_1 and A_2 red-cell membranes showed that whereas there was a line of identity between adjacent cells containing A_1 and A_2 preparations an additional band of precipitate appeared in relation to A_1, which was absent from A_2.

ANTI-A AND ANTI-B ANTIBODIES

Heterogeneity among anti-A and anti-B antibodies of the same general specificity.

Anti-A and anti-B antibodies display heterogeneity in a number of different ways. Many investigations have clearly demonstrated marked heterogeneity both in physical and chemical properties and in serological specificity. In fact, it is found, not surprisingly, that anti-A and anti-B antibodies follow the pattern which emerges from the general field of modern immunology in which it is shown that a whole spectrum of antibody molecules varying in molecular size, specificity and in affinity for the corresponding antibody, etc., arises following the stimulus afforded by a single antigen.

Evidence that anti-A and anti-B molecules are not all exactly alike has been obtained from experiments with animal red cells. For example, the existence of human anti-B molecules of differing specificities has been obtained by absorption experiments with the B-like antigen which is widely distributed in the animal kingdom. The major earlier work on this subject was that of Friedenreich and Witt (1933). Owen (1954) noted a number of different human anti-B fractions using the B antigen of opossum, rat, hamster and rabbit; and Dodd in 1957 and 1958 carried out absorption and elution experiments using the red cells of human group B, rabbit, pig and guinea pig.

For example, nearly all human anti-B sera can be shown, by repeated absorption with rabbit red cells (which have a B antigen), to contain rabbit reacting anti-B and non-rabbit reacting anti-B; the proportions of the two fractions vary considerably in individual sera, some sera containing a great deal of rabbit reacting anti-B while others contain very little. An extension of the number of animal species used for the experiments uncovers further differences, not only in the anti-B population of human sera but in the B antigen of the various animals.

A useful distinction between immune and so-called naturally occurring anti-A can be made with the red cells of pigs, some of which have an A-like antigen designated, A^p. Pig A^p cells are agglutinated by haemolytic IgM anti-A but not by the IgM anti-A which is naturally occurring (Winstanley et al 1957). They are also sensitised but not agglutinated by IgG anti-A, and can therefore be agglutinated by anti-globulin reagents (Konugres and Coombs 1958).

Quite a different approach to the study of heterogeneity of Anti-A and anti-B molecules has been made by Wurmser and co-workers (Filitti-Wurmser et al., 1954). They carried out thermodynamic studies and show differences in thermodynamic properties of the anti-B from individuals of different ABO genotype i.e. OO, AA and AO. Their results applied to agglutinins and not to any form of immune anti-B molecules. Moreover, they found a striking homogeneity of the iso-agglutinins in a given serum.

In addition Filitti-Wurmser and Jacquot-Armand (1960) working with immune antibodies of both anti-A and anti-B specificities have shown by similar thermodynamic experiments that there is heterogeneity in these immune antibody populations as shown by their combination with the corresponding antigen. This is in contra-distinction to the homogeneity displayed by the "natural" agglutinins.

Antibodies in group O sera that cross react with both A and B red cells.

Group O sera as well as containing anti-A and anti-B antibodies very frequently contain antibodies which cross react with both A and B red cells.

They are quite simple to demonstrate by preparing eluates from A and B red cells using selected group O sera as the source of antibody. Eluates from A cells as well as giving the expected agglutination with A cells also agglutinate cells of group B and conversely eluates from B cells agglutinate A cells as well as B. Further evidence of cross reactivity can be obtained by inhibition tests. Absorption of group O sera with group A cells or A group specific substance will often result in a reduction in titre against B cells while absorption with cells or substance of B specificity reduces the titre against A cells.

Immune sera are the best source of cross reacting molecules. The exact nature of these antibodies has been an interesting and controversial problem for many years. At one time (Dodd, 1952) it was considered that some antibody molecules in group O sera had both anti-A and anti-B combining sites giving a molecule with two different specificities.

In the light of later greater understanding of the immunology and biochemistry of ABO antigens and antibodies this idea has been superseded and there are now two main theories to explain this phenomenon. The first which now has most adherents and a weight of experimental evidence in its favour postulates that cross reacting antibodies are directed not exclusively against the A or B specific groupings on the molecule but also against some of the common structures of these molecules (Kabat, 1956; Schiffman and Howe, 1965). This concept would indeed appear reasonable for, as noted above (*see also* Fig. 16.2) the two sugars responsible for A and B specificity are identical save for the substituent at the carbon 2 position.

By means of precipitation experiments using group O sera in which the anti-B had been stimulated with B group specific substance Schiffman and Howe (1965) demonstrated that the terminal oligosaccharides responsible for A and B blood group specificity would both inhibit the precipitation of cross-reacting antibody irrespective of whether the precipitation was brought about by A or B substances. Moreover these workers showed that B substance after the removal of D-galactose by enzymatic action lost B specificity and acquired H; however neither this material or H substance combined with cross reacting antibodies.

Inclusion of the specific portion of the terminal oligosaccharide as well as common portions of the molecule in the combining areas of cross reacting antibody molecules finds support in the fact that these antibodies are usually (although not invariably) A preferring or B preferring according to whether the A or B antigen stimulated their production. This observation was made by Dodd (1952) and has subsequently been confirmed with many examples of immune group O sera (Lincoln and Dodd, 1969; Dodd and Lincoln, 1974).

The second theory to explain cross reacting antibodies is that A, B and AB people have a separate common antigen C on their red cells for which there is a third antibody anti-C present in group O serum. Since the work of the biochemists has disclosed the extreme similarity between the A and B antigens it seems somewhat unnecessary to invoke the existence of a hypothetical antigen C when there is a perfectly good alternative explanation of the phenomenon to hand!

A modern review of cross reacting antibodies by champions of the C-anti-C theory may be found in Wiener *et al.* (1973).

It has been suggested that the Matuhasi-Ogata phenomenon may explain cross reactivity. When for example group B, D negative red cells were incubated with serum containing anti-B and anti-D an eluate prepared from the group B cells was found to contain anti-D as well as anti-B. The appearance of the anti-D in the eluate was explained by non-specific antibody adhesion to antigen-antibody complex (Matuhasi et al., 1960). The Matuhasi-Ogata phenomenon has been studied in some detail by Allen et al., (1969). However the titres of the "compatible" antibody in their eluates are very low in comparison with most of the values obtained for cross reacting antibodies in group O sera. The so-called Mutahasi-Ogata phenomenon is probably better explained by the general "stickiness" of protein molecules. Bove et al. (1973) using iodine-labelled reagents found that red cells took up a certain amount of IgG non-specifically and when the IgG taken up non-specifically included a blood group antibody in relatively high concentration, an eluate prepared from the cells contained sufficient antibody to be detectable. These workers did not find that the appearance of the antibody in the eluate depended upon adhesion to an antigen-antibody complex.

A different approach to the problem was made by Matuhasi (1966) by which he claimed to confirm that group O serum does not contain an antibody capable of reacting with both A and B cells. A mixture of normal B cells and fluorescent A cells when exposed to group O serum gave agglutinates which were either fluorescent or non-fluorescent. No mixed agglutinates were seen. However mixed agglutinates might well not appear since, given a choice of both antigens, A preferring cross reacting antibodies might react preferentially with A cells and B preferring antibodies might react preferentially with B cells. In neither case therefore would mixed agglutinates necessarily be formed.

The size of the combining site of cross reacting antibodies has been a matter for speculation among workers and for some disagreement. Kabat (1956) thinks that the cross reacting antibody is directed towards a larger area of the corresponding A or B determinant and so do Dodd et al. (1967).

On the other hand, Franks and Liske (1968) from work on the mixed agglutination technique using buccal cells, consider that their results show that cross reacting antibodies cannot compete so successfully as the mono-specific antibodies in the same serum, for antigenic sites. They therefore are of the opinion that cross reacting antibodies have a small combining sera and a low affinity for the corresponding antigen.

From radioimmunoassay studies Holburn (1975) also concludes that cross reacting antibody binds to a smaller determinant than mono-specific anti-A and anti-B but favours an antibody with a high affinity for the corresponding antigen! A small site if true is surprising since the evidence points to the inclusion of both specific and common portions of the A and B oligosaccharides within the combining area of cross reacting antibodies.

The possible clinical significance of cross reacting antibodies has been considered. Rosenfield (1955) maintained that cross reacting antibodies crossed the placenta more readily than mono-specific anti-A and anti-B but it seems more likely that the immuno globulin class of the antibody is much the most important factor in determining whether or not, it will cross the placenta. IgG antibodies whether cross reacting or mono-specific will be capable of passing the placental barrier whereas IgM molecules of either type cannot do so. That cross reacting antibodies can be found in both IgG and IgM classes has been shown by Lincoln (1967) and Tilley *et al.* (1975).

Nevertheless, there is some evidence that cross reacting antibodies do have special serological properties. They seem particularly efficient at agglutinating A_x cells.

An interesting observation was made by Tilley *et al.* (1975) when investigating the uptake on to O cells of lipid fraction containing A or B activity. These authors found that the acquired A or B activity was best detected by cross reacting (anti-AB) antibody from group O sera and usually remained undetected when mono-specific anti-A or anti-B sera were used.

THE SEROLOGY OF THE LEWIS SYSTEM

The way in which the genes *Le* and *le* interact with the *A*, *B* and *H* genes is described earlier in this chapter.

Here we summarise what is known about the serology of the Lewis system which has also been touched upon in the introductory chapters of this book.

The genes *Le* and *le* express themselves as soluble antigens in the body fluids from whence they are adsorbed on to the red cell surface. It is now known that the Lewis substances in plasma, are glycosphingolipids but Lewis substances in saliva are glycoproteins. The original observation by Sneath and Sneath (1955) that red cells were able to take up Lewis substances from plasma was made when a patient who was Le (a−b+) was transfused with Le (a+b−) cells. The transfused cells acquired Le^b from the recipient's plasma and typed as Le (a+b+). These workers then performed *in vitro* experiments and found that the same phenomena could be observed in incubating Le (a+b−) cells in Le (a−b+) plasma. In addition when Le (a+b−) or Le (a−b+) cells were incubated with Le (a−b−) plasma, they lost their antigen to the plasma. However the Lewis substances in saliva are unable to transform red cells, possibly because they are glycoproteins.

The various Lewis phenotypes

The phenotype Le (a−b+)

The secretions of people belonging to this phenotype contain H and Le^b and a small amount of Le^a and also of course their corresponding A or B substances when these are present on the red cells. Their sera also contain predominantly Le^b substance with less Le^a and only traces of H.

The red cells of group A_1 Le (a−b+) individuals only react with certain examples of anti-Le^b. In fact there appear to be two kinds of anti-Le^b; (1) called anti-Le^{bH} which is neutralised by the salivas of all ABH secretors including Le (a−b−) individuals and (2) anti-Le^b sera not neutralised by secretor salivas; these anti-Le^b sera, termed anti-Le^{bL} react with A_1 Le (a−b+) individuals almost as strongly as with other groups.

A curious antibody anti-A_1 Le^b reacting only if A_1 and Le^b are present on red cells was described by Seaman *et al.* (1968) and called Siedler. The antibody was

Table 16.5 The Lewis phenotypes

Phenotype	Anti-Le^a	Anti-Le$^{b'}$	Anti-Le^c	Anti-Le^d	Content of Saliva	Genes present
(1) Le (a−b+)	−	+	−	−	H, Le^b, little Le^a	*H, Se, Le*
(2) Le (a+b−)	+	−	−	−	Much Le^a, no Le^b or H, little Le^c	*H, se, Le*
(3) (a) Le (a−b−)	−	−	−	+	H, No Le^a or Le^b, little Le^c	*H, Se, le*
(b) Le (a−b−)	−	−	+	−	No H, No Le^a or Le^b, some Le^c	*H, se, le*

inhibited only by saliva from A$_1$ Le (b+) individuals and therefore appears to require the presence of both A$_1$ and Le^b for its activity.

This antibody makes a useful distinction between true A$_1$ Le (b+) and the "pseudo" A$_1$ Le (a−b−) found to be negative with anti-Le^b merely because the latter is of the anti-Le^{bH} type. The finding of anti- A$_1$ Le^b in a blood group chimera which agglutinated the A$_1$ Le^b cells present in her twin brother but failed to agglutinate the cells she acquired from him in utero led Crookston *et al.* (1970) to postulate that the plasma of group A$_1$ Le (b+) subjects normally contains A$_1$ Le^b molecules. Those interested in the deductions drawn from the experimental findings should consult the original paper and also a confirmatory investigation in another patient published later (Swanson *et al.*, 1971).

The phenotype Le (a+b−).

People of this type are non-secretors and do not have ABH substances in their body secretions. They do have a great deal of Le^a substance in their serum and saliva. The phenotype may be recognised by testing the saliva against anti-Le^a precipitating serum made in rabbits (Glynn *et al.*, 1956). Only Le (a+b−) saliva induces precipitation; this is probably a quantitative effect.

The phenotype Le (a−b−)

Individuals of this type are homozygous lele and therefore have neither Le^a or Le^b although if they are secretors they have H in their secretions. They are, however, not without some kind of Lewis substance since antibodies against Le (a−b−) red cells exist. These are of two types, the first, anti-Le^d (Potapov, 1970) was made by injecting the saliva from an O Le (a−b+) secretor into a goat where in addition to a potent anti-Le^b a weaker antibody reacting only with the red cells of Le (a−b−) secretors was found. The second, anti-Le^c was found by Gunson and Latham (1972) as a cold agglutinin reacting solely with the red cells of Le (a−b−) non-secretors. Anti-Le^c although specific for the red cells of Le (a−b−) non-secretors and strongly inhibited by the saliva of such individuals is also inhibited, although less strongly by the saliva of Le (a−b−) secretors and Le (a+b−) non-secretors. Le (a−b+) salivas hardly inhibit anti-Le^c at all.

Watkins quoted by Gunson and Latham (1972) suggests that Le^c specificity may be explained by the addition of L-fucose to 'type II' chains while Le^d specificity may be accounted for by the addition of a second L-fucose residue by the H gene-controlled 2-fucosyltransferase. Thus it is unnecessary to postulate additional genes in order to accommodate Le^c and Le^d in the Lewis system.

An antibody anti-Le^x reacting with all blood samples except Le (a−b−) has been described by Andresen and Jordal (1949) and Sturgeon and Arcilla (1970). It has some of the properties of a mixture of anti-Le^a + anti-Le^b but appears to react strongly with a high proportion of cord bloods. It is difficult at present to fit this antibody into the Lewis scheme.

The frequencies of the various Lewis red cell phenotypes

There is considerable variation in Lewis types throughout the world and indeed even between different parts of the British Isles.

Table 16.6 Distribution of Lewis types of red cells within the British Isles*

Centre	Total tested	Le (a+b−) (percent)	Le (a−b+) (percent)	Le (a−b−) (percent)
London	213	49 (23.00)	134 (62.91)	30 (14.08)
Aberdeen	550	154 (28.00)	361 (65.63)	35 (6.36)
Belfast	644	173 (26.86)	421 (65.37)	50 (7.76)
Dublin	597	165 (27.63)	385 (64.48)	47 (7.87)

*Percentage of each cell type given in parenthesis.

Table 16.6 taken from Lincoln and Dodd (1972) is illustrative. The Le (a−b−) frequencies may be slightly augmented by examples of group A_1 secretors possessing Le^b which were not detected by the anti-Le^b used although at least a weak reaction was scored with most group A_1 secretors. Since the *Lele* and *Sese* genes segregate independently the secretor/non-secretor ratio, in this phenotype is the same as that for the general population.

It is worth noting that the phenotype Le (a−b−) may be as high as 46 per cent in West African Negroes and since individuals of this type are those which most frequently develop Lewis antibodies which may become active at 37°C they sometimes prove to be a cross matching problem.

The serological properties of Lewis antibodies

Anti-Le^a usually behaves as an agglutinin and agglutinates red cells suspended in saline almost always more strongly at 15°C than at 37°C. Occasionally the antibody requires antiglobulin for its detection.

Anti-Le^b but rarely occurs without anti-Le^a. Its temperature range is similar to anti-Le^a.

Lewis antibodies habitually bind complement and anti-Le^a causes at least some lysis of red cells at 37°C particularly if the cells are first enzyme treated.

Lewis antibodies are not known to cause haemolytic disease of the newborn, but this is no surprise since they are almost all IgM antibodies. However they are able to effect rapid destruction of transfused red cells and haemolytic transfusion reactions due to Lewis antibodies have been described.

REFERENCES

ABO

Allen, F.H., Isitt, P.D., Degnan, T.J., Jackson, V.A., Reihart, J.K., Knowlin, R.J., & Adebahr, M.E. (1969) Further observations on the Matuhasi-Ogata phenomenon. *Vox Sang,* **16,** 47.

Andresen, P.H., & Jordal, K. (1949) An incomplete agglutinin related to the L-(Lewis) system. *Acta, path. microbiol, scand,* **26,** 636.

Beranová, G., Prodanov, P., Hrubisko, M. & Smálik, S. (1969) A new variant in the ABO blood group system B_h. *Vox Sang.,* **16,** 449.

Bhatia, H.M., Undevia, J.V. & Sanghui, L.D. (1965) Second Indian family of weak B (B_3) *Vox Sang.,* **10,** 506.

Bhende, Y.M., Deshpande, C.K., Bhatia, H.M., Sanger, Ruth, Race, R.R., Morgan, W.T.J., & Watkins Winifred M. (1952) A new blood group character related to the ABO system. *Lancet,* **i,** 903-904.

Boorman, K.E., Dodd, B.E., Loutit, J.F. & Mollison, P.L. (1946) Some results of transfusion of blood to recipients with "cold" agglutinins. *Brit. med. J.* **1,** 751.

Boorman, K.E. & Zeitlin, R.A. (1958) A subgroup of B. Proc. VII Congress of the International Society of Blood Transfusion. pp. 716-720. Basle: Karger, and New York.

Bove, J.R., Holburn, A.M., & Mollison, P.L. (1973) Non-specific binding of IgG to antibody-coated red cells. (The Matuhasi-Ogata phenomenon). *Immunology,* **25,** 793.

Brain, P. (1966) Subgroups of A in the South African Bantu. *Vox Sang.* **11,** 686.

Cahan, A., Jack, J.A., Scudder, J., Sargent, Mary, Sanger, Ruth & Race, R.R. (1957) A family in which A_x is transmitted through a person of the blood group A_2B. *Vox Sang.,* **2,** 8.

Cameron, C., Graham, F., Dunsford, I., Sickles, G., Macpherson, C.R., Cahan, A., Sanger, R., & Race, R.R. (1959) Acquisition of a B-like antigen by red blood cells. Brit. med. J., **2,** 29.

Cartron, J.P., Gerbal, A., Hughes-Jones, N.C., & Salmon, C. (1974) Weak A phenotypes. Relationship between red cell agglutinability and antigen site density. *Immunology,* **27,** 723.

Chaves, M.A., Boorman, K.E., & Leak, M. (1975) A_{RV} A subgroup of A similar to A_{finn}, Abstracts XIV Congress of the International Society of Blood Transfusion, Helsinki p47.

Crookston, M.C., Tilley, C.A. & Crookston, J.H. (1970) Human blood group chimaera with seeming breakdown of immune tolerance. *Lancet,* **ii,** 1110.

Darnborough, J., Voak, D. & Pepper, R.M. (1973) Observations on a new example of the A_m phenotype which demonstrates reduced A secretion. *Vox Sang.,* **24,** 216.

Dodd, B.E. (1952) Linked anti-A and anti-B antibodies from group O sera. *Brit. J. exp. Path.,* **33,** 1.

Dodd, Barbara E. (1957) Further studies of antibody molecules having both A and B specificity. *Trans. 6th Congress of the European Society of Haematology.* No. 207 733. Karger.

Dodd, Barbara E. (1958) Further evidence for the heterogeneity of the anti-AB molecules of group O sera. *Proc. Seventh Congress International Society of Blood Transfusion.* No. 62 234. Karger.

Dodd, B.E. & Gilbey, B.E. (1957) An unusual variant of group A. *Vox Sang.,* **2,** 390.

Dodd, B.E. & Lincoln, P.J. (1974) The effect of elution on the reactivity of antibodies of the ABO system, including cross reacting antibodies, as demonstrated by use of red cells of various subgroups of A, and group B. *Brit. J. Haemat.,* **26,** 93.

Dodd, B.E., Lincoln, P.J. & Boorman, K.E. (1967) The cross reacting antibodies in group O sera, immunological studies and a possible interpretation of the observed facts. *Immunology,* **12,** 39.

Ducos, J., Marty, Y. & Ruffie, J. (1975) A family with one child of phenotype A_m providing further evidence for the existence of the modifier genes Yy. *Vox Sang.,* **28,** 456.

Economidou, J., Hughes-Jones, N.C., and Gardner, B. (1967) Quantitative measurements concerning A and B antigen sites, *Vox Sang.,* **12,** 321.

Fawcett, K.J., Eckstein, E.G., Innella, F. & Yokoyama, M. (1970) Four examples of Bh_m· blood in one family. *Vox Sang.,* **19,** 457.

Filitti-Wurmser, S., Jacquot-Armand, Y., Aubel-Lesure, G. & Wurmser, R. (1954) Physico-Chemical study of human iso-haemagglutination. *Ann. Eugen.,* **18,** 183.

Filitti-Wurmser, S. & Jacquot-Armand, Y. (1960) Etude Quantitative de l'héterogénétté des agglutinines anti-A ou anti-B immunes des sérums humains. *Rev. D'Hémat.,* **15,** No. 1.25.

Fischer, W. & Hahn, F. (1935) Über auffallende Schwäche der gruppenspezifischen reaktionsfähigkeit bei einem Erwachsenen. *Z. Immun. Forsch.,* **84,** 177-188.

Franks, D. & Liske, R. (1968) The specificity of the cross reacting antibodies in blood group O sera which produce mixed agglutination.*Ämmunology,* **14,** 433.

Friedenreich, V. (1936) Eine bisher unbekannte blutgruppeneigenschaft (A_3). *Z. Immun. Forsch.,* **89,** 409.

Friedenreich, V., and Witt, S. (1933) Ueber B-antigen und B-antikorper bei Menschen und Tieren Z. Immun. Forsch **78.** 152

Gardas, A. & Koscielak, J. (1971) A, B and H blood group specificities in glycoprotein and glycolipid fractions of human erythrocyte membrane. Absence of blood group active glycoproteins in the membranes of non-secretors. *Vox Sang.*, **20**, 137.

Garratty, G., Willbanks, E., and Petz, L. D. (1971) An Acquired B-antigen Associated with *Proteus vulgaris* infection. *Vox Sang.* **21**, 45.

Glynn, A.A., Glynn, L.E. & Holborow, E.J. (1956) The secretor status of rheumatic fever patients. *Lancet*, **ii**, 759.

Gold, R. (1964) Modified A antigen in three cases of acute leukaemia and one case of pre-leukaemia. *Sangre*, **9**, 131.

Gold, E.R., Tovey, G.H., Benney, W.E. & Lewis, F.J.W. (1959) Changes in the group A antigen in a case of leukaemia. *Nature (Lond.)*, **183**, 892.

Gundolf, F. & Andersen, J. (1970) Variant of group B lacking the B antigen on the red cells. *Vox Sang.*, **18**, 216.

Gunson, H.H. & Latham, V. (1972) An agglutinin in human serum reacting with cells from Le (a–b–) non-secretor individuals. *Vox Sang.*, **22**, 344.

Hakomori, S.I. & Strycharz, G.D. (1968) Investigations on cellular blood group substances. I. Isolation and chemical composition of blood group ABH and Le^b iso-antigens of sphingoglycolipid nature. *Biochemistry*, **7**, 1279.

Hearn, V.M., Race, C. & Watkins, W.M. (1972) α-N-acetylgalactosaminyl and α-galactosyltransferases in human ovarian cyst epithelial linings and fluids. *Biochem, biophys. Res. Commun.*, **46**, 948.

Holburn, A.M. (1976) Radioimmunoassay studies of the cross reacting antibody of human group O sera. *Brit. J. Haemat.* **32** 589.

Hrubisko, M., Calkovska, Z., Mergancová, O. & Gallova, K. (1966) Beobachtungen über varianten des blutgruppensystems ABO I studies der variante A$_m$. *Blut*, **13**, 137.

Hrubisko, M., Laluha, J., Mergancová, O., & Zákovicová, S. (1970) New variants in the ABOH blood group system due to interaction of recessive genes controlling the formation of the H antigen in erythrocytes: the Bombay like phenotypes O$_{Hm}$O$_{Hm}^B$ and O$_{Hm}^{AB}$. *Vox Sang.*, **19**, 113.

Ikemoto, S., Kuniyuki, M. & Furuhata, T. (1964) A finding of rare B$_m$ blood type in Japanese. *Proc. Jap, Acad.*, **40**, 362.

Jenkins, G.C., Brown, J., Lincoln, P.J. & Dodd, B.E. (1972) The problem of acquired B antigen in Forensic serology. *J. forens. Sci. Soc.*, **12**, 597.

Kabat, E.A. (1956) The blood group substances. P.267. New York: Academic Press.

Kobata, A. & Ginsburg, V. (1970) Uridine diphosphate N-acetyl-D-galactosamine: D-galactose α-3-N-acetylgalactosaminyltransferase, a product of the gene that determines blood type A in man. *J. biol. Chem.*, **245**, 1484.

Kogure, T. & Isaki, S. (1970) A family of B$_m$ due to a modifying gene. *Proc. Jap. Acad.*, **46**, 728.

Konugres, Angelyn & Coombs, R.R.A. (1958) Studies on human anti-A sera with special reference to so-called "immune" anti-A. Identification of the antibody detected by Witebsky's partial neutralisation tests as anti- A^P and the occurrence of the A^P antigen on human and animal red cells. *Brit. J. Haemat.*, **4**, 261.

Landsteiner, K. & Levine, P. (1930) Differentiation of a type of human blood by means of normal animal serum. *J. Immunol.*, **18**, 87.

Lanset, S., Ropartz, C., Rousseau P., Guerbet, Y. & Salmon, C. (1966) Une famille comportant les phénotypes Bombay ,O$_h^{AB}$ et O$_h^B$. *Transfusion (Paris)*, **9**, 255.

Levine, P., Robinson, E., Celano, M., Briggs, O. & Falkinburg, L. (1955) Gene interaction resulting in suppression of blood group substance B. *Blood*, **10**, 1100-1108.

Levine, P., Celano, M.J. & Griset, T. (1958) B$_w$. a new allele of the ABO locus. *Proc. VI Cong. Int. Soc. Blood Trans.* P. 132-135.

Levine, P., Uhler, M. & White, J. (1961) A$_h$ an incomplete suppression of A resembling O$_h$. *Vox Sang.*, **6**, 561.

Lincoln, P.J. (1967) Antigen-antibody studies in the ABO blood group system. Ph.D. Thesis. London University.

Lincoln, P.J. & Dodd, B.E. (1969) Antigen-antibody studies in the ABO blood group system with particular reference to cross reacting antibodies in group O sera. *Immunology*, **16**, 301.

Lincoln, P.J. & Dodd, B.E. (1972) Variation in secretor and Lewis type frequencies within the British Isles. *J. med. Genet.*, **9**, 43.

Lundberg, W.B. & McGinnis, M.H. (1975) Hemolytic transfusion reaction due to anti-A$_1$. *Transfusion*, **15**, 1.

Mäkelä, O. & Mäkelä, Pirjo (1955) A weak B containing anti-B. *Ann. Med. exp. Fenn.*, **33**, 33-40.

Marcus, D.M. (1969) The ABO and Lewis blood group systems. *New Engl. J. Med.*, **280**, 994.

Marcus, D.M. & Cass, L.E. (1969) Uptake of glycosphingolipids with Lewis blood group activity by human erythrocytes. *Science*, **164**, 553.

Matuhasi, T., Kumazawa, H. & Usui, M. (1960) Question of the presence of so-called cross reacting antibody. *J. Jap. Soc. Blood Transfus.*, **6**, 295.

Matuhasi, T. (1966) Evidence of monospecificity of anti-A and anti-B in group O serum. *Abstracts 11th Congr. Blood Transf.* Sydney p. 142.

Mohn, J.F., Cunningham, R.K., Pirkola, A., Furuhjelm, U. & Nevanlinna, H.R. (1973) An inherited blood group A variant in the Finnish population. I. Basic characteristics. *Vox. Sang.* **25**, 193.

Mohn, J.F., Cunningham, R.K., Bates, J.F. (1975) Qualitative distinction between subgroups A_1 and A_2. Abstracts XIV Congress International Society of Blood Transfusion, Helsinki p.96

Moores, P.P., Issitt, P.D., Pavone, B.G., McKeever, B.G. (1975) Some observations on "Bombay" bloods, with comments on evidence for the existence of two different O_h phenotypes. *Tranfusion*, **15**, 237.

Moreno, C., Lundblad, A. & Kabat, E.A. (1971) Immunochemical studies on blood groups. Ll. A comparative study of the reaction of A_1 and A_2 blood group glycoproteins with human anti-A. *J. exp. Med.*, **134**, 439.

Morgan, W.T.J. & Watkins, W.M. (1969) Genetics and biochemical aspects of human blood group A–, B–, H–, Le^{a-} and Le^{b-} specificity. *British Medical Bull.*, **25**, No. 1, 30.

Moullec, J., Sutton, E. & Burgador, M. (1955) Une variante faible de l'agglutinogène de groupe B. *Rev. Hémat.*, **10**, 574-582.

Nevanlinna, H.R. & Pirkola, A. (1973) An inherited blood group A variant in the Finnish population. II Population studies. *Vox Sang.*, **24**, 404.

Owen, R.D. (1954) Heterogeneity of antibodies of the human blood groups in normal and immune sera. *J. Immunol.*, **73**, 29.

Potapov, M.I. (1970) Detection of the antigen of the Lewis system, characteristic of the erythrocytes of the secretory group Le (a–b–). *Probl. Hemat. Blood Transfus.* **15**, 45.

Race, C. & Watkins, W.M. (1972) The enzyme products of the human A and B blood group genes in the serum of Bombay 'O_h donors. *FEBS Letters*, **27**, 125.

Race, R.R. & Sanger, R. (1975a) *Blood groups in man.* 6th ed. P. 22, Blackwell.

Race, R.R. & Sanger, R. (1975b) *Blood groups in man.* 6th ed. P.35 Blackwell.

Race, R.R. & Sanger, R. (1975c) *Blood groups in man.* 6th ed. P.32. Blackwell.

Reed, T.E. & Moore, B.P.L. (1964) A new variant of blood group A. *Vox Sang.*, **9**, 363.

Reviron, J., Jacquet, A. & Salmon, C. (1968) Une exemple de chromosome 'cis A_1B'. Etude immunologique et gènetique du phénotype induit. *Nouv Revue Franc Hémat.*, **8**, 323.

Rosenfield, R.E. (1955) AB hemolytic disease of the newborn: analysis of 1,480 cord blood specimens, with special reference to the direct antiglobulin test and to the role of the group O mother. *Blood*, **10**, 17.

Salmon, C., Borin, P. & André, R., (1958) La groupe sanguin A_m dans deux générations d'une même famille. *Rev. Hémat.*, **13**, 529.

Salmon, C., André, R. & Phillippon, J. (1961) Agglutinabilité normale des hématies A_1 tranfusées à 3 malades leucémiques de phénotype A *modifié. Revue fr Étud. clin. biol.*, **8**, 792.

Salmon, C., & Reviron, J. (1964) Trois phénotypes "B faibles" B_{80}, B_{60}, B_0 définis par leur agglutinabilité comparée à celle du phénotype normal "B_{100}". *Nouv. Rev. Franc. Hémat.*, **4**, 655.

Salmon, Ch., Lopez M., Cartron, J.P. & Bouguerra A. (1977) Quantitative and thermodynamic studies of erythrocyte ABO antigens. *Transfusion*, **16**, 580.

Sawicka, T. (1971) Glycosyltransferases of human plasma. *FEBS Letters*, **16**, 346.

Schachter, H., Michaels, M.A., Tilley, C.A., Crookston, M.C. & Crookston, J.H. (1973) Qualitative differences in the N-acetyl-D-galactosaminyl-transferases produced by human A_1 and A_2 genes. *Proc. nat. Acad. Sci. USA*, **70**, 220.

Schenkel-Brunner, H., Chester, M.A. & Watkins, W.M. (1972) α-L-fucosyl transferases in human serum from donors of different ABO, secretor and Lewis blood group phenotypes. *Eur. J. Biochem.*, **30**, 269.

Schenkel-Brunner, H., Probaska, R. & Tuppy, H. (1975) Action of glycosyl transferases upon "Bombay" (O_h) erythrocytes. Conversion to cells showing blood group H and A specificities. *Eur. J. Biochem.*, **56**, 591.

Schiffman, G. & Howe, C. (1965) The specificity of blood group A and B cross reacting antibody. *J. Âmmunol.*, **94**, 197.

Seaman, M.J., Chalmers, D.G. & Franks, D. (1968) Siedler; An antibody which reacts with A_1 Le (a–b+) red cells. *Vox Sang.*, **15**, 25.

Seyfried, H., Walewska, I. & Werblińska, B. (1964) Unusual inheritance of ABO group in a family with weak B antigens. *Vox Sang.*, **9**, 268.

Sneath, J.S. & Sneath, P.H.A. (1955) Transformation of the Lewis groups of human red cells. *Nature (Lond.)*, **176**, 172.

Solomon, J.M. & Sturgeon, P. (1964) Quantitative studies on the phenotype A_{el}. *Vox Sang.*, **9**, 476.

Springer, G.F., (1970) Importance of blood group substances in interactions between man and microbes. *Ann. New York Acad. Sci.,* **169**, 134.

Stratton, F., Renton, P.H. & Hancock, J.A. (1958) Red cell agglutinability affected by disease. *Nature (Lond.),* **181**, 62.

Sturgeon, P., Moore, B.P.L. & Weiner, W. (1964) Notation for two weak A variants, A_{end} and $.A_{el}$ *Vox Sang.,* **9**, 214.

Sturgeon, P. & Arcilla, M.B. (1970) Studies on the secretion of blood group substances 1. Observations on the red cell phenotype Le (a+b+x+). *Vox Sang.,* **18**, 301.

Sussman, L.N., Pretshold, H. & Lacher, M.J. (1960) A second example of blood group B_3. *Blood,* **16**, 1788.

Swanson, J., Crookston, M.C., Yunis, E., Azar, M., Gatti, R.A. & Good, R.A. (1971) Lewis substances in a human marrow-transplantation chimaera. *Lancet,* **i**, 396.

Tilley, C.A., Crookston, M.C., Brown, B.L. & Wherrett, J.R. (1975) ALe^b substances in glycosphingolipid fractions of human serum. *Vox sang.,* **28**, 25.

Van Loghem, J.J. & Van der Hart, M (1954) The weak A_4 occurring in the offspring of group O parents. Vox Sang. (O.S.) **4**, 69.

Van Loghem, J.J., Dorfmeier, H, & Van der Hart, M (1957) Two A antigens with abnormal serological properties. *Vox Sang.,* **2**, 16-24.

Watkins, W.M. (1974) Genetic regulation of the structure of blood group specific glycoproteins. *Biochem. Soc. Symp.,* **40**, 125-146.

Watkins, W.M. & Morgan, W.T.J. (1955) Some observations on the O and H characters of human blood and secretions. *Vox Sang., (O.S.),* **5**, 1.

Weiner, W., Lewis, H.B.M., Moores, P., Sanger, R. & Race, R.R. (1957) A gene *y,* modifying the blood group antigen A. *Vox Sang.,* **2**, 25-37.

Weiner, W., Sanger, R. & Race, R.R. (1959) A weak form of the blood group antigen A: an inherited character. *Proc. 7th Congr. int. Soc. Blood Transf.* P.720.

Wiener, A.S., Socha, W.W. & Gordon, E.B. (1973) Further observations on the serological specificity C of the ABO blood group system. *Brit. J. Haemat.,* **24**, 195.

Winstanley, D.P., Konugres, A. & Coombs, R.R.A. (1957) Studies on human anti-A sera with special reference to so-called "immune" anti-A. *Brit. J. Haemat.,* **3**, 341.

Yamaguchi, H., Okubo, Y. & Hazama, F. (1965) An A_2B_3 phenotype blood showing an atypical mode of inheritance. *Proc. imp. Acad. Japan.,* **41**, 316.

Yamaguchi, H., Okubo, Y. & Tanaka, M. (1970) A rare blood B_x analogous to A_x in a Japanese family. *Proc. Jap. Acad.,* **46**, 446.

Yamaguchi, H., Okubo, Y. & Tanaka, M. (1972) Co-occurrence of A_m^h and B_m^h blood in a Japanese family. *Proc. Jap. Acad.,* **48**, 629.

Yokoyama, M., Stacey, S.M. & Dunsford, I. (1957) B_x a new subgroup of the blood group B. *Vox Sang.,* **2**, 348-356.

Ziderman, D., Gompertz, S., Smith, Z.G. & Watkins, W.M. (1967) Glycosyltransferases in mammalian gastric mucosal linings. *Biochem. Biophys. Res. Common.,* **29**, 56.

Chapter 17. Rh Genes and Antigens. The Present Position

The Rh system is one of enormous complexity. In Chapters 7-12 we have explored it to the depth necessary for day-to-day work in the routine serological laboratory, while its role in haemolytic disease of the newborn is discussed in Chapter 26. Here we review briefly the accumulated collection made by numerous enthusiasts over the years of rare Rh variants, antibodies revealing compound antigens, rare complex antigens, suppressors and lastly the finding of LW and Rh_{null} which begin to illuminate the genetic pathway for Rh antigens.

Although many of the complexities described below are sufficiently uncommon for them to leave ordinary serological routine undisturbed, most of them have come to light through the more thorough investigation of blood samples which were originally tested for clinical reasons.

LESS COMMON ALLELES AT THE CDE LOCUS

C variants

C^w

This variant was discovered when a patient who was R_1R_1 made an antibody against transfused blood which was apparently of the same phenotype namely R_1R_1 (Callender and Race, 1946). The antibody agglutinated the blood of about 2 per cent of the population all of whom where C positive. The antigen responsible for the stimulation was named C^w, the full genotype of the transfused blood being C^wDe/CDe and the corresponding antibody, anti-C^w. Many anti-C^w sera have since been found and, in addition, the curious fact has come to light that the majority of anti-C sera have the specificity anti-C + anti-C^w (similarly anti-CD sera are mostly anti-D + anti-C + anti-C^w in specificity). Since the frequency of the C^w antigen is low (2 per cent), it would seem that the antigen C can stimulate the production of anti-C^w. An unusual C^w immunisation has been found by Leonard et al 1976 in which a much transfused patient of type C^wDe/cde developed anti-C. This antibody, as might be expected, did not have an anti-C component. Anti-C^w has caused a transfusion reaction and haemolytic disease of the foetus.

C^x

Another rare form of C is C^x (Stratton and Renton, 1954). This is an allele at the C locus and the specific antibody anti-C^x has been found. This antibody was responsible for a case of haemolytic disease of the newborn. The antibody is very rare and unlike anti-C^w is not normally found in anti-C sera. About one person in a thousand is C^x positive.

c^v and $C^u_{..}$

Other forms of C found, are c^v and C^u These differ from C^w and C^x in that they were not discovered through the finding of specific antibodies, but were differentiated by being agglutinated by some anti-C sera but not others.

It is possible that C^u is a real allele of C similar to D^u, but it is also possible to interpret it as being a depressed C, written (C). c^v is not a true allele, it is rather the expression of C in the $R^z r$ (CDE/cde) genotype which gives weak reactions with many anti-C plus anti-Ce antibodies because the latter component does not react with $R^z r$ cells (*see under* compound antigens).

D variants

D^u

We have dealt at some length with the subject of D^u in Chapters 9 and 10, as this Rh subtype is quite common and affects routine Rh typing. It was originally defined as a cell which reacted with some but not all anti-D sera in saline and albumin tests, but was positive with all anti-D sera by anti-human globulin technique. Such cells are also positive with most anti-D sera if they are first enzyme treated. Individuals of this D^u type are regarded as Rh positive; they do not make anti-D.

Subdivisions of the D antigen Rh^A Rh^B etc.

There is however another type of D variant in which part of the normal D antigen is missing. Such cells if negative with a particular anti-D are truly negative even by antiglobulin and enzyme techniques. Individuals of this kind may make an anti-D against the component of D which they themselves lack.

Many examples of individuals lacking a D component have now been described. They usually announce themselves through the finding of a D positive person possessing anti-D.

Tests with the various examples of these anti-D sera in parallel reveal differences between them in that they do not all give the same pattern of reaction; in fact, the results indicate that the D antigen is a complex one and these antibodies are specific for different parts of it. It is when a part of the D antigen is missing in a particular individual that an antibody to the missing fraction may be formed. Four different fractions with corresponding antibodies have been named Rh^A, Rh^B, Rh^C, Rh^D by Wiener and his co-workers (Wiener *et al.,* 1957; Unger *et al.,* 1959; Unger and Wiener, 1959; Sacks *et al.,* 1959). A further agglutinogen which was Rh positive but lacked all four factors Rh^A Rh^B Rh^C and Rh^D was described (Sussman and Wiener, 1964). The serum of this case contained an anti-Rh antibody which reacted with all Rh positives except the cells of the patient himself. In addition, a variant form of Rh^A termed Rh^α has been described (Unger and Wiener, 1959). Dr Wiener and his colleagues indicate missing components by a small letter thus:- Rh^c_1 Rh^b_2 etc. Most D positive individuals possess all the fractions and so do not form the antibodies. There are some racial variations; for instance Rh^A is absent rather more often in Negroes (8 out of 877 tested compared with 0 out of 942 Whites). It is found, not surprisingly, that ordinary anti-D sera from Rh negative people contain mixtures of these antibodies directed towards special groupings of the D molecule. It is, of course, necessary to carry out absorptions with red cells known to lack one or more of the fractions A, B, C or D in order to reveal the presence of the corresponding antibody in an anti-D serum or to test with the rare cells which only have one D antigen e.g. Rh^B. Once the antibodies, anti-D^A, etc., have been obtained in a pure form, they can be used to detect the presence or absence of the various factors in D positive individuals. So far it is found that there is much variety in the antibody mixtures which occur, but anti-Rh^B is a component of most anti-D sera.

Tippett and Sanger (1962) studied eighteen persons who appeared to be D positive and whose sera contained anti-D and showed that they fell into six broad categories. Since then many more examples have been found but it is still possible to assign them to one of the six classes. They are summarised in Table 17.1. Most of the anti-D antibodies made by such people require an enzyme technique for their detection.

Categories I to IV would probably be typed as Rh positive in routine tests, while categories V and VI might be confused with D^u.

The antigen Go^a Gonzales (Rh30)

Anti-Go^a, causing mild haemolytic disease was investigated by Alter et al. (1967). It was later discovered to be part of the Rh system (Lewis et al., 1967) and finally the antigen disclosed itself as an antigen of category IV (see Table 17.1). The Go^a antigen which is rare has so far only been found in Negroes.

The antigen D^W

An antigen, Wiel, was discovered to be part of the Rh system (Chown et al., 1962). Cells of the propositus and other examples were found to give reactions of category V (see Table 17.1) and all were positive with the original anti-D^W. The antigen is more frequent in Negroes than Whites; O in 13,000 Whites, 9 in 235 Negroes.

E variants

E^u and E^w

The E^u gene was described in 1950 by Ceppellini et al. It is an allele at the E locus and gives rise to an E antigen which is agglutinated by some anti-E sera but not others. Several families with E^u have been studied and they have all given the same pattern of reaction with a given set of antisera which suggests, although the number of examples is small, that E^u is a more uniform variant than D^u. No anti-E^u has been found.

The antigen E^w was discovered by the finding of an antibody which had been the cause of haemolytic disease (Greenwalt and Sanger, 1955). The mother's probable genotype was CDe/cde and the father's C^wDe/cDE^w while the affected child's was CDe/eDE^w. E^w is characterised by being agglutinated by some anti-E sera and not others but in contrast to E^u a specific anti-E^w exists. The allele is very rare, although several examples have now been found.

Table 17.1 Subdivision of the D antigen (after Tippett and Sanger, 1962; Tippett 1963)

Category	Reactions with anti-"D" sera found in						Remarks
	Rh negatives	Cat. II	Cat.III	Cat. IV	Cat. V	Cat. VI	
I	All +	+	+	+	+	+	Contains weak anti-D. Red cells positive with all anti-D's except own
II	All +	-	+	+	+	+	Cells Rh_o^d most members negroid serum anti-Rh^D
III	All +	+	-	+	+	+	
IV	96 per cent +	+	W	-	+	+	One member classified as $Rh_1^{ab}rh$ Negroid members Go(a+), Whites Go(a−)
V	74 per cent +	+	-	+	-	Some − Some W Some +	Founder member Rh_1^{cd}. Antibody—anti-Rh^c All cells D^w positive.
VI	35 per cent +	-	-	+	-	-	Heterogeneous—all white
"Normal" D Pos. cells	+	+	+	+	+	+	
"Normal" D Neg. cells	-	-	-	-	-	-	

Non-Caucasian E-e variants

hr[s]

An antibody was found in the blood of a Bantu woman which reveals more than one kind of hr" (Shapiro, 1960). He called the antibody anti-hr[s]. Her cells, and as found later those of a number of other Negroid types, lacked a component of the hr"(e) antigen. This component has been given the name hr[s] and the antibody anti-hr[s]. This antibody which was present in a pure form in the propositus is contained in most, if not all, anti-hr"(e) sera and seems to be the major or even the only component of some sera. Errors may arise in anti-hr"(e) typing, if an anti-hr"(e) which is pure anti-hr[s] is used for typing a blood which is hr"(e) positive but lacks the component hr[s].

hr[B]

Anti-hr[B] (Shapiro *et al.* 1972) detects yet another 'e' variant of which there seems to be a confusing number! It was found in a South African Negro woman (Mrs Bas) whose genotype appears to be $Cde^s/cD^{III}e$ (for explanation of D^{III} see D categories in Table 17.1).

VS or e[s]

This is another allele of e found mostly in Negroid bloods. The anti-serum anti-e[s] was originally called anti-VS (Sanger *et al.*, 1960). The antibody reacted with the cells of Negroid people of the phenotype V (ce[s]) and Cde[s]. (It should be pointed out that e[s] is not the same antigen as hr[s]).

The gene complex Cde[s]

Cde[s] has been sometimes called the Negroid r' but the Negroid characteristic lies with the e[s] rather than with the C component. Cde[s] gives a negative reaction with anti-C sera which are mainly anti-Ce presumably because the latter antibody will only react with the compound antigen formed when C is accompanied by the Caucasian type of e. (*See under* compound antigens).

An unexpected characteristic of Cde[s] is that it does appear to contain some c and should perhaps be written as Ccde[s].

e[i]

This allele of e was found by Layrisse *et al.* (1961) in a Chibcha Indian tribe where about 20 per cent of the gene complexes were cDe^i. The homozygotes are similar to the suppressed genotype $cD-/cD-$ but they give weak reactions with some anti-e sera. The D in cDe[i] is weaker than in cD— but stronger than the D in Negro cDe.

E[T]

Vos and Kirk (1962) found a naturally occurring antibody (which they called anti-E[T]) in the serum of an Australian aborigine of probable phenotype CcDEe which reacted with all White people with E but not with about one-third of E positive Australian aborigines.

COMPOUND ANTIGENS

Over the years there has been a gradual awareness that the individual Rh genes sometimes affect each other and may vary in their expression according to their partners.

A difference in the C and E antigens of the red cells of individuals whose genotypes contain the same Rh genes but in different combinations was shown by Race *et al.* (1954) in that when *C* and *E* were in the cis position, the antigen C was inhibited and when *C* and *E* were in the trans position, E was inhibited. Only certain antisera made this distinction; when other sera were used the antigens C and E appeared to be present in about the same strength in all the different genotypes tested.

Some of these position effects result in the production of compound antigens. For example, it seems that when *C* and *e* are in the cis position *i.e.* originating from one chromosome *e.g.* (as in *Cde/cde* and *CDe/cDE*) they can give rise to a compound antigen, Ce. On the other hand, when *C* and *e* are in the trans position such a compound antigen is not formed. The antibody corresponding to the Ce antigen is anti-Ce. This antibody, however, does not behave as does a mixture of anti-C+ anti-e which will agglutinate C and e wherever these are found; on the contrary it will only agglutinate the red cells of individuals who have *C* and *e* in the cis position. In standardising Rh antisera it is important to test whether they are of this type.

It is now thought that the antigen originally designated f (Rosenfield *et al.*, 1953) is the compound antigen formed by the genes *ce* when they are in the cis position. This is consistent with the original observation that anti-f reacted with *cde*, *cDe* and *cD^u e*, but not with, for example, cells of the genotype *CDe/cDE* where *c* and *e* are in trans. The antibody is therefore anti-ce. There are some difficulties concerning this antibody since the gene complex *cD*- (see below) reacts with anti-ce where a negative is expected. Moreover the gene complex r^L which has depressed c and e activity, nevertheless gives a normal reaction with anti-ce. These two anomalies can be explained if f is a compound antigen of only part of the ce complex (Boorman and Lincoln 1962) cf r^G and r^M.

Antibodies to the compound antigens CE and cE are also known (Tippett *et al.*, 1961; Keith *et al.*, 1965).

The compound antigen V *or* ce^s

This factor was discovered by means of serum from a *cde/cde* patient who had received many transfusions (De Natale *et al.*, 1955). The antigen V is found only in people with the gene complexes *cDe*, *cD^u e* or *cde*. It is almost exclusively a Negroid antigen. Only 2 English families possess it; they have no history of African ancestry. Not all workers agree that V is a Negroid compound antigen ce^s. Rosenfield *et al.* (1973) consider V to be a product of the *Ee* locus rather than a cis product involving *c*, and there is a hint of *V* travelling with *CDe* in one solitary family.

The antigens r^G *and* r^M

It is probable that the antigens r^G and r^M are also compound antigens arising not from interaction of whole genes but from those portions of the D and C and C and E genes which are adjacent. Boorman and Lincoln (1962) expanded this idea and showed that it would explain many of the observed reactions of these antigens.

r^G. Allen and Tippett (1958) investigated the red cells of a White Boston blood donor Mrs Crosby which although apparently Rh negative, reacted with most anti-CD sera. The genotype proposed for Mrs Crosby was $r^G r$ and anti-CD sera were assumed to have an anti-G component. Anti-G was isolated from anti-CD sera by elution using the cells of Mrs Crosby. Tests with anti-G showed that all common gene complexes except cde and cdE contained G.

The existence of G explains how cde/cde women, never transfused but immunised by a foetus can make apparent anti-CD although their husbands lack C. The antibody is in fact anti-D + G and does not contain anti-C.

The finding of the very rare genotype $r^G r^G$ (the outcome of a first cousin mating) by Levine et al. (1961) showed that r^G was negative with anti-c and weakly positive with some anti-C made in D positive people. The $r^G r^G$ was negative with two anti-ce sera. Several examples of Negro $r^G r$ have been reported. Further work on the $r^G r^G$ cells has led Rosenfield et al. (1975) to the conclusion that r^G resembles a mutant r' in which only e is expressed normally.

r^M The antigens expressed by this complex are depressed G accompanied by some kind of weak C and E so that $r^M r$ for example may be written $(C)d(E)/cde$, the brackets denoting weakness of the enclosed gene.

DEPRESSED ANTIGENS

$\bar{\bar{R}}^N$ and (C)D(e)

In 1960 Rosenfield et al. found in a Negro family an Rh gene complex producing weak C and e antigens with a normal D. Distinct from this Negroid $\bar{\bar{R}}^N$ is a complex ($(C)D(e)$) found in Whites which is not identical with the Negroid $\bar{\bar{R}}^N$ because not only does it display a different pattern of reaction with anti-C and anti-e sera but is negative with antibodies which have been found to be anti-$\bar{\bar{R}}^N$.

About 1 per cent of American Negroes have $\bar{\bar{R}}^N$ and it occurs as a great rarity in Whites. It has been shown to be inherited in a straight-forward fashion.

The White $(C)D(e)$ (Broman et al., 1963) was found to be of two kinds one producing normal and the other an elevated D antigen. In 1971 Giles and Skov found an antibody specific for the complex without the elevated D.

Rh33 or R_o^{Har}

Giles et al. (1971) were alerted to this rare antigen complex by finding that the red cells of a German donor when tested for Rh antigens, only reacted with anti-c. Further tests showed reactions with a few anti-D and weak reactions with anti-e but no C or E antigens were detectable. The cells were positive with anti-ce (f). A second example was recognised in an English blood donor whose cells reacted with a few anti-D and anti-CD sera. The cells had normal c and weak e.

An antibody, anti-Rh33 was separable from one anti-D. The donor of this antibody was Cde/cde, had never been transfused and although she had made anti-D in response to five pregnancies her anti-Rh33 agglutinin was negative with her husband's CDe/cDE cells.

A number of further examples of Rh33 have been discovered; the family of one of them showed Rh33 to be inherited in a straightforward way through three generations, the gene complex producing the antigen being a modified *cDe*.

Be^a *(Berrens)*

Anti-Be^a was described in 1953 by Davidsohn *et al.* but twenty years passed before it was discovered that the corresponding antigen (Be) belongs to the Rh system.

In the original family and in two others the antibody was responsible for haemolytic disease of the newborn.

Ducos *et al.* (1974) demonstrated in the Kos family that Be^a belongs to the Rh system. In three generations of the family the Be(a+) members have an unusual *cde* complex resulting in weak e, c and ce antigens whereas two Be (a−) members have no such abnormality.

SUPPRESSIONS

−D−

There are rare individuals in whom all or some of the expected Rh antigens are missing. The first to be described (Race *et al.*, 1951) lacked all trace of *C−c* or *E−e* products and possessed only *D*. It is written −D−. The propositus was the offspring of a consanguineous marriage. There are now about 23 examples of individuals who are −D−/−D−, sixteen of which certainly and three more probably are the product of consanguineous marriages. This is a very high rate compared with that found in other families who lack common antigens *e.g.* p, p^k and O$_h$. Its cause is as yet unknown

The red cells of people homozygous or heterozygous for −D− have more D than ordinary DD or Dd cells. The antigen sites on a few examples have been counted (see Table 17.2). The increase in D sites and their distribution leads to the ability of −D− cells to be agglutinated in a saline suspension by incomplete anti-D sera. Most such sera will agglutinate the homozygous −D− cells suspended in saline but to distinguish the heterozygote, incomplete anti-D sera have to be specially selected because some will agglutinate in a saline suspension *cDe/cDE* cells which are also strong in D.

The −D− gene complex has to be remembered in the interpretation of exclusion by the Rh system in paternity tests (*see* Chapter 29).

−D−/−D− people are readily immunised and present transfusion problems. The lack of products of *Cc* and *Ee* genes seem to remove a restraining influence on the immune response which has a tendency to go wild!

In some examples separable specific antibodies, particularly anti-e can be demonstrated. Others cross react. For example, antibodies directed against both C and c have been found and sometimes there appears to be a single antibody reacting with all Rh antigens except D.

Rh$_{null}$

As the name infers red cells of this type have no Rh antigens at all. The first such propositus was an Australian aboriginal woman, Mrs E.N. discovered by

Voss *et al.* (1961). It is most likely that the condition arises from the lack of a common gene necessary for the synthesis of an Rh precursor substance. Levine *et al.* (1962) found that the cells of Mrs E.N. were negative with anti-LW (see below).

Mrs E.N. had no family but the finding of further examples of Rh_{null} provided the opportunity for family studies which revealed that there are two kinds of Rh_{null}.

One kind appears to be the result of a silent gene or amorph at the Rh locus (Ishimori and Hasekura, 1967), the other kind, of which there are more examples, seems to be caused by a regulator gene which is not part of the Rh complex locus (Levine *et al.*, 1965; Senhauser *et al.*, 1970). In the amorph type of Rh_{null}, family studies may show, for example, that an apparently *cDE/cDE* parent has an apparent *Cde/CDe* child. The actual genotypes are in fact, parent *cDE/---* and child *CDe/---*.

The regulator type of Rh_{null} reveals itself when either the parent or child of the propositus has normal Rh genes *i.e.* both *C* and *c* or both *E* and *e* thus indicating that the normal Rh genes are present in the Rh_{null} person although they are unable to express themselves. In fact, a hint of the presence of D on the cells of one. Rh_{null} individual of the regulator type was obtained by the ability to elute anti-D from the red cell surface.

Antibodies found in Rh_{null} people. When antibodies are found in Rh_{null} people they are of various kinds and most appear to have been made in response to transfusion or pregnancy. The antibody in some reacts with all cells tested including suppressed types such as $-D-/-D-$ but not with Rh_{null}. One Rh_{null} male donor has been reported to have an antibody which has arisen without known stimulus. This antibody did not react with $-D-/-D-$ cells and therefore lacked anti-D and anti-LW components. Rh_{null} individuals with Rh antibodies of other specificities are known *e.g.* anti-e and anti-C.

The red cell membrane of the Rh_{null} cell. The Rh_{null} condition of the regulator type is associated with some defect of the red cell surface. This was first noticed by Schmidt *et al.* in 1967; these workers also drew attention to the fact that normal reactivity with anti-s and anti-U sera was disturbed. Almost concurrently it was observed that the defect of the red cell membrane was accompanied by a haemolytic anaemia, occasionally severe but often mild enough to remain undetected unless special tests are performed.

The anaemia is associated with a high reticulocyte count, shortened survival time of the individual's own cells, an abnormally high concentration of foetal haemoglobin and an increased strength of i antigen, also stomatocytes are seen.

A detailed investigation of the reaction of anti-S, anti-s and anti-U with a variety of Rh_{null} cells of the regulator type has been made by Race and Sanger (1975). This showed suppression of S, s and U reactions but this was only apparent when the antiglobulin test was used. With anti-S and anti-s sera which reacted with Rh_{null} cells in saline no false negatives were seen. Race and Sanger consider this difference in reactivity may result from a less firm attachment of these antibodies to the defective cell membrane with consequent loss of antibody during the washing stage of the antiglobulin test.

It has been pointed out that since Nicholson *et al.* (1971) have shown that Rh antigens are an integral part of the red cell wall, it is not surprising that the Rh_{null} condition should be responsible for a defect in the wall structures. We think that this association might equally well be expressed the other way round *i.e.* the Rh_{null} condition may be a consequence of a defect in the cell wall structure.

C^wD-

Besides the lack of e, this gene complex is characterised by an increased activity of D and weakened C^w. A family in which five members were homozygous for C^wD- was found by Gunson and Donohue (1957). Like most other families with suppressed antigens the parents of the propositus were consanguineous. The propositus had an antibody which was compatible only with C^wD-/C^wD- cells and two examples of $-D-/-D-$. There were no separable components.

$cD-$

The first example of a family with three members homozygous for this gene complex was described by Tate *et al.* (1960). Since then a number of similar families have been found. Some of the reactions of the cells with various antisera are puzzling.

The D antigen in the heterozygote is more than that expected from one D gene; the *c* gene product is weak to the point of being negative with a few otherwise good anti-c sera. Some anti-ce sera give positive reactions while others are negative. The positive reactions are unexpected since the compound antigen ce is surely absent.

The original propositus and some other individuals found later had an antibody for all cells tested except those homozygous for $-D-$, $cD-$, C^wD- and Rh_{null}.

$(C)D^{iv}-$

A woman whose third child died of haemolytic disease of the newborn was found to be homozygous for this very rare gene complex (Salmon *et al.*, 1969). Her serum reacted with all red cells but her own and those homozygous for $-D-$. Her fourth child was successfully treated with $-D-/-D-$ blood.

$(C)D^{IV}-$cells have a depressed C and D as in Tippett's category IV. Some anti-Ce sera were positive although the e antigen is almost certainly absent.

THE LW ANTIGEN

It has now come to be realised that the anti-Rhesus antibody made originally in rabbits and guinea pigs by Landsteiner and Wiener (1940) is not the same as the human anti-Rh (anti-D) which is of such clinical importance. The similarity of the two antibodies is caused by the fact that they belong to systems interrelated somewhere along their genetic pathways. The antigen in human red cells detected by the Rhesus monkey antibody is now termed LW in honour of Landsteiner and Wiener. The knowledge that the human and monkey antibodies were different allowed a number of unexplained findings to fall into place.

For example in 1942 Fisk and Foord reported that all newborn babies whether

Rh positive or Rh negative as defined by human anti-Rh sera, were positive with guinea pig anti-Rh serum. Later the guinea pig serum was shown to be anti-LW.

Moreover Murray and Clarke (1952) made the unexpected observation that heat extracts of Rh negative red cells were capable of stimulating the formation of what seemed to be anti-D in guinea pigs. This antibody was also later identified as anti-LW. The fact that the D antigen can be expressed in the absence of LW was first shown by Levine *et al.* (1963) when they found two individuals with Rh positive LW negative red cells whose serum contained anti-LW. Rh negative cells were shown to have less LW antigen activity than Rh positive cells, but LW negative cells do not react with anti-LW even if they are Rh positive. Levine and his colleagues (1961) contributed the additional evidence that the anti-D like antibody of the guinea pig still agglutinated D positive cells even after the D sites were blocked with incomplete anti-D.

Finally, examples of anti-LW made in humans appeared and it was found that Rh_{null}'cells were negative with both human and animal anti-LW.

That the genes responsible for LW and Rh were distinct was established from family studies (Tippett 1963; Swanson and Matson 1964; Swanson *et al.*, 1974).

Further distinctions in the LW system emerged when it was found that there are apparently two kinds of LW antibody, and two kinds of LW positive red cells. One antibody is anti-LW + LW$_1$ (analogous to anti-A+A$_1$) and the other is anti-LW$_1$ (similar to anti-A$_1$). Anti-LW$_1$ distinguishes two different LW antigens, LW$_1$ and LW$_2$. Most people are LW$_1$ (Swanson *et al.*, 1974).

Table 17.2 summarises all the Rh variants mentioned in this chapter.

Table 17.2 A summary of Rh variants

Type	Name	Corresponding antibody	Occurrence	Remarks
Alleles of CDE locus	*C variants*			
	C^w	Anti-C^w	2 per cent	Most anti-C sera contain anti-C^w.
	C^x	Anti-C^x	0.1 per cent	Anti-C^x not normally found in anti-C sera.
	c^v	None		Not true allele but weak expression of C in R$_z$r.
	C^u	None		Agglutinated by some anti-C sera and not others.
	D variants			
	D^u	None		Much variation in reactivity with anti-D sera. Individuals do not form anti-D.

Table 17.2 A summary of Rh variants   contd

Type	Name	Corresponding antibody	Occurrence	Remarks
	Rh^A Rh^B Rh^C Rh^D	Anti-Rh^A Anti-Rh^B Anti-Rh^C Anti-Rh^D		Individuals lack some component of D antigen and can make antibody to portions which they lack.
	Go^a	Anti-Go^a	Negroid	Has portion of Tippett's D^{iv} antigen missing.
	D^w	Anti-D^w	More frequent in Negroids.	Probably belongs to Tippett's category D^v.
	D^I to D^{VI}			see table 17.1
	E variants E^u	None	Caucasians	Agglutinated by some anti-E sera and not by others.
	E^w	Anti-E^w		Agglutinated by some anti-E sera and not by others.
	hr^s	Anti-hr^s	hr^s antigenic component more often lacking in Bantu than in Whites.	Only few individuals lack the hr^s component of e. Anti-hr^s present in most anti-e sera.
	e^s	Anti-e^s	More common in Negroes than Caucasians.	Originally called VS.
	hr^B	Anti-hr^B	Negroid	Variant of e.
	e^L	None	20% in Columbian Indians.	Weak reactions with some anti-e sera. D stronger than in Negroid cDe.
	E^T	Anti-E^T	Common component of E.	30% Australian aborigines who have E lack E^T.
Compound antigens	Ce	Anti-Ce	Formed by *C* and *e* in cis	
	f	Anti-f	Formed by *c* and *e* in cis	
	CE	Anti-CE	Formed by *C* and *E* in cis	
	cE	Anti-cE	Formed by *c* and *E* in cis	
	$V(ce^s)$	Anti-$V(ce^s)$	Most Negroid	May be allele of Ee rather than compound antigen.
	r^G	Anti-G	G antigen in all complexes except *cde* and *cdE*.	Possible compound antigen of adjacent portions of D and C.
	r^M	None		Has depressed G, C and E antigens.

Table 17.2 A summary of Rh variants   contd

Type	Name	Corresponding antibody	Occurrence	Remarks
Depressed antigens	R^N	Anti-R^N	1% American Negroes	Weak C and e. Normal D. Not same as White (C)D(e).
	(C)D(e)	Anti-(C)D(e)	Found in Caucasians	Some with normal D, others elevated D. Negative with anti-R^N.
	Rh33(R_o^{Har})	Anti-Rh33	Caucasians but rare	Weak with anti-e. Reacts with some anti-D's. Normal c antigen.
	Be^a (Berrens)	Anti-Be^a	Caucasian but rare	Weak c, e and ce antigens.
Suppressed Antigens	−D−	None	Caucasian and Negroid examples.	No Cc or Ee antigens. Elevated D activity. Complex antibodies formed.
	Rh_{null}	None	Caucasian and Australian aboriginal examples.	One type caused by regulator gene independent of Rh locus, other type, less common produced by silent gene at Rh locus. Often have antibodies reacting with all cells except Rh_{null}.
	$C^wD−$	None	Caucasian but very rare.	Enhanced D, weakened C^w
	cD−	None	Caucasian but rare	Slight enhancement of D, weakened c.
	$(C)D^{iv}−$	None	Caucasian but very rare.	D as in category IV C depressed.

PROPOSED GENETIC PATHWAYS

Tippett (1972) has proposed the genetic pathways shown in Fig. 17.1 to show how they may give rise to the four known types of individual summarised as follows:-

(a) Those with ordinary Rh and LW antigens (the great majority).

(b) The LW negative who has normal Rh antigens.

(c) The Rh_{null} amorph type.

(d) The Rh_{null} regulator type recognised when a parent or child of the propositus has both C and c or both E and e antigens.

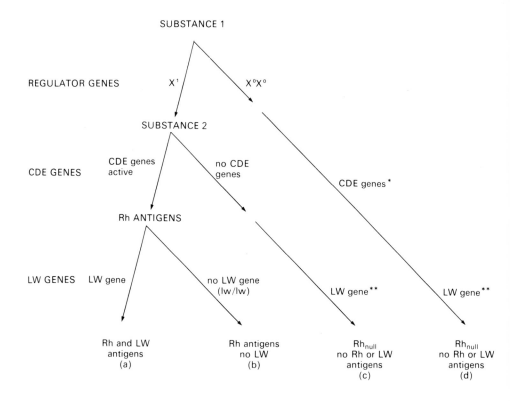

Fig. 17.1 Possible pathways for the synthesis of Rh and LW antigens. Notes: *, these may also be very rare types with no CDE genes; **, may also be very rare types with no *LW* gene (*lw/lw*).

A precursor substance 1 is postulated which in the presence of a common allele X^1, independent of the Rh locus, is converted into substance 2. By means of normal *CDE* and *LW* genes, substance 2 is used for the synthesis of Rh antigens and also for LW (a).

It is further proposed that Rh_{null} people of the regulator type are homozygous for a rare allele X^0 which suppresses the formation of substance 2. Thus even though *CDE* and *LW* genes *are* present no Rh or LW antigens are formed (d). Individuals of the amorph type of Rh_{null} have substance 2 but in the absence of *CDE* genes, are unable to convert it into Rh and LW antigens (c).

Finally in the absence of the *LW* gene *i.e.* in individuals of genotype *lw/lw*, no LW antigen is present although the *CDE* genes are capable of functioning normally (b).

A CHEMICAL APPROACH TO THE D ANTIGEN

Knowledge of the chemical composition of Rh antigens is as yet at a very early stage. Rh substances are not detectable in any appreciable amount in body fluids, so this source which has been so rewarding in the study of A, B, H and Lewis substances is not available for the chemical study of Rh.

Attempts to extract Rh active structures from red cell membranes with organic solvents or detergents have failed; what little is known of the properties of Rh antigens has so far been derived from work on intact red cells or dried red cell membranes.

It has been found that Rh antigens are more heat labile than A and B antigens. Their pH stability also differs in that the Rh activity of dried red cell membranes is unstable below pH 5.8 and above pH 9.2 (Green, 1965). These characteristics are suggestive of a protein rather than carbohydrate antigen. However evidence that carbohydrate structures might be connected with D specificity was obtained for the fact that the antigenicity is readily destroyed by treatment of red cells with dilute periodate at a concentration so low that even A and B antigens, which are known to be carbohydrate, are not destroyed.

The role of sialic acid in Rh specificity has been considered but evidence for this has been equivocal. It has been suggested that Rh activity may depend on membrane protein.

A further significant finding was made by Green (1968, 1972) who extracted Rh-positive cell membrane with 100 per cent butanol. At this concentration butanol does not solubilize protein or carbohydrate. However it destroyed the D activity of the membranes. The butanol extract did not have Rh activity but was capable of restoring Rh activity when added back to the extracted membranes. Moreover lipid fraction from Rh negative cells was also capable of restoring D activity to D positive butanol-extracted membranes. The reaction appears to depend on the presence of phospholipids with at least one unsaturated fatty acid since non-phosphorus containing fatty acids and fully saturated phospholipids both failed to restore activity. Support for this view comes from the rather different approach of Hughes-Jones and co-workers (1975) who experimented with phospholipase A_2. Red cell stromata when treated, with this enzyme which catalyses the removal of the unsaturated fatty acid from the 2-position of phospholipids, showed a loss of activity of the Rh antigens c, D and e. A further finding of interest was that anti-D bound to the red cells protected the D antigen from inactivation by phospholipase A_2.

Rh ANTIGEN SITES

The distribution of Rh antigen sites, particularly D has been studied by a number of workers. The method of Nicholson et al. (1971) was that of sensitising D positive cells with ^{125}I-labelled anti-D after which the cells were lysed. The membranes were spread flat, stained with a ferritin labelled goat anti-human IgG reagent which stained only the upper exposed surface of the cell membrane, and the distribution of the ferritin particles was examined using the electron microscope.

The results suggested that the D sites are present as single molecular entities distributed in an 'aperiodic and random two dimensional array'.

Table 17.3 Rh antigen sites

Type of site	Cell type	Approximate number of sites
D	CcDEe	33,300 − 38,500
	−D−	110,000 − 202,000
c	cc	70,000 − 85,000
	Cc	37,000 − 53,000
e	ee	18,200 − 24,400
	Ee	13,400 − 14,500
E	EE	4890 − 5560 (1)
		22,400 − 25,600 (2)
	Ee	450 − 2890 (1)
		5800 − 11,800 (2)

(1) and (2) are results from two different examples of anti-E.

Similar studies were undertaken by Romano *et al.* (1975) using a gold labelled anti-IgG reagent. These experiments confirmed the findings of Nicholson and co-workers. The work was extended to include simultaneous labelling of D and c sites and showed that in the cells used which were ccDEE the D and c sites were very close to each other.

The same investigation included evidence that enzyme (papain) treatment of the cells prior to lysis produces a clustering of the antigen sites. It is of significance that −D− cells showed a clustered distribution of D sites without enzyme treatment. This fact provides part at least of the reason why IgG anti-D is capable of agglutinating untreated −D− cells suspended in saline.

Table 17.4 Various Rh notations

Numerical	CDE	Rh-Hr	Numerical	CDE	Rh-Hr	Other
Rh 1	D	Rh_o	Rh 18		Hr	
Rh 2	C	rh'	Rh 19		hr^s	
Rh 3	E	rh″	Rh 20	VS, e^s		
Rh 4	c	hr'	Rh 21	C^G		
Rh 5	e	hr″	Rh 22	CE		
Rh 6	f, ce	hr	Rh 23	Wiel, D^w		
Rh 7	Ce	rh_i	Rh 24	E^T		
Rh 8	C^w	$rh^{w'}$	Rh 25			LW
Rh 9	C^x	rh^x	Rh 26			'Deal'
Rh 10	V, ce^s	hr^v	Rh 27	cE		
Rh 11	E^w	rh^{w2}	Rh 28		hrH	
Rh 12	G	rh^G	Rh 29			'Total Rh'
Rh 13		Rh^A	Rh 30			Go^a
Rh 14		Rh^B	Rh 31		hr^B	
Rh 15		Rh^C	Rh 32			$\bar{\bar{R}}^N$
Rh 16		Rh_D	Rh 33			$R_o^{'Har}$
Rh 17		Hr_o	Rh 34			Bas
			Rh 35			1114

Clustering of D sites after enzyme treatment of cells was observed also by Voak *et al.* (1974). Rh antigen sites have been counted (Hughes-Jones *et al.,* 1971). The results are assembled in Table 17.3. There are fewer sites for Rh by comparison with A_1, A_2 and B (*see* Table 16.1). The exception is D in the $-D-$ pheno-type when since it suffers no competition from *Cc* and *Ee* alleles, achieves a count of 110,000-202,000 sites in the homozygote.

Rh notation

In Table 17.4, we give the numerical notation suggested by Rosenfield *et al.* (1962) and the corresponding CDE and Rh-Hr nomenclature.

REFERENCES

Allen, F.H. & Tippett, P.A. (1958) A new Rh blood type which reveals the Rh antigen G. *Vox Sang.,* 3, 321.

Alter, A.A., Gelb, A.G., Chown, B., Rosenfield, R.E. & Cleghorn, T.E. (1967) Gonzales (Go^a) a new blood group character. *Transfusion (Philad)*, 7, 88.

Boorman, K.E. & Lincoln P.J. (1962) A suggestion as to the place of r^G and r^M on the Rh system. *Ann., Hum., Genet.,* 26, 51.

Broman, B., Heiken, A., Tippett, P.A. & Giles, C.M. (1963) The DC(e) gene complex revealed in the Swedish population. *Vox Sang.,* 8, 588.

Callender, S.T. & Race, R.R. (1946) A serological and genetical study of multiple antibodies formed in response to blood transfusion by a patient with lupus erythematosus diffusus. *Ann., Eugen., (Lond.),* 13, 102.

Ceppellini, R., Ikin, E.W. & Mourant, A.E. (1950) A new allele of the Rh gene E. *Boll., 1st Sieroter Milanese,* 29, 123.

Chown, B., Lewis, M. & Kaita, H. (1962) A 'new' Rh antigen and antibody. *Transfusion (Philad),* 2, 150.

Davidsohn, I., Stern, K., Strauser, E.R. & Spurrier, W. (1953) Be, a new 'private' blood factor. *Blood,* 8, 747.

De Natale, A., Cahan, A., Jack, J.A., Race, R.R. & Sanger, R. (1955) V, a new Rh antigen common in Negroes, rare in White people. *J.A.M.A.,* 159, 247.

Ducos, J., Marty, Y., Ruffié, J., Gavin, J., Teesdale, P. & Tippett, P. (1974) In preparation. See also Race, R.R. & Sanger, R. (1975) Blood Groups in Man 6th ed., p. 204.

Fisk, R.T. & Foord, A.G. (1942) Observations on the Rh agglutinogen of human blood. *Amer. J. clin. Path.,* 12, 545.

Giles, C.M., Crossland, J.D., Haggas, W.K. & Longster, G. (1971) An Rh gene complex which results in a 'new' antigen detectable by a specific antibody anti-Rh$_{33}$. *Vox Sang.,* 21, 289.

Giles, C.M. & Skov, F. (1971) The *CDe* rhesus gene complex; some considerations revealed by a study of a Danish family with an antigen of the rhesus gene complex *(C)D(e)* defined by a 'new' antibody. *Vox Sang.,* 20, 328.

Green, F.A. (1965) Studies on the Rh (D) Antigen. *Vox Sang.,* 10, 32.

Green, F.A. (1968) Phospholipid requirement for Rh antigenic activity. *J. Biol. Chem.,* 243, 5519.

Green, F.A. (1972) Erythrocyte membrane lipids and Rh antigen activity. *J. biol. Chem.,* 247, 881.

Greenwalt, T.J. & Sanger, R. (1955) The Rh antigen E^w. *Brit. J. Haem.,* 1, 52.

Gunson, H.H. & Donohue, W.L. (1957) Multiple examples of the blood genotype C^wD-/C^wD- in a Canadian family. *Vox Sang.,* 2, 320.

Hughes-Jones, N.C., Gardner, B. & Lincoln, P.J. (1971) Observations of the number of available c, D and E antigen sites on red cells. *Vox Sang.,* 21, 210.

Hughes-Jones, N.C., Green, E.J. & Hunt, V.A.M. (1975) Loss of Rh antigen activity following the action of phospholipase A$_2$ on red cell stroma. *Vox Sang.,* 29, 184.

Ishimori, T. & Hasekura, H. (1967) A Japanese with no detectable Rh blood group antigens due to silent Rh alleles or chromosomes. *Transfusion (Philad),* 7, 84.

Keith, P., Corcoran, P.A. Caspersen, K. & Allen, F.H. (1965) A new antibody; anti-Rh (27) (cE) in the Rh blood group system. *Vox Sang.,* 10, 528.

Landsteiner, K. & Wiener, A.S. (1940) An agglutinable factor on human blood recognised by immune sera for rhesus blood. *Proc. Soc. exp. Biol. (N.Y.),* **43**, 223:

Layrisse, M., Layrisse, Z., Garcia, E. & Parra, J. (1961) Genetic studies of the new Rh chromosome $Dce^if(Rh_0^i)$ found in a Chibcha tribe. *Vox Sang.,* **6**, 710.

Leonard, G. L., Ellsior, S. S., Reid, M. E., Sanchez, P. D., and Tippett, P. (1976) An unusual Rh immunisation. Vox. Sang. **31**. 275.

Levine, P., Celano, M.J., Wallace, J. & Sanger, R. (1963) A human D-like antibody. *Nature, (Lond.),* **198**, 596.

Levine, P., Rosenfield, R.E. & White, J. (1961) The first example of the Rh phenotype r^Gr^G. *Amer. J. hum. Genet.,* **13**, 299.

Levine, P., Celano, M., Fenichel, R., Pollack, W. & Singher, H. (1961) A 'D-like' antigen in rhesus monkey, human Rh positive and human Rh negative red blood cells. *J. Immunol.,* **87**, 747.

Levine, P., Celano, M., Vos, G.H. & Morrison, J. (1962) The first human blood - - -/- - - which lacks the D-like antigen. *Nature (Lond.),* **194**, 304.

Levine, P., Celano, M.J., Falkowski, F., Chambers, J., Hunter, O.B. & English, C.T. (1965) A second example of - - -/- - -blood, or Rh$_{null}$ blood. *Transfusion (Philad.),* **5**, 492.

Lewis, M., Chown, B., Kaita, H., Hahn, D., Kangelos, M., Shepeard, W.L. & Shackleton, K. (1967) Blood group antigen Go^a and the Rh system. *Transfusion (Philad),* **7**, 440.

Murray, J. & Clarke, E.C. (1952) Production of anti-Rh in guinea pigs from human erythrocytes. *Nature (Lond.),* **69**, 886.

Nicholson, G.L., Masouredis, S.P. & Singer, S.J. (1971) Quantitative two-dimensional ultra structural distribution of Rh$_0$(D) antigenic sites on human erythrocyte membranes. *Proc. Nat. Acad. Sci.,* **68**, 1416.

Race, R.R., Sanger, R., Levine, P., McGee, R.T., Van Loghem, J.J. Van der Hart, M. & Cameron, C. (1954) A position effect of the Rh blood group genes. *Nature (Lond.),* **174**, 460.

Race, R.R., Sanger, R. & Selwyn, J.G. (1951) A possible deletion in a human Rh chromosome; A serological and genetical study. *Brit. J. Exp. Path.,* **32**, 124.

Race, R.R. & Sanger, R. (1975) Blood groups in Man. P.225 Oxford: Blackwell.

Romano, E.L., Stolinski, C. & Hughes-Jones, N.C. (1975) Distribution and mobility of the A, D and c antigens on human red cell membranes. Studies with a gold-labelled anti-globulin reagent. *Brit. J. Haemat.,* **30**, 507.

Rosenfield, R.E., Vogel, P., Gibbel, N., Sanger, R. & Race, R.R. (1953) A new Rh antibody, anti-f. *Brit. Med. J.,* **i**, 975.

Rosenfield, R.E., Haber, G.V., Schroeder, R. & Ballard, R. (1960) Problems in Rh typing as revealed by a single Negro family. *Amer. J. hum. Genet.,* **12**, 147.

Rosenfield, R.E., Allen, F.H., Swisher, S.N. & Kochwa, S. (1962) A review of Rh serology and presentation of a new terminology. *Transfusion (Philad),* **2**, 287.

Rosenfield, R.E., Allen, F.H. & Rubinstein, P. (1973) Genetic model for the Rh blood group system. *Proc. Nat. Acad. Sci.,* **70**, 1303.

Rosenfield, R.E., Levine, P. & Heller, C. (1975) Quantitative Rh typing of r^{G}r^G with observations on the nature of G (Rh12) and anti-G. *Vox Sang.,* **28**, 293.

Sacks, M.S., Wiener, A.S., John, E.F., Spurling, C.L. & Unger, L.J. (1959) Isosensitization to the new blood factor RhD with special reference to its clinical importance. *Ann. Int. Med.,* **51**, 740.

Salmon, C., Gerbal, A., Liberge, G., Sy, B., Tippett, P. & Sanger, R. (1969) La complexe genique D^{iv}(C)− *Rev. fr Transf.,* **12**; 239.

Sanger, R., Noades, J., Tippett, P., Jack, J.A. & Cunningham, C.A. (1960) An Rh antibody specific for V and R^{is} *Nature (Lond.),* **186**, 171.

Schmidt, P.J., Lostumbo, M.M., English, C.T. & Hunter O.B. (1967) Aberrant U blood group accompanying Rh$_{null}$. *Transfusion (Philad),* **7**, 33.

Senhauser, D.A., Mitchell, M.W., Gault, D.B. & Owens, J.H. (1970) Another example of Rh$_{null}$. *Transfusion (Philad)* **10**, 89.

Shapiro, M. (1960) Serology and Genetics of a new blood factor hr^s. *J. For. Med.,* **7**, 96.

Shapiro, M., LeRoux, M. & Brink, S. (1972) Serology and genetics of a new blood factor hr^B *Haematologia,* **6**, 121.

Stratton, F. & Renton, P.H. (1954) Haemolytic disease of the newborn caused by a new Rh antibody, anti-C^x. *Brit. Med. J.,* **i**, 962.

Sussman, L.N. & Wiener, A.S. (1964) An unusual Rh agglutinogen lacking blood factors Rh^A, Rh^B, Rh^C and Rh^D. *Transfusion(Philad),* **4**, 50.

Swanson, J. & Matson, G.A. (1964) Third example of a human 'D-like' antibody or anti-LW. *Transfusion (Philad),* **4**, 257.

Swanson, J.L., Miller, J., Azar, M. & McCullough, J.J. (1974) Evidence for heterogeneity of LW antigen revealed in family study. *Transfusion (Philad)*, **14**, 470.

Tate, H., Cunningham, C., McDade, M.G., Tippett, P.A. & Sanger, R. (1960) An Rh gene complex *Dc*–. *Vox Sang.*, **5**, 398.

Tippett, P. & Sanger, R. (1962) Observations on subdivision of the Rh antigen D. *Vox Sang.*, **7**, 9.

Tippett, P.A., Sanger, R., Dunsford, I. & Barker, M. (1961) An Rh gene complex r^M in some ways like r^g. *Vox Sang.*, **6**, 21.

Tippett, P. (1963) Serological study of the inheritance of unusual Rh and other blood group phenotypes. *Ph.D. Thesis*, London University.

Tippett, P. (1972) A present view of Rh. *Pathologica*, **64**, 29.

Unger, L.J. & Wiener, A.S. (1959) Observations on blood factors Rh^A, Rh^α., Rh^B and Rh^C. *Amer. J. Clin. Path.*, **31**, 95.

Unger, L.J., Wiener, A.S. & Weiner, L. (1959) New antibody (anti-Rh^B) resulting from blood transfusion in Rh positive patient. *J.A.M.A.*, **170**, 1380.

Voak, D., Cawley, J.C., Emmines, J.P. & Barker, C.R. (1974) The role of enzymes and albumin in haemagglutination reactions, a serological and ultra structural study with ferritin-labelled anti-D. *Vox Sang.*, **27**, 156.

Vos, G.H., Vos, D., Kirk, R.L. & Sanger, R. (1961) A sample of blood with no detectable Rh antigens. *Lancet*, **i**, 14.

Vos, G.H. & Kirk, R.L. (1962) A naturally-occurring anti-E which distinguishes a variant of the E antigen in Australian aborigines. *vox Sang.*, **7**, 22.

Wiener, A.S., Geiger, J. & Gordon, E.B. (1957) Mosaic nature of Rh_o factor of human blood. *Exper. Med. & Surg.*, **15**, 75.

H

Chapter 18. A further look at MNSs, P, Lutheran, I, Kell and Duffy together with other systems

Blood group systems often appear uncomplicated when first discovered. A common sequence is the finding of a single antibody detecting a red cell antigen and afterwards the finding of a second antibody antithetical in its reactions to the first. It is then postulated that the two antibodies are detecting antigens produced by a pair of allelic genes (*e.g.* Fy^a, Fy^b; Jk^a, Jk^b). The ABO system was an exception and was probably the least simple at the time of its discovery.

Experience has shown that the simple beginnings are almost always followed by further discoveries which have revealed complexities which have not always been easy to unravel. This state of affairs lasts until the system seems to crystallise and to take its final form - an unwise conclusion to draw as the history of several systems illustrates. The P system, for example, has developed in four main stages:- in 1927 the discovery of a single antigen (although variable in strength) and its corresponding antibody; in 1955 the recognition that Tj^a belonged to P; in 1959 an extension to include P^k and in 1965 a further extension to include Luke.

As new antibodies are found each necessitates careful investigation including family studies to determine whether it belongs to one of the known systems or is independent of them.

Families with rare genes or displaying unusual genic effects, although in some respects collector's pieces, have yet contributed vitally to the understanding of various blood group systems. (For example "Bombay" bloods and Rh null cells.)

Antigens which segregate with a well recognised system but are not alleles at the same locus are always a puzzle (see associations with MNSs). Such associations may be phenotypic as well as genetic.

The following chapter adds rather more depth to the accounts given of the MNSs, P, Lutheran, I, Kell and Duffy systems in Chapter 13 and introduces the reader to short descriptions of others such as Scianna, Colton, Dombrock, Xg etc.

It is hoped that the material here together with the reference pages listed separately for each system will provide sufficient information for workers requiring a basic knowledge of these systems.

RARE *MNSs* ALLELES AND ASSOCIATES

The complexity of the MNSs system is obvious from a glance at Tables 18.1 to 18.3. Variants which appear to be the products of alleles at the MN or Ss loci are shown in Table 18.1. These are characterised by their failure to react with some or all of the regular anti-MNSs antisera. In many cases a specific antibody has been found. A second category (Table 18.2) is composed of antigens closely associated with the MN and Ss loci but not, in the main, affecting the expression of the M, N, S, s antigens with which they are associated. They are detected by the finding of specific antisera and family studies then reveal that the gene for the rare antigen in question is segregating with the *MNSs* gene. The Miltenburger

Table 18.1 Rare alleles at the MN or Ss Locus

Antigens	Characteristics	Occurrence	Antibodies
M^g	Anti-M and Anti-N negative	0 in 61,128 English 0 in 44,000 Boston 0.153 per cent in Swiss	Anti-Mg fairly common
M^c	Intermediate between M and N. NM^c positive with anti-M_1 negative with anti-M′	several families	No specific antibody.
M_1	Variable reaction with anti-M	17 per cent Negro M is M_1 3 per cent White M is M_1	Anti-M_1 is a component of some human anti-M sera.
M^k	Absence of M, N, S, s and Mg. Weak reaction with a few rabbit anti-N	5 in 3894 Swiss	No anti-M^k found
M^v	Positive with a rare "anti-N like" antibody	1 in 400M Whites	Anti-M^v is human "anti-N" reacting with 1 in 400M.
N_2	Weak or negative with anti-N often associated with a positive direct anti-human globulin test	Very rare, 1 in 3894 Swiss	No specific antibody.
T_m	Antigen variable in strength—usually with N	20 per cent Whites 30 per cent N.Y. Negroes	Anti-T_m fairly rare. (Reactions similar to those expected of an anti-N_1)
S_j	All S_j positives are also T_m positive	2 per cent Whites 4 per cent Negroes	Anti-S_j very rare.
S_u	Has no S or s	1 per cent Negro, rare in Whites	Anti-U (reacts with all S+ or s+ and some S−s− cells).
S_2	Reacts with some anti-S sera	One family	No specific antibody.
M^z	NM^z negative with anti-M_1 positive with anti-M′. Inherited as $M^z s$ Produces M and N	One family	No specific antibody. Anti-M differs from anti-M_1 only in its reactions with M^z and M^c
M′	Produces M and N. M stronger than M^c or M^z. N reacts with all anti-N	A few families	No specific antibody.
M^a	lack facet M^A of M	A few families	Anti-M^A differentiates M^a and M^A
N^a	lack facet of N	10-30 per cent Melanesians	Anti-N^A differentiates N^A and N^a

group of antigens really belongs in Table 18.2 but because it is more complex we have given it a table of its own (Table 18.3).

Alleles at the MN and Ss loci

Short notes about some of the more important and interesting variants are given below. Even shorter notes of the remaining known variants that appear to be true alleles are to be found in table 18.1.

M^g

This is an exceedingly rare allele, except in Switzerland. It is selected for a short description owing to its great interest and the fact that it has a specific antibody which is by no means as rare as the antigen. The antigen M^g does not react with anti-M or anti-N. The M^g propositus (Allen *et al.,* 1958) was a patient requiring blood and by chance the serum of his selected donor contained anti-M^g.

When M^g pairs with M, a single dose M reaction is obtained on typing with anti-M and a negative reaction with anti-N; blood of type M^gN appears to be NN but gives only a single dose reaction with anti-N sera. The presence of M^g could theoretically give rise to false exclusions in cases of doubtful paternity; it is unlikely to do so in practice however, both on account of its rarity and the fact that anti-M^g should always be fairly readily obtainable for the confirmation of relevant results. Among English people, 23 examples of anti-M^g were found out of 703 individuals tested, although tests on 61,128 English donors did not reveal a single example of the M^g antigen! In Switzerland, however, the frequency of M^g is 0.153 per cent and this has enabled family studies to be carried out even to the finding of one family in which each parent had M^g and a child was produced who was homozygous for M^g and, of course, negative with anti-M (Metaxas *et al.,* 1966) but was weakly positive with anti-N giving a slightly stronger reaction with anti-N than do MM cells.

Nordling *et al* (1969) showed that M^g was associated with physico-chemical changes to the red cell surface.

M_1

An antigen M_1 has been distinguished by an anti-M_1 component of some anti-M sera. Originally anti-M_1 was found to be a component of 6 out of 20 human anti-M sera. It was not found in rabbit anti-M and anti-N sera (Jack *et al.,* 1960). Almost all examples of anti-M_1 have been found in N individuals in which anti-M is also detectable at low temperatures. Absorption of these sera by M cells which are negative with anti-M_1 results in a gradual removal of anti-M_1.

Anti-M_1 detects a qualitative difference in the M antigen (Race and Sanger, 1975) and the frequency of M_1 in Whites is 3 per cent in American Negroes 26 per cent and in Bantu 50 per cent. Tests for M_1 have been difficult because all the antisera contained anti-M+ anti-M_1. Now however a monospecific anti-M_1 made in an MN person has been found by Giles and Howell (1974) in a British patient. This serum gave a lower frequency for M_1 in Negroes (16.7 per cent) which the authors think may be because some false positives may have been obtained in the earlier results through the variable reaction of the anti-M component of the anti-M + M$_1$ sera.

M^k

M^k is remarkable for the absence of any sign of M, N, Mg, S or s activity (Metaxas and Metaxas-Bühler, 1964; Henningsen, 1966).

Less than a dozen families with M^k have been found. These announced themselves either by discrepancies in family studies, for example by exclusions against the mother, or in dosage experiments in which the expected double dose activity was a single dose reaction owing to the silent M^k gene (Sturgeon et al., 1970; Metaxas, et al., 1970).

No anti-M^k antibody appears to exist and it seems likely no M^k antigen, since Nordling et al. (1969) have shown that the condition is almost certainly due to a marked shortage of sialic acid on M^k cells. The existence of an operator gene, which switches off all activity at the MN and Ss sites, has been invoked, rather than a true allele (Sanger, 1970). Alternatively Metaxas et al. (1971) suggest M^k may be an amorph whose presence leaves unconverted a necessary basic substance for production of the MNSs antigens. Whatever the cause, the condition is inherited as a dominant.

The discovery of further examples of M^k and two "new" alleles M^z and M^r are illustrative of the rewards which may be expected through testing large numbers of blood samples with "dosing" anti-M and anti-N sera. (Metaxas et al. 1968). These workers selected a pair of human sera (anti-M and anti-N) which would only agglutinate red cells of type MM and NN and these were used in conjunction with normal rabbit antisera. Any cell sample whose reactions with the rabbit sera were M + N− or M−N+ and which were not agglutinated by the appropriate "dosing" serum, was presumed to be heterozygous at the MN locus and to possess one of these rare alleles. In their investigation on 3895 blood donors (Swiss) 15 such samples were found and in each of these a rare allele was demonstrated: M^g in six cases, M^k in five and one example each of M^e, M^z, M^r and N_2 (see Table 18.1).

M^v

This antigen was disclosed by the finding of an anti-N which agglutinated 1 in 400 M samples from White people (Gershowitz and Fried, 1966). The antibody appeared to result from the immunisation of an MM mother by an MM^v foetus. The anti-N and anti-M^v components of the serum could not be separated but later (in an AB control serum!) Crossland et al. (1970) found anti-M^v without anti-N.

M^v produces an antigen which behaves like M and yet the M^vM foetus stimulated an antibody in the MM mother which possessed as well as anti-M^v, an anti-N component. Moreover M^v is more like N in the frequency of its association with S and s.

M^a and N^a

These rare variants appear to lack a part of the normal M or N antigen and in this respect they are similar to the variants of the RhD antigen.

Konugres *et al.* (1966) found anti-M in the serum of a child who was MN; the antibody did not react with the childs' own cells. The childs' antigen was designated M^a and the antibody anti-M^A. Similarly Booth (1971) found in two Melanesian blood donors an Anti-N which failed to agglutinate between 10 per cent and 30 per cent of NN Melanesians of different ethnic groups. The antiserum was called anti-N^A, the positive N cells, N^A and those which were negative, N^a.

U or S^u

In 1953 an antibody was described by Wiener et al which agglutinated the red cells of 1100 White persons tested but was negative with 12 out of 989 New York Negroes. It was later shown by Greenwalt *et al.* (1954) that blood samples negative with anti-U were also negative with anti-S and anti-s. Anti-U therefore became to be thought of as anti-S + anti-s or more accurately anti-Ss as absorption and elution failed to separate the components.

The picture is more complicated because not all S-s- Negroid people are U−. The reactions are variable and sometimes weak. In random Negroes about 84 per cent are U− and 16 per cent U+ (Francis and Hatcher, 1966).

Various explanations have been offered as a background for the S−s− phenotype but the favourite seems to be that it is the homozygous expression of a

Table 18.2 Antigens associated with MNSs

Antigens	Characteristics	Occurrence	Antibodies
Hu	Associated with N	7 per cent Am. Negroes 22 per cent W. Africans Rare Whites	Anti-Hu made in rabbits.
He	Associated variously with NS, Ns, MS and Ms according to ethnic origin	2.7 per cent W. Africans 0 in 1,500 Whites	Anti-He made in rabbits.
Vr		3 in 12,000 Dutch	Anti-Vr.
Ri^a		3 in 17,013 English	Anti-Ri^a (one example in same serum as anti-St^a).
St^a	Variously aligned with NS, Ns, Ms	20 in 17,013 English 14 in 220 Japanese 6 in 414 Chinese	Anti-St^a (several found).
Mt^a	Aligned with Ns	28 in 11,907 Whites 3 in 318 Thais	Anti-Mt^a probably naturally occurring. Immune in rabbits.
Cl^a	Aligned with Ms in two families		Anti-Cl^a (found in 0.45 per cent of blood donors).
Ny^a	Aligned with Ns in 12 families	10 in 5931 Norwegians	Anti-Ny^a.
Sul	Aligned with Ns in one family	0 in 4935 mixed races	Anti-Sul.
Far	Aligned with Ns in one family	0 in 14,000 French	Anti-Far
Z	Aligned with Ss in one family	61 per cent Europeans 36 per cent Melanesians	Anti-Z "naturally occurring"

rare allele at the Ss locus and for this reason it is now designated S^u although with the proviso that it is heterogeneous. Family studies have shown that there is not a suppressor gene at work, since S−s−individuals do not have S+s+ parents or children. Their MN genes are expressed normally.

So far there is no example of a White S−s− blood but the phenotype S−s−U− has been found in four sibs of an Indian family in Natal (Moores, 1972).

Anti-S^u although rare is a clinically very important antibody. The first example caused a transfusion death and another example was responsible for a stillbirth due to haemolytic disease. Auto-anti-S^u has been identified in cases of acquired haemolytic anaemia.

Associated antigens (*See* Table 18.2)

Of the antigens associated with MN, Hu and He have been known for many years. Anti-Hu was produced in rabbits after injection with the blood of a Negro, Mr Hunter (Landsteiner, *et al.,* 1934). All blood samples giving positive reactions belonged to groups N or MN. Another Negro antigen, He, was found by Ikin and Mourant (1951). Anti-He was made in rabbits also.

The other rare antigens shown in Table 18.2 were brought to light when antibodies were found in human sera. They are all dominant characters and all but one appear to have no effect on the MNSs antigens with which they segregate. The exception is St^a. It may have an effect on the M antigen since two rare types M^z and M^r were both found to be St(a+). St^a is also associated with changes in the red cell surface. (For further details of these rarities see Race and Sanger, *Blood Groups in Man,* 6th ed.).

The Miltenburger sub-system

Cleghorn (1966) proposed four classes of what he termed the Miltenburger sub-system. This name was preferred since the serum of Mrs Miltenburger contained the first example of the antibody now known to give most positive reactions. A fifth class has been added following the finding of an English Miltenburger type (Crossland *et al.,* 1970). Each class gives a different pattern of reaction with the type sera and all but class V are positive with anti-Mi^a (Miltenburger); *see* Table 18.3.

The Miltenburger antigens are all rare in white races although slightly more common in Switzerland than in Britain, the two countries in which large series have been tested.

M and N antigens associated with a direct positive anti-globulin reaction

Four families have been described in which a direct positive anti-globulin reaction is inherited as a dominant character. In two families, the phenomenon segregated with a weak N (Jensen and Freiesleben, 1962; Jeannet *et al.,* 1964), in one with a weak M (Jacobowicz *et al.,* 1949) and in the fourth the segregation could not be determined.

None of the anti-globulin positive individuals showed any sign of anaemia. The globulin sensitising the cells appeared to be IgM since anti-IgG, anti-IgA

Table 18.3 Miltenburger phenotypes as defined by the five main types of antisera

Class	Propositii	Types of antisera					Approx. frequency in Whites	Effect on associated MNSs reactions
		Verweyst anti-Vw	Milten burger anti-Mi[a]	Murrell anti-Mur	Hill anti-Hill	Hut anti-Hut		
I	Graydon Miltenburger Verweyst	+	+	−	−	−	1 in 1755	None
II	Hutchinson	−	+.	−	−	+	1 in 1552	None
III	Murrell	−	+	+	+	+	1 in 10,020	s antigen neg. with some anti-s.
IV	Hopper	−	+	+	−	+	1 in 50,101	S antigen neg. with some anti-S.
V	Mrs R	−	−	−	+	−	0 in 50,000 English 3 in 6202 Swiss	N antigen weak. s increased when aligned with Ns. M antigen weak. s increased when aligned with Ms.

and anti-complement reagents did not produce a positive reaction. Papain treatment of the cells abolished the reaction but neuraminidase had no effect on some examples. It is thought that the basic abnormality is an alteration in red-cell sialic-acid metabolism.

The biochemistry of M and N

M and N specific substances reacting with human or rabbit anti-sera are not found in body fluids and so red cells are the source from which these substances have been isolated by a phenol extraction procedure. The chemical composition of the glycoproteins from M, N or MN red cells is not detectably different. The characteristic feature of the carbohydrate component is the high sialic acid content. The sialoglycopeptides with M and N activity released from whole erythrocytes by treatment with trypsin or pronase contain up to 37 per cent of sialic acid.

The structures on the glycoprotein molecules that carry M and N specificities have not yet been isolated and characterised.

Treatment of red cells or isolated M and N substances with neuraminidase results in loss of M and N activity and since sialic acid is the only component of the glycoprotein released by this enzyme it would seem that sialic acid is involved in both M and N determinants although, it has been pointed out that changes in molecular configuration when negatively charged sialyl groups are removed, may underly the loss of M and N activity. Removal of sialic acid from N-active glycoprotein results in loss of activity towards human and most rabbit anti-N sera but does not eliminate the activity measured by the anti-N lectin from Vicia graminea. The activity of this reagent is destroyed by galactose oxidase and by β-galactosidase which indicates that the combining sites of Vicia are complementary to β-galactosyl structures. The fact that both sialic acid and β-galactosyl residues are implicated in N-specificity suggests a branched structure for the determinant with these two sugars as non-reducing terminal units.

The cross-reactivity of anti-N with M cells and isolated M substances suggests the presence of a small amount of N-active substance in MM cells. Moreover, the substances isolated from group M cells show some N activity whereas substances isolated from N cells appear to be free of M activity. The occurrence of latent N structures in M substances suggested to several workers that an N-like substance is the precursor substance in the MN system.

Thus the genes controlling MN are envisaged as being M and m, where M controls the changes in the basic substrate and m is inactive. In NN individuals the precursor substrate appears unchanged. In MN individuals partial conversion to M would occur and in MM individuals the conversion would be at the maximum. The mechanism is thought to involve the addition of N-acetylneuraminic acid units to certain chains in the basic N substance. Biosynthetic pathways have been proposed by Springer and Huprikar, 1972.

However a different interpretation of the cross reactivity between N and M based on other experimental findings which do not favour N as the precursor of M is proposed by Dahr and Uhlenbruck, 1975. These workers suggest that amino acid heterogeneity at the N terminal and another position on the polypeptide chain could be responsible for M and N specificity and that certain amino acids common to both M and N substances could account for the cross reactivity.

THE PECULIARITIES OF P

In December 1955 (Sanger 1955) the P system which had remained undisturbed since its discovery in 1927 was shown to be directly related to the Jay system of blood groups (Levine *et al.,* 1951).

The Jay system was defined by an antibody called anti-Tj^a reacting with an antigen Tj^a found in almost all human red cells. The anti-Tj^a was characterised by its power to haemolyse red cells strongly at room temperature. Only fourteen persons belonging to the $Tj^{a\cdot}$ negative group (members of only eight families) were found between 1951 and 1962. The anti-Tj^a sera have all contained potent antibodies active at room temperature and at 37° C, and have been incriminated in causing miscarriages. The antibodies are probably naturally occurring since no case of a Tj^a negative person without anti-Tj^a in their serum has so far been encountered.

The realisation that Tj^a was part of the P system came when six unrelated $Tj(a-)$ people were all found to be negative with anti-P_1.

Subsequently it was found that if anti-Tj^a sera were absorbed by P_2 cells (the old P negative type) anti-P_1 was left. Anti-Tj^a therefore appeared to be a mixture of two antibodies, anti-P and anti-P_1.

The expanded P system is given below:-
Antibodies   Anti-P_1 (previously anti-P)
                Anti-P + Anti-P_1 (previously anti-Tj^a)

Antigens P_1 (previously P) $\Big\}$ previously Tj^a
               P_2 (previously p)
               p (previously Tj^b)

Therefore the old P positive group (including P strong, P medium and P weak) contains three genotypes P_1P_1 (29 per cent), P_1P_2 (50 per cent) and P_1p (v. rare). The old P negatives can be split into 3 genotypes P_2P_2 (21 per cent), P_2p (v. rare) and pp (v.rare).

The phenotype P^k

This phenotype was disclosed and shown to belong to the P system when a sample of blood was found to contain an anti-Tj^a-like antibody although the cells of the propositus which were expected to behave like p cells did not give the expected negative reaction with known anti-Tj^a sera. This finding suggested that a third antibody was present in anti-Tj^a sera. This antibody afterwards called anti-P^k, can be isolated from the serum of some p people by absorption with P_1 cells. The antibody which is regularly present in the serum of P^k people is anti-P with which P^k cells do not react. Most P^k people have the P_1 antigen (phenotype P_1^k) but some lack P_1 (phenotype P_2^k). P^k is unusual in not being inherited as a straight forward dominant character. In fact all the parents tested of P^k people lack the antigen. Family studies show that P^k is unlikely to be part of the P locus nor is it closely linked to it but seems to be involved somewhere along the same biochemical pathway. A full account of the genetics of P and P^k including a discussion of the possible biosynthesis of this complicated system is to be found in Blood Groups in Man (Race and Sanger, 1975).

Table 18.4 The reactions of P phenotypes including P^K with the various P antibodies

Phenotype	Approx. frequency	Anti-P_1	Anti-P, P_1, P^K (Anti-Tj^a)	Anti-P	Anti-P^K
P_1	75%	+	+	+	−
P_2	25%	−	+	+	−
p	Very rare	−	−	− or w	−
P_1^k	Very rare	+	+	−	+
P_2^k	Very rare	−	+	−	+

The reactions of the various P antigens and antibodies are shown in Table 18.4.

The antigen P^k is very rare even in Finnish people in whom the first examples were found (Matson *et al.*, 1959; Kortekangas *et al.*, 1959). Many thousands of samples have been tested in Finland and Britain without finding an example of P^k. However five families have been found in Japan (Nakajima & Yokota 1977).

P^k although so rare on red cells could be demonstrated on cultured fibroblasts of all of nine P_1 and ten P_2 people tested but it was absent from the fibroblasts of seven p people (Fellous *et al.*, 1972). These authors put forward the theory that P^k is an almost universal 'public' gene prevented from expressing itself on the red cells by regulator genes which they call *Ff*. F when present in single or double dose, FF or Ff suppresses P^k on the red cells. The genotype *ff* which is very rare allows P^k to appear on the red cells.

Further information was obtained from mouse-man hybrid cultures involving samples from P_1 or P_2 people. It was found that P^k could be lost from a clone of cells whether or not PP_1 remained. This fact was taken to confirm that P^k is genetically independent of the P locus. However P^k was not found after PP_1 disappeared which suggested that the PP_1 genes act earlier than P^k (Fellous *et al.*, 1974).

Luke

In 1965, Tippett *et al.* advanced the P system still further with work on the Luke phenotypes. The Luke antibody, found first in the serum of a Negro with Hodgkin's disease, is like anti-P in its failure to react with the cells of p and P^k people but in addition it fails to react with the cells of about 2 per cent of P_1 and P_2 people. It seems that so far only three examples of this antibody have been found and these give graded reactions of (+), weak and negative.

The weak and negative reactions were significantly more common with P_2 than with P_1 cells and with A_1 either in A_1 or A_1B. Family studies suggest that the strongest (although still rather weak) Luke (+) character is dominant while Luke negative is recessive and although connected with P_1 yet segregates independently of the P system.

Relationship of P with Lutheran

In 1974, Crawford *et al.* found that the rare dominant inhibitor of the Lutheran antigens Lu^a and Lu^b (see Lutheran section below) also inhibits the P_1 antigen although the P antigen is not affected. A family has been found in which the presence of the inhibitor has resulted in what appeared to be a $P_2 \times P_2$ mating with a P_1 child (Contreras and Tippett, 1974).

P_1 substance

Substances with blood group activity P do not occur in a water-soluble form in human secretions, but are found in sheep hydatid cyst fluids (Cameron and Staveley, 1957). These workers found that patients with hydatid disease had potent anti-P_1 antibodies in their sera.

Morgan and Watkins (1964) and Watkins and Morgan (1964) extracted active P_1 substance from hydatid cyst fluids of sheep and showed that it was a glycoprotein composed of 50-55 per cent reducing sugar, 20-25 per cent hexosamine and 10-15 per cent of amino acids. The immuno-dominant sugar responsible for P_1 activity is α-D-galactose.

Injection of P_1 substance coupled to the O antigen of *Shigella shigae* into rabbits produced powerful anti-P_1. Such antisera are invaluable in confirming P weak individuals whose red cells are not always agglutinated by human naturally occurring anti-P_1 antibodies.

The nature of the P_1 determinant has been further elucidated by Cory *et al.* (1974) and a striking similarity has been found between the P_1 —active trisaccharide described and the carbohydrate structure isolated by Naiki and Marcus (1974) from P^k red cells, thus indicating a close relationship between P_1 and P^k determinants.

FURTHER FACTS ABOUT THE Ii SYSTEM

As mentioned in Chapter 13, at birth the I antigen is poorly developed and there is a gradual increase in I development until the adult strength is reached at about 18 months. It has been suggested that, whereas, in most blood group systems the genes put the stamp of specificity on a basic substrate, the I genes seem to function by assisting the development of i into I. In fact some cold auto-agglutinins relating to the Ii system found in Melanesians appeared to be antibodies directed to a developing I antigen and were accordingly designated anti-I^T (Booth et al., 1966).

Two types of i have been distinguished, i_1 is the weaker and so far only found in White people, while i_2, a little stronger is confined mainly to Negroes. Both are distinct from the i of cord cells. Later (Marsh *et al.,* 1971) found two types of I antigen were definable, I^F present in foetal cells and i adults, and I^D (developed) the antigen of normal adults.

Red cells from adults show a wide range of normal activity with anti-i and anti-

I both auto or allo-antibodies. Anti-I is found commonly as an auto-antibody but as an allo-antibody it is rare because of the rarity of ii people.

Rosse and Sherwood (1970) noted the significant fact that cord cells and adult i cells in spite of their weak agglutinability by anti-I, absorbed almost as much of this antibody as normal adult I cells. This finding suggests that a structural difference at the surface of the cells rather than lack of I antigen sites may account for the difference between i and I cells.

Relationship with the ABO system

The relationship with the ABO system is not genetic. Pedigrees have shown that the locus for Ii is not part of or closely linked to the locus for ABO (Race and Sanger, 1975).

There is however abundant evidence for some kind of association through the finding of many antibodies which will react with red cells only if these are carrying I and another antigen of the ABH or Lewis systems. Of these the commonest is anti-HI which occurs in the serum of A_1 or more particularly A_1B individuals. It used to be called anti-H until it was shown that the antibody reacted only with cells carrying both H and I specificities. There is probably a whole spectrum of antibodies of this specificity, at one end recognising mainly H and at the other, mainly I.

Tippett et al, (1960) described anti-IA and Tegoli et al. (1967) showed that anti-IB antibodies existed while Tegoli et al. (1971) found anti-ILe[bH].

From chemical studies it has been deduced that the I gene is involved in the development of A, B, H, Le[a] and Le[b] and that I may be a precursor of these substances (Feizi et al., 1971). If this is true, O_h cells might be expected to contain extra I, but the evidence for this at the present time is equivocal.

Anti-I and P

An antibody reacting only when I and P_1 are together, anti-IP_1, was described by Issitt et al. (1968). This antibody was inhibited to a certain extent by hydatid cyst fluid but not so markedly as anti-P_1 by itself.

An anti-IP_1 is not a suitable antibody for P_1 typing the cells of the newborn since they lack all but a trace of I and anti-IP_1 requires the presence of I and P_1 on the red cells if it is to work properly.

Inhibition of anti-I

Many anti-I sera are not inhibited by saliva but a few have been found which are strongly inhibited, not only by saliva but by human milk. In addition there seems to be plenty of I substance in the saliva of infants at birth and in adult i individuals.

Relationship to clinical medicine

Jenkins et al. (1965) have investigated a case of leukaemia with weakened A in which I was also depressed. However the i reaction was stronger than in the average adult cell, so that the reciprocal relationship between I and i was maintained. In other haematological disorders i is increased but the I is not decreased.

Schmidt *et al.* (1965) have stimulated the interest of other besides blood group specialists with their experiments on mycoplasma strains; 18 out of 25 strains of these organisms inhibited anti-I agglutination. Agglutination by anti-Le[a], anti-Le[b] and anti-A[1] was not so inhibited. Mycoplasma have been demonstrated in association with leukaemia which may explain the inagglutinability by anti-I of red cells of patients with leukaemia.

Anti-I has been shown to be the auto-antibody concerned in most cases of "cold-type" autoimmune haemolytic anaemia (see Chapter 27). Anti-i has been shown to be the cold auto-agglutinin present in some cases of infective mononucleosis.

A significant observation was made by Hillman and Giblett (1965). They reported that the i reactivity of normal adults can be increased by submitting their marrow to the stress of repeated phlebotomy so that the intra-marrow maturation time of cells is gradually decreased. Although the i increases, there is no change in the strengh of the I or H antigens.

THE LUTHERAN SYSTEM

As already seen in Chapter 13 knowledge of the Lutheran system advanced along a familiar path, the finding of one antibody anti-Lu[a] followed, albeit after a long interval, by a second antibody, anti-Lu[b] which detected a second allele.

These two antibodies between them define three genotypes, $Lu^a Lu^a$, $Lu^b Lu^b$ and $Lu^a Lu^b$ which account for virtually the whole of the general population. The familiar pattern continued with the finding of red cells negative with both antisera and therefore Lu(a–b–), Crawford *et al.*, (1961). After which an antibody anti-Lu[a]Lu[b] (anti-Lu3) was found; this reacted with all but cells of the phenotype Lu(a–b–), Darnborough *et al.* (1963).

The phenotype Lu(a–b–) is of two types, one dominant and the other recessive as shown by family studies. The types are distinguishable serologically. The appropriate Lutheran antisera (anti-Lu[b], anti-Lu[a]Lu[b], anti-Lu[b]) can be taken up and eluted from Lu(a–b–) cells of the dominant type but not from cells of the recessive type (Tippett, 1971). The recessive type is thought to be due to homozygosity for a "silent" allele.

The dominant type of Lu(a–b–) requires some kind of inhibitor gene to explain its activity. Family studies have shown the independence of the inhibitor gene from the Lutheran locus (Taliano *et al.*, 1973). These authors suggested the term In(Lu) for the rare allele responsible for inhibition and in(Lu) for the common allele.

An association between Lu(a–b–) of the dominant type and Auberger was established. In the Crawford family the 7 Lu(a–b–) members were Au(a–) whereas the 6 members who were not Lu(a–b–) were all Au(a+). In 1974 Crawford, *et al.* found that In(Lu) inhibits P[1] and i as well as Lutheran and Au[a] antigens.

Further extensions of Lutheran

A flood of antibodies which have been given numbers, anti-Lu4, Lu5 etc and are now reaching Lu20, have disclosed themselves as being in some way related to Lutheran by giving consistently negative reactions with Lu(a-b-) cells whether these are of the dominant or recessive type. They also are negative with their own cells but positive with the cells of most of the other possessors of these antibodies. Many of the antibodies are of the 'public' type. They are summarised by Race and Sanger (1975a).

The antigens distinguished by two of these antibodies, Lu9 and Lu6, in family studies show clearly their relationship with the Lutheran locus and strongly suggest that the Lutheran locus is turning out to be of similar pattern to Rh. For example Lu9 is not an allele at the Lu^a Lu^b site because Lu(a+b+) can also be Lu9 positive. It would seem therefore that the relationship of Lu9 to Lutheran is like C to D or E in the Rh system (Molthan *et al.,* 1973). Lu6 was shown to be an allele of Lu9 after two unrelated people and two relatives of one of them, who all were negative with anti-Lu6 (which is a rare state), where found to be positive with anti-Lu9. An antibody anti-Lu6 has been described by Marsh (1972) and Wrobel *et al.* (1972).

The other antigens defined by the Lutheran numbered antibodies mentioned above have been described by Race and Sanger (1975b) as para-Lutheran antigens as their place in the system is so far little understood. The owners of these antibodies themselves appear to have normal Lutheran antigens of phenotype Lu(a-b+).

Mention should be made of the antigen Lu12 (Mrs Much) defined by the corresponding anti-Lu12 since there is evidence that this antigen is not controlled by the Lutheran locus. The Lutheran genes of the Much family did not segregate but the secretor genes did and showed that the Much antigen was not close to the secretor locus which in turn is close to the Lutheran locus (Sinclair *et al.,* 1973).

Lutheran antibodies

Anti-Lu^a is characterised by producing morula-like agglutinates with plenty of free cells. Anti-Lu^b may give the same pattern of agglutination but usually to a less marked extent and is often best detected by the anti-globulin technique. Anti-Lu^b, probably because it is more often an incomplete antibody, is of greater clinical significance than anti-Lu^a both in relation to transfusion and haemolytic disease of the newborn. Compatible donors are difficult to find for recipients with anti-Lu^b since they have to be selected from the 0.02% of the population who are Lu^aLu^a.

FURTHER KELL TYPES

The Kell system has become one of great complexity and so numerous have become the antigens and antibodies associated with it that a system of numbers has been introduced.

As well as *K(K1)* and *k(K2),* three further allelic pairs have been identified,

Kp^a(K3) and Kp^b(K4), Js^a(K6) and Js^b *(K7)*, *Coté (K11)* and *Wk^a(K17)*. These are briefly described below.

Kp^a (K3) and Kp^b (K4)

A "new" antigen was reported by Allen and Lewis in 1957. It occurred in about 2 per cent of the population and family studies suggested that it was associated with the Kell system. It was designated Kp^a. Later the same workers (Allen *et al.,* 1958) described an antibody to a high frequency antigen and found that each of the few negatives obtained was Kp^a positive. They had therefore discovered an allele for Kp^a which they termed Kp^b. Only two Kp^b negatives were found in testing 5,500 unrelated people.

In 1957, Chown *et al.* discovered a phenotype negative with the four Kell antisera (anti-K-k-Kp^a-Kp^b) known at that time. The phenotype K-k-Kp(a–b–) was given the notation K_o. The propositus had an antibody (anti-Ku(K5)) which reacted with all cells except K_o (*see also* Corcoran *et al.,* 1961).

Js^a (K6) and Js^b (K7)

It was some years before it was realised that this pair of alleles belonged to the Kell system and at first they were described under the name of Sutter. Giblett (1958) found an antibody, anti-Js^a which reacted with about 20 per cent of Negro donors but not with 240 White people. Subsequently one White person was found to be positive out of many hundreds tested.

An antibody giving antithetical reactions to anti-Js^a was found by Walker *et al.,* (1963). Interest in this system grew when Stroup *et al.* (1965) showed that K-k-Kp(a–b–) persons were also Js(a–b–). This was too much of a coincidence and stimulated these workers to undertake lengthy family studies which provided good evidence that Sutter should be considered part of the Kell system.

Coté (K11) and Wk^a (K17)

The antibody termed anti-Coté (later anti-K11) was discovered by Guévin *et al.* (1971). It reacted with all cells tested except K_o cells, the maker's own cells and those of two of her eight sibs.

Three years later a second team of workers (Strange *et al.,* 1974) recorded Wk^a (Weeks), yet another antigen which was shown to have a relationship with the Kell system. The antibody was stimulated by transfusion, the recipient having been transfused with blood from a certain Mr Weeks. The frequency of Wk^a was found to be 0.3 per cent. No Wk^a positive was found to be K positive. Family studies placed the antigen in the Kell system and showed it going with k. Wk^a and Coté were shown to be alleles when two unrelated Coté negative individuals were found to be strongly Wk^a positive.

The antigen Ul^a (K10)

Anti-Ul^a defines an antigen having a frequency of 2.6 per cent among Helsinki blood donors but which is almost non-existence among other tested populations (Furuhjelm *et al.,* 1968).

After a long investigation and many families studies, it was concluded that Ul^a was part of the Kell locus or in very close linkage with the system (Furuhjelm *et al.,* 1969). Both known examples of anti-U1[a] were found in much transfused patients.

Other Kell associates

Two individuals with depressed Kell antigens may give a clue to the genetic background of the system although there is no convincing proof that either of them is controlled from the Kell locus. The first of these, McLeod, was found by Allen *et al.* (1961). The cells of the propositus reacted weakly with anti-Ku, anti-K and anti-Kp[b]. They were negative with anti-K and anti-Kp[a]; their reaction was also unusually weak with anti-Js[b].

The McLeod phenotype can therefore be written:- K–kw Kp(a-bw) Js (a-bw). A second individual Claas (Van der Hart and Van Loghem, 1968) was found to have cells which behaved like those of McLeod. An antibody found in his serum anti-KL (anti-K9) did not react with his own cells or those of McLeod but did react with all other cells tested *including* cells of the type K_o. Absorption and elution tests suggested that the Claas antibody was directed at the whole Kell complex of antigens. It is important in revealing that Ko cells do have some type of Kell antigen. Further examples of anti-KL have been found.

Anti-KL has been shown to possess two separable antibodies. One is directed against an antigenic determinant present on red cells of common Kell types. The second antibody is almost antithetical in its reaction and is directed against an antigen present on K_o cells which appears to be in minimal amount on red cells of common Kell type. Marsh *et al.* (1975) have named this second component anti-Kx (anti-K15). Both KL and Kx antigens are missing from cells of the McLeod type. Anti-Kx is useful in detecting K_o in heterozygotes. These individuals cannot be identified by dosage studies with ordinary Kell antibodies but with anti-Kx they give reactions intermediate between K_o and K1.

Para Kell antigens
Boc (K12), Sgro (K13) and San (L14)

These are detected by antibodies to very high frequency or public antigens but which are all negative with K_o cells, the maker's own cells and sometimes those of the sibs. These antibodies react weakly with cells have depressed Kell antigens of the McLeod type (Heistø *et al.,* 1973; Marsh *et al.,* 1974). A further antigen of this type K18 has been found by Marsh *et al.* (1975). None of them have been proved to be alleles at the Kell locus.

Kell antigens on leucocytes

Marsh *et al.* (1975) by comparative titrations before and after absorption with buffy coat preparations have shown no loss of activity of anti-K, anti-k, anti-Kp[b], anti-Js[b], anti-Ku, anti-K12, anti-K13, anti-K16 or anti-K18 but leucocyte-platelet preparations were found to have a marked absorptive capacity for anti-Kx. Most of the activity was found to reside in the neutrophils.

White cell preparations from at least fifty people have been tested and all showed a capacity for absorbing anti-Kx and it seems that, unlike red cells, it is a regular constituent of normal neutrophils.

The relationship between chronic granulomatous disease (CGD) and the Kell system

Giblett *et al.* (1971) in studying patients with CGD disease found that too many of them had red cells of the K_0 or McLeod types. Such patients tended to have Kell antibodies, such as anti-Ku, anti-KL or anti-Kp^b, all of which are antibodies to high frequency antigens and therefore selecting donors for these patients became a difficulty.

Marsh *et al.* (1975) found four unrelated children with CGD, three boys and one girl. Leucocytes of the girl absorbed anti-Kx to the same extent as normal control cells but the cells of the three boys did not absorb the antibody.

In the course of their study they established evidence that four patterns of leucocyte and red cell distribution of the Kx antigen exist:-

(1) Normal people of ordinary Kell type in which red cells and white cells have Kx.
(2) Healthy McLeod type in whom the white cells have Kx but the red cells do not.
(3) CGD McLeod type in whom both types of cell lack Kx.
(4) CGD, ordinary Kell type, in whom the white cells lack Kx but the red cells do not.

A further discussion of the inheritance of Kx, its possible place in the Kell system and a possible genetic pathway in the Kell blood group system may be read in the original paper. Later studies are to be found in Marsh *et al* (1976).

THE EXPANSION OF THE DUFFY SYSTEM

Tests with two antisera anti-Fy^a and anti-Fy^b disclosed a phenotype Fy (a–b–) which is common in Negroes but rare in Whites (Sanger *et al.*, 1955). The symbol *Fy* is used for the responsible gene.

It now appears that there are two types of Fy, one of these (Fy) corresponds to the common Negroid gene and results in no detectable antigen on the red cells, while the other (Fy^x) which is commoner than Fy in Whites gives a weak reaction with anti-Fy^b sera (Lewis *et al.,* 1972). In fact it is best detected by absorption and subsequent elution with anti-Fy^b. Fy^x although considered to be a weak form of Fy^b does seem to be the product of a separate allele.

The Negroid Fy gene is one of the most useful in distinguishing between Negro and White bloods as it has a frequency of over 90 per cent in West Africans, 80 per cent in New York Negroes and less than 3 per cent in Europeans.

There are other anthropological differences related to the Duffy system, for instance the Fy (a–b–) phenotype occurs in Yemenite Jews while Japanese, Koreans and Newfoundland Eskimos have a very high frequency of Fy^a.

Other unusual Duffy alleles

Fy 3

Anti-Fy3 was found in a White woman who typed as Fy (a–b–) but whose cells did not give the reaction of Fy^x (Albrey *et al.*, 1971). Her antibody reacted with all common Duffy phenotypes and with two examples of Fy (a–bw) *i.e.* $Fy^x Fy^x$. It did not react with her own cells or with the Fy (a–b–) of Negroes. In addition it did not react with the cells of a second individual who made a similar antibody. The pattern of reaction is that which would be expected of anti-$Fy^a Fy^b$ but cannot be directed towards these antigens because its activity is enhanced rather than abolished by enzymes.

Two non-Negroid FyFy individuals have made anti-Fy3 whereas the many Negroid FyFy individuals have failed to do so.

Fy4

Anti-Fy4 was found in a Fy (a+b+) Negro girl with sickle cell anaemia who had received frequent blood transfusions over a period of 6 years (Behzad *et al.*, 1973). This antibody reacted with all samples of type Fy (a–b–), most Negroid Fy (a+b–) or Fy (a–b+) types but with none of type Fy (a+b+). In reacting with all Fy (a–b–) bloods the antibody appears to correspond to the anti-Fy^c suggested by Sanger *et al.* (1955). Like anti-Fy3, anti-Fy4 reacts best by anti-globulin on papain treated cells. It has been suggested that antigen detected may be the product of an allele of Fy3.

Fy5

Anti-Fy5 occurred in a Negro of type Fy (a–b–) Fy–3. The antibody at first seemed to be anti-Fy3 for it reacted with all cells with Fy^a and Fy^b but failed to react with Fy (a–b–). However the antibody did react with the cells of one of the people who had made anti-Fy3.

The reaction could be detected both by anti-globulin and papain techniques.

Colledge *et al.* (1973) who discovered anti-Fy5 found that it did not react with Rh_{null} cells and was only weakly reactive with –D– cells of normal Fy types. From their data they argue that the most likely explanation of the relationship with Rh is that the Fy5 determinant is formed by interaction of Rhesus and Duffy gene products.

A second example of anti-Fy5 has been found by DeNapoli *et al.* (1976). The antibody also failed to react with Rh_{null} cells of both the amorph and regular types. All of nine examples of –D– cells reacted weakly.

SID GROUPS (Sd^a) INCLUDING Cad ("SUPER SID")

A characteristic of the agglutination produced by this antigen and its corresponding antibody is that only a proportion of cells are agglutinated even when the reaction is a strong one. In this it resembles the agglutination observed with anti-Lu^a. The reaction is variable and when the first anti-Sd^a antibodies were found the main difficulty was in distinguishing the weak positives from true negatives. An improved typing technique was devised by Renton *et al.* (1967) who found that more clear cut reactions could be obtained using anti-globulin with either a powerful anti-IgM or anti-complement component.

About 91 per cent of English people are Sd (a+) but of those only 10 per cent react strongly with anti-Sd^a

Sd^a is found in saliva and in most other secretions, the highest concentration being found in urine. In fact the presence or absence of Sd^a in urine gives a truer estimate of the antigen frequency; about half the individuals whose red cells are Sd (a–) secrete Sd^a in the urine (Morton *et al.*, 1970). Of the 4 per cent of people who are true Sd^a negatives about half have an IgM anti- Sd^a in their sera.

In 1968, a low incidence antigen termed Cad was described by Cazal *et al.* Three members of a family had cells which were polyagglutinable to the extent of being agglutinated by eighty normal sera. None of the three cells was agglutinated by serum of the other Cad positive members of the family. Cad red cells, even when group O, were found to be agglutinated by *Dolichos biflorus* and snail anti-A. In these respects they behave like Tn cells.

In 1971, Sanger *et al.* showed that Cad is in fact a strongly reacting Sd^a ("Super Sid"). Race and Sanger (1971) suggested that the polyagglutinability might be due to anti- Sd^a present in the sera of most people but only detectable by the strongest Sd^a +++ cells as found in the Cad family, and this idea gained further support from the work of Springarm *et al.* (1974).

The reason that Dolichos reacts with Sd (a++) cells as well as A$_1$ is probably because it is reacting with a terminal N-acetyl-D-galastosamine present both in Sd (a++) and A$_1$.

Red cell Sd^a alters through pregnancy and there are too many Sd (a–) people among pregnant women. The change does not influence the presence of Sd^a in the urine and the antigen re-appears on the red cells soon after delivery (Morton *et al.*, 1970).

Anti-Sd^a has caused a haemolytic transfusion reaction (Petermans and Cole-Dergent (1970) in a male patient who received many units of blood for a bleeding gastric ulcer. A cell survival study with 50 Cr labelled strong Sd (a+) red cells resulted in some of the cells being eliminated rapidly while the rest survived normally. It was suggested that this phenomenon could be an expression of the uneven antigen distribution, the red cells with the most antigen being destroyed rapidly in the circulation. Surface counting for radio-activity showed that the

Table 18.5 Distinctions between T, Tn and Cad cells

	Cells		
Reaction with:	T	Tn	Cad
Normal serum	+	+	+
Serum + papain-treated cells	+	–	+
Arachis extract (peanuts)	+	–	–
Dolichos extract	–	+	+
Bauhinia (anti-N diluted out)		+	–

cells were sequestered in the liver rather than the spleen.

This is perhaps a not inappropriate place in which to insert a table showing useful distinctions between T, Tn and Cad cells (Table 18.5).

THE Bg AND CHIDO ANTIGENS

These should more properly be considered white cell antigens but they are found, although in a less active state, on red cells too; they also have in common their presence in a soluble form in plasma.

We have selected them for a short description because they often cause practical difficulties in cross matching. Moreover the Bg antibodies in particular have a habit of turning up as contaminants in blood grouping reagents, particularly anti-D. This has been known to give rise to the typing of D negative individuals as D^u and as a result Rh immunoglobulin has been withheld after delivery of an Rh positive infant.

The Bg antigens discovered and investigated independently by a number of workers were variously named Ot, Ho, Bennett-Goodspeed-Sturgeon or Donna.

The relationship between them was established some years later by Seaman *et al.* (1967) using the AutoAnalyser which greatly enhanced some of the rather feeble reactions obtained by manual methods. Thus by manual methods the antigen which they called Bg^a gave only 2-3 per cent positive reactions while by AutoAnalyser the frequency of positives was increased to 30 per cent.

Two other associated Bg antigens, Bg^b and Bg^c are less common than Bg^b

The association with leucocytes was seen when Morton *et al.* (1969) found that Bg^a corresponded to HL-A7 (B7). Later the same workers allocated Bg^b to W17 (BW17) and Bg^c to W28 (A28) (Morton *et al.*; 1971).

It has also been shown that Bg (a–) red cells can be converted to Bg (a+) cells by incubation in Bg (a+) plasma.

Chido began life as a few "nebulous" antibodies (Harris *et al.*, 1967). Out of 2000 New York donors only two or three convincing negatives were found. However after it was shown by Middleton (1972) that Chido positive people had Chido substance in their plasma, Chido typing was found to be more reliable by inhibition test using plasma rather than by agglutination tests on red cells. Using this method Middleton and Crookston (1972) found 11 of 639 (1.7 per cent) Toronto donors to be Chido negative. Children who lacked the antigen on their red cells possessed Chido in their plasma to the same degree as in adults.

Chido has been shown to be genetically independent of ABO, MNSs, Rh, Duffy, Kidd and ABH secretion.

The outcome of a large investigation reported by Middleton *et al.* (1974) shows a clear linkage between Chido and HLA.

DOMBROCK

This system is defined by two rare antibodies, anti-Do^a and anti-Do^b. The first example of anti-Do^a was found by Swanson *et al.* in 1965. The antibody is detectable by anti-human globulin, but requires specially selected ahg reagents. Many otherwise excellent reagents are unsuitable for detecting this antibody. This fact should be borne in mind when, on clinical grounds, an antibody is suspected to be present since testing with a number of different reagents might reveal anti-Do^a

Anti-Do^b was discovered by Molthan *et al.*, 1973 and with the two antisera the following frequencies have been calculated for Northern Europeans:- $Do^a Do^a_,$ 0.1764, $Do^a Do^b$ 0.4872 and $Do^b Do^b$ 0.3364 (Tippett, 1967).

AUBERGER GROUPS

So far only two examples have been found of the antibody which defines the antigen Au (named after Madame Auberger whose serum contained the first example of the antibody), (Salmon *et al.,* 1961). In both cases, the antibody was one of a mixture of antibodies of different specificities, all presumably immune since their owners were many times transfused. It is likely therefore that Au is a weak antigen. In both sera the anti-Au reacted best by anti-globulin technique using cells pretreated with papain. About 82 per cent of French and English people are Au (a+). Serological association with most other major systems has been eliminated.

One of the most interesting facts about Au^a is its relationship to In(Lu) the inhibitor gene responsible for the dominant type of Lu (a–b–). This gene appears to inhibit the activity of the Au antigen as well as Lu^a and Lu^b (see Lutheran groups above). However, it has been shown that Au^a is controlled from a locus independent of the Lutheran locus.

SCIANNA

The group name Scianna includes two antigens Sm and Bu^a, originally thought to be unrelated but now known to be the products of alleleic genes, one very common Sm, (Scl) and one very rare Bu^a (Sc2), (Schmidt *et al.,* 1962; Anderson *et al.,* 1963). The two antibodies were investigated together by Lewis *et al.* (1974), after finding that an Sm negative person was Bu (a+) and 1000 unrelated Caucasians were tested. These workers found 983 $Sc^l Sc^l$ and 17 $Sc^l Sc^2$ individuals. The rare $Sc^2 Sc^2$ was, not surprisingly, absent from this series.

Scianna has been shown to be independent of most major systems. The original anti-Scl was probably stimulated by pregnancies. It reacted by anti-globulin technique. The first example of anti-Sc2 was stimulated in a male patient after transfusion. Four other examples were accidentally produced in the sera of Rh negative volunteers who were injected with Rh positive blood with the intention of producing anti-D (Seyfried *et al.,* 1966).

DIEGO

The antigen Di^a (Layrisse *et al.,* 1955; Levine *et al.,* 1956) when first found appeared to be very rare since over 2000 white persons were tested without a further example apart from the family of the propositus. When South American Indians were tested, however, as many as 36 per cent of some tribes were Di^a positive.

The antigen is found among most Mongolian peoples but not in Eskimos in whom it would also be expected to occur.

In 1967 Thomson *et al.* discovered the antithetical antibody anti-Di^b. So far no Di (a–b–) people have been found.

Diego has been shown to be independent of all other systems except Lutheran which awaits the finding of suitable family material.

Anti-Di^a is a possible although rare cause of haemolytic disease of the newborn. Anti-Di^b has caused a transfusion reaction.

THE COLTON SYSTEM

The Colton blood groups, which began with the finding of an antibody (anti-Co^a) defining a high frequency antigen Co^a (Heistø et al., 1967), has gone the way of many systems; an antithetical antibody anti-Co^b has been discovered (Giles et al., 1970) followed by a Co (a–b–) type and an anti-Co^{a}Co^b antibody (Rogers et al., 1974).

The genotype frequencies of Europeans are as follows:- $Co^a Co^a$ 0.9137, $Co^a Co^b$ 0.0843 and $Co^b Co^b$ 0.0020. The antibodies of the system all appear to be immune and stimulated by transfusions and/or pregnancies. They are best detected by anti-globulin technique with papain treated red cells.

The Co^b antigen would appear to be a weak antigen (probably weaker than Co^a), if the number of antibodies of other specificities (indicating a high degree of immunisation) found with each example of anti-Co^b may be taken as a criterion.

The anti-Co^{a}Co^b was found in the serum of a French Canadian woman whose red cells were Co (a–b–). It reacted with all cells except her own and those of two of her four sibs who were also Co (a–b–).

No anti-Co^a or anti-Co could be eluted from Co (a–b–) cells first treated with these antibodies, nor, using absorption and elution could the anti-Co^{a}Co^b be separated into anti-Co^a and anti-Co^b components.

En GROUPS

The first example of a rare antibody, subsequently termed anti-En^a, was reported by Darnborough et al., (1969) to a meeting of the British Society of Haematology in 1965. A second example was found in Finland (Furuhjelm et al., 1969). The antibody detects an antigen En^a which is a dominant character found in most people. No random En (a–) person was discovered in testing 12,500 English and 8800 Finnish individuals (Darnborough et al., 1969; Furuhjelm et al., 1973).

En (a–) red cells have been shown to have an abnormal cell envelope in that there is more than a 50 per cent reduction in sialic acid content (the name En derives from envelope). This has the same effect as enzyme treatment of the cells and they behave in the manner characteristic of such cells. For example they are agglutinated in a saline suspension by incomplete anti-D and their M and N activity is depressed although the S and s reactions are normal or even enhanced. Even the heterozygotes, $En^a En$, have this capacity to be agglutinated in saline with selected incomplete anti-D sera. A puzzling fact is that the En^a of normal cells is not depressed as might be expected, by treatment with neuraminidase or proteolytic enzymes. En (a–) cells give enhanced reactions with seed extracts and non-immune animal sera (Furuhjelm et al., 1969). En (a–) cells have the great distinction, unlike all other human cells tested, of giving a negative reaction when mixed with the plasma of a coelacanth (Tippett and Teesdale, 1973)!

The few anti-En^a sera found so far have been immune as a result of transfusion and in one case perhaps also of pregnancy. They agglutinated cells suspended in saline but the agglutination was improved if anti-globulin or enzyme techniques were used.

THE SEX-LINKED BLOOD GROUP Xg

This blood group system which came to light through the finding of an antibody afterwards called anti-Xg^a (Mann et al., 1962) is unique in that it is controlled by an X-linked locus. The first anti-Xg^a appeared in a much transfused male patient.

The Xg phenotype gene and genotype frequencies for 6,784 unrelated Northern Europeans, taken from Race and Sanger (1975a) are as follows:-

	Xg (a+)	Xg (a−)	Total
Males	2304 65.6%	1209 34.4%	3513
Females	2900 88.7%	371 11.3%	3271

These figures can be used to calculate the gene frequencies:

Xg^a 0.659
Xg 0.341

Expected genotype and phenotype frequencies calculated from these gene frequencies:

Males	Females
Xg^a 0.659 Xg 0.341	$Xg^a Xg^a$ 0.434 $\Big\}$ 0.884 $Xg^a Xg$ 0.450 $Xg\ Xg$ 0.116

The many family studies that have now been completed show without doubt that the locus for Xg is on the X chromosome. Figure 18.1 shows how Xg^a can be inherited when (a) the father, (b) and (c) the mother are Xg^a positive. Several points about sex-linked inheritance are illustrated by these pedigrees.

If the father is Xg^a positive he cannot pass Xg^a to his sons since they have to inherit his Y chromosome, but he must pass Xg^a to his daughters as they have to inherit his X chromosome (pedigree 1).

If the mother is Xg^a positive she can either be $Xg^a Xg$ as in pedigree 2 or $Xg^a Xg^a$ as in pedigree 3. When she is $Xg^a Xg$ she as an equal chance of passing Xg^a to her sons or daughters; as her husband is Xg^a negative half the children will be Xg^a positive and half Xg^a negative—if her husband was Xg^a positive (not shown in

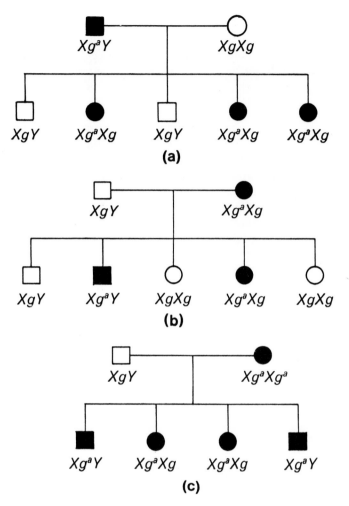

Fig. 18.1 Families showing inheritance of Xg^a.

pedigree 2) the daughters in the family would be Xg^a positive but the sons would have an equal chance of being either Xg^a positive or negative.

When the mother is Xg^aXg^a as in (3) all the children are Xg^a positive.

There are a few exceptions! These constitute four Xg (a−) daughters of Xg (a+) fathers [(see Sanger et al., 1971), who do not consider these particular exceptions carry much weight as two were trisomic children and in the other two non-paternity had not been specifically excluded] and the very rare occurrence of Xg (a+) sons of Xg (a−) mothers. The most favoured explanation of these latter exceptional families is mosaicism as was shown in one particular case in which the peripheral blood of a phenotypically normal mother was found to be XO/XX, the two cell lines being in the proportion of 1 to 2. The mother and husband were phenotypically Xg (a−) but one son and one daughter were Xg (a+). The mother's genotype was considered to be Xg^aXg but there was evidence that her red cells were derived from a predominantly XO line, not carrying Xg^a (Buckton *et al.,* 1971). The karyotype of the marrow showed about 90 per cent of the cells to be XO and it is known that if only 10 per cent of erythrocytes carry Xg^a they are not detectable.

Anti-Xg^a

Anti-Xg^a reacts by anti-globulin technique but not by saline, albumin, trypsin, papain, ficin, bromelin or capillary methods (Mann *et al.,* 1962). Moreover only certain anti-globulin reagents give positive results. For this reason some anti-Xg^a antibodies may escape detection. The inclusion of anti-complement globulin in the tests has been shown to be important by Cook *et al.* (1963) who also observe that the titre of anti-Xg^a declines very rapidly after stimulation. The Xg^a antigen is presumably not a good stimulator of antibodies since about 20 per cent of transfusions would be expected to give the recipient the opportunity of making anti-Xg^a. On the other hand, experience has shown that when anti-Xg^a does appear it is usually unaccompanied by other antibodies, a fact which does not accord with the more usual finding that the individual who responds to one weak antigen has usually responded to several others as well with the result that his serum contains a mixture of antibodies.

Most examples of anti-Xg^a have been found in males which is not unexpected since the male sex has a higher proportion of Xg (a–).

The cells of the Xg^a positive male (Xg^aY) react as strongly with anti-Xg^a as do the cells of the Xg^aXg^a female. Between 5 and 10 per cent of Xg^aXg females give rather weak reactions. Even in the strong reactors many free cells are seen.

Xg^a in other tissues

Xg^a has been sought but not found in serum, saliva and on spermatozoa. It has been detected on cultured fibroblasts (Fellous *et al.,* 1974) and also in man-man, man-mouse and man-hamster hybrids. The antigen is also detected in some lymphoid cell cultures when a micro-complement fixation method is employed.

Xg^a has been found on the red cells of gibbons (Gavin *et al.,* 1964) and from its distribution in the two sexes appears to be an X-linked dominant character. It was not found in some other species including chimpanzees, gorillas, baboons and orangutang.

Xg in the study of human genetics

The contribution of Xg to the Lyon hypothesis

The theory of Lyon, now experimentally established, asserts that one of the two X chromosomes in each somatic cell of the female is inactivated at a very early stage in embryonic development and it is a matter of chance whether it is the paternal or the maternal X which is inactivated in any given cell. However once an X is inactivated it remains inactive in all the descendants of that cell.

At the time of the discovery of Xg there was doubt whether the inactivation applied to man and it was hoped that evidence would be obtained from a study of

Xg. For if true in the average $Xg^a Xg$ female half the red cells should be Xg (a+) and half Xg (a–).

However before reliable results could be obtained a special technique had to be devised to overcome the difficulty mentioned above of the considerable number of cells normally left unagglutinated by anti-Xg^a. This was achieved by Gorman *et al.* in 1963 and these workers went on to show that the red cells of $Xg^a Xg$ females did not consist of a mixture of Xg (a+) and Xg (a–) cells. A number of other pieces of evidence have now accumulated in support of the fact that the Xg locus is not subject to the Lyon inactivation effect and is now thought that the early inactivation of the X chromosome does not involve all its loci and that the Xg locus is among those which escape.

Xg and Sex-chromosome aneuploidy

Normally in somatic cells the chromosomes are present in pairs. Any abnormality such as one chromosome missing or chromosomes in threes, fours etc, is called aneuploidy.

Xg can sometimes make a contribution to pinpointing the particular cell division at which the accident responsible for sex-chromosome aneuploidy has occurred.

The accidents are of two kinds:-

(1) Two X chromosomes which should part at meiosis and each go to separate nuclei, stay together so that one daughter nucleus has two X and the other none. This phenomenon is called non-disjunction.

(2) Anaphase lag. This most often affects the Y chromosome which fails to reach the spindle poles at the anaphase stage of cell division and may get into the same daughter cell as the X or fail to get into either daughter cell.

Individuals exhibiting the syndrome of Klinefelter and Turner are examples of such abnormalities.

Klinefelter's Syndrome

These are males with more than one X chromosome and occasional abnormality of Y and they may be of the following types: (a) *XXY*, (b) *XXXY*, (c) *XXXXY*, (d) *XXYY*, (e) *XX* males, (f) *XXY* mosaics.

Two examples selected from many described in the literature will serve to illustrate how Xg^a typing may give information as to the origin of the extra chromosomes and also may indicate at which of the meiotic divisions the accident has occurred.

(1) Father Xg (a+), mother Xg (a–) and Klinefelter *XXY* son Xg (a+). This Xg^a result shows that the extra X of the son must be of paternal origin, and that the father must have some sperm carrying both *X* and *Y*.

This fixes the non-disjunction as happening in the father who thus contributed an *X* and a *Y* to the son. Moreover if *X* and *Y* go into one sperm the only opportunity for this is at the 1st meiotic division since it is at this division the X and Y normally part and go into separate cells.

(2) A boy on chromosomal analysis of his leucocytes was found to be *XXYY*.

His red cells and those of his father were Xg (a+). The mother's cells were Xg (a−). The second X of the son is thereby shown to be of paternal origin and must have arisen by non-disjunction at the first meiotic division of spermatogenesis. The extra Y probably originated by non-disjunction at the second meiotic division (Pfeiffer *et al.*, 1966).

Turner's Syndrome

Individuals with this syndrome are females with various abnormalities of their gonads. They are infertile. They usually lack the whole of one X chromosome or less commonly the short arm of one X. Such patients, as would be expected from possessing only one X, show the male Xg distribution. A number of the Turner families investigated for Xg groups make it clear whether the single X is of maternal or paternal origin.

For example, father Xg (a+), mother Xg (a−), Turner daughter (XO) Xg (a+). This shows the daughter's X to be of paternal origin.

A second example in which the father was Xg (a+) and the mother Xg (a−), daughter Xg (a−), shows the daughter's X to be maternal in origin. This finding is of particular interest since it had been believed before this that the paternal X was always the missing one. Both these Turner families are from Lindsten *et al.* (1963).

The Xg blood group system in relation to X-chromosome mapping

Information about the distance between genes on a chromosome is derived from studying families in which the linkage between two characters can be followed through several generations (linked genes are those whose loci are carried within a measureable distance of each other on the same chromosome). When two different genes are on the same chromosome and are fairly close to each other, the two characters controlled will be seen travelling together through the generations but occasionally at meiosis crossing over between the genes occurs and the two characters will be found apart in some of the children. These children are termed recombinants. The frequency of the occurrence of recombinants can be taken as an index of the distance between genes on a chromosome. For example, if 6 per cent of children are seen to be cross overs the recombination frequency is said to be 0.06 and this is expressed as centimorgans which in this example are 6. Recombination frequencies greater than 0.15 have to be corrected for double cross-overs.

The study of suitable cross-over families has made possible a tentative map of the human X chromosome and when the Xg blood group system was discovered it was hope that it would greatly facilitate the measurement of linkages and mapping of the position of characters on the X chromosome. This hope has not been realised to the extent at first anticipated. Only three definite linkages with Xg are established, X-borne ichthyosis, ocular albinism and retinoschisis and there is a probable linkage with Fabry's disease (α-galactosidase deficiency). Direct linkage with Xg has been excluded for G6PD, Haemophilia (factor VIII deficiency). Christmas disease (factor IX deficiency), colour blindness and Duchenne's muscular dystrophy. This means that the latter conditions are not within measurable distance of Xg and its known linkages.

Race and Sanger (1975b) suggest that the shortage of proved linkages to *Xg* may be because this locus occupies a terminal position on the chromosome and there is some reason for thinking that it might be situated at the terminal end of the short arm of the chromosome.

There are, therefore, two clusters of linkages on the *X,* one around colour vision and one around *Xg* but as yet the length of the chromosome between the two clusters is unknown.

REFERENCES

MNSs system

Allen, F.H., Corcoran, P.A., Kentqn, H.B. & Breare, N. (1958) M^g a new blood group antigen in the MNSs system. *Vox Sang.,* **3,** 81.
Booth, P.B. (1971) Anti-N^{1}A^1 An antibody sub-dividing Melanesian N. *Vox Sang.,* **21,** 522.
Cleghorn, T.E. (1966) A memorandum on the Miltenburger blood groups. *Vox Sang.,* **11,** 219.
Crossland, J.D., Pepper, M.D., Giles, C.M. & Ikin, E.W. (1970) A British family possessing two variants of the MNSs blood group system. M^v and a new class within the Miltenburger complex. *Vox Sang.,* **18,** 407.
Dahr, W. & Uhlenbruck, G. (1975) Immunochemistry of the MN system. 6th Internationale Tagung der Gesellschaft für forensische Blutgruppenkunde.
Francis, B.J. & Hatcher, D.E. (1966) MN blood types. The S–s–U+ and the M$_1$ phenotypes. *Vox Sang.,* **11,** 213.
Gershowitz, H. & Fried, K. (1966) Anti-M^v, a new antibody of the MNS blood group system. 1. M^v. a new inherited variant of the M gene. *Amer. J. hum. Genet.* **18,** 264.
Giles, C.M. & Howell, P. (1974) An antibody in the serum of an MN patient which reacts with M$_1$ antigen. *Vox Sang.,* **27,** 43.
Greenwalt, T.J., Sasaki, T., Sanger, R., Sneath, J. & Race, R.R. (1954) An allele of the S(s) blood group genes. *Proc. Nat. Acad. Sci. (Wash.),* **40,** 1126.
Henningsen, K. (1966) Exceptional MNSs and Gm-types within a Danish family. Causal relationship or coincidence? *Acta genet.,* **16,** 239.
Ikin E.W. & Mourant, A.E. (1951) A rare blood group antigen occurring in Negroes. *Brit. Med. J.,* **i,** 456.
Jack, J.A., Tippett, P., Noades, J., Sanger, R. & Race, R.R. (1960) M$_1$, a subdivision of the human blood group antigen M. *Nature (Lond.),* **186,** 642.
Jacobowicz, R., Bryce, L.M. & Simmons, R.T. (1949) The occurrence of unusual positive Coombs reactions and M variants in the blood of a mother and her first child. *Med. J. Aust.,* **2,** 945.
Jeannet, M., Metaxas-Bühler, M. & Tobler, R. (1964) Anomalie héréditaire de la membrane érythrocytaire avec test de Coombs positif et modification de l'antigène de groupe N. *Vox Sang.,* **9,** 52.
Jensen, K.G. & Freiesleben, E. (1962) Inherited positive Coombs reaction connected with a weak N-receptor (N$_2$). *Vox Sang.,* **7,** 696.
Konugres, A.A., Brown, L.S. & Corcoran, P.A. (1966) Anti-M^A and the phenotype M^{a}N, of the blood group system MN (A new Finding) *Vox Sang.,* **11,** 189.
Landsteiner, K., Strutton, W.R. & Chase, M.W. (1934) An agglutination reaction observed with some human bloods, chiefly among Negroes. *J. Immunol.,* **27,** 469.
Metaxas, M.N. & Metaxas-Bühler, M. (1964) M^k an apparently silent allele at the MN locus. *Nature (Lond.),* **202,** 1123.
Metaxas, M.N., Metaxas-Bühler, M. & Edwards, J.H. (1970) MNSs frequencies in 3,895 Swiss blood donors. *Vox Sang.,* **18,** 385.
Metaxas, M.N., Metaxas-Bühler, M. & Ikin, E.W. (1968) Complexities of the MN locus. *Vox Sang.,* **15,** 102.
Metaxas, M.N., Metaxas-Bühler, M., & Romanski, J. (1966) Studies on the blood group antigen Mg. 1. Frequency of Mg in Switzerland and family studies. *Vox Sang.,* **11,** 157.
Metaxas, M.N., Metaxas-Bühler, M. & Romanski, Y. (1971) The inheritance of the blood group gene M^k and some consideration on its possible nature. *Vox Sang.,* **20,** 509.
Moores, P. (1972) Four examples of the S–s–U-phenotype in an Indian family. *Vox Sang.,* **23,** 452.

Nordling, S., Sanger, R., Gavin, J., Furuhjelm, U., Myllyla, G. & Metaxas, M.N. (1969) M^k and M^s, some serological and physiochemical observations. *Vox Sang.,* **17,** 300.

Race, R.R. & Sanger, R. (1975) *Blood Groups in Man.* 6th Ed. P. 123 Oxford: Blackwell.

Sanger, R. (1970) *Genetics of Blood Groups in Blood and Tissue Antigens,* ed Aminoff, D. N.Y. Acad. Press. Pp. 17-31.

Springer, G. F., & Huprikar, S. W. (1972) On the biochemical and genetic basis of the human blood group MN specificities. *Haematologia* **6,** 81-92.

Sturgeon, P., Metaxas-Bühler, M., Metaxas, M.N., Tippett, P. & Ikin, E.W. (1970) An erroneous exclusion of paternity in a Chinese family exhibiting the rare MNSs gene complexes M^k and Ms^{III} *Vox Sang.,* **18,** 395.

Wiener, A.S., Unger, L.J. & Gordon, E.B. (1953) Fatal hemolytic transfusion reaction caused by sensitisation to a new blood factor, U. *J. Amer. Med. Ass.,* **153,** 1444.

P system

Cameron, G.L. & Staveley, J.M. (1957) Blood group P substance in hydatid cyst fluids. *Nature (Lond.),* **179,** 147.

Contreras, M. & Tippett, P. (1974) The Lu (a–b–) syndrome and an apparent upset of P_1 inheritance. *Vox Sang.,* **27,** 369.

Cory, H.T., Yates, A.D., Donald, A.S.R., Watkins, W.M. & Morgan, W.T.J. (1974) The nature of the human blood group P_1 determinant. *Biochem. Biophys. Res. Comm.,* **61,** 1289.

Crawford, M.N., Tippett, P. & Sanger, R. (1974) Antigens Au^a, i and P_1 of cells of the dominant type of Lu (a–b–). *Vox Sang.,* **26,** 283.

Fellous, M., Gerbal, A., Tessier, C., Frezal, J., Dausset, J. & Salmon, C. (1974) Studies on the biosynthetic pathway of human P erythrocyte antigens using somatic cells in culture. *Vox Sang.,* **26,** 518.

Fellous, M., Tessier, C., Gerbal, A., Salmon, C., Frezal, J. & Dausset, J. (1972) Genetic dissection of P biosynthesis pathway. *Bull. Europ. Soc. Hum. Genet.* November. P.31.

Kortekangas, A.E., Noades, J., Tippett, P., Sanger, R. & Race, R.R. (1959) A second family with the red cell antigen P^k. *Vox Sang.,* **4,** 337.

Levine, P., Bobbitt, O.B., Waller, R.K. & Kuhmichel, A. (1951) Isoimmunisation by a new blood factor in tumour cells. *Proc. Soc. exp. Biol.* (N.Y.), **77,** 403.

Matson, G.A., Swanson, J., Noades, J., Sanger, R. & Race, R.R. (1959) A new antigen and antibody belonging to the P blood group system. *Amer. J. hum. Genet.,* **11,** 26.

Morgan, W.T.J. & Watkins, W.M. (1964) Blood group P_1 substance (I) Chemical properties. *Proc. 9th Congr. Int. Soc. Blood Transf.* P. 225. Mexico, 1962.

Naiki, M. & Marcus, D.M. (1974) Human erythrocyte Panel P^k blood group antigens: identification as glycosphingolipids. *Biochem. Biophys. Res. Commun.,* **60,** 1105.

Nakajima, H. & Yokota, T. (1977). Two Japanese families with P^k members. *Vox Sang* **32,** 56.

Race, R.R. & Sanger, R. (1975). *Blood Groups in Man.* P.163. Oxford: Blackwell.

Sanger, R. (1955) An association between the P and Jay systems of blood groups. *Nature,* 176, 1163.

Tippett, P., Sanger, R., Race, R.R., Swanson, J. & Busch, S. (1965) An agglutinin associated with the P and the ABO blood group systems. *Vox Sang.,* **10,** 269.

Watkins, W.M. & Morgan, W.T.J. (1964) Blood group P_1 substance (II) Immunological properties. *Proc. 9th Congr. Int. Soc. Blood Transf.* P. 230. Mexico, 1962.

Ii system

Booth, P.B., Jenkins, W.J. & Marsh, W.L. (1966) Anti-I^Ta new antibody of the I blood group system occurring in certain Melanesian sera. *Brit. J. Haemat.,* **12,** 341.

Feizi, T., Kabat, E.A., Vicari, G., Anderson, B. & Marsh, W.L. (1971) Immunochemical studies on blood groups. XLVII. The I antigen complex-precursors in the A, B, H, Le^a and Le^b blood group systems—hemagglutination-inhibition studies. *J. exp. Med.,* **133,** 39.

Hillman, R.S. & Giblett, E.R. (1965) Red cell membrane alteration associated with marrow stress. *J. clin. Invest.,* **44,** 1730.

Issitt, P.D., Tegoli, J., Jackson, V., Sanders, C.W. & Allen, F.H. Jr (1968) Anti-IP_1: antibodies that show an association between the I and P blood group systems. *Vox Sang.,* **14,** 1.

Jenkins, W.J., Marsh, W.L. & Gold, E.R. (1965) Reciprocal relationship of antigens I and i in health and disease. *Nature (Lond.),* **205,** 813.

Marsh, W.L., Nichols, M.E. & Reid, M.E. (1971) The definition of two I antigen components. *Vox Sang.,* **20,** 209.

Race, R.R. & Sanger, R. (1975) Blood Groups in Man. 6th ed. P.450. Oxford: Blackwell.

Rosse, W.F. & Sherwood, J.B. (1970) Cold reacting antibodies: differences in the reaction of anti-I antibodies with adult and cord red cells. *Blood,* **36,** 28.

Schmidt, P.J., Barile, M.F. & McGinnes, M.H. (1965) Mycoplasma (pleuropneumonia-like organisms) and blood group I. Association with neoplastic disease. *Nature (Lond.),* **205,** 371.

Tegoli, J., Cortez, M., Jensen, L. & Marsh, W.L. (1971) A new antibody anti-ILe[bH] reacting with àn apparent interactive product of the I, Le, Se and H genes. *Vox Sang.,* **21,** 397.

Tegoli, J., Harris, J. O., Issitt, P.D. & Sanders, C.W. (1967) Anti-IB, an expected 'new' antibody detecting a joint product of the I and B genes. *Vox Sang.,* **13,** 144.

Tippett, P., Noades, J., Sanger, R., Race, R.R., Sausais, L., Holman, C.A. & Buttimer, R.J. (1960) Further studies of the I antigen and antibody. *Vox Sang.,* **5,** 107.

Lutheran

Crawford, M.N., Greenwalt, T.J., Sasaki, T., Tippett, P., Sanger, R. & Race, R.R. (1961) The phenotype Lu(a-b-) together with unconventional Kidd groups in one family. *Transfusion (Philad.),* **1,** 228.

Crawford, M.N., Tippett, P. & Sanger, R. (1974) The antigens Au[a], i and P$_1$ of cells of the dominant type of Lu(a-b-). *Vox Sang.,* **26,** 283..

Darnborough, J., Firth, R., Giles, C.M., Goldsmith, K.L.G. & Crawford, M.N. (1963) A 'new' antibody anti-Lu[a] Lu[b] and two further examples of the genotype Le (a-b-). *Nature (Lond.),* **198,** 796.

Marsh, W.L. (1972) Anti-Lu5, anti-Lu6 and anti-Lu7. Three antibodies defining high frequency antigens related to the Lutheran blood group system. *Transfusion (Philad.),* **12,** 27.

Molthan, L., Crawford, M.N., Marsh, W.L., & Allen, F.H. (1973) Lu9, another new antigen of the Lutheran blood group system. *Vox Sang.,* **24,** 468.

Race, R.R. & Sanger, R. (1975a) Blood *Blood Groups in man.* P.275. Oxford: Blackwell.

Race, R.R. & Sanger, R. (1975b) *Blood Groups in man.* P.274. Oxford: Blackwell.

Taliano, V., Guevin, R.M. & Tippett, P. (1973) The genetics of the dominant inhibitor of the Lutheran antigens. *Vox Sang.,* **24,** 42,

Tippett, P. (1971) A case of suppressed Lu[a] and Lu[b] antigens. *Vox Sang.,* **20,** 378.

Sinclair, M., Buchanan, D.I., Tippett, P. & Sanger, R. (1973) Another antibody related to the Lutheran blood group system (Much). *Vox Sang.,* **25,** 156.

Wrobel, D.M., Moore, B.P.L., Cornwall, S., Wray, E., Øyen R. & Marsh, W.L. (1972) A second example of Lu(-6) in the Lutheran system. *Vox Sang.,* **23,** 205.

Kell

Allen, F.H. Jr. & Lewis, S.J. (1957) Kp[a] (Penney) a New antigen in the Kell blood group system. *Vox Sang.,* **2,** No. 2, 81.

Allen, F.H. Jr., Lewis, S.J. & Fudenberg, H. (1958) Studies of anti-Kp[h], a new antibody in the Kell blood group system. *Vox Sang.,* **3,** No. 1.

Allen, F.H., Krabbe Sissel, M.R. & Corcoran, P.A. (1961) A new phenotype (McLeod) in the Kell blood group system. *Vox Sang.,* **6,** 555.

Chown, B., Lewin, M. & Hiroko, K. (1957) A new Kell blood group phenotype. *Nature (Lond.),* **180,** 711.

Corcoran, P.A., Allen, F.H.Jr., Lewis, M. & Chown, B. (1961) A new antibody, anti-Ku (anti-Peltz), in the Kell blood group system. *Transfusion* **1,** No. 3, 181.

Furuhjelm, U., Nevanlinna, H.R., Nurkka, R., Gavin, J., Tippett, P. Gooch, A. & Sanger, R. (1968) The blood group antigen Ul[a] (Karhula) *Vox Sang.,* **15,** 118.

Furuhjelm, U., Nevanlinna, H.R., Nurkka, R., Gavin, J., & Sanger, R. (1969) Evidence that the antigen Ul[d] is controlled from the Kell complex locus *Vox Sang.,* **16,** 496.

Giblett, Eloise R. (1958) Js, a new blood group antigen found in Negroes. *Nature (Lond.),* **181,** 1221.

Giblett, E.R., Klebanoff, S.J., Pincus, S.H., Swanson, J., Park, B.H. & McCullough, H. (1971) Kell phenotypes in chronic granulomatous disease: a potential transfusion hazard. *Lancet,* **i,** 1235.

Guévin, R.M., Taliano, V. & Waldmann, O. (1971) The Coté serum, an antibody defining a new variant in the Kell system. *Amer. Ass. Blood Banks Program 24th Annual Meeting.* P.100.

Hart, Mia, V. D. & Loghem J.J. Van. (1968) A new antibody associated with the Kell blood group system. *Vox Sang.,* **15,** 456.

Heistø, H., Guevin, R.M., Taliano, V., Mann, J., MacIlroy, M., Marsh, W.L., Tippett, P. & Gavin, J. (1973) Three further antigen-antibody specificities associated with the Kell blood group system. *Vox Sang.,* **24,** 179.

Marsh, W.L., Jensen, L., Oyen, R., Stroup, M., Gellerman, M., McMahon, F.J. & Tsitsera, H. (1974) Anti-K13 and the K-13 phenotype, a blood group variant related to the Kell system. *Vox Sang.,* **26,** 34.

Marsh, W. L., Øyen, R., and Nichols, M. E., (1976) Kx Antigen, The McLeod Phenotype, and chronic granulomatous disease. Further studies. *Vox Sang,* **31,** 356.

Marsh, W.L., Øyen, R., Nichols, M.E. & Allen, F.H. (1975) Chronic granulomatous disease and the Kell blood groups. *Brit. J. Haemat.,* **29,** 247.

Strange, J.J., Kenworthy, R.J., Webb, A.J. & Giles, C.M. (1974) Wkª (Weeks) a new antigen in the Kell blood group system. *Vox Sang.,* **27,** 81.

Stroup, M., MacIlroy M., Walker, R. & Aydelotte, J.V. (1965) Evidence that Sutter belongs to the Kell blood group system. *(Philad.) Transfusion* **5,** 309.

Walker, R.H., Argall, C.I., Steane, E.A., Sasaki, T.T. & Greenwalt, T.J., (1963) Anti-Jsᵇ, the expected antithetical antibody of the Sutter blood group system. *Nature (Lond.),* **197,** 295.

Duffy

Albrey, J.A., Vincent, E.E.R., Hutchinson, J., Marsh, W.L., Allen, F.H., Gavin, J. & Sanger, R. (1971) A new antibody, anti-Fy3 in the Duffy blood group system. *Vox Sang.,* **20,** 29.

Behzad, O., Lee, C.L., Gavin, J. & Marsh, W.L. (1973) A new anti-erythrocyte antibody in the Duffy system: anti-Fy4. *Vox Sang.,* **24,** 337.

Colledge, K.I., Pezzulich, M. & Marsh, W.L. (1973) Anti-Fy5, an antibody disclosing a probable association between the Rhesus and Duffy blood group genes. *Vox Sang.,* **24,** 193.

DiNapoli, J., Garcia, A., Marsh, W.L. & Dreizen, D. (1976) A second example of anti-Fy5. *Vox Sang.,* **30,** 308.

Lewis, M., Kasta, H. & Chown, B. (1972) The Duffy blood group system in Caucasians. *Vox Sang.,* **23,** 523.

Sanger, R., Race, R.R. & Jack, J. (1955) The Duffy blood groups of New York Negroes. The phenotype Fya-b- *Brit. J. Haem.,* **1,** 370.

Sdᵃ and Cad

Cazal, P., Monis, M., Caubel, J. & Brives, J. (1968) Polyagglutinabilité héréditaire dominante: antigène privé (Cad) correspondant à un anticorps public et à une lectine Dolichos biflorus. *Rev, franc. Transfus.,* **11,** 209.

Morton, J.A., Pickles, M.M. & Terry, A.M. (1970) The Sdª blood group antigen in tissues and body fluids. *Vox Sang.,* **19,** 472.

Petermans, M.E. & Cole-Dergent, J. (1970) Haemolytic transfusion reaction due to anti-Sdª. *Vox Sang.,* **18,** 67.

Renton, P.H., Howell, P., Ikin, E.W., Giles, C.M. & Goldsmith, K.L.G. (1967) Anti-Sdª-a new blood group antibody. *Vox Sang.,* **13,** 493.

Sanger, R., Gavin, J., Tippett, P., Teesdale, P. & Eldon, K. (1971) Plant agglutinin for another human blood group. *Lancet,* **i,** 1130.

Race, R.R. & Sanger, R. (1971) Quoted in *Blood Groups in Man* (1975) P.399. Oxford: Blackwell.

Springarm, S., Chiewsilp, P., Tubrod, J. & Sriboonruang, N. (1974) Cad receptors in Thai blood donors. *Vox Sang.,* **26,** 462.

Chido

Harris, J.P., Tegoli, J., Swanson, J., Foster, N., Gavin, J. & Noades, J. (1967) A nebulous antibody responsible for cross matching difficulties (Chido). *Vox Sang.,* **12,** 140.

Middleton, J. (1972) Anti-Chido: a cross matching problem. *Can. J. med. Technol.,* **34,** 41.

Middleton, J. & Crookston, M.C. (1972) Chido-substance in plasma. *Vox Sang.,* **23,** 256.

Middleton, J., Crookston, M.C., Falk, J.A., Robson, E.B., Cook, P.J.L., Batchelor, J.R., Bodmer, J., Ferrara, G.B., Festenstein, H., Harris, R., Kissmeyer-nielsen, F., Lawler, S.D., Sachs, J.A. & Wolf, E. (1974) Linkage of Chido and HL-A. *Tissue Antigens,* **4,** 366-373.

Morton, J.A., Pickles, M.M. & Sutton, L. (1969) The correlation of the Bgª blood group with the HL-A7 leucocyte group: demonstration of antigenic sites on red cells and leucocytes. *Vox Sang,* **17,** 536.

Morton, J.A., Pickles, M.M., Sutton, L. & Skov, F. (1971) Identification of further antigens on red cells and lymphocytes. *Vox Sang.,* **21,** 144.

Seaman, M.J., Benson, R., Jones, M.N., Morton, J.A. & Pickles, M.M. (1967) The reactions of the Bennett-Goodspeed group of antibodies with the Auto-Analyser. *Brit. J. Haemat.,* **13,** 464.

Dombrock

Molthan, L., Crawford, M.N. & Tippett, P. (1973) Enlargement of the Dombrock blood group system: the finding of anti-Do^b. *Vox Sang.,* **24,** 382.
Swanson, J., Polesky, H.F., Tippett, P. & Sanger, R. (1965) A "new" blood group antigen, Do^a. *Nature (Lond.),* **206,** 313.
Tippett, P. (1967) Genetics of the Dombrock blood group system. *J. med. Genet.,* **4,** 7.

Auberger

Salmon, C., Salmon, D., Liberge, G., André, R., Tippett, P. & Sanger, R. (1961) Un nouvel antigène de groupe sanguin erythrocytaire présent chez 80% des sujets de race blanche. *Nouv. Rev. franc. Hémat.,* **1,** 649.

Scianna

Anderson, C., Hunter, J., Zipursky, A., Lewis, M. & Chown, B. (1963) An antibody defining a new blood group antigen, Bu^a. *Transfusion (Philad.),* **3,** 30.
Schmidt, R.P., Griffiths, J.J. & Northman, F.F. (1962) A new antibody, anti-S, reacting with a high incidence antigen. *Transfusion (Philad.),* **2,** 338.
Seyfried, H., Frankowska, K. & Giles, C.M. (1966) Further examples of anti-Bu^a found in immunised donors. *Vox Sang.,* **11,** 512.
Lewis, M., Kaita, H. & Chown, B. (1974) Scianna blood group system. *Vox Sang.,* **27,** 261.

Diego

Layrisse, M., Arends, T. & Dominguez, S.R. (1955) Nuevo grupo sanguineo encondrado en descendientes de Indios. *Acta Medice Veneczolano,* **3,** 132.
Levine, P., Robinson, E.A., Layrisse, M., Arends, T. & Dominguez, S.R. (1956) The Diego blood factor. *Nature (Lond.),* **177,** 40.
Thompson, P. R., Childers, D.M. and Hatcher, D.E. (1967) Anti-Di^b, first and second examples *Vox. Sang.* **13,** 314.

Colton

Giles, C.M., Darnborough, J., Aspinall, P., Fletton, M.W. (1970) Identification of the first sample of anti-Co^b. *Brit. J. Haemat.,* **19,** 267.
Heisto, H., Van der Hart, M., Madsen, G., Moes, M., Noades, J., Pickles, M.M. Race, R.R., Sanger, R. & Swanson, J. (1967) Three examples of a new red cell antibody, anti-Co^a. *Vox Sang.,* **12,** 18.
Rogers, M.J., Stiles, P.A. & Wright, J. (1974) A new minus-minus phenotype. Three Co(a–b–) individuals in one family AABB abstracts. *Transfusion (Philad.),* **14,** 508.

En

Darnborough, J., Dunsford, I., & Wallace, J.A. (1969) The En^a antigen and antibody. A genetical modification of human red cells affecting their blood grouping reactions. *Vox Sang.,* **17,** 241.
Furuhjelm, U., Myllyla, G., Nevanlinna, H.R., Nordling, S., Pirkola, A., Gavin, J. Gooch, A., Sanger, R. & Tippett, P. (1969) The red cell phenotype En(a –) and anti-En^a: serological and phys:o-chemical aspects. *Vox Sang.,* **17,** 256.
Furuhjelm, U., Nevanlinna, H.R. & Pirkolá, A. (1973) A second Finnish En(a–) propositus with anti-En^a. *Vox Sang.,* **24,** 545.
Tippett, P. & Teesdale, P. (1973) Limited blood group tests on samples from two coelacanths, *(Latineria chalumnae). Vox Sang.,* **24,** 175.

Xg

Buckton, K.E., Cunningham, C., Newton, M.S., O'Riordan, M.L. & Sanger, R. (1971) Anomalous Xg inheritance with a probable explanation, *Lancet,* **i,** 371.
Cook, I.A., Polley, M.J. & Mollison, P.L.·(1963) A second example of anti-Xg^a. *Lancet,* **i,** 857.
Fellous, M., Bengtsson, B., Finnegan, D. & Bodmer, W.F. (1974) Expression of the Xga antigen on cells in culture and its segregation in somatic cell hybrids. *Ann hum. Genet.,* **37,** 421.

I

Gavin, J., Noades, J., Tippet, P., Sanger, R. & Race, R.R. (1964) Blood group antigen Xg[a] in gibbons. *Nature,* **204,** 1322.

Gorman, J.G., di Re, J., Treacy, A.M. & Cahan, A. (1963) The application of −Xg[a] antiserum to the question of red cell mosaicism in female heterozygotes *J. Lab. clin. Med.,* **61,** 642.

Lindsten, J., Bowen, P., Lee, C.S.N., McKusick, V.A., Polani, P.E., Wingate, M., Edwards, J.H., Hamper, J., Tippett, P., Sanger, R. & Race, R.R. (1963) Source of the X in XO females: the evidence of Xg. *Lancet,* **i,** 558.

Mann, J.D., Cahan, A., Gelb, A.G., Fisher, N., Hamper, J., Tippett, P., Sanger, R. & Race, R.R. (1962) A sex linked blood group. *Lancet,* **i,** 8.

Pfeiffer, R.A., Körver, G., Sanger, R. & Race, R.R. (1966) Paternal origin of an XXYY anomaly. *Lancet,* **i,** 1427.

Race, R.R. & Sanger, R. (1975a) *Blood Groups in Man* 6th ed. P.579. Oxford: Blackwell.

Race, R.R. & Sanger, R. (1975b) *Blood Groups in Man* 6th ed. P.610. Oxford: Blackwell.

Sanger, R., Tippett, P. & Gavin, J. (1971) The linked blood group system Xg: tests on unrelated people and families of Northern European ancestry *J. Med. Genet.,* **8,** 427.

Chapter 19. The HLA System

This chapter concerns the most complex system of antigens known in Man. However, it is important to realise that it is only one of a number of antigen systems which are expressed on leucocytes and platelets.

The HLA human leucocyte system is of greatest concern to the transplantation immunologist, since differences in HLA types between a grafted organ and the person who receives it are associated with rejection of the organ or with a reaction of grafted blood cells (immuno-competent lymphocytes) against the patient (graft-versus-host disease).

The system is also important, however, to the blood group serologist, since HLA antibodies can lead to reactions against transfused blood, and these antibodies can also lead to *in vitro* reactions between patients' sera and cells from donor blood. HLA antibodies can also form troublesome contaminants in blood group typing sera.

Before discussing the practical aspects of the system, the detection of antibodies and tissue typing, we will briefly discuss some features of interest in the theoretical background to the system.

Thorsby (1974) is a recent review on the subject.

Genetic background and nomenclature

The expression of the HLA antigens on the surface of the cell is controlled by a region of chromosome 6, which is schematically shown in Figure 19.1. This region has been called the HLA supergene by Ceppellini on account of its complexity. At the present time it seems that the region is subdivided into four loci, at each of which there are many alleles. Allelic genes at three of these loci

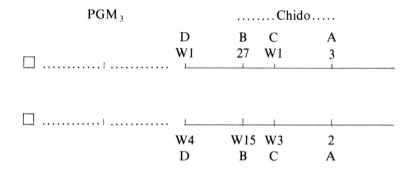

Fig. 19.1 Diagrammatic representation of chromosome 6 showing HLA loci.

Table 19.1—New W.H.O. nomenclature for HLA system (July 1975)

The previous nomenclature is also included for comparison

New	Old	New	Old	New	Old	New	Old
HLA-A	LA	HLA-B	4 Series	HLA-C	AJ	HLA-D	MLC
HLA-A1	HL-A1	HLA-B5	HL-A5	HLA-CW1	T1 AJ	HLA-DW1	27a, "J"
A2	HL-A2	B7	HL-A7	CW2	T2 170	W2	7a
A3	HL-A3	B8	HL-A8	CW3	T3 UPS	W3	8a
A9	HL-A9	B12	HL-A12	CW4	T4 315	W4	15a
A10	HL-A10	B13	HL-A13	CW5	T5	W5	–
A11	HL-A11	B14	W14			W6	–
A28	W28	B18	W18			W107	12a
A29	W29	B27	W27			W108	–
AW23	W23	BW35	W5				
AW24	W24	BW40	W10				
AW25	W25	BW15	W15				
AW26	W26	BW16	W16				
AW30	W30	BW17	W17				
AW31	W31	BW21	W21				
AW32	W32	BW22	W22				
AW33	W19.6,Mal1,Fe55	BW37	TY				
AW34	Malay2,10.35 etc	BW38	W16.1 (DA31)				
AW36	MO*,LT	BW39	W16.2				
AW43	BK	BW41	Sabell, LK				
		BW42	MWA				

control the expression of antigens which can be detected using serological methods (mainly lymphocytotoxicity). The fourth locus has allelic genes which govern the presence on the cell surface of antigens which are not serologically detectable: at present these are investigated using the technique of mixed lymphocyte culture and the antigens themselves are termed "lymphocyte defined" (LD) as opposed to the "serologically defined" (SD) antigens produced by genes at the other three loci.

Figure 19.1 illustrates the possible complexity of the antigenic make-up of an individual. Each individual possesses a pair of No. 6 chromosomes, like the other autosomes of the body, and each chromosome has four HLA loci. At each locus, any one of a number of alleles which belong to the corresponding series may be present (Table 19.1 shows a list of some of the alleles present at each locus). If the individual is heterozygous at all four loci, he will have as many as eight HLA antigens, six of which can be detected serologically. All of these antigens will be found on the surface of at least some of the different kinds of cells making up that individual. The exact distribution of all the antigens has not yet been determined, but those of the first and second series are very widely distributed, and those of all series are found on lymphocytes.

The tissue type of the person depicted in Fig. 19.1 would be written:-

A3   B27   CW1   DW1
A2   BW15   CW3   DW4

Two other known loci on chromosome 6 are shown on the diagram. These are PGM 3 which occurs somewhere between HLA-D and the centromere, and Chido, the exact location of which is unknown but it occurs somewhere in association with the HLA-A, B and C regions.

The nomenclature of the HLA system has recently been revised, the main advantage of the present system being that the antigen designation itself shows to which locus the controlling genes belong. Thus HLA A2 can be seen to belong to the A locus, and HLA DW4 to the D locus, and so comparisons between donor and recipient tissue types are more easily made. Note that the inclusion of "W" in a designation indicates that the antigen has been accepted at workshops, but is not yet well enough defined to justify the allocation of a definitive number.

Table 19.1 gives the 1975 nomenclature for the HLA system and also the previous nomenclature. The region is now called HLA (hyphen is dropped). LA or first locus is now HLA-A, 4 or second locus is now HLA-B. AJ or third locus is HLA-C and the MLC locus is HLA-D.

Crossing-over between the loci

The relationship of the four loci to each other and their distance apart on the chromosome was established by the study of separation and recombination at meiosis. The recombination rate between the HLA-A and -B loci is in fact quite high, probably about 1 per cent. This fact has to be borne in mind in theoretical considerations, particularly relating to linkage disequilibrium, which is such a feature of the system (*see below*). Crossing over must also be considered in paternity investigations.

Linkage disequilibrium

This is the name given to the non-random associations of the antigens of the HLA-A and -B loci. The most striking cases are the associations of A1 with B8, and A3 with B7. Thus when a person has A1, he or she is very likely also to have B8, and similarly A3 goes with B7. Since the tendency for the two series to separate is so high, there must be some mechanism which tends to keep certain of the antigen combinations in existence. At present this mechanism is unknown.

Linkage disequilibrium is apparently even more marked between the B and C loci than between the A and B loci and also occurs between the B and D loci.

It should be noted that linkage disequilibrium also occurs in red cell systems *e.g.* the MNSs system, although it is not referred to as such. Thus the gene controlling the M antigen tends to occur on the same chromosome as the gene controlling the S antigen. Here there is no measurable recombination rate because the two loci are so close together, and no special mechanism need exist to maintain the disequilibrium, although it is of course interesting to speculate how it arose in the first instance.

Some of the associations which have been seen to exist between particular HLA-A and HLA-B antigens and certain diseases may also be the result of linkage disequilibrium between the genes controlling these antigens and genes governing susceptibility to the diseases.

Example

Linkage disequilibrium may be illustrated using figures from the Fourth International Workshop 1970, for the HLA antigen combinations in particular haptotypes—(*i.e.* the individual chromosomes).

Total chromosomes with HLA-A1 numbered 159 per 1000
"   "   "   HLA-B8 numbered   92 per 1000
If A1 and B8 had been randomly associated (linkage equilibrium) there would have been:

$$\frac{159}{1000} \times \frac{92}{1000} \times 1000 = 14.6 \text{ chromosomes with both 1 and 8.}$$

The actual number observed was 67.
For HLA-A3 and B7 the figures were:
Total chromosomes with HLA-A3   163
"   "   "   "   B7   125

giving an expected number with A3 and B7 of 20.
The number actually observed was 40.

Cross-reactivity

The prevalence of this feature is of paramount importance for the serologist, and has led to many difficulties in the definition of antigens. There is a marked tendency for HLA antigens to stimulate the production of antibodies which react not only with the stimulating antigen, but also with one or more other antigens at the same locus. Thus immunisation with the HLA-A2 antigen often gives rise to a serum which reacts also with AW28, and in fact, sera which react strongly with A2 and are negative with AW28 cells are quite hard to find. Often the cross-reacting component is much less strong than the stimulating component, but since HLA typing involves very sensitive techniques which are liable to be influenced by slight variations in experimental conditions, the cross-reactivity can show itself to such an unpredictable degree that the serum may be of little use for typing purposes.

Racial differences

There are striking differences in the antigen distributions between different races and these differences were the subject of the 5th International Histocompatibility Workshop (1972). Moreover, sera which have been defined by testing with one population sometimes give different reactions in a second population. Clearly this presents great difficulties when antisera are being used in mixed populations. This is one reason why two people who are being investigated for compatibility in HLA type should always be tested with the same battery of antisera used by exactly the same techniques.

Association with disease

Some diseases are associated with particular HLA types to an extraordinary degree. Thus practically all (about 95 per cent) of people with ankylosing spondylitis (a.s.) have the B27 antigen. This degree of correlation allows tissue typing to aid diagnosis of this disease. It is important however to bear in mind that about 10 per cent of individuals without a.s. have B27 and that 5 per cent of individuals with a.s. do not. This very striking association between HLA type and disease has stimulated a vigorous search for other possible disease associations. A discussion of this whole subject is to be found in a paper by McDevitt and Bodmer 1974.

Presence of HLA antigens on red cells

This is of importance because it interferes with red cell antibody detection and identification.

Some HLA antigens have now been detected on red cells, where they may be the cause of weak and poorly reproducible reactions with sera containing HLA antibodies. They particularly occur with saline RT, anti-human globulin and especially AutoAnalyser techniques. Because the HLA types of the donors of the red cells used are usually unknown, and because of the weakness and variability of the reactions, it is usually impossible to identify their specificity, and they can greatly complicate life for the serologist. They can be particularly troublesome in red cell typing reagents because they are usually difficult to remove by absorption. For the AutoAnalyser operator they add to the number of antibodies which, once detected, cannot satisfactorily be worked out by manual methods.

Some antigen-antibody reactions which were originally thought to be caused by true red cell antigen-antibody systems are now seen to be due to HLA antigens. The best understood is the Bennett-Goodspeed group of antigens. (Morton *et al.,* 1971.)

The antigens of this group have been shown to be associated with HLA antigens in the following way:-

HLA B 7   positive individuals have red cells possessing Bg^a

    B 17   "   "   "   "   "   " Bg^b

    A28   "   "   "   "   "   " Bg^c

This correlation was established after Seaman *et al.* (1967) had succeeded in making the reaction of the Bennett-Goodspeed antibodies more intense by the use of the AutoAnalyser.

Other antigens which have been correlated with HLA types are Chido, where Chido negative individuals tend to have an excess of HLA B12 and BW35 antigens, and Rodgers where Rg(a–) individuals are HLA A1, B8, or HLA A1, BW35 (James *et al.,* 1976). Here the Ch and Rg alleles may be associated with HLA alleles as a result of linkage disequilibrium, Chido having already been shown to be closely linked with HLA (Middleton *et al.,* 1974).

Tissue typing and screening for HLA antibodies

Unfortunately most antisera are not monospecific and it is usually necessary to use at least 2-3 sera to define each specificity. Some are more readily defined than others but certain specificities can only be assessed in the most advanced laboratories. In one such laboratory 120 highly selected sera are used to type each individual and even then resort has to be made on occasions to a further 60 sera.

The specificity of the sera is in principle assessed in the same way as for red cell antisera: the sera are screened against a panel of reference cells containing all known HLA specificities. A newly formed HLA laboratory has the problem of not having established a reference cell panel (which needs in the first instance to be typed with well defined sera) and is therefore limited in its ability to test unknown immune sera for the presence of specific HLA antibodies.

Pregnant women may develop antibodies in response to foetal HLA antigens, and so their sera should be tested against a reference panel of cells which ideally should contain all the HLA specificities. If a random panel is used for screening, many specificities, particularly the less frequent ones, may not be represented and the corresponding antibodies may be missed. This is particularly unfortunate as these are the sera usually in very short supply.

In order to increase their screening capacity, some laboratories will ask more advanced centres to test their cell panel for the less clearly defined specificities. Facilities for freezing lymphocytes in liquid nitrogen also make possible the screening of each batch of sera with selected cells thus eliminating the need for continually bleeding donors for fresh cells.

B cell antigens

Recently serologically defined antigens controlled by gene(s) in the HLA complex, apparently separate from the HLA-A, -B and -C loci, have been identified on B cells but not T cells. This association is analogous to the so called

Ia antigens in the H-2 complex of mice. The immunogenetics of these antigens have not yet been elucidated but preliminary data suggests a close association with these antigens and the HLA-D locus. This association is the main subject of the Histocompatibility Workshop in 1977.

These antigens may well prove to be more relevant to histo-compatibility than those controlled by the HLA–A, –B and –C loci.

TECHNIQUES

Technique 19.1 The Lymphocytotoxic test

This test is based on the following principles:-

Live lymphocytes when mixed with a serum containing the appropriate HLA antibodies become sensitised by these antibodies. If complement is then added and the cell/serum/complement mixture is incubated, the sensitised lymphocytes are killed by the action of complement. The difference between live and dead lymphocytes can be distinguished by phase contrast microscopy, or by ordinary bright field microscopy if a dye such as Trypan blue is used which stains only dead cells.

If phase contrast microscopy is used in conjunction with a dye, the distinction between live and dead cells is facilitated. The results are expressed as a percentage of dead cells.

The lymphocytotoxic test is used routinely for both tissue typing and screening for anti-HLA cytotoxic antibodies. The modification described below is that of Festenstein *et al.* (1976).

Lymphocytes can be readily separated from peripheral blood by heavy density barrier centrifugation on Ficoll/Triosil (F/T) reagent.

One method is to gently layer about 8 ml of blood on 2-3 ml F/T and centrifuge at 3000 r.p.m. for 15 minutes. Alternatively, 2 ml of blood and 1 ml of F/T is used and centrifuged at 5000 r.p.m. for 5 minutes. In general 1 ml of blood provides 1 $\times$ 10⁶ lymphocytes.

The lymphocyte layer at the interphace between the serum and the F/T reagent can be readily harvested, washed and resuspended to a concentration of about 1.5×10^6/ml cells. Most buffered physiological solutions can be used, CFT diluent can be used although it may be slightly toxic and therefore increases the sensitivity of the test.

The serum plates are prepared by dispensing 1μl aliquots of 60 different sera on to a 'Terasaki' plate (Falcon microtest plates). It is convenient to prepare about 80 plates at one time which are then stored at –40°C. Before dispensing the sera the plates are covered in light liquid paraffin to prevent subsequent evaporation. 1μl of the cell suspension is added to each of the 60 different sera on the plate and incubated for ½ hour at room temperature. 5μl of complement are added and the test incubated for a further one hour at room temperature. Pooled serum freshly frozen from selected rabbits is used as a source of complement. The test cells are then observed with an inverted, preferably phase contrast, microscope—killing can be assessed either directly with phase contrast or by the dye uptake (Trypan blue or Eosin) of the dead cells.

Notes

Defibrinated or heparinised blood is most commonly used for lymphocyte preparations. The advantage of defibrinated blood is that platelets are removed and cannot contaminate the lymphocyte suspension—platelets separate with the lymphocytes on the Ficoll-Triosil reagent and, since they carry HLA antigens, may interfere with the lymphocytotoxicity test.

The disadvantage of defibrinated blood is that it requires a certain expertise to carry it out without damaging the cells or allowing the blood to clot. To avoid this problem blood can be collected into 3.8 per cent sodium citrate (10 parts blood : 1 part citrate). It is then recalcified with 20 per cent calcium gluconate (0.3 - 5 ml of blood). After which one drop of thrombin (diluted 1:50) is added and the blood is defibrinated at leisure. This is particularly useful for blood samples collected at other hospitals. Usually a satisfactory suspension can be obtained from a specimen 24-hours old *but at no time should the blood sample (or the lymphocytes) be refrigerated.*

The sensitivity of the test is largely dependent on the amount of complement and the length of incubation. Most centres that previously used less complement for a shorter incubation period have now switched to the National Institute of Health technique, because of the numerous false negative results obtained. This is of particular importance in the cross-match between lymphocytes of a kidney donor and the patient's serum. To obtain reproducible results it is also important to check that the rabbit serum is potent as a source of complement but not toxic.

Technique 19.2 Agglutination technique (for further details see Van Rood *et al.,* 1970)

Solutions:

EDTA	- 5 per cent Na_2 EDTA in 0.9 per cent NaCl.
Dextran	- Dextraven 110 (outdated is satisfactory)
Toluidine blue	- 0.2 per cent in distilled water ⎫ mix equal volumes
Sodium chloride	- 1.8 per cent ⎬ just before use. ⎭

Leucocyte suspension

Add 1.8 ml blood to 0.2 ml EDTA solution in a siliconed tube and mix gently. Add 0.5 ml dextran and mix gently again. Incline the tube at 45° to horizontal and incubate at 37°C for ½ hour. Remove the plasma layer after this time, taking about ¾ of the plasma. Check that the cell count is within the limits of 3000 and 10,000 per mm³ and use immediately.

Test

Add 2 μl of leucocyte suspension to each well containing 2μl of serum. Incubate for 2 hours at 37°C. Add 1 μl of 0.1 per cent Toluidine blue and examine for agglutination after 5 minutes at laboratory temperature.

The sera being tested must be free of particulate matter.

Technique 19.3 Complement Fixation Test using platelets

In this test platelets are incubated with serum suspected of containing antibodies, together with a known amount of complement. At the end of the incubation period, sheep cells sensitised with haemolytic antibody are added, and the mixture incubated again. If the complement originally added is still present, the cells are lysed: if the complement has become fixed to the cell surface as a result of antigen-antibody reaction, then there is no lysis of the sheep cells. Thus lysis indicates a negative result, and absence of lysis a positive one.

The complement fixation test is not used routinely. It is a relatively difficult and prolonged test to perform and not all the HLA-A, B and C specificities defined on lymphocytes are established on platelets.

REFERENCES

Festenstein, H., Sachs, J.A. & Wolf, E. (1976) Personal communication.

Histocompatibility Testing (1970) *Joint Report of Fourth International Histocompatibility Workshop.* Copenhagen: Munksgaard.

Histocompatibility Testing (1972) Report of Fifth International Histocompatibility Workshop, Copenhagen: Munksgaard.

James, J., Stiles, P., Boyce, F. & Wright, J. (1976) The HLA type of Rg (a–) individuals. *Vox Sang.,* **30,** 214.

McDevitt, H. O., and Bodmer, W. F., (1974) HL-A, immune response genes and disease. Lancet, **i.** 1269.

Middleton, J., Crookston, M.C., Falk, J.A., Robson, E.B., Cook, P.J.L. Batchelor, J.R., Bodmer, J., Ferrara, G.B., Festenstein, H., Harris, R., Kissmeyer, Nielsen, F., Lawler, S.D., Sachs, J.A., & Wolf, E. (1974) Linkage of Chido and HLA. *Tissue Antigens,* **4,** 366.

Morton, J.A., Pickles, M.M., Sutton, L. & Skov, F. (1971) Identification of further antigens on red cells and lymphocytes. *Vox Sang., (Basel),* **21,** 141.

Seaman, M.J., Benson, R., Jones, M.N., Morton, J.A. & Pickles, M.M. (1967) The reactions of the Bennett-Goodspeed group of antibodies with the Auto-Analyser. *Brit. J. Haemat.,* **13,** 464.

Thorsby, E. (1974) The major human histocompatibility system. *Transplant Rev.,* **18,** 51-129.

Van Rood, J.J., Van Leeuen, A.S., Zweerus, R. (1970) The 4a and 4b antigens. Do they or don't they? Histocompatibility testing 1970, P.93. Copenhagen: Munksgaard.

Chapter 20. Serum Allotypes

The development of more and more refined methods for the separation of serum proteins has made possible the discovery of differences between individuals which follow inherited patterns. These serum proteins can be grouped together into systems which are just as authentically blood group systems as those involving the red cell antigens which form the principle subject of this book.

Some of these serum components and the techniques for their identification are beyond our present scope; these are therefore dealt with quite shortly and details of methods are not given. The following systems are included: Gm; Km(Inv); haptoglobins; Gc; Ag; Lp; and serum transferases. We have chosen to describe three of these systems, *i.e.* Gm, haptoglobins and Gc groups in more detail than the others since they are used fairly extensively. Details of techniques for the identification of allotypes of each of these three are given.

Gm typing will be most familiar to students of red cell types since Gm allotypes can be identified by methods similar to those used for red cell typing. Haptoglobins are usually determined by means of starch gel electrophoresis and Gc types by immuno-electophoresis in agar. A summary of the serum allotypes mentioned in this chapter is given in Table 20.1.

Table 20.1 Summary of serum allotypes

System	Globulin fraction	Common Genes	Common phenotypes in Caucasians	Method of detection
Gm	IgG (heavy chains)	Gm^1 (Gm^a) Gm^2 (Gm^x) Gm^{12} (Gm^b)	Gm (1, 2, 12) Gm (1,–2, 12) Gm (–1, –2, 12)	Inhibition of agglutination of globulin coated red cells by anti-Gm
Inv	IgG, IgA, IgM (light chains)	$Inv\ 1$ $Inv\ 2$	Inv (–1, 2) Inv (1, 2) Inv (1, –2)	Inhibition of agglutination of globulin coated red cells by anti-Inv.
Gc	α_2	Gc^1 Gc^2	Gc 1 Gc 2–1 Gc 2	Immuno-electrophoresis in agar
Ag	β_1 lipoprotein	Ag^a Ag	Ag (a+) Ag (a–)	Agar gel precipitation.
Lp	β_1 lipoprotein	Lp^a Lp	Lp (a+) Lp (a–)	Agar gel precipitation.
Haptoglobins	α_2	Hp^1 Hp^2	Hp 1 Hp 2–1 Hp 2	Starch gel electrophoresis.
Transferrins	β_1	TfC TfB TfD	C BC CD	Starch gel electrophoresis.

Gm GROUPS

These owe their identification to an observation by Grubb (1956), Grubb and Laurell (1956) that, at quite high dilution, the serum of a small proportion of people (mostly sufferers from rheumatoid arthritis) agglutinated D positive cells, first sensitised by incomplete anti-D. Grubb noticed that this agglutination could be inhibited by the serum of about 60 per cent of Swedish people. Other studies showed that the ability to inhibit was inherited as a Mendelian dominant character.

Further investigations showed that it was probable that the inhibitor was located in the gamma globulin fraction of the serum, hence the name Gm (a+) for the phenotype of the inhibitory sera and Gm (a–) for that of the non-inhibitory sera. It is now known that the agglutinating activity of the rheumatoid sera (often called Ragg) is due to anti-Gm antibodies reacting with a specific determinant (antigen) on the anti-D immunoglobulin molecule which has been used for sensitising the red cell. The principle underlying the phenomenon is very similar to that governing the anti-human-globulin (Coombs) test. The anti-human globulin (in this case anti-Gm) agglutinates red cells sensitised by antibody globulin which thereby acts as the corresponding globulin antigen. Antibodies of any specificity are suitable for sensitising the red cell; Anti-D is selected because it is so readily available. An anti-D suitable for the agglutination of cells by a particular anti-Gm antibody must of course originate from individuals who themselves possess the corresponding Gm antigen. For example, Grubb's original antibody which is now called anti-Gm (1) agglutinates only cells sensitised with anti-D from individuals who are Gm (1) positive and therefore their anti-D molecules have the Gm (1) antigen.

It follows also that Gm (1) positive individuals cannot themselves form anti-Gm (1) but this antibody has to be sought in the serum of Gm (1) negative people.

The agglutination by anti-Gm (1) of red cells sensitised by the appropriate anti-D is inhibited if the anti-Gm (1) serum is first mixed with serum which has Ig molecules with Gm (1). Hence an inhibition test (*see below*) is used for Gm typing unknown samples.

The complexity of the Gm system

Gradually a large number of Gm antigens have been found. One of the first of these was discovered by Harboe and Lundevall (1959) by the finding of an anti-Gm antibody of the Ragg type which was inhibited by a Gm antigen contained in some sera which were Gm (1) positive and by none of the sera which were Gm (1) negative. The percentage of positives (termed Gm(x)) among Norwegians was 26 and of negatives was 74. Gm(x) is now Gm (2) and the corresponding antibody anti-Gm(2) (*see* Table 20.2). With few exceptions, Gm^1 and Gm^2 are inherited together.

A further allele of Gm, Gm^b (Gm^5) which appeared antithetical to Gm^a (Gm^1) was found by Harboe (1959). The anti-D used to disclose this type was from an individual of type Gm (–1–2). Only 1 out of 65 sera of the Ragg type contained anti-Gm (5). When this system was used in an inhibition test against unselected

Table 20.2 Nomenclature of Gm system and relation to Ig subclasses

| Nomenclature | | IgG subclass |
Alphabetical	Numerical	
a	1	1
x	2	1
f	3, 4	1
b or b^1	5, 12	3
c^3	6	3
r	7	1
e	8	?
p	9	1
b^5	10	3
b^0	11	3
b^3	13, 25	3
b^4	14	3
s	15	3
t	16	3
z	17	1
Rouen 2	18	1
Rouen 3	19	?
San Francisco 2	20	1
g	21	3
y	22	1
n	23	2
c^5	24	3
Pa	–	3

sera, 81.5 per cent were positive including all of 46 Gm (1) negatives. Although Gm (1) and Gm (5) have an antithetical relationship in Europeans showing that their genes behave like alleles, in African Negroes they are almost always inherited as a unit.

It is perhaps helpful to compare Gm and Rh inheritance. For example the Rh antigenic complex cDe is common in Negroes but uncommon among Caucasians. Similarly the Gm antigens (1), (3) and (5) are but rarely inherited from a single parent in Caucasians but in Orientals they are not infrequently inherited together.

However, whereas each red cell bears the antigenic end product of each gene in the complex this is not so for the Gm serum allotypes. Only one gene of a complex can be expressed on any single immunoglobulin molecule. For example an individual of the phenotype Gm (1, 5) will have some IgG molecules carrying Gm (1) and some carrying Gm (5). The Gm antigens are found on the heavy chains of IgG molecules but are absent from IgA and IgM. Most are situated on the Fc portion but Gm (3) and Gm (17) occur on the Fd fragment (see Fig. 20.1).

A particular Gm antigen is associated with one particular IgG subclass. Of the common types it can be seen from Table 20.1 that Gm (1) and Gm (2) occur on IgG1 molecules whereas Gm (5) occurs on IgG3. These two subclasses of heavy chains share practically all the Gm types between them, there being no Gm antigens associated with IgG4 and only one so far described for IgG2, and since IgG1 molecules considerably outnumber those of IgG3, those Gm antigens

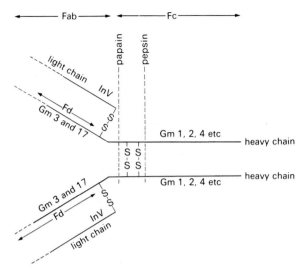

Fig. 20.1 Diagram showing the position of Gm-InV markers on the immunoglobulin molecule.

situated on IgG1 chains will be more serologically active than antigens on IgG3.

Table 20.2 lists the Gm antigens giving both numbered and alphabetical nomenclatures and the IgG chains to which the various types are related. It will be seen that a few types originally given different numbers have now been shown to have the same specificity.

Gm frequencies

Tables 20.3 and 20.4 show the frequencies of some of the principle Gm antigens and phenotypes in the United Kingdom. These figures are taken from Brazier and Goldsmith 1968.

There are wide racial variations. For example, in Negroes Gm (1) is hardly

Table 20.3 Frequencies of single Gm and Inv(Km) antigens

	Gm(1)	Gm(2)	Gm(4)	Antigen Gm(10)	Gm(11)	Gm(12)	Inv(1)	Inv(2)
Percentage positive	58.3	22.5	88.7	88.7	88.7	88.7	17.6	16

Table 20.4 Frequencies of some individual Gm phenotypes

	Gm(1)	Gm(1,2)	Phenotype Gm(1,4,10,11,12)	Gm(1,2,4,10,11,12)	Gm(4,10,11,12)
Percentage positive	5.4	5.9	30.4	16.6	41.7

polymorphic since almost 100 per cent of Negroid people have Gm (1). Gm (2) on the other hand is very rare in Negroid populations.

Anti-Gm sera

The Gm system is a life's work for interested specialists and many of the anti-Gm sera are rare. Anti-Gm (1), anti-Gm (2) and anti-Gm (5) are the most readily available. Techniques 20.3 and 20.4 described below are suitable for any of these antibodies.

It is strongly recommended that beginners obtain a known anti-Gm typing serum, preferably anti-Gm (1), from a specialist laboratory, together with a selected anti-D for use with it. Suitable dilutions of the anti-Gm for typing purposes are usually 1 in 5 or 1 in 10 but preliminary tests are done to determine the lowest dilution of the antiserum that still gives strong agglutination of the sensitised cells.

Rheumatoid arthritic (Ragg) sera suitable for typing come usually from patients with long histories of the disease. The sera should be treated at 63°C for 10 minutes as this destroys the R.A. factor and prevents agglutination of saline controls.

More satisfactory reagents can be prepared from the occasional healthy donor who possesses anti-Gm antibodies (SNagg). This is because rheumatoid agglutinators are less specific than the anti-Gm sera from normal persons in that they are often inhibited by high concentrations of serum negative for the corresponding Gm factor. They also tend to be less sensitive than SNagg sera and are inhibited by only low dilutions of sera containing their specific Gm factor. Other sources of satisfactory anti-Gm sera are rabbits or monkeys immunised with human gamma globulin. These anti-Gm sera show a specificity and sensitivity similar to the SNagg type of antibodies.

The immune response to Gm antigens

Children seem to be particularly liable to form Gm antibodies following transfusion. Allen and Kunkel (1963) found Gm antibodies with various specificities in 17 out of 24 children mostly with thalassaemia major who had received multiple transfusions and Stiehm and Fudenberg (1965) found similar antibodies in 11 out of 32 children who had been exchange transfused at birth for haemolytic disease of the newborn.

In adults more prolonged stimulation seems necessary. The stimulus afforded by Gm type differences between mother and child results in Gm antibody formation particularly in the infants. The finding of a maternal Gm antibody made against a foetal Gm antigen is much less common.

Technique No. 20.1. The coating of red cells

Only a few anti-D sera are suitable and these will be found among those of high titre. For Gm (1) typing, such anti-D sera must of course originate from individuals who are themselves Gm (1).

The red cells used are preferably of probable genotype *CDe/CDe* or *CDe/cDE* and must be of group O so they are ABO compatible with all test sera. For sensitisation of these cells by anti-D, the proportion of cells to anti-D serum is found by trial and error. The cells are incubated with the serum for $3/4$ to 1 hour at 37°C and then washed three times. They should give strong rapid agglutination with an anti-human globulin reagent.

Technique No. 20.2. Screening of sera for Gm antibodies

Each serum to be tested is diluted 1 in 5 with saline. If Ragg sera are being screened several dilutions *e.g.* (1 in 10, 1 in 50) may be required owing to the fact that these sera have much higher titres and often show a prozone phenomenon. Equal volumes of suitably diluted serum and a 2 per cent suspension of the sensitised red cells are mixed, left at room temperature for 1 hour and read for agglutination. Strong positives can be titrated. Normal uncoated group O cells mixed with each serum is an essential control since a serum may contain an atypical antibody which agglutinates the test cells. It will be appreciated that only cells coated with anti-D from a Gm (1) positive individual will detect the presence of anti-Gm (1) antibodies. Similarly, anti-Gm (5) will have to be looked for with Gm (5) sensitised cells and anti-Gm (2) with Gm (2) sensitised cells. It is advisable to use more than one example of the relevant anti-D.

Technique No. 20.3. Gm typing using anti-Gm (1)

Equal volumes of serum to be Gm (1) typed including known Gm(1) positive and negative controls and anti-Gm(1) each diluted 1 in 5 are mixed and left at room temperature for about 30 minutes. A drop of each mixture is placed on a tile and a drop of sensitised D positive cells added to each. The tile is gently rocked for several minutes and the tests read as for agglutination.

Controls
(1) The test cells + anti-human globulin.
(2) The test cells + anti-Gm (1).
(3) The test cells with each test serum at a dilution of 1/5.

The same technique is suitable for other Gm antibodies *e.g.* anti-Gm (2) and anti-Gm (5).

Technique No. 20.4. The dis-agglutination technique for Gm typing

This method is sometimes used instead of technique No. 20.3. Unit volumes of anti-Gm (1) diluted 1 in 5 are delivered on to a tile allowing one volume for each serum to be Gm typed plus controls. A volume of Gm (1) sensitised red cells is added to each, immediately mixed and the tile is rocked gently until agglutination of the sensitised cells is well developed. Then an equal volume of each serum to be typed is added to the agglutinated red cells and the mixture is thoroughly stirred. The agglutination disperses and is only reformed if the test sera lack the corresponding Gm (1) component. The controls required are the same as those for technique No. 20.3.

Km GROUPS (FORMERLY INV)

In 1961 Ropartz *et al* described Inv, another system of inherited serum antigens which in contrast to those of the Gm system are related to the light chains of the globulin molecule and are found associated with IgG, IgA and IgM immuno-globulins (see Fig. 20.1). The name has now been changed to Km for Kappa marker.

Three types have been recognised, Km (1), Km (2) and Km (3) but these appear to arise from two allelic genes since Km (1) and Km (2) travel together and are allelic to Km (3). So far there is no biochemistry to support a distinctive Km (2) gene. No linkage has been found between Km and Gm.

Only occasionally are individuals Km (1 –2) and no examples of Km (–1 2) seem to exist. Km (–1 –2) is the commonest in all races tested. The figures given by Brazier and Goldsmith 1968 for the various phenotypes in the United Kingdom are as follows:-

	per cent
Km (1 –2)	1.6
Km (1 2)	16.0
Km (–1 –2)	82.4

For most practical purposes, the Km typing of individuals is done only with anti-Km (1) since anti-Km (2) is rare and only one or two examples of anti-Km (3) are known. Of those tested, most Km (–1 –2) people are Km (3) positive.

Km antibodies seem to occur exclusively in the sera of normal individuals. Patients who have received multiple transfusions are occasionally a source of Km antibodies. The typing method for Km is exactly the same as that for Gm except that the anti-D must be selected from people of the appropriate Km type. Km(1) has now been found in saliva and semen (Davie & Kipps, 1976).

HAPTOGLOBINS

These are haemoglobin-binding proteins found with the α_2 globulins (see frontispiece). Their major function appears to be the prevention of loss of haemoglobin and thus of iron from the body. They can be separated by means of starch gel electrophoresis and characteristic patterns obtained (Smithies, 1955). These patterns are the result of two genes called for convenience *Hp1* and *Hp2*. Most individuals can be classified into one of three phenotypes: Hp1, Hp2-1, Hp2. In developing the bands after electrophoresis the haemoglobin binding capacity of haptoglobin is utilised and the fact that benzidine forms a blue coloured compound in the presence of haemoglobin. The three main groups are easily distinguishable. Hp1 forms a single thick band which lies next to the free haemoglobin on its cathodic side. Hp2-1 and Hp2 both form a cluster of lines well to the cathodic side of the Hp1 band and they are readily distinguishable from each other. The Hp1 component of the Hp2-1 type occupies the same position as the corresponding band of the Hp1 but is not so pronounced. This band is absent from Hp2. Hp2-1 has in addition a broad band lying at the extreme anodic side of its cluster. This band stains more intensely than any of the

Hp2 bands. A photograph of typical results is shown in Fig. 20.2. The bands here are developed by the phenolphthalein staining (Kastlemeyer) method (see below). It is of interest to note that the Hp2-1 pattern is different from that obtained by mixing haptoglobins of the two homozygous types. In England the frequencies of the common phenotypes are as follows:-

Hp 1	18 per cent
Hp 2–1	49 per cent
Hp 2	33 per cent

A number of variants have been observed. For example Hp2-1 (modified) is found in about 10 per cent of Negroes. This resembles the normal Hp2-1 in the mobilities of the components but there is relatively more of the fast moving component as in Hp1 and relatively less of the components in the slower moving cluster. Another rare variant HpCa has zones similar to those of both Hp2-1 and Hp2, the latter components being present in greater concentration than the Hp2-1 components.

There is also a silent allele Hp^0 which occurs with varying frequency among different races. In Britain it has a gene frequency of 0.003 (Cook *et al.*, 1969) but it can have a much higher frequency, *e.g.* in Negroes. Its existence provides the reason for extreme caution when attempting to base an exclusion of paternity on a second order exclusion within the haptoglobin system (see chapter 29).

Haptoglobin components are not fully developed at birth and it is recommended that in testing for this system in cases of doubtful paternity the infants should be at least 4-6 months old. Haptoglobins are occasionally absent from healthy adults and also from individuals in whom a haemolytic process is taking place.

Technique No. 20.5. The determination of haptoglobin types

Reagents

The starch for the gel is "Starch hydrolysed" obtained from the Connaught Laboratories, Toronto.

Tris-citrate buffer for gel pH 8.6–8.8. 9.15 g Tris and 1.05 g citric acid are each dissolved in distilled water and the final volume adjusted to 1 litre. The pH is checked.

Poulik's borate buffer for electrophoresis bath. pH 7.8–8.0. 27.8 g boric acid and 3.0 g NaOH are each dissolved in distilled water and the final volume adjusted to 1.5 litres. The pH is checked. The borate buffer can be used for several "runs".

Preparation of starch gel

The gel is prepared by making a 13 per cent solution of starch in the gel buffer; 100 ml of starch solution makes a mould of 11 × 11 cm, suitable for about eight samples. A piece of perspex about ½–1 cm in thickness, upon which a frame may be constructed with perspex rods, forms a suitable mould. The gel should cover an area of about 11 × 11 cm and be about 7-mm thick.

The starch-buffer mixture is gently heated in a buchner flask over a blue flame with continuous shaking. The solution first becomes very viscous and then, as boiling point is approached, it becomes fluid again. Gentle heating should be continued for 1-2 minutes. The flask is then evacuated at about 500 mm Hg for 30 seconds to boil and de-gas the solution. A water pump if reliable, or a high vacuum pump may be used. Afterwards the starch solution is quickly poured into the mould and left to set in a draught free atmosphere at room temperature for 2-3 hours, or the setting may be hastened by placing at 4°C.

Application of samples to the gel

The samples, to which a little haemoglobin A is added to make them pink (haemolysed red cells from the donors of the serum samples may be used, unless they are coloured people deficient in Hb A), are taken up into pieces of 3M Whatman paper (about 4×3 mm). The papers should be thoroughly impregnated with the test serum but any excess serum should be dabbed off on tissue; if the papers are too wet there may be diffusion and blurring of the bands.

The gel is cut through its whole depth and across the width about 2 cm from the end that is intended for the cathode. The cut off piece is gently moved so that the impregnated papers can be inserted in a row at right angles to the surface and at such a depth that they do not project above the surface level of the gel. A distance of approximately 5 mm should be left between each specimen. The slit is then closed and the preparation is ready for electrophoresis.

Electrophoresis

This is carried out at 6 V/cm measured across the gel for 3-4 hours in the bridge buffer described above. For wicks, three layers of surgical gauze are suitable. These are stretched across the width of the gel at each end and should make good even contact overlapping the gel about 1½ cm. The free ends should dip well under the buffer solution in the bath. The whole wicks are immersed in the buffer solution before being placed in position. Care must be taken that they do not become dry during the run. The voltage across the gel is checked using an avometer and adjustment to the voltage reading on the power supply made to maintain the correct voltage across the gel. It is a good plan to run for the first 30 minutes at 100 V on the power pack. By this time the 'borate line' should have passed through the origin. The voltage is then increased to 400 on the power pack and electrophoresis is continued for a further 2-3 hours or until the 'borate line' has moved to within 1 cm from the anodic wick contact.

Slicing and staining of gel

At the end of the run the gel is sliced horizontally. A dermatome such as the Allen and Hanbury's Improved dermatome is suitable; the blade should pass steadily through the gel in one movement along its length. A piece of perspex of about half the thickness of the gel placed at each side parallel to its length is of assistance in making a clean cut at the right depth. The sliced gel is opened like a book and the freshly made benzidine or phenol phthalein solution is painted on in generous amount. Immediately after which any excess fluid is quickly blotted off. The haemoglobin bands should begin to appear after a few seconds and be fully developed within a few minutes. Reading should take place immediately the

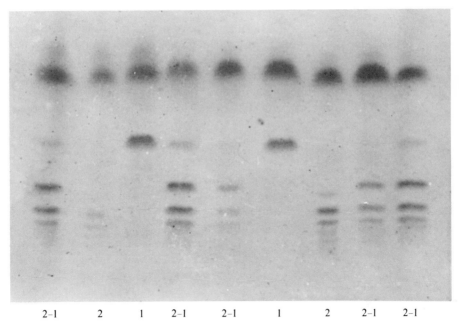

| 2-1 | 2 | 1 | 2-1 | 2-1 | 1 | 2 | 2-1 | 2-1 |

Fig. 20.2 Haptoglobin patterns in starch gel.

bands are clearly seen as there is gradual fading after 5-10 minutes. The appearance is as in Fig. 20.2.

Preparation of benzidine solution for development of Hp bands

Great care must be exercised in the handling of benzidine; the powder must not be inhaled and rubber gloves must be worn. 5 ml glacial acetic acid is diluted with 5 ml distilled water in a test tube. Approximately 25 mg benzidine and 200 mg barium peroxide are added and the whole mixed. With experience these amounts may be judged by eye. It will be found that the powders do not completely dissolve. The solution is freshly prepared immediately before use. All benzidine contaminated glassware and perspex must be carefully washed separately in plenty of running water and must not be added to other dirty glassware.

Although some workers still prefer benzidine staining it has been superceded in some laboratories by other staining methods one of which, the Kastlemeyer, is described below.

Phenolphthalein staining for haptoglobins (Kastlemeyer)

Phenolphthalein becomes colourless in alkaline solution but in the presence of hydrogen peroxide and an oxidising agent such as the peroxidase of haemoglobin a deep pink colour develops. It is therefore suitable for staining the various haptoglobin components as these are conjugated with haemoglobin.

Preparation of reagent. 2 g of phenolphthalein and 20 g of potassium hydroxide are boiled slowly in 100 ml of distilled water, using a reflux condenser and adding 10-20 g of powdered or granulated zinc during the process. Boiling is continued until the solution becomes colourless; this takes one hour approximately. When cool, the solution should be apportioned out into dark bottles; alternatively it is convenient to store the stock solution in the freezer at $-20°$C. Some of the zinc is added to keep the solution in the reduced form. A part of this stock solution is made up for use as required by adding an equal volume of methyl alcohol and 2 or 3 drops of hydrogen peroxide (10-volume strength). It is painted generously over the starch gel.

THE Gc SYSTEM

This system was first described by Hirschfeld (1959). He recognised three different precipitation patterns in the α_2 globulin of human serum, by a method of immuno-electrophoresis. Family studies showed the patterns to be genetically controlled and two simple codominant genes were postulated. The gene Gc^1 gives in double dose the genotype $Gc1$-1 which after immuno-electrophoresis shows as a mono-centric arc near the anode. Gc^2 gives in double dose the genotype $Gc2$-2 with a similar arc nearer to the cathode while the heterozygote $Gc2$-1 is characterised by a double arc similar to a bird's outstretched wings. These patterns are shown diagramatically in Figure 20.3. The heavy line of the α_2 macroglobulin is shown also as this forms an essential marker.

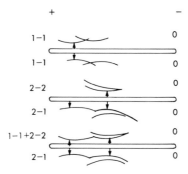

Fig. 20.3 Diagram representing the Gc patterns obtained by immuno-electrophoresis in agar.

The distribution of Gc phenotypes is fairly uniform among Caucasians. Gc 1 - 53.1 per cent, Gc 2-1 - 40.3 per cent, Gc 2-6.6 per cent. Family studies have shown the system to be a reliable genetic marker and a useful tool in cases of doubtful paternity in which the system offers about a 15 per cent chance of excluding a man wrongly accused.

Technique No. 20.6. The determination of Gc types

Preparation of Buffer solutions

	For agar	For tank
Barbituric acid (diethyl)	3.32 g	2.76 g
Sodium barbitone	21.02 g	17.52 g
Calcium lactate	3.07 g	0.768 g

Distilled H_2O	2 litre	2 litre
Merthiolate (1 per cent)	2 ml	2 ml

The pH of the buffers must be checked; they should give a pH reading of 8.6. With the addition of merthiolate they may be stored in a cool place for weeks. Tank buffer can be used for more than one electrophoretic run if it is removed from the bath, filtered and the pH checked.

Preparation of agar

The following are convenient quantities.

6 g agar (Oxoid or Difco) are added to 300 ml distilled H_2O and melted in a boiling water bath, with occasional stirring. It is important that the agar is completely dissolved. 200 ml agar buffer and 100 ml distilled H_2O are mixed and warmed to 60°C and then added to the melted agar. Finally 6 ml of merthiolate is added. The agar is then bottled and stored at room temperature.

Preparation of agar slides

An appropriate quantity of prepared agar is melted in a boiling water bath. A thermometer is inserted into the agar. It will be found that the agar is completely melted at about 90°C.

Glass slides 8 cm × 8 cm are convenient and these must be absolutely grease free and are therefore polished with spirit immediately before use.

The melted agar is quickly distributed across the slides using a generous 10 ml of agar per slide. The operation must be carried out on a completely level surface, for example on a levelling table. The slides are left for 30 minutes on the bench before use. It is recommended that they are poured immediately before being required, and not stored overnight.

Equipment can be obtained especially designed for punching out the circular wells and troughs required for Gc determinations. Three pairs of circular wells (2 mm in diameter) are punched about ¾ inch from the cathodic end of the slide (*see* Fig. 20.3). Then a longitudinal trough is cut in a central position between each pair of wells. The distance between each well and the central trough should be 4-5 mm. The centres of the circular wells are removed by suction. The same pipette as that used for punching the holes, attached to a water suction pump is convenient. The agar is not removed from the trough at this stage.

Setting up the tests

Serum samples to be tested are placed one in each circular well using a fine capillary pipette. Care must be taken not to overfill. Controls of known Gc types 1, 2 and 2-1 are included with each run. It is advisable to mix an equal quantity of amido schwarz with one of the controls as this facilitates the assessment of how far the samples have run during the course of the electrophoresis. A good deal of trial and error may be required before the optimum conditions for the electrophoretic run are found. Wicks consisting of two layers of Whatman paper No. 3 may be used. Care must be taken that these are pressed evenly along the length of the tray holding the slides. The wicks must be well immersed in the tank buffer before use and must not be allowed to become dry during the run. 6-7 V/cm across the gel for 1½ - 2 hours will probably be found to be satisfactory running conditions.

After electrophoresis, the troughs are scooped out. This can be done with a short metal or wooden stick after cutting the agar at each end of the trough. Each trough is then filled with anti-Gc serum and the slides are placed in a moist chamber at 37°C for 18 -24 hours. (Anti-Gc sera may be obtained commercially.) The tests are then read against a dark background using oblique light. Special viewing boxes can be constructed for this purpose. The Gc lines are those which lie nearest to the trough. The Gc lines may be developed further if necessary by submerging the slide in 1 per cent tannic acid for 5 - 10 minutes after differentiation in 2.5 per cent NaCl for several hours to get rid of general background protein.

A permanent record can be made by photographing the results immediately or the slides may be stained as follows:

Amido schwarz staining

All purpose stain 10B amido black is used. 0.5 g of the dye is dissolved in 100 ml of a solution consisting of 90 ml methanol (99.8 per cent) and 10 ml of glacial acetic acid (99.7 per cent). The slides are immersed for 20 - 24 minutes and differentiated in methanol-glacial acetic acid solution of the same strength as that in which the stain is dissolved. Differentiation requires from 3 to 5 washes of 5 - 10 minutes duration using fresh solution for each washing.

OTHER SYSTEMS

Ag System

In 1961 Allison and Blumberg found that sera from certain individuals who had received many transfusions, formed allo-precipitins against donor serum proteins. Only a certain proportion of human sera formed precipitates in agar gel against such a serum from a multi-transfused individual. The "new" polymorphism was found to be associated with ß-lipoproteins and the system was termed Ag and the first found antibody anti-Ag. The technique for detection of Ag antisera and antibody is by agar gel diffusion and micro-diffusion tests on microscope slides are satisfactory. As usual further research showed the system to be a complicated one and it is now thought that there are five antibody specificities. These have been called anti-Ag(x), anti-Ag(y), anti-Ag(a₁), anti-Ag(z) and anti-Ag(t) with corresponding antigens Ag(x), Ag(y), Ag(a₁), Ag(z) and Ag(t).

Not all the theoretically possible combinations of these antigens have been found. The combinations observed could be accounted for by postulating complex genes similar to the Rh system.

Hirschfeld (1968) has carried out extensive studies comparing the reactions of 28 allo-precipitin sera against a large series of unrelated individuals. He found only 13 of the theoretically possible phenotypes which would be expected using the five antisera. No Ag(x–y–) was found nor has been since this investigation.

The percentage of various phenotypes was as follows:-

$Ag(x-y+a_1-z-t+)$ 28
$Ag(x+y+a_1+z-t+)$ 24
$Ag(x-y+a_1+z+t+)$ 17
$Ag(x-y+a_1+z-t+)$ 11
$Ag(x+y+a_1+z+t+)$ 7
$Ag(x+y-a_1+z-t+)$ 5

Another seven phenotypes had frequencies ranging from 0.4 to 3.5 per cent. Ag^x and Ag^y with gene frequencies in Europe of 0.206 and 0.794 respectively have been applied to paternity testing (Bradbrook et al., 1971). However sera containing reliable anti-Ag^x and anti-Ag^y alloprecipitins are not readily obtainable and are found mainly among polytransfused patients with thalassaemia.

Lp System

This is also a ß-lipoprotein variant but it is independent of Ag. Berg (1963) immunised rabbits with purified human ß-lipoprotein. After appropriate absorption an antibody was left which divided the population into two types Lp(a+) and Lp(a–). The method of detection is by precipitation after double diffusion in agar (Berg, 1963).

Serum Transferrins

These are iron binding proteins composed of $ß_1$ globulins of which there are a number of variants. There are also racial differences. A few Caucasians have a faster migrating variant B, while approximately 12 per cent of Negroes have been found to be heterozygous for a slow moving variant D. The different types are detectable by starch gel electrophoresis (Giblett, 1962).

REFERENCES

Allen, J.C. & Kunkel, H.G. (1963) Antibodies to genetic types of gamma globulin after multiple transfusions. Science, 139, 418.
Allison, A.C. & Blumberg, B.S. (1961) An isoprecipitation reaction distinguishing human serum protein types. Lancet, 1, 634.
Berg, K. (1963) A new serum type system in Man—the Lp system. Acta path. microbiol. scand., 9, 369.
Bradbrook, I.D., Grant, A. & Adinolfi, M. (1971) Ag(x) and Ag(y) antigens in studies of paternity cases in the United Kingdom. Hum. Hered., 21, 493.
Brazier, D.M. & Goldsmith, K.L.G. (1968) Frequency of certain Gm and Inv factors in the United Kingdom. Nature, 219, 193.
Cook, P.J.L., Gray, J.E., Brack, R.A., Robson, E.B. & Howlett, R.M. (1969) Data on haptoglobin and D group chromosomes. Ann. Hum. Genet., 33, 125.
Davie, M. J., and Kipps, A. E. (1976) Km(1) [Inv(1)] typing of saliva and semen. Vox. Sang. 31, 363.
Giblett, E.R. (1962) The plasma transferrins, in Progress in Medical Genetics, 2nd ed. A.G. Steinberg. Grune & Stratton: New York.
Grubb, R. (1956) Agglutination of erythrocytes coated with 'incomplete' anti-Rh by certain rheumatoid arthritic sera and some other sera. The existence of human serum groups. Acta path. microbiol. scand., 39, 195.
Grubb, R. & Laurell, A.B. (1956) Hereditary serological human serum groups. Acta path. microbiol. scand., 39, 390.

Harboe, M. (1959) A new haemagglutinating substance in the Gm system, anti-Gm[b]. *Acta path. microbiol. scand.,* **47,** 191.

Harboe, M. & Lundevall, J. (1959) A new type in the Gm system. *Acta path. microbiol. scand.,* **45,** 357.

Hirschfeld, J. (1959) Immuno-electrophoresis demonstrating quantitative differences in human sera and their relation to haptoglobins. *Acta path. microbiol. scand.,* **47,** 160.

Hirschfeld, J. (1968) The Ag system—comparison of different isoprecipitin sera. *Series haematologica,* **i,** 1, 38.

Ropartz, C., Lenoire, J. & Rivat, L. (1961) A new inheritable property of human sera; the Inv factor. *Nature (Lond.),* **189,** 586.

Smithies, O. (1955) Zone electrophoresis in starch gels; group variations in the serum proteins of normal human adults. *Biochem. J.,* **61,** 629.

Stiehm, E.R. & Fudenberg, H.H. (1965) Antibodies to gamma globulin in infants and children exposed to isologous gamma-globulin. *Pediatrics,* **35,** 229.

Further Reading

Giblett, E.R. (1969) Genetic markers in human blood. Oxford: Blackwell.

Van Loghem, E. (1973) Genetic studies on human immunoglobulins, in *Handbook of Experimental Immunology,* 2nd ed. Ed. Weir, D.M. Oxford: Blackwell.

PART III

PRACTICAL APPLICATION OF BLOOD GROUP THEORY

SECTION 1. Autoanalysis and antibody identification

"Things flow about so here!"

Lewis Carroll, THROUGH THE LOOKING GLASS

Chapter 21. Automation

Enthusiasm for the application of mechanised methods to blood grouping presumably stemmed from the hope of introducing greater reliability and also of avoiding some of the tedium of grouping endless numbers of donor samples. It therefore came as some surprise to find that an even more important achievement resulting from the development of the automated techniques was an increase in sensitivity in the detection of blood group antibodies.

The first type of machine to arrive on the scene was the Technicon Auto Analyser continuous flow system which was adapted from machines designed to automate clinical chemistry procedures.

A much later arrival was the Groupamatic, a machine which, using plastic trays with reaction wells, automates a procedure which is essentially the same as that used in manual agglutination tests.

As yet, the fully automated Groupamatic machines are in limited use in the United Kingdom and consequently this type of machine will receive only short consideration in this chapter.

The available machines appear to have one or more of the following advantages over existing manual techniques.

1. Speed of operation.
2. Increased sensitivity.
3. More accurate quantification.
4. Applicability to computerised record keeping.

THE AUTOANALYSERS

Blood grouping AutoAnalysers are built on the continuous flow principle.

The reagents are measured by peristaltic pumps which work by means of rollers compressing the pump tubes. The quantity of reagents delivered depends on the flow rates through the tubes, which is governed only by the diameter of the tubing since the rollers move over the tubing at constant speed. The design of the pump allows many pump tubes to be accommodated, and in modern systems a single pump can be used for the whole system.

The reagents necessary for the reaction are mixed and pass into the manifold, which is a system of glass tubing and coils in which the reaction takes place. An important feature of the system is that the stream is broken up into segments by the injection of air bubbles at regular intervals. The liquid/air interface of the air bubbles cleans the walls of the tubing and ensures that there is maximum forward movement of the liquid, thus reducing mixing between samples. The extent to which sample mixing or "carry-over" can be reduced is the limiting factor in efforts to speed up the rate at which samples can be tested.

In the machine, agglutination has to be brought about in the minimum time and preferably at laboratory temperature. Rouleaux formers, to bring the sensitised red cells close together and thus facilitate agglutination are important aids to this end, together with the use of enzymes in some instances. Thus, the finding that some macromolecular substances induce rouleaux of red cells and that such aggregation of unsensitised cells can be dispersed has been of the utmost importance in the development of automated techniques.

Polyvinylpyrrollidone (PVP) was used in the early machines in conjunction with bromelin. Other means of inducing rouleaux include the use of methyl cellulose in place of PVP and the use of Polybrene (hexadimethrine bromide) under conditions of low ionic strength and acid pH. The sampling rates for Auto Analysers vary with the function of the machine—120 per hour on grouping machines, 20 per hour for antibody quantification.

The antibody detection AutoAnalyser (one and two channel machines)

The actual reagents and the design of the manifold differ according to the reaction being measured, but a schematic diagram of the flow system for a single channel antibody detection machine using bromelin and methyl cellulose is shown in figure 21.1.

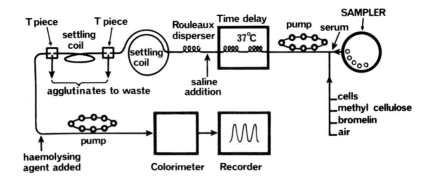

Fig. 21.1 Diagrammatic representation of the general layout for a single-channel AutoAnalyser.

The sample enters the machine via the sampling probe and is mixed with the red cells which are supplied continuously together with the bromelin and methyl cellulose. Air is introduced to divide the flow into segments and as the mixture moves through the coils there is continuous gentle movement of the red cells and this is conducive to antigen-antibody reaction.

After passing through the reaction coil the rouleaux which have been induced largely by the methyl cellulose are dispersed by the injection of saline into the system so that only true agglutinates remain. The flow then enters a settling coil where the agglutinates sediment by gravity. Agglutinates and a small constant portion of unagglutinated cells are removed by a T-junction. A second settling coil followed by another T-junction ensures that all the agglutinates are removed.

The remaining (unagglutinated) cells are haemolysed by detergent added to the flow system at this stage. The optical density of the haemolysate is then measured in a continuous flow colorimeter at 550 nm and the results recorded on a chart moving at approximately 0.5 inches/min. Hence it is the haemoglobin concentration after the specifically agglutinated cells have been removed, that is measured. The depth of fall from the baseline (which represents 100 per cent red cells unagglutinated) is proportional to the number of agglutinated cells removed *i.e.* the strength of antigen/antibody reaction. A section of typical chart is shown in Figure 21.2. The chart has been inverted so that the baseline is at the bottom of the paper and the positive reactions appear as peaks.

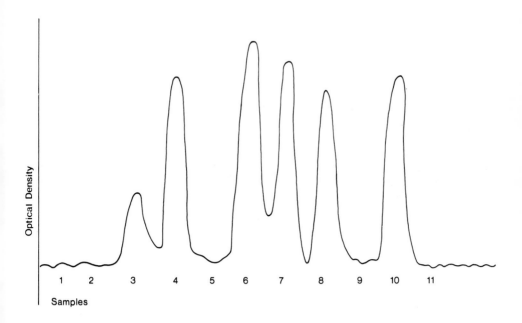

Fig. 21.2 Typical print-out from a single-channel AutoAnalyser.

Applications of 1 and 2 channel AutoAnalysers

Antibody detection

Using the AutoAnalyser for antibody screening usually achieves greater sensitivity than the appropriate manual techniques. The efficiency of the AutoAnalyser for the detection of antibodies varies depending upon specificity of antibody and the system used. For instance the two widely used techniques, the bromelin/methylcellulose system (BMC) and low ionic strength polybrene system (LISP) do not detect antibodies equally well. The relative merits of the two systems and also comparison with manual techniques has been the subject of many studies. The LISP system has been shown to be very suitable for antibody screening because of its great sensitivity in the detection of most red cell antibodies. Perrault and Högman (1971) found that except for certain haemolysing antibodies, LISP was in no instance less sensitive than manual techniques but that anti-s, $-Fy^a$, $-Jk^a-Jk^b$ and $-K$ were less sensitively detected by BMC than by the appropriate manual method.

If maximum sensitivity is to be achieved red cells from a single donor must be used in the machine and this creates the problem of finding suitable donors possessing antigens for all the relevant antibodies. The addition of a second channel to the machine using cells from a second donor increases the number of available antigens. Pooling of cells is sometimes advocated but is not a recommended practice since it dilutes the antigens and leads to weaker agglutination with many antibodies.

One of the outcomes of the increased sensitivity is the finding of antibodies which will not react at all by manual techniques and whose identification can only be carried out using a panel of cells on the AutoAnalyser. A supply of sufficient suitable cells for the identification of "machine-only" antibodies can prove to be difficult.

Quantification of antibodies

The most widely used method for quantification is the BMC method. However it is generally recognised that there are serious theoretical and practical difficulties which must be taken into account when interpreting the results and it should always be remembered that the high degree of precision with which the results are often expressed can be misleading. One advantage of the technique, claimed by some workers, has been that the final reading of the agglutination is objectively measured and does not depend on a subjective assessment as in manual titrations.

It is considered that under the conditions used in the AutoAnalyser virtually all the antibody is bound to the red cells so that differences in binding constant have less effect on the results (Rosenfield, *et al.,* 1964). This is in contrast to manual titration where at the end point, the agglutination is caused by the few antibodies with the highest binding affinity and the titre of the serum is dependent upon the proportion of such antibody molecules present. However, Gunson *et al.* (1974a) have shown that the ambient temperature of the manifold after addition of the rouleaux dispersing reagent can affect the amount of agglutination obtained because antibody molecules of lower binding capacity may be readily eluted at ambient temperatures.

Where quantification is carried out using enzyme treated cells to obtain a high degree of sensitivity, it is well to consider that at least some of the detected antibodies may have little clinical significance mainly because the enzyme activates antibodies which have a low affinity for the corresponding antigen and these are clinically less damaging.

Reagents used in the machine, such as red cells, bromelin, bovine albumin and AB serum, are of biological origin and are subject to considerable variation. Bromelin, being crude extract of pineapple stem, is not easy to control except by careful testing with red cells, which is not often carried out in practice. In bovine albumin occasionally there may be inhibitors present which markedly depress anti-D agglutination, and every batch must be standardised (*see* Appendix II). Likewise the AB sera may contain antibodies which can only be detected using the AutoAnalyser.

No doubt the interaction of all these reagents is complex, and the control of them in practice is a compromise between the ideal and the possible.

The accurate preparation of high dilutions of the potent anti-D sera for quantification has proved difficult in practice and substantial improvements in reproducibility have been reported (Gunson *et al.*, 1972) upon adopting the use of an automatic diluter.

To obtain a measurement of anti-D in a serum in terms of quantity of antibody the unknown serum has to be compared with a standard anti-D using a calibration curve. A laboratory reference serum of which there is a good supply can be used provided this has been standardised with an international anti-D standard (*e.g.* 1st British Standard for Anti-D (Rho) antibodies).

About three to five dilutions of the standard anti-D must be tested on the AutoAnalyser at least at the beginning and the end of the day's run, and a graph prepared showing the change in optical density for known anti-D concentrations.

The reproducibility of the AutoAnalyser offers great advantages in the quantification of antibodies such as anti-D. Using a common standard the concentration of anti-D estimated on the same sample by different laboratories was found to agree within ±25 per cent by Moore (1969) although reports from other workers have differed by much more than this. A more recent reappraisal by Moore and Fernandez (1972) using bromelin and PVP claims a reproducibility of anti-D estimates as ±6 per cent for triplicate tests in the same laboratory on successive days. Gunson *et al.* (1972) found the overall reproducibility of their bromelin methyl cellulose system using a standard pooled anti-D serum and an automatic diluter was ±14 per cent but more recently (Gunson *et al.*, 1974b) have shown that with certain antisera the variation is greater than this.

Estimates of the lowest detectable concentrations of antibodies not surprisingly vary from worker to worker. Limits of detection of anti-D achieved by Perrault and Högman (1971) running the BMC and LISP techniques in parallel show the BMC system less sensitive (0.002-0.004 μg/ml) than the LISP system (0.0002-0.0004 μg/ml) while Moore and Fernandez (1972) detected a similar amount (0.0004 μg/ml) using the PVP/bromelin technique.

Results obtained in our own and some other laboratories while agreeing with the limits of the degree of sensitivity of the BMC system differ for the LISP system in that less sensitivity is achieved.

K

It is interesting to note that in spite of the claims that the AutoAnalyser achieves far greater sensitivity than manual methods, the minimum quantity detected by the BMC is not very much less than the minimum quantity (0.003 - 0.004 μg/ml) detectable by papain manually in our own laboratory!

In making comparisons of sensitivity between the automated techniques and the manual techniques it is not valid to compare (as some workers seem to!) an automated technique using an enzyme with the manual ahg technique, a corresponding manual enzyme technique must be compared.

Other uses of the AutoAnalyser

Other uses to which the AutoAnalyser has been successfully applied include cell-bound antibody detection and quantification, syphilis testing and the detection of Australia antigen. In forensic serology, it is used in the detection of antibody in the eluates from stains.

Cell typing AutoAnalysers (8 to 15 channel machines)

Machines designed to type red cells are based on the same principles as the antibody detection machines described above, but are composed of more channels. Although they are designed for typing, some channels may be used for antibody screening and syphilis testing.

Samples to be tested are centrifuged to separate cells and plasma before being loaded into the sampler tray in numerical order. Cells and plasma are sampled simultaneously by a double probe at the rate of about 120 per hour. The probe is reverse flushed after each sample to reduce contamination of one sample by another. Donor plasma and red cells are distributed to the various channels and mixed with the appropriate test serum or cells. A 15 channel machine might be used as follows:-

ABO grouping:	anti-A, anti-B, group O serum
(7 channels)	A_1, A_2, B and O cells.
Rh typing:	
(4 channels)	2 anti-D, anti-D+C, anti-D+E
Antibody Screening:	
(2 channels)	OR$_1$ R$_2$ K− cells, O rr K+ cells
Syphilis test:	
(1 channel)	Carbon coated with antigen
Control	
(1 channel)	Own cells + AB serum.

The main difference between this machine and the antibody machine is the way in which the results are recorded, in that a portion of test material is decanted onto a moving belt of filter paper and is subsequently interpreted by visual examination. The time lapse between sampling and the test appearing on the filter paper is about 15 minutes.

Using this method large agglutinates can be satisfactorily distinguished on the filter paper but the difference between weak positive and negative reactions is not always easy to detect.

Comments

Such machines are only useful where large numbers of samples have to be tested. Although they have been widely adopted in the Transfusion Centres they do not appear to have greatly reduced the number of personnel required for testing donor blood, but they do relieve the tedium of manual testing.

They are usually used in conjunction with manual testing which in all cases remains the final arbiter when doubtful results are obtained. Routines vary from laboratory to laboratory. Some Centres are prepared to issue blood which has been grouped only on the machine and never tested (even on previous occasions) by manual techniques. Other Centres are prepared to issue blood on machine testing only provided the donor has been tested manually on a previous donation. A major drawback of these machines is the lack of machine readable sample identification and automatic print-out of results in both machine readable and human readable forms. Correct correlation of results from the filter paper with the appropriate sample is an essential requisite of the method and various procedures have been adopted by laboratories to meet this *e.g.* insertion of coloured saline at intervals or simply a saline blank. Difficulty in reading is experienced if the flow rates vary in the different channels because the tests do not arrive on the filter paper from all the channels at precisely the same time.

Moore *et al.* (1972) consider the main advantages of the machine to be consistent accuracy and precision and report the results of testing 69,492 samples on a 15 channel AutoAnalyser where no D typing errors and only one early ABO error were encountered, although 29 out of 1079 samples were incorrect as far as their D^u status was concerned and 49 errors occurred in the antibody screening channel.

In a recent paper Jenkins *et al.* (1975) report their experience of the 8 channel AutoAnalyser for typing hospital patients as opposed to a donor population. These authors found some ABO anomalies which would probably have been caught if A_2 cells had been used in a 9th channel but also there were some D negative patients typed as D positive, not by malfunction of the machine but from incorrect reading on the filter paper.

THE GROUPAMATIC

This French machine works on a completely different principle from the AutoAnalyser. Red cells and serum react in shallow plastic cups, the bottoms of which are concave. If there is agglutination, the red cells tend to collect in the centre of the cup, whereas unagglutinated cells cover the bottom of the cups more evenly. The difference in light transmission between the centre and the periphery of the cup is read photo-electrically. The machine has automatic sample identification, automatic censoring of doubtful reactions, automatic recognition of incorrect instrument function, electronic conversion of the result to an output signal and is suited to computerisation. It has 12 channels and is capable of testing 360 samples per hour but in practice, the testing rate is sometimes much less, since some operators test all samples twice, and the ones which give discrepant results, three times. The number of samples which need manual testing is considerable—up to 15 per cent according to Freiesleben *et al.* (1975). This machine has been adapted for a wide range of tests, including A_1 and A_2 sub-grouping, detection of immune anti-A and anti-B, and Australia antigen and antibody detection. These latter tests can be done using the AutoAnalyser but a colorimeter read-out is needed.

The experience gained from some 600,000 routine tests on the Groupamatic has been reported by Garretta *et al.* (1975), who carry out the majority of their routine serological procedures on such a machine.

Although this machine appears to overcome some of the difficulties of the AutoAnalysers its high cost would appear to limit its use to only the largest of transfusion centres.

* * * * * *

The invasion of the serology laboratory by the AutoAnalysers was thought to herald the replacement of people by machines but this has not been so and there are aspects where the ultimate answer comes from the manual technique and not the machine. Moreover it has been found that temperament is not confined to serologists and to a great extent a kindly working relationship has to be established between the serologist and his machine, who like horse and rider have to love one another!

TECHNIQUES

Technique 21.1 Bromelin-methyl cellulose method (BMC)

Stock Solutions
   Tween:10 ml in 100 ml distilled H_2O (10 per cent)
   Triton:50 ml in 1 litre distilled H_2O (5 per cent)
   Methyl cellulose:3 g in 100 ml saline (3 per cent) Store at 4°C for up to 7 days.

Solutions for a day's run
   Methyl cellulose:10 ml stock + 90 ml saline
   Bromelin: 0.2g bromelin + 20 ml buffered saline pH 5.5 (10 ml 0.1M phosphate buffer pH 5.5 + 90 ml saline). Shake vigorously, stand for 10 minutes then spin and take off supernatant.
   Triton:100 ml stock Triton + 900 ml distilled H_2O.
   Tween/saline:2 ml stock Tween + 1 litre saline.
   Albumin/saline wash: 15 ml 30 per cent bovine albumin + 2 ml stock Tween + 1 litre saline.
   Red cells: Wash three times, filter to remove small clots and make up to 20 per cent using following diluent; 20 ml 30 per cent bovine albumin + 15 ml AB serum + 15 ml saline.
   Cell suspension constantly stirred and kept in crushed ice during run.

Daily running and cleaning

Saline and/or reagents are run through tubes at beginning of the day for ½ to 1 hour.

At the end of the day, saline is run through all lines for 15 minutes.

Decon (approximately 2 per cent) is left in system overnight.

Technique 21.2. Low ionic strength—Polybrene method (LISP)

Stock Solutions

Polybrene: 1g in 10 ml of 0.9 per cent NaCl

Glucose: 100 g in 2 litre of distilled H_2O

Citric acid: 21.04g in 100 ml of distilled H_2O

Sodium citrate: 29.41g in 100 ml of distilled H_2O

Solutions for a day's run

Polybrene:	0.1 ml stock Polybrene + 100 ml 0.9 per cent saline (pH 6.4 - 6.5)
Acid/glucose:	0.5 ml stock citric acid + 200 ml stock glucose (pH 2.9)
Sodium citrate:	100 ml stock sodium citrate + 400 ml distilled H_2O (pH 8.2)
Triton X-100:	0.8 ml Triton + 400 ml distilled H_2O
Red cells:	These are washed 3 times in 1.3 per cent buffered saline (pH 7.0 - 7.2). To 6.5 ml of these packed cells are added 15 ml AB serum and 15 ml 1.3 per cent buffered saline (pH 7.0 - 7.2). The cell suspension is stirred continuously while standing in crushed ice.
Wash:	1.3 per cent buffered saline + 4 drops tween 20 per litre.

Daily running and cleaning

O.05 M NaOH is run through all tubes for ½ - 1 hour at beginning of the day followed by 0.9 per cent saline (containing 1 ml Tween 20 per litre) in all tubes except Triton line which has distilled water.

The reagents are pumped through all lines for about 1 hour before cells and samples.

At the end of the day all lines are washed through with 5 per cent Decon in all tubes except the saline wash line, until tubes clear. Decon is left in the system overnight.

REFERENCES

Freiesleben, E., Madsen, G. & Sørensen, H. (1975) Experiences with automated blood grouping using a Groupamatic 360C in connection with a reply and recording system adapted to a hospital Transfusion Service. *ISBT Helsinki Abstracts*, P.32.

Garretta, M., Gener, J., Muller, A., Matte, C. & Moullec, J. (1975) The Groupamatic System for routine Immunohaematology. *Transfusion*, **15**, 422.

Gunson, H.H., Phillips, P.K. & Stratton, F. (1972) Manipulative and inherent errors in anti-D quantitation using the AutoAnalyzer. *J. clin. Path.* **25**, 198.

Gunson, H.H., Phillips, P.K. & Stratton, F. (1974a) The effect of ambient temperature on the anti-D assay using the AutoAnalyzer. *J. clin. Path.,* **27,** 356.

Gunson, H.H., Phillips, P.K. & Stratton, F. (1974b) Observations on the reproducibility of the bromelised test cell anti-D assay using the Auto-Analyser. *Vox Sang.,* **26,** 334.

Jenkins, G.C., Fewell, R.G., Lloyd, M.J., Brown, J., Judd, J., Lane, R.S. & Jenkins, W.J. (1975) Mechanised blood grouping: a hospital trial using an 8-channel grouping machine. *J. clin. Path.,* **28,** 860.

Moore, B.P.L. (1969) Automation in the blood transfusion laboratory. *Canad. med. Ass. J.,* **100,** 381.

Moore, B.P.L. & Fernandez, L. (1972) Reappraisal of an auto-analyser haemagglutination system for anti-D quantification. *Scand. J. Haemat.,* **9,** 492.

Moore, B.P.L. Humphreys, P. & Lovett-Moseley, C.A. (1972) *Serological and Immunological Methods.* 7th ed. P.279. Toronto: Canadian Red Cross Society.

Perrault, R. & Högman, C. (1971) Automated red cell antibody analysis. A parallel study 1. Detection and quantitation. *Vox Sang.,* **20,** 340.

Rosenfield, R.E., Szymanski, I.O. & Kochwa, S. (1964) Immunochemical studies of the Rh system: III Quantitative haemagglutination that is relatively independent of source of Rh antigens and antibodies. *Cold. Spr. Harb. Symp. quant. Biol.,* **29,** 427.

Chapter 22. Identification of Antibodies and Mixtures of Antibodies

The various blood group systems have been described separately, but obviously when an unidentified antibody is discovered they must all be considered together, since the antibody may belong to any of them.

Apart from the detection of anti-A and anti-B agglutinins (serum grouping technique No. 2.2) routine antibody tests are designed mainly to detect Rh antibodies. (*See* Chapters 8 and 11) This is because Rh antibodies are the most common cause of transfusion reaction and haemolytic disease of the newborn. Nevertheless, in some cases a pattern of reaction which is not characteristic of any of the Rh antibodies will be obtained in the routine testing. Evidence for the presence of other atypical antibodies may also be found in other cases in which it has been deemed necessary, in the absence of any trace of Rh antibodies, to seek further for a serological cause of a clinical syndrome. Cold agglutinins will not normally be detected unless especially sought. However, occasionally their presence will be advertised by an anomalous result occurring in serum grouping tests for ABO agglutinins.

The detection and identification of Rh antibodies has already been considered in detail in Chapter 11. It is, therefore, unnecessary to reconsider them here. In this chapter we are concerned with the detection and identification of other atypical antibodies and also mixtures of antibodies belonging to different blood group systems.

Choice of Standard Red Cells

It is essential that any laboratory undertaking the identification of atypical antibodies has a good panel of standard cells which have been tested for as many blood group systems as possible. These, of course, should all be of group O to avoid interference by the reaction of anti-A and/or anti-B. It should not be too difficult to select approximately twelve different red cell standards which will not only detect most of the comparatively common known antibodies but also distinguish between them. An example of a useful panel is shown in Table 22.1. These standard red cells should be used whenever the routine Rh antibody test has given anomalous results or in those cases in which the routine Rh antibody test is negative but there are clinical reasons for suspecting the presence of an atypical antibody. In addition if the antibody is reacting with most or all standard cells the rare homozygotes must be included, *e.g.* Lu^{a}Lu^a, KK, Vel negative, etc. If the antibody reacts with one cell only then knowledge of the rare antigens it contains will be helpful, *e.g.* Wr^a, Sw^a or V^w, etc. Many laboratories find it convenient to use a commercially produced panel of cells which will include cells which have a selection of the rarer antigens.

Investigation of the Serum

It is suggested that the unknown serum be tested with the selected standard cells and the patient's own cells by some or all of the standard antibody detection methods. The investigation of the serum by all these methods in parallel is described in technique No. 22.1. (For typical results see table 22.1)

An idea as to which methods will be the most profitable to use in any particular case may be gained from the results of the routine antibody tests that have already been done. If, for example, the antibody seems to be more readily detectable by ahg technique, then in further tests with the enlarged panel of red cells, saline and papain techniques might well be omitted. Similarly, if the presence of a cold agglutinin is suspected, tests with cells suspended in saline at 15°C are appropriate.

Table 22.2 will be found a useful reference table containing most of the known antibodies classified under three sections according to the frequencies of their corresponding antigens.

Interpretation of Results

The temperature of reactivity, the techniques which have to be employed to show the presence of the antibody and the frequency of positive reactions obtained, are all guides to identity (see Table 22.2). For example, an antibody reacting better at 37°C than at a lower temperature is not a cold antibody. This observation makes it unlikely that the antibody is anti-P_1, anti-H, anti-HI, anti-M, anti-N, anti-Le^a, anti-Le^b, anti-Lu^a etc. An antibody reacting by indirect anti-human globulin test at 37°C with approximately 1 in 10 of the samples of red cells used, is likely to be anti-K. Other similar deductions which give a line on the specificity of an antibody may be made.

A convenient method of recording the results obtained with a panel of known cells is shown in Table 22.1. The arrangement of the results in this fashion makes it easy to see whether the pattern of reactions given by the serum being tested corresponds to a known antigen-antibody system. The findings will fall into one of five categories which will be considered separately; namely (a) clear-cut positive and negative reactions; (b) indeterminate reactions; (c) positive reactions with all standard cells but negative with own cells; (d) positive reactions with all cells including own; (e) negative reactions throughout.

Clear-cut Positive and Negative Reactions.

When clear-cut reactions are obtained an inspection of a protocol similar to that shown in Table 22.1 will usually suggest the identity of the antibody; but *see also* Table 22.2.II. For example, the unknown serum St. reacts with all P_1 positive cells, giving stronger reactions at room temperature than at 37°C, thus suggesting that the antibody detected is anti-P_1. Its range of reaction is also typical of anti-P_1. The second unknown antibody reacts only by indirect anti-

Table 22.1 Identification of antibodies by testing with a selected panel of standard red cells

Standard red cells (all group O)	Rh type	Antigens in red cells															Unknown serum St.					Unknown serum Mc.				
																	R.T.			37°C		R.T.			37°C	
		C	D	E	c	e	M	N	S	P_1	Lu^a	K	Le^a	Le^b	Fy^a	Jk^a	Sal.	Sal.	Alb.	Ahg	Pap	Sal.	Sal.	Alb.	Ahg	Pap
LB	rr	–	–	–	+	+	–	+	+	+	–	–	–	+	+	+	v	w	–	–	–	–	–	–	–	–
ML	rr	–	–	–	+	+	+	+	+	+	+	–	–	+	–	–	v	–	–	–	–	–	–	–	–	–
RS	rr	–	–	–	+	+	+	+	+	+	–	+	+	–	+	–	w	–	–	–	–	–	–	–	+++	–
RL	R_1R_1	+	+	–	–	+	+	–	+	+	+	–	–	+	+	+	v	–	–	–	–	–	–	–	–	–
RZ	R_1R_1	+	+	–	–	+	–	+	–	–	–	–	–	+	+	+	–	–	–	–	–	–	–	–	–	–
BH	R_1r	+	+	–	+	+	+	+	+	+	–	–	–	+	+	–	v	w	–	–	–	–	–	–	–	–
LP	R_1r	+	+	–	+	+	+	+	+	–	–	–	+	–	–	+	–	–	–	–	–	–	–	–	–	–
CL	R_1r	+	+	–	+	+	+	+	+	+	–	–	–	+	+	+	+	–	–	–	–	–	–	–	–	–
RB	R_2R_2	–	+	+	+	–	+	+	+	+	–	–	+	–	–	+	v	–	–	–	–	–	–	–	–	–
DM	R_2R_2	–	+	+	+	–	+	–	+	–	–	–	–	+	+	+	–	–	–	–	–	–	–	–	–	–
MP	R_2r	–	+	+	+	+	+	+	–	–	–	–	–	+	+	+	v	w	–	–	–	–	–	–	–	–
JRL	R_2r	+	+	+	+	+	+	+	+	+	+	+	–	+	+	+	–	–	–	–	–	–	–	–	+++	–
Own St.	R_1r	+	+	–	+	+	+	–	+	+	–	–	–	+	–	+	–	–	–	–	–	–	–	–	–	–
Own Mc.	rr	–	–	–	+	+	+	–	+	+	–	–	–	+	+	+	–	–	–	–	–	–	–	–	–	–

Table 22.2 Section I. Antibodies for frequent antigens

(For references not given in this table, see under appropriate blood group systems, especially chapters 13 and 18.)

Antibody	Antigen or system	Approximate Frequency of antigen	Frequency of antibody	Usual technique and temperature	Remarks	References
Anti-At[a]	August	Almost universal	Rare	ahg 37°C	Immune to pregnancy or transfusion IgG	Applewhaite et al. (1967)
Anti-Chido	Chido	98 per cent	Rare	ahg 37°C	Antibodies tend to give variable reactions with red cells. Chido is plasma antigen. Linked with HL-A	
Anti-Co[a]	Colton	99.7 per cent	Rare	ahg or ahg-papain 37°C		
Anti-Cs[a]	Cs[a]	97.5 per cent	Rare	ahg 37°C	Marked variation of strength of antigen - probably a white cell antigen	Giles et al. (1965)
Anti-Di[b]	Diego	100 per cent in White and Negroes and Eskimos	Rare	ahg 37°C	See also Section II	
Anti-Dp	Dupuy	Very frequent	Rare	ahg and enzyme		Frank et al. (1970)
Anti-e	Rh	97 per cent	Fairly common	ahg and papain 37°C	Also found as auto antibody in some haemolytic anaemia cases	
Anti-El	Eldridge	Very frequent	Rare	ahg and enzyme		Schmidt et al. (1967)
Anti-En[a]	En	Almost universal	Rare	Saline, alb., ahg and enzyme	En(a-) cells give unusual reactions for MN and Rh	

Anti-Ge	Gerbich	Very frequent no random Ge neg found. Ge neg common in Melanesians	Rare	Some ahg 37°C others saline RT	3 types of antibody anti-Ge 1, 2, 3 anti-Ge 1, 2 anti-Ge 1	Rosenfield et al. (1960)
Anti-Gnᵃ	Gonsowski	Very frequent	Rare	ahg		Fox and Taswell (1969)
Anti-Goᵇ Anti-Gyᵃ Anti-H	Rh Gregory ABO	Very frequent Very frequent Very frequent	Rare Rare Common	ahg 37°C ahg 37°C Saline 4°C or 15°C Sometimes papain 37°C	Reacts best with GpO cells and least well with Gp, A₁B cells. Weak with cord cells. Inhibited by secretor saliva	Swansen et al. (1966)
Anti-HI	ABO and I	Very frequent in adults. Cord cells, weak or negative	Common	Saline 4°C or 15°C	Reactions similar to anti-H. Also negative with Oii and hhI cells. Usually not inhibited by secretor saliva	
Anti-Hy	Holley	Very frequent all Hy-negatives are negroid	Rare	ahg.37°C	Related to Gregory (Gyᵃ) Transfusion reactions Stimulated by pregnancy and transfusions	Schmidt et al. (1967) Moulds et al. 1975.
Anti-I	I	Very frequent in adults. Not found in infants	Common	Saline 4°C or 15°C. Can also be ahg or papain 37°C.	Often found as auto-antibody in "cold"-type haemolytic anaemia. Not inhibited by secretor saliva	
Anti-Iᵀ	I		Found as cold auto agglutinin in Melanesians.	Saline, cold	Strong with cord cells. Less strong with adult I cells. Weak with adult i cells.	
Anti-i	I	Weak with almost all adult cells. Strongly positive with all cord cells	Rare	Saline, cold	Also found as auto-antibody associated with infectious mononucleosis	

Antibody	Antigen or system	Approximate Frequency of antigen	Frequency of antibody	Usual technique and temperature	Remarks	References
Anti-Inb(?)	In			18 and 37°C Sal, alb., and ahg, weak or neg by enzyme.		Giles (1975).
Anti-Jra	Jra	Very frequent	Rare	ahg	Potential transfusion reaction	Stroup and MacIlroy (1970)
Anti-Jsb(K7)	Kell	100 per cent Whites 99 per cent Negroes	Rare	ahg 37°C		
Anti-k(K2)	Kell	99 per cent	Rare	ahg 37°C		
Anti-KL(K9)	Kell	Very frequent	Rare	ahg 37°C	KL negative persons lack K and may have traces only of k, Kpb and Jsb	
Anti-Kna	Knops Helgeson	Very frequent	Rare	ahg	Antigens may be primarily HL-A.	Helgeson et al. (1970)
Anti-Kpb(K4)	Kell	Very frequent	Rare	papain		
Anti-KU(K5)	Kell	Very frequent	Rare	ahg or papain 37°C		
Anti-Coté(K11)	Kell	Very frequent	Rare	ahg 37°C		
Anti-Bφc(K12)	Para Kell	Very frequent	Rare	ahg		
Anti-Sgro(K13)	Para Kell	Very frequent	Rare			
Anti-San(K14)	Para Kell	Very frequent	Rare	ahg		
Anti-Lan	Lan	Very frequent	Rare	ahg most reliable	All examples IgG	Van der Hart et al. (1961)
Anti-Lu2 (Anti-Lub)	Lutheran	Very frequent	Rare	Saline or ahg	Causes haemolytic disease	
Anti-Lu3 (Anti-LuaLub)	Lutheran	Very frequent	Rare	ahg	Reacts with all but the very rare Lu(a-b-) cells	

	Para Lutheran	Antibodies to 'public' antigens				
Also Anti-Lu 4, 5, 7, 8, and 11 Anti-Luke	Luke	98 per cent negative with p and pᵏ and 2 per cent P₁ and P₂	Rare	ahg or ahg on enzyme treated cells.	Genetically independent of P.	
Anti-P	P	Very frequent	Rare (all p people have these antibodies.)	Saline, R.T. or 37°C	Often occurs with anti-P₁ and Pᵏ, originally called anti-Tjᵃ.	
Anti-P,P₁Pᵏ (anti-Tjᵃ)	P	Very frequent	Rare	Saline, R.T. or 37°C	Haemolytic antibody. Associated with abortions	Roelcke (1969)
Anti-Pr	Pr	Not polymorphic (100 per cent pos)		Cold auto-aggs. Neg with enzymes	Not found in healthy people. Sub groups found using animal cells.	Roelcke et al (1976)
Anti Rg	Rg	97 per cent	One example so far	ahg but serum inhibition more reliable ahg 37°C	Antigen present in cells and serum	Longster and Giles (1976)
Anti-Scl (formerly Sn)	Scianna	Very frequent	Rare			
Anti-T	T	Very frequent	Very frequent	Saline, R.T.	Only reacts with cells that have been modified by bacteria to expose T receptor.	
Anti-Tn	Tn	Very frequent	All adult sera	Saline R.T.	Not caused by infection	
Anti-U	MNSs	Very frequent	Rare	ahg 37°C	All U-negative persons are S- s-	
Anti-Vel	Vel	Very frequent	Many examples	Saline 37°C better by ahg with anti-IgM	May also haemolyse Vel positive cells. Transfusion reactions.	Sussman and Miller (1952)
Anti-Ytᵃ	Yt	99.8 per cent	Rare	ahg 37°C	Variation in strength of reaction. May be white cell antigen. Antibody stimulated by transfusion but no reaction.	Eaton et al. (1956)
Anti-Ykᵃ	York	Very frequent	Many examples			Moltham et al. (1969)

Table 22.2 Section II. Antibodies for antigens of frequency less than 95 per cent to about 1 per cent

Antibody	Antigen or System	Approximate frequency of antigen	Frequency of antibody	Usual technique temperature	Remarks	References
Anti-A	ABO	42 per cent (S. England) (A+AB)	Found in sera of all A negative persons	Saline R.T. (also active 37°C)		
Anti-A[1]	ABO	34 per cent (S. England) (A[1] and A[1]B)	Typical component of all anti-A sera Atypical. In about 25 per cent of A[2] and A[2]B sera	Saline R.T. (also active 37°C) Saline 4°C may also be active R.T. and very rarely at 37°C		
Anti-Au[a]	Auberger	82 per cent (French and English)	Rare	ahg 37°C	Relationship between dominant Lu (a-b-) type and Auberger	Salmon et al. (1961) Tippett (1963)
Anti-B	ABO	10 per cent (S. England) (B and AB)	Found in sera of all B negative persons	Saline R.T. (also active 37°C)		
Anti-Bg[a]	Bg. Also HLA	29 per cent	Fairly common	Saline or ahg	Antibodies usually weak and give variable positive frequency	
Anti-Bg[b]	Bg. Also HLA (formerly HO)	2 per cent	Not uncommon	ahg 37°C	Sera may contain mixtures e.g. anti-Bg[a] + anti-Bg[b]	
Anti-Bg[c]	Bg Also HLA2 positive in 300		Not uncommon	ahg 37°C	Anti-D sera should be tested with R' cells for possible presence of anti-C. (See also anti-G.)	
Anti-C	Rh	63.5 per cent	Commonly found with anti-D in Rh negative persons. More rarely in Rh positives and then often in association with anti-e	Saline and papain 37°C (also ahg 37°C)		

Antibody	System	Frequency	Rarity	Technique	Notes
Anti-c	Rh	80 per cent	Fairly rare	ahg alb and papain 37°C	Found in R_1R_1 persons often in association with anti-E
Anti-C^x	Rh	Varies with race from 2-9 per cent	Rare, less uncommon as a component of anti-C and anti-CD sera	Saline ahg and papain 37°C	
Anti-CE	Rh	15 per cent	Rare	Saline or papain 37°C	
Anti-Ce	Rh	63 per cent	Rare—pure but a component of many anti-C sera	Saline, ahg and papain 37°C	
Anti-cE	Rh	31 per cent	Rare	ahg or papain 37°C	
Anti-ce	Rh	64 per cent	Rare alone found in many anti-c and anti-e sera	ahg or papain 37°C	
Anti-ce^s	Rh	Rare in whites, up to 40 per cent in negroes	Rare	ahg and papain 37°C	
Anti-Ce^s	Rh	Rare in whites, common in negroes	Rare	ahg and papain 37°C	
Anti-Co^b	Colton	8 per cent	Rare	ahg 37°C and even better papain ahg	
Anti-D	Rh	85 per cent	Common	Saline, alb., ahg and/or papain 37°C	
Anti-Di^a	Diego	Found in Mongolian races and South American Indians. Varies 2.5 per cent-36 per cent	Rare	ahg 37°C	
Anti-Di^b	Diego	In Mongoloid races allelic to Di^a distribution	Rare	ahg 37°C	
Anti-Do^a	Dombrock	Europeans 66 per cent American Negroes and Indians lower Thais 13 per cent	Rare	ahg 37°C	ahg sera have to be especially chosen

Antibody	Antigen or System	Approximate frequency of antigen	Frequency of antibody	Usual technique temperature	Remarks	References
Anti-Do[b] Anti-Donna	Dombrock (see anti-Bg[a])	82 per cent	Rare			
Anti-E	Rh	30 per cent	Common	Saline, alb., ahg papain 37°C	Often detectable only by pap. tech. especially if naturally occurring	
Anti-E[1]	Rh	30 per cent Whites 20 per cent Australian Aborigines	Rare	Saline R.T.		
Anti-e[s]	Rh	35-45 per cent negroes	Not uncommon often with other Rh antibodies	ahg and papain 37°C		
Anti-f (see anti-ce)	Rh	16 per cent	Rare alone found in most anti-c and anti-e sera	Papain and ahg 37°C		
Anti-Fy[a]	Duffy	Whites 66 per cent	Fairly common	ahg 37°C	Inactivated by papain	
Anti-Fy[b]	Duffy	Whites 80 per cent	Fairly rare	ahg 37°C	Inactivated by papain	
Anti-G	Rh	85 per cent	Common in anti-CD sera	Saline, alb., ahg and/or papain		
Anti-In[a]	In	3 per cent	Rare	18°C and 37°C Sal, alb and agh. weak or neg by enzyme	Found with other immune antibodies	Badakere et al (1974)
Anti-IP_1	I and P	75 per cent	Rare	Saline, cold		
Anti-Jk[a]	Kidd	76 per cent (higher in Negroes)	Not uncommon	Saline, cold, ahg., and/or ahg on enzyme treated cells		
Anti-Jk[b]	Kidd	71 per cent (lower in Negroes)	Rare	As anti-Jk[a]	Some sera behave as if they were detecting more than one antigen	

Antibody	System	Frequency	Commonness	Technique	Notes
Anti-Js^a (K6)	Kell	20 per cent in Negroes	Rare	ahg 37°C	
Anti-K (K1)	Kell	9 per cent	Common	ahg 37°C	Often found in association with other immune antibodies
Anti-Kp^a (K3)	Kell	2 per cent	Rare	ahg 37°C	
Anti-Le^a	Lewis	22 per cent	Common	Saline cold /or ahg, ahg and complement and papain 37°C	
Anti-Le^b	Lewis	Varies with ABO group and serum used	Common	Saline cold occasionally ahg 37°C (or ahg and complement)	
Anti-Le^X	Lewis	90 per cent	Rare	As for anti-Le^a	Positive with cells of all persons who secrete Le^a
Anti-Lu^a	Lutheran	8 per cent	Rare	Saline R.T. or rarely ahg 37°C	
Anti-LW	Rh	85 per cent (give +ve reactions) rr cells are negative but absorb the antibody	Rare	ahg or papain	Genetically independent of Rh
Anti-M	MNSs	78 per cent	Common	Saline R.T. can also be ahg 37°C	
Anti-M^1	MNSs	22.6 per cent of group M. 4 per cent group MN	Rare	Saline R.T.	Not identical with anti-M$_1$
Anti-M$_1$	MNSs	About 5 per cent in Whites. About 20 per cent in Negroes	Found in many human anti-M sera	Saline ph 6.5 R.T.	
Anti-N	MNSs	72 per cent	Fairly uncommon	Saline R.T.	
Anti-P$_1$	P	79 per cent	Very common	Saline or papain R.T.	Can very rarely be active by ahg at 37°C

Antibody	Antigen or system	Approximate Frequency of antigen	Frequency of antibody	Usual technique and temperature	Remarks	References
Anti-Rh_A Rh_B, etc.	Rh	Same as D except for very rare cells	Rare	Papain 37°C		
Anti-S	MNSs	55 per cent (varies with MN type)	Fairly common	ahg 37°C or saline R.T.		
Anti-s	MNSs	98 per cent (varies with MN type)	Rare	ahg 37°C		
Anti-Sd^a	Sid	91 per cent	About 1 per cent of normal donors	Saline R.T. or ahg with anti-IgM	Reactions variable. Sd^a present in urine	
Anti-S	MNSs	2 per cent Whites 4 per cent Negroes	Rare (found with anti-Tm)	Saline R.T.	All S_j +ves were Tm+ also	
Anti-St^a	MNSs	Very rare Whites but 14 in 220 Japanese	Rare	Saline R.T.		
Anti-Ul^a (K10)	Related to Kell	2.6-5 per cent in Finns	Rare	ahg 37°C		
Anti-V(Ce') Rh	Rh	Very rare in Whites Up to 40 per cent in Negroes	Rare	ahg 37°C papain		
Anti-VS(e') Rh	Rh	Very rare in Whites reacts with Negroes up to about 60 per cent	Rare	ahg 37°C	React with all V+ and most R^1 Negroes	
Anti-Xg^a	Xg	Males 67.5 per cent Females 89.4 per cent	Rare	ahg 37°C	Sex linked	
Anti-Yt^b	Yt	8 per cent	Rare	ahg 37°C	Previously called Marriott	Boorman et al. (1975).
Anti-Zt^a	Zt^a	3 per cent	Rare	ahg		

Table 22.2. Section III. Antibodies for Rare Antigens

Antibody	Antigen or system	Frequency of antigen	Frequency of antibody	Usual technique and temperature	Remarks	References
Anti-An[a]	Ahonen	Rare	Rare		No evidence of stimulation. Cross matching difficulty	Furuhjelm et al. (1972)
Anti-Be[a] (Berrens)	Rh	Rare	Rare	ahg 37°C	Causes haemolytic disease. Antibody has been produced by immunisation of volunteers	
Anti-Becker	Becker	Rare	Rare	ahg 37°C	Haemolytic disease	Elbel and Prokop (1951)
Anti-Bi	Biles	Rare	Rare	ahg 37°C	Stimulated by pregnancy	Wadlington et al. (1961)
Anti-Bp[a]	Bishop	Rare	Rare	Saline R.T.	Slightly more common in AIHA sera than in normal sera.	Cleghorn (1964) unpublished.
Anti-Sc2 (formerly Bu[a])	Scianna	Rare	Rare	ahg 37°C	Antibody can be produced by immunisation.	
Anti-Bx[a]	Box	Rare	Rare			Jenkins and Marsh (1961)
Anti-By	Batty	Rare	Rare	ahg and papain 37°C	Liable to occur in AIHA sera. Doubtful case of very mild haemolytic disease.	Simmons and Were (1955) Cleghorn (1960)
Anti-C[x]	Rh	Rare	Rare in normal sera	Saline and ahg 37°C Albumin 37°C	Less rare in AIHA sera	
Anti-Chr[a]	Chr[a]	Rare	Rare			Kissmeyer-Nielsen (1955)
Anti-Cl[a]	MNSs	Rare	Rare	Saline R.T. papain 37°C	Probably identical with Tippett's Category V.	
Anti-D[w]	Rh	Very rare in Whites. 4 per cent in Negroes.	Rare			

Antibody	Antigen or system	Frequency of antigen	Frequency of antibody	Usual technique and temperature	Remarks	References
Anti-Di[a]	Diego	Mainly confined to Mongolians	Rare	ahg 37°C		
Anti-E[w]	Rh	Rare	Rare	ahg 37°C	Haemolytic disease.	
Anti-Evans	Maybe Rh	Very rare	Rare	ahg 37°C	Haemolytic disease.	
Anti-Gf	Griffiths	Rare	Rare	Papain 37°C		Cleghorn et al. (1966) unpublished.
Anti-Go[a]	Rh	Very rare	Rare	ahg 37°C	Related to Tippetts category IV	
Anti-Good	Good	Rare	Rare	ahg 37°C	Severe haemolytic disease	Frumin et al. (1960)
Anti-Gr	MNSs	Rare	1 per cent of normal sera	Saline R.T.		
Anti-He	MNSs	2.7 per cent West Africans. 0 per cent Whites	Rare	Saline R.T.	Can be made in rabbits	
Anti-Heibel	Heibel	Rare	Rare	ahg 37°C	Haemolytic disease	Ballowitz et al. (1968)
Ani-Hey	Hey	Rare	Rare		Found in routine screening	Yvart et al. (1974)
Anti-Hill	MNSs	Very rare. Reacts with Mi[a], Vw, Mu+, Hill+ cells only	Rare	ahg 37°C		
Anti-Hov	Hov	Rare	Rare		Found with anti-Fy[a] in a mother	Szaloky et al. (1973)
Anti-Ht[a]	Hunt	Rare	Rare	ahg 37°C	Haemolytic disease	Jahn and Cleghorn (unpublished 1962)
Anti-Hu	MNSs	Rare in Europe 22 per cent Africans	Rare	Saline R.T.	Made in rabbits	

Antibody	System			Technique	Comments	References
Anti-Je[a]	Jensen	Rare	Rare	Saline R.T.		Skov (1972)
Anti-Jn[a]	Jn[a]	Very rare	Very rare	Saline, cold		Kornstad et al. (1967)
Anti-Js[a] (K6)	Kell	Very rare in all but Negroes	Very rare	ahg 37°C		
Anti-Kamhuber	Kamhuber	Rare	Rare	ahg 37°C	Transfusion reaction	Speiser et al. (1966)
anti-Kx (K15)	Kell	Rare	Rare	ahg	Is a component of anti KL and can be eluted from Ko cells stimulated by transfusion	
Anti-Levay	Levay	Very rare	Very rare	Saline R.T.		Callender and Race (1946)
Anti-Ls[a]	LewisII	Very rare	Rare	Saline R.T.		Cleghorn and Dunsford (Unpublished, 1963)
Anti-M[a]	MNSs	Very rare	Very rare	Saline R.T.	Possibly lacks some portion of the M antigen	
Anti-M[g]	MNSs	Very rare	Common	Saline R.T.		
Anti-M[k]	MNSs	Very rare (cells are M-N-S-s-)	Very rare	Saline R.T.	Antibody very weak	
Anti-Mi[a]	MNSs	Very rare	Fairly common	Saline R.T.	Sometimes found in haemolytic anaemia sera. Often found as anti-Mi[a]+V[w]	
Anti-Mt[a]	MNSs	Very rare	Very rare	Saline R.T.		
Anti-Mur.	MNSs	Very rare	Very rare	Saline R.T.		
Anti-Ny[a]	MNSs	Rare	Rare	Saline R.T.		
Anti-Or	Orris	Rare	Rare			
Anti-P[k]	P	Extremely rare	Occurs with anti-P and Anti-P$_1$	Saline R.T. and 37°C		Cleghorn et al. un-published 1964)
Anti-Pt[a]	Peters	Rare	Rare		Often found with anti-Wr[a] and/or anti-Vw	Pinder et al. (1969)

Antibody	Antigen or system	Frequency of antigen	Frequency of antibody	Usual technique and temperature	Remarks	References
Anti-Rd	Radin	Very rare	Very rare	ahg 37°C	Haemolytic disease	Rausen et al. (1967)
Anti-Raddon	Raddon	Very rare	Rare	ahg 37°C		Lockyer and Tovey(Unpublished 1967)
Anti-Re^a	Reid	Rare	Rare		IgG caused slight HDN	Guévin et al. (1971)
Anti-Ri^a	MNSs	Very rare	Rare	Saline R.T.	Found with other antibodies to private antigens	Kornstad (1974)
Anti-Rl^a	Rosenlund	Rare	Rare			
Anti-Rm	Rm	Very rare	Rare	ahg 37°C	Haemolytic disease	Van der Hart et al. (1954)
Anti-St^a	MNSs	20 in 17,000 Whites 14 in 220 Japanese	Rare	Saline R.T.		
Anti-Stobo	Stobo	2 in 3000 Scots	Fairly rare		Probably part of Bg System	Wallace and Milne (1959)
Anti-Sul	MNSs	Rare	Fairly common	Saline R.T.		
Anti-Sw^a	Swann	Rare	Fairly common in pathological sera, AIHA etc.	ahg 37°C	Found in cross-matching	Cleghorn (1959 and 1960)
Anti-Tm	MNSs	Very rare	Rare	Saline R.T.		
Anti-To^a	Torkildsen	Rare	Rare	Saline R.T.		Kornstad et al. (1968)
Anti-Tr^a	Traversu	Rare	Rare	Saline R.T.	When antibody found it is usually associated with anti-Wr^a	Cleghorn (unpublished 1962) Kornstad (1974)
Anti-Ven	Ven	Rare	Rare	ahg 37°C	Haemolytic disease	Van Loghem et al. (1952)
Anti-Vr	MNSs	Rare	Very rare	ahg 37°C		
Anti-Vw	MNSs	Rare	Common	ahg 37°C	(See also Gr)	

Antibody	Name			Technique	Notes	References
Anti-Wb	Webb	Very rare	Rare	Saline R.T.		Simmons and Albrey (1963)
Anti-Wiel Anti-Wr[a]	Rh Wright	Rare Rare	Rare Common	Papain 37°C ahg and Papain 37°C often saline R.T. also	Haemolytic disease and transfusion reactions	Holman (1953) Cleghorn (1960)
Anti-Wu	Wulfsberg	Very Rare	Rare	Saline 18°C & 37°C and enzyme Neg. by alb and ahg	Cross-match problem	Heisto (1966) Kornstad et al (1976).
Anti-Wk[a] (K17)	Kell	Rare	Rare		Antithetical with anti-Côté (K11)	

human globulin technique with cells which are **K** positive, thus suggesting that it is anti-**K**.

The results of tests with such a known panel of standard cells do not necessarily prove conclusively the specificity of a particular antibody, although the probability that it is of the specificity suggested is high.

A relatively simple statistical method of confirming the specificity of a particular antibody is that of analysing the results by means of Fisher's exact method for 2×2 tables to estimate the probability of these reactions occurring by chance.

As an example, the serum St. from Table 22.1 is considered. The results are arranged as follows:

Known cells	Serum	St		
	+	−	
P_1 pos.	8a	0b	8
P_1 neg.	0c	4d	4
	8	4	12N

If the squares are lettered a, b, c, d, and the total number of red cells tested is N, the probability of the reaction not being due to an anti-P_1 antibody can be determined from the general formula:-

$$\text{probability} = \frac{\underline{/a+b}\underline{/c+d}\underline{/a+c}\underline{/b+d}}{\underline{/N}\underline{/a}\underline{/b}\underline{/c}\underline{/d}}$$

$$= \frac{\underline{/8}\underline{/4}\underline{/8}\underline{/4}}{\underline{/12}\underline{/8}\underline{/0}\underline{/0}\underline{/4}}$$

$$= \frac{1}{495}$$

(This formula is only applicable if b or c = o) This means that the antibody is almost certainly anti-P_1, since a probability of $\frac{1}{20}$ is usually taken as the level of significance for this type of comparison, although if the level were as low as $\frac{1}{20}$ further tests would be planned in the hope of improving the probability.

Clear-cut results which do not conform to any particular antibody pattern are probably due to the serum containing a mixture of antibodies and it should be investigated as shown below. There is, of course, always the exciting but rather remote possibility that a hitherto undescribed antigen-antibody system is being detected. The establishment of a new system is a long and complicated research project and as such is outside the scope of this book.

Indeterminate Results.

The difficulty of correctly identifying a weakly reacting antibody must be realised. It is nearly always useless to contemplate identification of specificity unless the reactions obtained are in the V to + range. The use of a more sensitive technique e. g. 22.4 may enhance the reaction to give clear cut positive and negative results. There is also the question of dosage to be considered and the possibility that the unknown antibody is reacting only with red cells containing a double dose of the corresponding antigen. It is occasionally possible to identify such an antibody.

Antibodies may increase in titre as the result of immunisation and therefore in certain circumstances (*e.g.* during pregnancy) it is worth testing a later sample in the hope of identifying the antibody.

Positive Reactions with all Standard Cells but Negative with Own Cells.

A positive reaction obtained with all the red cells tested with the exception of the patient's own is indicative of the presence of either: (1) a type of antibody which reacts preferentially with group O cells or (2) an antibody corresponding to an antigen of high frequency, *see* Table 22.2.I, or (3) a mixture of antibodies.

If the antibody is of the cold type it is likely to be anti-I, anti-HI or possibly a mixture of anti-Le^a and anti-Le^b. Testing with several examples of group O Le(a–b–) red cells will reveal whether or not the third alternative is correct. If the reactions with these red cells are positive, proving that an anti-Le^a + anti-Le^b mixture is not involved, titrations against red cells in saline of group O, several examples of group A$_1$ and at least one group A$_2$ should be performed using the master titre technique (No. 3.4). Anti-H and anti-HI agglutinins are usually found in persons of groups A$_1$ or A$_1$B but occasionally occur in group B. In the latter eventuality it will only be possible to titrate with red cells of group O and group B, since A$_1$ and A$_2$ cells will react with the patient's own anti-A. If the values obtained are appreciably higher with cells of groups O and A$_2$ than with cells of group A$_1$ then the antibody is almost certainly of the anti-HI or anti-H type. A distinction between the two broad classes of such antibodies can be made by the saliva inhibition method, where those inhibited by secretor saliva are said to be anti-H and those not so affected anti-HI. However, the anti HI found occasionally in non-secretors is also inhibited by secretor saliva.

Anti-I and anti-HI are both cold agglutinins which are characterised by their poor reactivity with cord bloods.

If the unidentified antibody has a wide thermal range yet reacts better below 37°C, it may be anti-Tj^a (now known to be anti-P + anti-P^k + anti-P$_1$). This can be confirmed by absorbing a portion of serum with P$_2$ red cells which should then leave an anti-serum reacting with all P$_1$ cells. A potential anti-Tj^a serum should be sent, for further confirmation, to a laboratory known to have the very rare Tj^a negative red cells.

Other rare antibodies, the presence of which might have to be considered, are, anti-U and anti-Vel. This again would mean consultation with a laboratory having the appropriate red cells negative with these antibodies.

The chief "warm" antibodies to be considered are anti-e and anti-k. With the panel of standard red cells shown in Table 22.1, the presence of anti-e would be immediately suggested by the finding of a negative reaction with cells DM and RB which are of phenotype R$_2$R$_2$. However, the investigator might not be fortunate enough to obtain cells of this phenotype, in which case positive reactions would be found in all tests. For further identification of anti-e *see* Chapter 11.

Over 200 random red cell samples might have to be tested before a negative reaction could be obtained if the antibody was anti-k. Therefore if its presence is suspected, red cells known to be of type KK should be obtained and in addition the cells of the donor of the serum typed with anti-K and anti-k.

The numerous other possibilities can be seen on Table 22.2 Section 1. It should be noted that antibodies giving 100 per cent reactions with one ethnic group *e.g.* Whites, may give a quite different frequency if tested with another *e.g.* Negroid.

Positive Reactions with all Cells Including Own.

In this category the following alternatives have to be considered:

(1) Optimum reactions obtained by saline technique at room temperature indicate the presence of cold auto-antibodies or pan-agglutinins (*see* Chapter 14 and techniques 14.1 and 14.2). It should be borne in mind that auto-agglutinins may mask the presence of other specific antibodies so that the serum must be re-tested after their removal by absorption with the patient's own cells (technique No. 22.2). If the direct ahg test is positive this may be a case of cold type AIHA (auto-immune haemolytic anaemia) and the auto-antibody is probably anti-I.

(2) Reactions obtained by indirect anti-human globulin test at 37°C suggest a case of "warm type" autoimmune haemolytic anaemia and tests should proceed as outlined in Chapter 27.

(3) It is by no means unusual to obtain positive reactions with all red cells including the patient's own by enzyme technique. In some cases the phenomenon seems to be associated with the presence of cold auto-antibodies but this is not always so. It is thought that the effect may be due to virus infection in the patient but no clinical significance has as yet been attached to it. Absorption with the patient's own enzyme treated red cells sometimes unmasks an antibody of blood group specificity which is often found to be one of the Rh antibodies. Such an absorbed serum, therefore, should be tested for Rh antibodies (*see* Chapter 11) before embarking upon tests with the enlarged panel of standard cells.

(4) That the reaction may be due to pseudo-agglutination will probably be suspected from the characteristic appearance of the clumps under the microscope. In such circumstances, the anti-human globulin technique is used.

Negative Reactions Throughout (*see* Tables 22.2 and 3).

If the further investigation of the serum was instigated by the occurrence of anomalous results in routine Rh and ABO antibody testing, then the finding of negative reactions with the whole panel of group O red cells is most unlikely, the exception being an anomalous reaction with A_1 cells in routine serum grouping which might be due to anti-A_1 (α_1). This antibody will normally have been identified before tests are made against a panel of group O cells (*see* Chapters 2 and 4) but if not it can now be done.

If the further testing has been undertaken on clinical grounds alone and not because reactions suggestive of atypical antibody formation have been found, then negative results throughout may occur. In these circumstances it has to be decided whether the clinical reasons are strong enough for a further investigation to be planned or whether the search for antibodies should be given up at this stage.

Re-testing the serum with the same panel of cells by the ahg plus enzyme technique (No. 22.4) and/or agh plus complement technique (No. 22.5) may be of value. The other methods of enhancing serological reactions *in vitro* can also be used, including the AutoAnalyser with an enzyme and or a low ionic strength system. Moreover, if the serum being investigated is the maternal serum in a case suspected to be one of haemolytic disease of the newborn, it should be tested against the red cells of infant and husband (*see* Chapter 26) or if it is from a suspected case of haemolytic transfusion reaction, cross matched with the red cells of the donors concerned. (Technique No. 23.3.)

To complete the identification of any atypical antibody the red cells of the patient in whose serum the antibody (or antibodies) occurs should be typed and shown not to contain the corresponding antigen. Indeed it is often worth while, if the necessary typing sera can be spared, to type the patient's cells for as many known blood group antigens as possible at the outset of the investigation. A knowledge of which antigens are absent from the red cells will provide a guide to which antibodies can be formed in the serum so that the selected panel of standard cells may be suitably modified. Of course, if the antibody being identified is in the serum of a patient with auto-immune disease it may well be directed towards an antigen the patient possesses.

After the identity of a rare antibody has been established an effort should be made to secure the serum for typing purposes if it is of suitable strength. The principles underlying the selection, standardisation and preparation of such sera are essentially the same as those for Rh typing sera (Chapter 12). The minimum titration values acceptable will depend to a great extent upon the frequency with which a particular antibody is found. Almost any example of a very rare antibody is probably of value for typing although negative reactions will have to be interpreted with caution.

Identification of Mixtures of Antibodies

One of the most difficult serological undertakings is the identification of mixtures of antibodies. These often belong to different blood group systems. It is by no means an uncommon task, since individuals who have reached the stage of producing one atypical antibody readily produce others. If difficulty in identifying the specificity of a serum is experienced, the possibility of the occurrence in it of several antibodies of differing specificity must be considered.

There are several pointers which suggest that more than one antibody has been formed. A different distribution of positive and negative reactions at different temperatures indicates a mixture of "warm" and "cold" antibodies. An example of this might be a serum containing anti-D and anti-P$_1$. In this case the anti-D would be readily identified by performing the tests at 37°C, for at this temperature anti-P$_1$ is rarely active. At 37°C, therefore, the reactions would pattern as anti-D. Tests at room temperature would reveal the anti-P$_1$ but the anti-D might also be active, although not so strongly as at 37°C; therefore it would be essential to confirm the specificity of the anti-P$_1$ by confining the room temperature tests to red cell samples which were D negative. However, if the anti-D did not react in a saline medium no interference with the anti-P$_1$ would be experienced since the latter antibody is an agglutinin and is tested for by saline technique. Any such mixture of the agglutinin form of one antibody and the incomplete form of another can be readily disentangled and identified even if both have the same temperature range.

A further point concerns the identification of mixtures of antibodies when the components vary in strength and the antiglobulin test is being used as the method of detection, reading the tests on a tile. Cells sensitised by a potent incomplete antibody will agglutinate very quickly after the addition of the anti-globulin while the weakly sensitised cells will take perhaps as long as 10-15 minutes to become agglutinated. Thus if the tests are discarded after agglutination caused by the stronger antibody has developed, the presence of the weaker antibody may be missed.

Here also, noting the antigens missing from the red cell samples which are negative with the serum under test may aid the detection of the components of a mixture. For instance, a serum containing a mixture of anti-M and anti-P$_1$ could not be differentiated by testing at various temperatures or by different techniques since both are cold agglutinins and react in a saline medium. Nevertheless a clue to their identity could be obtained by noting that the only red cells negative with the serum in question did not contain either M or P$_1$. This principle can also be applied to the identification of mixtures containing more than two antibodies. The greater the number of antibodies the larger should be the panel of known red cells.

Titration of the unknown serum against various standard red cells will often reflect a mixture of antibodies since different cells will give different titration values. However, there are other reasons for titration variation of which dosage is a common one. Nevertheless, if the dosage phenomenon can be ruled out, any gross discrepancy in the titre of a serum against different red cells is most likely to be due to the presence of more than one antibody in the serum. An example of this is given in Table 22.3 where the values obtained suggest a mixture of anti-P$_1$ and anti-M. Note that the titre of the anti-M is that given by the P$_1$ negative M red cells and that of the anti-P$_1$ by the P$_1$ positive N cells. The titration against P$_1$ negative MN cells suggests that the anti-M may show slight dosage.

If one component of a mixture is very much weaker than another it can probably be diluted out so that the specificity of the stronger component can be directly demonstrated. Alternatively absorption of portions of the serum with various selected red cells may result in a series of absorbed sera containing each of the components separately.

One of the most satisfactory methods of actually· isolating and thereafter

Table 22.3 Elucidation of a mixture of antibodies by means of titration

Red cells	Serial dilution						
	1	2	4	8	16	32	64
Type MP$_1$−	V	+	(+)	−	−	−	−
Type NP$_1$+	V	V	++	+	(+)	w	−
Type MNP$_1$−	+	w	−	−	−	−	−
Type MP$_1$+	V	V	V	+	(+)	w	−
Type NP$_1$−	−	−	−	−	−	−	−

identifying the individual antibodies in a mixed serum is the elution technique. The selection of the optimum temperature for absorption and the most suitable elution technique often makes possible the separation of one antibody from a serum containing a mixture of several. The Rubin's elution technique is particularly successful when eluting IgG Rh antibodies and Landsteiner's technique, while a good all purpose technique, is perhaps the preferred technique when dealing with ABO antibodies.

In connection with elution it has to be appreciated that because of the existence of cross reacting antibodies and antibodies to compound antigens, antibodies may be removed and recovered together.

A serum thought to contain anti-S + anti-Fy^a + anti-Kell for example could be divided into three parts and treated as follows:

Part 1 absorbed with S +K−Fy (a−) red cells and an eluate made in an attempt to obtain pure anti-S.

Part 2 absorbed with S − K+Fy(a−) red cells and an eluate made which would contain any anti-K component.

Part 3 absorbed with S− K−Fy(a+) red cells and an eluate made to recover any anti-Fy^a.

TECHNIQUES

Technique No, 22.1. The full investigation of a serum for atypical antibodies
A full investigation should include the following techniques:

(a) Saline, incubating the serum-cell mixtures at 15-18°C.
(b) Saline, incubating the serum-cell mixtures at 37°C.
(c) Albumin at 37°C.
(d) Indirect anti-human globulin at 37°C.
(e) Papain or other enzyme technique.

Techniques (b)-(e) are carried out in exactly the same manner as for anti-Rh testing (techniques 8.1-5). Technique (a) is identical with (b), except that the tests are left at 15-18°C instead of at 37°C.

The serum is tested by each method against a panel of standard red cells and the patient's own cells. (See Table 22.1.) A weak incomplete anti-D set up against

D positive and D negative cells should be included as a control for albumin, indirect anti-human globulin and enzyme techniques.

The serum to be investigated is then run, in one manipulation, into every tube in which it is required followed by the appropriately prepared standard cells.

The results are recorded as shown in Table 22.1.

Technique No. 22.2. The removal of auto-antibodies from a serum

(a) The Removal of Agglutinins.

The red cells used for the absorption are the patient's own red cells. These should be freed from auto-agglutinins (technique No. 14.1) prior to being mixed with the patient's serum. Preferably "warm separated" red cells may be used.

The serum is then mixed with an equal volume of packed washed red cells and left for 1 to 2 hours (or overnight) at 0–4°C.

The mixture is then centrifuged at this temperature and the supernatant absorbed serum collected. This is re-tested against some or all of the panel of twelve standards and the patient's own cells by saline technique at room temperature. If a reaction is obtained with all or almost all of them including the patient's own cells, then the absorption has not been successful and must be repeated. Negative reactions with all red cell samples indicates that the auto-agglutinin has been removed completely and that there was no additional specific antibody present in the serum. Positive reactions with some of the standard cells and not others suggests that a specific antibody has been unmasked and this must be investigated.

(b) The Removal of Auto-antibodies requiring enzyme treated cells.

This technique is essentially similar to *(a)* except that packed enzyme treated cells are used for the absorption which, therefore, takes place for 1 hour at 37°C instead of in the cold.

The absorbed serum is tested against selected enzyme treated red cells including the patient's own. If there is still a reaction with the patient's cells a re-absorption may have to be carried out.

Technique No. 22.3. Elution of antibody by the Landsteiner technique

The selected red cells are carefully washed three times in saline and packed. The optimum proportion of serum to cells for the absorption stage may have to be found by trial and error. A ratio of serum to cells of 5:1 is often suitable. It is not always appreciated that if the red cell concentration is too high it is difficult to obtain a satisfactory recovery of antibody in the eluate. This mixture is left for 1½-2 hours at the optimum temperature of reactivity for the particular antibody that it is desired to recover in the eluate (0-4°C for ABO and cold agglutinins and 37°C for Rh antibodies, etc.).

The red cells are then carefully washed at least four times in a large volume of saline (6-8 ml.) at 4°C. This can be achieved using ice cold saline and precooled centrifuge buckets, or alternatively the washing can be carried out in a cold room or using a thermostatically controlled centrifuge.

After the red cells are thoroughly washed, a volume of saline equal to the volume of serum used for absorption is added to them and they are placed in a water bath at 56°C for 10 minutes. During this time the suspension is continuously agitated. The tube is then centrifuged maintaining the temperature at 56°C and the supernatant saline which contains the eluted antibody is removed as quickly as possible. It may be an advantage to elute into 0.3 per cent albumin especially if the eluate is to be stored before testing.

The key to success in the preparation of eluates lies in the meticulous washing of the cells after the absorption stage and in the maintenance of the various temperatures necessary to keep the antibody in the attached or free state according to whichever is appropriate at the time.

Technique No. 22.4. Detection of antibody by indirect anti-human globulin on enzyme treated cells

The chosen standard red cells are first enzyme treated. They are then used to test the serum by the indirect anti-human globulin technique (technique No. 8.3b).

Technique No. 22.5. Detection of antibody by anti-human globulin with albumin

In this method the cells are incubated with the serum in the presence of bovine albumin before proceding with the indirect ahg technique. Three volumes of 30 per cent albumin and 4 volumes of serum are mixed with one volume of 5 per cent red cells. The mixture is incubated at 37°C for 30-45 minutes. From this point the procedure is as in technique No. 8.3b.

Technique No. 22.6. Detection of antibodies by indirect anti-human globulin plus complement

The source of complement for this technique can be fresh human or animal serum. If human serum is chosen it must not contain antibodies which would agglutinate the test cells. It should be used undiluted. Animal complement is diluted 1 in 5 or 1 in 10 at which dilutions it will not usually agglutinate red cells. It is however advisable to check this on each batch before use.

The anti-human globulin should be either one of wide specificity used at a suitable dilution for the detection of complement, or an anti-complement globulin. The test is set up as for indirect test (technique No. 8.3b) but before incubation one unit volume of complement-containing serum is added to each tube. Control tubes are also set up, one for each of the standard cells used, containing equal volumes of complement, saline and standard cells. After this the procedure is as for indirect anti-human globulin.

Technique No. 22.7. The "build-up" antiglobulin technique

If there is only a low affinity between an antibody and its corresponding antigen the antibody molecules will be washed off the cells during the washing stage of an ahg test. However sometimes sufficient antibody molecules remain attached to the red cell for a positive ahg test to be obtained by layering on to the red cell firstly the low affinity antibody then the antiglobulin, followed by further globulin-anti-globulin layers. The method described is a modification of that used by Coombs *et al* (1951) when studying the properties of Ox red cells.

Method

Two volumes of the serum containing the low affinity antibody are incubated for 1 hour at 37°C with 4 volumes of a 2 per cent suspension of red cells possessing the corresponding antigen. Red cells lacking the antigen are included with each batch of tests to act as negative control.

The supernatant is removed, the cells are washed three times and then 2 volumes of anti-human globulin are added to each tube. After standing on the bench for a few minutes the tubes are lightly centrifuged. The cells are gently resuspended and a very small aliquot is taken out, placed on a slide and examined microscopically for agglutination. (This is the 1st ahg test and normally no agglutination is observed.)

The remaining bulk of the red cells are washed once and then 2 volumes of AB serum diluted 1/50 are added as a source of globulin. After a further period of incubation (½ to 1 hour) at 37°C the cells are again washed three times. A second addition of anti-globulin is made as in the procedure just described (2nd ahg test). The "building up" process is repeated once more (3rd ahg test).

Comment. Some antibodies will agglutinate the appropriate red cells after a 3 stage globulin-antiglobulin lattice has been built up, while others require only 2 applications of antiglobulin before agglutination occurs (Casey *et al.*, 1972).

REFERENCES

Applewhaite, E., Ginsberg, V., Gerena, J., Cunningham, C.A. & Gavin, J. (1967) A very frequent red cell antigen At[a]. *Vox Sang.*, 13, 444.

Badakere, S.S., Parab, B.B. & Bhatia, H.M. (1974) Further observations on the In[a]. (Indian) antigen in Indian populations. *Vox Sang.*, 26, 400.

Ballowitz, L., Fielder, M., Hoffman, C. & Pettenkofen, H. (1968) 'Heibel' a new rare human blood group antibody, revealed by haemolytic disease of the newborn. *Vox Sang.*, 14, 307.

Boorman, K.E., Benton, J., Dodson, S. & Walker, G.V. (1975) Zt[a], a new blood group antigen. *Abstracts ISBT* (Helsinki) P.45.

Callender, S.T. & Race, R.R. (1946) A serological and genetical study of multiple antibodies formed in response to blood transfusion by a patient with lupus erythematosus diffusus. *Ann. Eugen. (Lond.),* 13, 102.

Casey, F.M., Dodd, B.E. & Lincoln, P.L. (1972) A study of the characteristics of certain Rh antibodies preferentially detectable by enzyme technique. *Vox Sang.*, 23, 493.

Cleghorn, T.E. (1959) A 'new' human blood group antigen, Sw[a]. *Nature*, 184, 1324.

Cleghorn, T.E. (1960) The inheritance of the antigen Sw[a] and evidence for its independence of other blood group systems. *Brit. J. Haem.*, 6, 433.

Cleghorn, T.E. (1960) The frequency of the Wr[a], By and Mg blood group antigens in blood donors in the South of England. *Vox Sang.*, 5, 556.

Coombs, R.R.A., Gleeson-White, M.H. & Hall, J.G. (1951) Factors affecting the agglutinability of red cells, II. The agglutination of bovine red cells previously classified as inagglutinable, by the building up of an anti-globulin-globulin lattice on the sensitised cells. *J. exp. Path.*, 32, 195.

Eaton, B.R., Morton, J.A., Pickles, M.M. & White, K.E. (1956) A new antibody anti-Yt[a], characterising a blood group of high incidence. *Brit. J. Haemat.*, 2, 333.

Elbel, H. & Prokop, O. (1951) Ein neues erbliches Antigen als Ursache gehaufter Fehlgeburten. *Zeitschr. für Hygiene,* **132,** 120.

Fox, J.A. & Taswell, H.F. (1969) Anti-Gn[a], a new antibody reacting with a high incidence erythrocyte antigen. *Transfusion (Philad.),* **9,** 265.

Frank, S., Schmidt, R.P. & Baugh, M.(1970) Three new antibodies for high incidence antigenic determinants (anti-El, anti-Dp and anti-So). *Transfusion (Philad.),* **10,** 254.

Frumin, A.M., Porter, M.M. & Eichman, M.F. (1960) The Good factor as a possible cause of haemolytic disease of the newborn. *Blood,* **xv,** 5, 681.

Furuhjelm, U., Nevanlinna, H.R., Gavin, J. & Sanger, R. (1972) A rare blood group antigen, An[a] (Ahonen). *J. Med. Genet.,* **9,** 385.

Giles, C.M. (1975) Antithetical relationships of anti-In[a] with the Salis antibody. *Vox Sang.,* **29,** 73.

Giles, C.M., Huth, M.C., Wilson, T.E., Lewis, H.B.M. & Grove, G.E.B. (1965) Three examples of a new antibody, anti-Cs[a] which reacts with 98 per cent of red cell samples. *Vox Sang.,* **10,** 405.

Guévin, R.M., Taliano, V., Fiset, D., Bérubé, P. & Kaita, H. (1971) L'Antigène Reid, un nouvel antigène privé. *Rev. fr. Transf.,* **14,** 455.

Hart, M.v.D., Bosman, H. & Loghem, J.J. Van (1954) Two rare human blood group antigens. *Vox Sang.,* **4,** 108.

Hart, M.v.D., Moes, M., Veer, M.v.D. & Loghem, J.J. Van (1961) Ho and Lan-two new blood group antigens. *Proceedings of VIIIth European Congress Haematology.*

Heisto, H. (1966) Personal communication to Race, R.R. & Sanger, R. *Blood Groups in Man.* 6th ed. P.436. Oxford: Blackwell.

Helgeson, M., Swanson, J. & Polesky, H.F. (1970) Knops-Helgeson (Kn[a]), a high frequency erythrocyte antigen. *Transfusion (Philad.),* **10,** 137.

Holman, C.A. (1953) A new rare human blood group antigen (Wr.[a]). *Lancet,* **ii,** 119.

Jenkins, W.J. & Marsh, W.L. (1961) Auto immune haemolytic anaemia; three cases with antibodies specifically active against stored red cells. *Lancet,* **ii,** 16.

Kissmeyer-Nielsen, F. (1955) A new rare blood group antigen Chr[a]. *Vox Sang.,* **5,** 102.

Kornstad, L. (1974) Personal communication to R.R. Race and R. Sanger, Blood groups in Man. 6th ed. P.435. Oxford: Blackwell.

Kornstad, L., Kout, M., Larsen, A.M.J. & Ørjasacter, H. (1967) A rare blood group antigen, Jna. *Vox Sang.,* **13,** 165-170.

Kornstad, L., Øyen R., Cleghorn, T.E. (1968) A new rare blood group antigen To[a] (Torkildsen) and an unsolved factor, Skjelbred. *Vox Sang.,* **14,** 363.

Kornstad, L., Howell, P., Jørgensen, J., Heier Larsen, A.M., & Wadswoth, L.D (1976) The rare blood group antigen Wu. *Vox Sang.,* **31,** 337.

Loghem, J.J. Van & Hart, M. v.D. (1952) Een zeldzaam voorkomende bloedgroep (Ven). *Bull. van het Centraal Laboratorium van de Bloedtransfusiedicast van het Nederlandse Rode Kruis,* **2,** 225.

Longster, G. & Giles, C.M., (1976) A new antibody specificity, anti-Rg[a], reacting wth a red cell and serum antigen. *Vox Sang.* **30** 175.

Moltham, L., Crawford, M.N., Giles, C.M., Chudnoff, A. & Eichman, M.F. (1969) A new antibody Yk[a] (York) and its relationship to anti-Cs[a]. *Transfusion (Philad.),* **9,** 281.

Moulds, J.J., Polesky, H.F., Reid, M. & Ellisor, S.S. (1975) Observations on the Gya and Hy antigens and the antibodies that define them. *Transfusion (Philad.),* **15,** 270.

Pinder, L.B., Staveley, J.M., Douglas, R. & Kornstad, L. (1969) Pt[a] a new private antigen. *Vox Sang.,* **17,** 303.

Rausen, A.R., Rosenfield, R.E., Alter, A.A., Hakim, S., Graven, S.M., Appollon, C.J., Dallman, P.R., Dalziel, J.C., Konugres, A.A., Francis, B., Gavin, J. & Cleghorn, T.E. (1967) A new infrequent red cell antigen Rd (Radin). *Transfusion, (Philad.),* **7,** 336.

Roelcke, D. (1969) A new serological specificity in cold antibodies of high titre: anti-HD. *Vox Sang.,* **16,** 76.

Roelcke D., Ebert, W., & Geisen H.P. (1976) Anti-Pr₃: Serological and immunochemical identification of a new anti-Pr sub-specificity. *Vox Sang.,* **30,** 122.

Rosenfield, R.E., Haber, G.V., Kissmeyer-Nielsen, F., Jack, J.A. Sanger, R. & Race, R.R. (1960) Ge a very common red cell antigen. *Brit. J. Haem.,* **6,** 344.

Salmon, C., Salmon, D., Liberge, G., André, R., Tippett, P. & Sanger, R. (1961). Un nouvel antigène de groupe sanguin erythrocytaire present chez 80 per cent des sujets de race blanche. *Nouv. Rev. France. Hemat.,* **1,** 649.

Schmidt, R.P., Frank, S. & Baugh, M. (1967) New antibodies to high incidence antigenic determinants (anti-So, anti-El, anti-Hy and anti-Op). *Transfusion, (Philad.),* **7,** 386.

L

Simmons, R.T. & Albrey, J.A. (1963) A new blood group antigen Webb (Wb) of low frequency found in two Australian families. *Med. J. Aust.,* **1,** 8.

Simmons, R.T. & Were, S.O.M. (1955) A 'new' family blood group antigen and antibody (By) of rare occurrence. *Med. J. Aust.,* **ii,** 55.

Skov, F. (1972) A new rare blood group antigen, Je^a. *Vox Sang.,* **23,** 461.

Speiser, P., Küböck, J., Mickerts, D., Pausch, V., Reichel, G., Lauer, D., Poremba, I., Doering, I., & Hamacher, H. (1966) Kamhuber, a new human blood group antigen of familial occurrence, revealed by severe transfusion reaction. *Vox Sang.,* **11,** 113.

Stroup, M., & MacIlroy, M., (1970). Jr. five examples of an antibody defining an antigen of high frequency in the Caucasian population. *23rd Ann. Meet. AABB San Francisco,* P.86.

Sussman, L.N. & Miller, E.B. (1952) Un nouveau facteur sanguin, Vel. *Rev. D'Hem.,* **7,** 368.

Swanson, J., Zweker, M. & Polesky, H.F. (1966) A new public antigenic determinant Gy^a (Gregory). Transfusion (Philad.), **7,** 304.

Szaloky, A., Sijpesteijn, N.K. & Hart, M.V.D. (1973) A new blood group antigen, Hov. *Vox Sang.,* **24,** 535.

Tippett, P. (1963) Serological study of the inheritance of unusual Rh and other blood group phenotypes. *Ph.D. Thesis. University of London.*

Wadlington, W.B., Moore, W.H. & Hartmann, R.C. (1961) Maternal sensitisation due to Bi, a preserved 'new private' red cell antigen. *Amer. J. Dis. Ch.,* **101,** 623.

Wallace, J. & Milne, G.R. (1959) A 'new' human blood group antigen of rare frequency. *Proc. 7th Congr. Int. Soc. Blood Transf.,* 587.

Yvart, J., Gerbal, A. & Salmon, C. (1974) A new 'private' antigen, Hey. *Vox Sang.,* **26,** 41.

Section 2. Blood Transfusion

"Nothing like blood, sir, in hosses, dawgs and men".

W.M. Thackeray

Chapter 23. The Choice of Blood for Transfusion and Cross Matching Tests

Blood transfusion has developed so rapidly since the second World War that it comes as something of a shock to realise that its history goes back into the remote past. In ancient thinking the words "blood" and "life" were almost interchangeable and many endeavours were made to transfer the healthy life blood of a young man to the aged and infirm. In most cases this was done by the recipient drinking the blood; the results were, of course, rather disappointing!

As early as the sixteenth century it was realised that the transference should be from blood vessel to blood vessel, but it is not known whether such an exchange was in fact performed. Harvey's discovery of the circulation of the blood in the early seventeenth century gave a new impetus to the interest in transfusion and Lower actually kept alive, dogs, which had been exsanguinated, with blood from other dogs, transferred by connecting the carotid artery of the one to the jugular vein of the other by means of quills. The success of this venture led to attempts to transfuse Man. Animals (sheep and lambs) were used as donors, but the experiments were discontinued when the fourth recipient died. It is interesting to note that this patient had three transfusions in all, the first symptomless, the second showing typical symptoms of a haemolytic transfusion reaction and the third resulting in the patient's death.

During the latter half of the nineteenth century experiments started again, sometimes using animal blood, sometimes human, but the results were so often serious or even fatal that transfusion was abandoned. Then in 1901 Landsteiner discovered the ABO blood group system although it was not until some fifteen years later that it was universally accepted that blood grouping and direct compatibility tests were a necessary prelude to transfusion. It was then realised that if the recipient had agglutinins active at 37°C in his serum and the transfused blood had the corresponding agglutinogen, the blood would be destroyed *in vivo* and a haemolytic transfusion reaction would result.

The possibility of the destruction of the recipient's red cells by transfused

307

antibody was not considered to be a real danger because of the dilution factor. For this reason, up to about 1940, group O blood was considered safe for transfusion to all groups and was called Universal Donor Blood. Nowadays it is realised that transfusion with homologous blood, *i.e.* blood of the same type as the recipient, is to be preferred, not only because the transfusion of antibodies may be dangerous, but also because the number of potential donors is doubled; an important point when the demand for blood is steadily increasing. The titre of anti-A and anti-B antibodies in most donor blood is not dangerous so that in emergency, one unit of group O can be given with little risk, but in massive transfusions of group O blood to patients of other groups the quantity of antibody transfused becomes considerable* and may even result in the destruction of almost all the recipient's own red cells. In particular, it has been shown that exchange transfusion of infants suffering from haemolytic disease should be performed with blood of the infant's own ABO group.

The discovery of the ABO blood groups was, however, merely the beginning. Today many blood group systems are known, by means of which some hundreds of types of blood can be differentiated. Should they all be taken into consideration in choosing blood for transfusion? It is obvious that they cannot be and except in special cases only two systems are in fact considered, ABO and Rh.

When blood is transfused there are many dangers present, two of which are directly concerned with the antigen content of the transfused blood, the first being that of sensitisation, the second that of incompatibility.

In the first case the recipient does not possess the antigen found in the transfused blood nor the corresponding antibody, but the transfusion acts as a sensitising dose so that antibodies are produced in response to the transfusion or to a subsequent stimulus by the same antigen. Blood for transfusion cannot be chosen to exclude every possibility of sensitisation but fortunately most of the blood group systems are not strongly antigenic in Man and can usually be disregarded. The main exception is the Rh system, and here the problems of sensitisation must be faced. In the ABO system (where antibodies occur naturally) and in other systems whenever atypical antibodies active at 37° C have been formed the problem is not that of sensitisation but of incompatibility.

A consideration of the two systems, ABO and Rh, gives an idea of the factors involved and how best to arrive at the objective, the safe transfusion of blood.

The ABO blood group system is still the most dangerous. This is because the antibodies are naturally occurring and over 95 per cent of all recipients will have anti-A and/or anti-B in their serum. On the other hand ABO blood grouping is a straightforward procedure and the simplest of cross-matching techniques will detect any incompatibility. Most of the mistakes which occur are clerical rather than technical. Too much trouble cannot be taken to ensure that samples are correctly labelled and that compatibility labels with the patient's full name, etc., are attached to the bottles to be transfused (*see* below). On the technical side, the grouping of both recipient and donor blood should be performed on red cells and serum independently by either tube technique (No. 2.2) or moist chamber slide

---

*This is true even if donors with high titre antibodies, in particular haemolysins, are excluded.

technique (No. 2.1). The controls must never be omitted; this simple precaution would have prevented many mistakes which resulted in incompatible blood being transfused.

The final test which is performed after the careful grouping of both donor and recipient is the cross-match. This test involves incubating the patient's serum with the red cells of the prospective donors at room temperature and 37°C by techniques appropriate to the detection of antibodies which might be present in the patient's serum and which might cause an incompatible transfusion.

However meticulously the grouping of donor and patient has been carried out prior to transfusion, and however thorough the search has been for atypical antibodies in the patient's serum, *the cross-match (or direct match) should never be omitted.* The red cells that are in actual fact going to be given to the patient are the most important ones to include in any antibody detection test.

The ideal cross-matching technique for detecting any ABO incompatibility is the incubation of equal parts of the recipient's serum with 2-3 per cent suspension of donor red cells in saline at room temperature, either in a precipitin tube for 2 hours, or on a slide in a moist chamber for 30 minutes. ABO agglutination is depressed in bovine albumin and a false negative reaction may be obtained. When the time available for cross-matching is less than that recommended it is worth mixing recipient's serum and donor red cells for even as little as 5 minutes—a negative reading will not mean that the blood is necessarily compatible but if the reaction is positive, a tragedy can be averted.

In considering the Rh blood group system it must be remembered that the most antigenic of the Rh agglutinogens is D. Both anti-D and the other Rh antibodies rarely, if ever, occur naturally, being immune antibodies produced in response to stimulation by the corresponding antigen. This can occur either by transfusion, injection of blood or during pregnancy. The antibodies are active at 37°C and are, therefore, capable of causing severe and even fatal transfusion reactions.

Ideally Rh negative patients should never be transfused with Rh positive blood. When Rh negative blood is in short supply the claims of: (a) persons who already have an Rh antibody; (b) Rh negative women who are not past the child-bearing age, and (c) infants suffering from haemolytic disease of the foetus have to be given priority. It is exceedingly important that girls and young women who are Rh negative should only receive Rh negative blood, as their sensitisation may not only expose them to a possible incompatible transfusion reaction in the future, but also their Rh positive children, even the first, might suffer from haemolytic disease of the newborn.

If it is necessary to give Rh positive blood to an Rh negative person a search for even a trace of Rh antibody in the recipient's serum should be made. We would suggest that the serum is tested against a panel of Rh positive and Rh negative cells by anti-human globulin and by papain techniques. A papain technique should be included in the cross-match, as there may be Rh antibodies present which are not detectable by the anti-human globulin technique.

While the problem of sensitisation and antibody formation is seen most clearly in the immunisation of Rh negative individuals to the D antigen the other antigens must not be forgotten. The transfusion of Rh positive blood to Rh positive recipients may result in the production of anti-C, anti-E, anti-c, anti-e— the production of anti-c and anti-e can also be stimulated by the transfusion of Rh positive persons with Rh negative blood, a reminder that it is not always safe to use Rh negative blood even in emergency.

TESTING OF RECIPIENTS

It is preferable to test the recipient at least one day before the transfusion is given. In the case of patients known to be for major surgery this preliminary testing can be done on a sample taken at the out-patient clinic.

Taking of Sample and Documentation

A sample of about 10 ml of venous blood should be labelled with the patient's full name, date of birth (a much better aid than age to the establishment of identity), serial number, the ward and the date on which the sample was taken. Such a label, completed in every detail, should be attached to the sample at the patient's bedside before there is any chance of confusion with blood from another patient. Hospitals will work out their own error proof system of identifying patients and samples. The identity disc attached to the patient's wrist is almost certainly the best source of accurate information. Patients themselves may be too ill or too nervous to answer even simple questions of identity accurately. When a patient is required to confirm his identity he should not be asked whether he is John Smith but the questioner should ask "What is your name?" "Your date of birth?" etc.

Case notes attached to the patient's bed are not necessarily a reliable source of information without prior checking; patients are sometimes put into a different bed and their case notes left behind to be changed over later. More than one transfusion tragedy has occurred because a sample was incorrectly labelled.

Pretransfusion tests

Tests on Patients Requiring a Single Transfusion
(no previous transfusions or abnormal obstetric history)

The ABO group and Rh(D) type of the patient is determined and the serum screened for antibodies. The cells used for the screening test should be capable of detecting those antibodies most likely to be found in the recipient's serum. It is not often possible to find the required antigens in one individual so the screening is either carried out with cells from two donors separately or to reduce the work entailed, the cells may be pooled. It is undesirable to use a pool of cells of more than two people since this considerably reduces the sensitivity of the tests and weak antibodies may go undetected. The most important antigens to include are all the Rh antigens so R_1R_2 cells are used and these cells should have as many as possible of the following antigens, Fy^a, Fy^b, K, Jk^a, M, N, S, s and Le^a. Another useful addition when possible is C^w.

We recommend that the screening tests should include saline at 18°C, anti-human globulin and an enzyme technique preferably papain at 37°C. The albumin addition technique should also be included in laboratories not thoroughly experienced at the anti-human globulin technique. Blood of the same ABO group and Rh(D) type as the patient is selected and cross-matched (technique No. 23.4). In the rare event of incompatibility with blood of any of the prospective donors being found, the antibody causing this should be identified before a further cross-match is attempted. Only if there is little time available is it necessary to find compatible blood without identifying the causative antibody—a large pretransfusion sample should be taken so that the antibody may be identified later.

Tests on Patients Requiring a Further Transfusion

The ABO groups and Rh(D) type will almost certainly be known at this stage. Since a previous transfusion has been given which may have sensitised the patient, the screening tests outlined above must be repeated on a fresh sample taken from the patient. This sample is also used for the cross-match. On no account may the sample taken prior to the first transfusion be used as the cross-match sample for the second. If no atypical antibodies are found blood (of the same ABO group and Rh(D) type as the patient) is cross-matched. In the event of atypical antibodies being found, these should if possible be identified before the blood is selected.

Tests on Patients for Multiple Transfusions*

In addition to the tests already cited above, it is often rewarding to perform a full Rh sub-typing on patients likely to need many transfusions. Even if it is not possible to give them blood of their own Rh sub-type a knowledge of the Rh antigens possessed by the patient will form a guide to the Rh antibodies that might be formed as a result of repeated transfusion.

Ideally this sub-typing is carried out on blood taken from the patient before any transfusions are given but sometimes this is not possible and the patient will already have donor red cells mixed with his own. In order that these donor red cells may interfere as little as possible with the sub-typing results the sample for this determination is taken as long after the previous transfusion as is practicable. Even with this precaution the typing may prove difficult (but *see* technique No. 23.1).

Here again any atypical antibodies found either as a result of the antibody tests or during cross-matching, should be identified before blood is transfused.

Tests on Patients with Transfusion or Obstetric History Suggestive of Antibody Formation

The ABO grouping, full Rh sub-typing and antibody tests recommended above are the first step in the investigation of these cases. Any atypical antibody which may be present will in most instances be revealed at this stage and can then be identified. If no atypical antibody is found, an additional search against a larger panel of standard cells according to technique No. 22.1 will be necessary.

---

*Haemolytic anaemias form a special case and are dealt with in Chapter 27.

Tests on Patients whose Serum Protein Balance is Disturbed, e.g. those with Multiple Myelomatosis

In these cases an abnormality in plasma protein balance develops which results in a strong tendency for the patient's serum to cause pseudo-agglutination of all red cells including his own.

ABO grouping and Rh typing of such patients can only be carried out on well washed red cells. Serum ABO grouping is usually not possible by normal agglutination techniques, it can however be done by the anti-human globulin technique using patient's serum and standard A_1, A_2, B and O red cells.

The pseudo-agglutination has a characteristic appearance (*see* Fig. 1. 1a) and with experience becomes readily recognisable. The clumps of red cells seem to glow, there being less refraction of the light than with true agglutination where the clumps are almost opaque. However, pseudo-agglutination may mask true agglutination and, therefore, no opinion should be pronounced on the result of any test in which it appears. the indirect anti-human globulin test for antibodies can be used, as interference from pseudo-agglutination will not be encountered.

Tests on Patients who Have Received Dextran

These patients are in a similar category to those described above. The presence of dextran in the plasma results in heavy pseudo-agglutination which may mask the presence of true agglutination. The testing can usually be done on a pre-dextran sample but where this has not been taken the procedure is the same as for patients with an altered protein balance.

Tests on Patients with Atypical Antibodies

The methods employed for the identification of atypical antibodies have already been described in some detail (*see* Chapters 11 and 22). The identification should be completed before blood is chosen for the transfusion. It is because this may take some time that it is recommended that wherever possible testing should take place at least 24-hours pre-transfusion. It is often the practice to transfuse a patient whose serum contains an atypical antibody before that antibody has been identified. It is argued that from the practical point of view the identity does not matter if a careful cross-match is carried out. This is in fact only true if the atypical antibody is a fairly strong one. To rely entirely upon a cross match to detect a weak atypical antibody is to court danger, however carefully the tests are done. This is particularly true if the atypical antibody in the patient's serum is one that shows dosage. Anti-c, for instance, is characterised by showing marked dosage, therefore a weak anti-c might react with all rr (ccddee) cells with two doses of "c", whereas some R_1r (CcDee) red cells with one dose of "c" might be negative. A weak unidentified anti-c, therefore, might appear compatible with blood of phenotype R_1r but would in fact be incompatible *in vivo*.

If an atypical antibody is properly identified the blood selected for transfusion can be typed with a stronger example of the same antibody from the laboratory's collection of typing sera and this danger eliminated. When the antibody is too weak to identify no such check is possible; in which case it must be realised that if the antibody shows any activity at 37°C, although the blood appears to be compatible *in vitro* on the results of the cross match, it may in fact be incompatible *in vivo*. The clinician must be warned of this possibility so that he can take the necessary steps, *i.e.* giving the transfusion slowly, watching for clinical symptoms and also, if desired, withdrawing a sample after about 50 ml of blood has been given to be examined for haemoglobin pigments (*see* Chapter 25).

In some cases patients may have an enzyme reactive auto-antibody which reacts with their own cells and with all test and/or donor cells. In such cases the patient's serum should be absorbed with his own enzyme treated cells until there is no reaction. The absorbed serum can then be used for the cross-match by the enzyme technique.

Tests on Patients Undergoing Hypothermia

When patients are operated upon for heart defects under profound hypo-thermia, they also receive massive transfusions of blood, using a heart-lung machine.

This means that for a period of time, recipient and donor bloods are in contact at about 10°C. At this temperature the vast majority of patients have cold antibodies, auto-antibodies, anti-H, anti-I, anti-P_1, and anti-A_1, etc. If the normal saline cross-matching technique is performed at 10°C strong positive reactions are encountered in many cases, often with all bloods tested including the recipient's own blood. A different cross-matching technique (No. 23.4) has been devised for these cases using mixtures of whole blood (Batchelor *et al.*, 1966). This gives results which are closely correlated with the degree of agglutina-tion that is found on the pump and shows that in almost all cases these cold antibodies are not causing agglutination in the conditions found in the actual transfusion. If this cross-matching technique gives strong positive results attempts must be made to find more compatible blood or the patient must not be cooled to 10°C but to a temperature at which the cross-match is compatible.

This test has been done by us for several years for three units where operations under conditions for hypothermia are regularly carried out. If the special cross match is even weakly positive, and the antibody is an allo-antibody of known specificity, *e.g.* anti-A_1, anti-P_1 etc. blood is chosen compatible with that antibody. In two cases which were inadvertently cooled further than had been expected there were signs of blood destruction. In one there was evidence of intravascular destruction and in the other haematuria following the operation. Obviously these are complicated cases and there may be other reasons for the observed findings but the clinicians felt that the transfused blood was implicated. In the first case the "whole blood" cross match was positive at 8°C with all cells including the patient's own and in the second case, (also at 8°C), A_1 cells gave a positive reaction.

Changes in Blood Group Systems in Malignancy

Changes in blood group antigens or antibody content may occur in cases of malignancy so that grouping of such patients occasionally presents particular problems. Sometimes there is a lack of the allo-antibodies (anti-A and/or anti-B); this is usually because the patient has little or no gammaglobulin in his serum. Electrophoresis of his serum will confirm that the gammaglobulin is absent. On the other hand occasionally more antibody is formed, *e.g.* anti-B has been found in A_1B, etc. Sometimes an excess of blood group substances occurs in the serum which may lead to neutralisation of the anti-A and anti-B grouping sera unless the patient's cells are carefully washed several times. Anti-I antibodies are common especially in cases of leukaemia.

The commonest change in red cells is that they become poly-agglutinable due to the exposure of the T antigen on the cells, anti-T occurring in all adult human sera. Other changes which may occur are reduction in strength of the A agglutinogen, the acquiring of a pseudo-B antigen by A cells and alteration in strengths of the Rh antigens.

If anomalies occur during the testing of the cells or serum of patients with malignancy, if at all possible, the blood groups should be fully investigated possibly by a specialist laboratory before transfusion is undertaken.

CHOICE OF BLOOD

Choice of ABO group

The ABO system is potentially the most dangerous in causing incompatible blood transfusions because over 95 per cent of all recipients have anti-A and/or anti-B. On the other hand, ABO grouping is a straightforward procedure and a simple cross-matching routine will detect incompatibility.

Ideally recipients should receive at all times blood of their own ABO group but in emergencies, which may be clinical or due to shortage of blood in the blood bank, it may not always be possible to adhere to this.

Group O recipients

Whatever the circumstances there is no choice but to transfuse these recipients with group O blood.

Group A recipients

Normally group A recipients should receive group A blood. If because of exceptional circumstances, group O blood has to be given, it has to be remembered that the anti-A of group O donors is likely to be more potent than the anti-B and hence the A recipient is more at risk than a B recipient from such donor antibodies. It is inadvisable to give more than one or two units of such blood even if "high titre" donors have been screened out before the blood is selected.

The problem of subgroups of A is concerned with the advisability of giving A_1 blood to group A_2 recipients since other subgroups are rarely encountered.

Anti-A_1 occurs as a cold agglutinin in 1-2 per cent of group A_2 and about 26 per cent of group A_2B individuals, but only in a few instances does it become active at $37°C$ and cause abnormally rapid destruction of A_1 cells. Therefore routine A_1/A_2 subtyping of potential donors and recipients is not warranted but if antibody screening suggest a strong anti-A_1 active at room temperature, then post transfusion samples should be checked in case the anti-A_1 becomes immune and active at $37°C$.

Group B recipients

Since group B donors form but 8 per cent of the donor population, recipients of group B are more likely than those of group A, of occasionally receiving group O, but as far as possible they should receive blood of their own group.

Subgroups of B are very rare but it is well to note that they may constitute a cross-matching problem since they have anti-B in their plasma.

Group AB recipients

When group AB donors are unavailable either group A or group B blood can be used but group A blood is likely to be more available and its anti-B will probably be weaker than the anti-A in group B blood. It is not advisable to change from group A to B or vice versa when giving more than one unit as a continuous transfusion.

The remarks concerning A_2 given above apply to recipients of group A_2B.

As explained above, transfusing group AB patients with group O blood should be avoided at all times.

Consideration of Rh type

Ideally all D-negative individuals should receive D-negative (*i.e.* Rh negative) blood. The classes of patients taking priority when Rh negative blood is in short supply have been discussed above.

Occasionally it is necessary to consider Rh antibodies other than anti-D. Table 23.1 gives the choice of blood for patients with various Rh antibodies. Note that in

Table 23.1 The type of blood to choose for transfusion to patients whose sera contain Rh antibodies

Atypical antibody present	Type of blood to give*
Anti-D Anti-CD Anti-DE	rr (*cde/cde*)
Anti-C in D-positive patient	R_2r (*cDE/cde*) or R_2R_2 (*cDE/cDE*)
Anti-C in D-negative patient	rr (*cde/cde*)
Anti-E in R_1R_1 (*CDe/CDe*) patient (also anti-Ec)	R_1R_1 (*CDe/CDe*)
Anti-E in R_1r (*CDe/cde*) patient	R_1R_1 (*CDe/CDe*) or R_1r (*CDe/cde*)
Anti-E in D-negative patient	rr (*cde/cde*)
Anti-c	R_1R_1 (*CDe/CDe*)
Anti-e (also anti-Ce)	R_2R_2 (*cDE/cDE*)

*Probable genotype in brackets.

the case of anti-E occurring in a patient of R_1R_1 (CCDee) it is safer to assume the presence of anti-c with the anti-E even if this is not apparent at the time of the transfusion.

Other Systems

Atypical antibodies which are completely inactive at 37°C can usually be ignored when selecting blood for transfusion. However, before it is concluded that a cold antibody detectable by saline technique at room temperature is inactive at 37°C, the indirect anti-human globulin test with the addition of complement (technique No. 23.2) should be performed as activity at 37°C demonstrable by this technique is accompanied by a diminished survival *in vivo* of red cells containing the corresponding antigen. The transfusion reactions due to such antibodies are usually mild, the main effect of the incompatibility being a failure to achieve full benefit from the transfused blood.

If the atypical antibodies are active at 37°C they must be taken into account and the appropriate blood selected *e.g.* K negative blood for patients with anti-K, $Fy^{a'}$ negative blood for those with ani-Fy^a etc.

Some patients may form mixtures of antibodies. When complicated mixtures are found it may take some time to find compatible blood not only because it is advisable to identify the antibodies but also compatible donors may be difficult to obtain.

When blood which is really rare is required for patients whose antibody is incompatible with all but a handful of donors scattered throughout the world an international panel of donors of rare types has to be consulted. The British National Blood Transfusion Service holds a record of these donors. An international blood bank of rare donors is held at the Central Laboratory of the Netherlands Red Cross Blood Transfusion Service in Amsterdam. The units of blood stored there at a temperature of –196°C maintain their efficiency for at least 5 years, the red cell survival rate comparing favourably with that of fresh blood.

CROSS-MATCHING (OR DIRECT-MATCHING) OF BLOOD FOR TRANSFUSION

Non-emergency Transfusions

Serum from the recipient should be tested against the cells of the donor by technique No. 23.3 which includes:

(1) Saline tube technique at R.T. 18°C.
(2) Saline tube technique at 37°C.
(3) Albumin Addition technique at 37°C.
(4) Indirect anti-human globulin technique at 37°C.
(5) Papain technique at 37°C (in special cases and especially where Rh positive blood is being given to an Rh negative recipient).

In cases where an atypical antibody has been detected by another technique this must also be included as part of the cross-match.

Moreover, the indirect anti-human globulin plus complement method (technique No. 23.2) should be included wherever cold agglutinins are present in the recipient's serum. The testing of the recipient's serum with his own red cells by each of the techniques employed should be included as a negative control. The reasons for selecting each particular method are given below so that the dangers that may arise from omitting any of the tests may be appreciated.

(1) *Saline Tube Technique at 18° C.* This is the optimum temperature and medium for the detection of ABO incompatibility and potent cold agglutinins.

(2) *Saline Tube Technique at 37° C.* This is the optimum temperature and medium for the detection of "warm" agglutinins (complete antibodies).

(3) *Albumin Addition Technique at 37° C.* This is a good technique for the detection of most Rh incomplete antibodies although a few of them may show a prozone. Incomplete antibodies of other blood group systems may not show up well by this method. It is an easier technique at which to become proficient than the indirect anti-human globulin but may be omitted in a laboratory experienced in the latter technique.

(4) *Indirect anti-human globulin at 37° C.* This technique should never be omitted. It is highly efficient in the detection of all kinds of incomplete antibodies.

(5) *Papain Technique at 37° C.* This is a most sensitive antibody detection technique. It is not included in all cross-matching because there is a tendency to give positives due to auto-antibodies and it is exremely sensitive so that weak cold antibodies are detected, for example anti-P_1 or anti-Lewis, whose presence does not constitute a transfusion hazard. Some Rh antibodies detected by this technique will not be detectable by any other method.

THE *IN VIVO* SIGNIFICANCE OF *IN VITRO* FINDINGS

In the foregoing it has been assumed that the cross-matching test outlined will detect all clinically important antibodies and that any antibody so detected would have adverse effects *in vivo*. This is in the main true but it may be of interest to consider what is known of the correlation between *in vivo* and *in vitro* findings. When blood is transfused into a recipient there may be one of three main patterns of survival: (1) The blood may be very rapidly destroyed, in which case there is almost invariably a pre-existing antibody and it is usually easily detectable by one of the methods recommended as part of a normal cross-match. (2) The blood may survive normally for a time, then an immune response may occur in the recipient to a transfused antigen and then cells carrying that antigen will be eliminated more rapidly. In this case the pre-transfusion cross match will be negative but an antibody will usually be demonstrable *in vitro* at, or soon after the time at which the abnormally rapid destruction of the incompatible cells takes place. (3) The blood may survive normally.

It has been shown that all antibodies which have haemolytic characteristics *in vitro* will destroy red cells, some rapidly (*e.g.* anti-A, anti-B) when the destruction is mainly intravascular, and some more slowly (anti-Le[a] and Le[b]) where the destruction is mainly extra-vascular. Most agglutinating antibodies whether or not they bind complement cause extravascular destruction of cells, mainly in the liver. These antibodies are usually detected by saline technique at 37°C and also at room temperature. Antibodies detectable by anti-human globulin technique ("incomplete" antibodies) will cause extravascular destruction, mainly in the liver if they bind complement and in the spleen if they do not. (Rh antibodies fall into the latter category) (*see also* Chapter 25). Antibodies detectable only by enzyme techniques do not usually cause immediate destruction of transfused cells, but in many cases the second pattern of survival is seen where the cells survive normally for some hours or even days and then an immune response occurs in the recipient and the cells are eliminated. At this stage the antibody is usually detectable by anti-human globulin as well as enzyme techniques.

Lewis antibodies deserve a special mention. Recipients whose sera contain these antibodies active at 37°C will lyse Le[a] or Le[b] positive incompatible cells. If, however, plasma which contains Lewis substances is given prior to transfusion the recipient's antibodies will be neutralised. This is only a temporary phenomenon as an immune response usually takes place and even more potent antibodies may be produced. Blood given during the neutralisation phase often survives normally however as after some days in the circulation of an Le (a–b–) recipient they will lose their Lewis antigens and become phenotypically Le (a-b-). A classic case was reported by Mollison *et al.* (1963) and this technique has been used successfully by us when it was necessary to give Lewis positive blood to a Le (a–b–) recipient.

Deliberate studies of *in vivo* survival corresponding to various *in vitro* results have been made, the best method being labelling a small quantity of cells with [51]Cr. For comparative studies a sample of the patient's own cells labelled with ^{32}P is usually used. Such studies have not only been informative in studying the *in vivo* effect described above where there was an antibody incompatible at 37°C with the transfused cells but they have also yielded evidence with regard to the importance (or lack of it) of cold agglutinins active at temperatures between 29°C and 37°C. It has been shown that antibodies which are not reactive at 30°C rarely, if ever, cause abnormal destruction. If they react definitely at 30°C and only weakly or not at all at 37°C *in vitro* they usually only destroy a portion of the transfused cells. The degree of destruction correlates with the thermal range and with the strength of the antigen and antibody. In one case with an anti-HI weakly active at 37°C by anti-human globulin test and more strongly at 30°C as a saline agglutinin, over 80 per cent of group O cells were eliminated rapidly but A_2 cells showed no significant destruction (Mollison, 1959; Mollison 1972). In practice, however, if specific antibodies, *e.g.* anti-A_1, anti-P_1, anti-HI, anti-M are detected at room temperature it is usual for blood compatible with the antibodies to be chosen even though they may have no 30 - 37°C activity *in vitro*. If it is necessary to give blood incompatible at room temperature (*e.g.* to a patient who has anti-e and anti-P_1 for whom it may not be possible to obtain enough e-negative P_1 negative blood in emergency) the tests should be repeated at 30°C and 37°C by saline and anti-human globulin techniques (using the two stage test with the addition of complement technique No. 22.6). If these tests are negative the blood can be given.

TECHNIQUES

Technique No. 23.1. Typing of patients with transfused blood in their circulation

For these cases the typing sera used should be the most potent available. The setting up of the tests with the appropriate anti-sera in no way differs from the methods already described. A negative reaction can be interpreted as applying to both recipient and donor, as can a strong positive reaction with practically no free cells. When, however, the red cells of one react with a particular anti-serum, while those of the other do not, a "mixed blood" picture is obtained (*see* Fig. 23.1). The full interpretation of a "mixed blood" picture can only be made with a

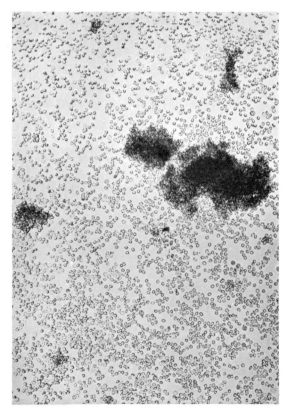

Fig. 23.1 "Mixed blood" appearance.

knowledge of the history of the case. For instance where Rh negative blood has been given in an emergency to a patient of Rh type unknown a "mixed blood" picture with anti-D serum on a post-transfusion sample clearly indicates that the recipient is Rh positive as the unagglutinated cells must be those of the Rh negative donor. In a more involved case, where it is desired to ascertain the full Rh sub-type of a patient for multiple transfusion who has already received Rh positive blood—the position is complicated if the Rh sub-type of the donor also is unknown. The proportion of agglutinated to free cells is the only guide as to which cells belong to the recipient and which to the donor and where large amounts of blood have been transfused even this fails. If difficulty is experienced in judging the proportion of agglutinated to free cells, mixtures of known constitution should be made and used as a standard for comparison.

In cases where the proportions are almost equal, the problem can ony be resolved by waiting until the circulation is relatively free from donor cells. If in the interim period it is essential to give further transfusions, the blood used must all be of the same sub-type as that first transfused. How this clarifies the position can be seen from the following protocol:

Table 23.2 Typing of patient with transfused blood in circulation

Sample	Date	Anti-A	Anti-B	Anti-C	Anti-D	Anti-E	Anti-c	Conclusion
Recipient	12/2/68	–	–	C	C	MB*	C	Mixture of O, R_1r and OR_1R_2
1st donor	15/4/68	–	–	C	C	–	C	OR_1r
2nd donor	15/4/68	–	–	C	C	–	C	OR_1r
3rd donor	15/4/68	–	–	C	C	–	C	OR_1r
Recipient	8/5/68	–	–	C	C	MB*	C	Mixture of O, R_1r, (donors) and OR_1R_2 (recipient)

*Mixed blood.

The O R_1r blood in sample dated 8/5/68 has come from the April transfusion—blood transfused before 12th February, 1968, would no longer be in the recipient's circulation on 8th May, 1968. The reaction with anti-E is, therefore, due to the recipient's own red cells being E positive and the recipient has been typed as O R_1R_2.

Technique No. 23.2. The investigation of a cold agglutinin for 37° C activity by the indirect anti-human globulin plus complement technique

Apart from the following modifications this technique is identical with technique No. 22.6 to which reference should be made for all practical details.

The serum containing the cold agglutinin is tested against cells which: (a) give a positive, and (b) give a negative reaction by saline technique at room temperature. The separate reagents including the complement are warmed to 37°C before being mixed. The tests are maintained at 37°C during the washing stage but the actual reading can be done at room temperature.

Technique No. 23.3. Cross-matching

First the necessary arrangement of tubes in racks is made to cover the whole cross-matching procedure, allowing for the testing of the patient's serum against

red cells from each proposed donor and his own cells by the following techniques:

(a) Saline tube technique incubating at room temperature.
(b) Saline tube technique incubating at 37°C.
(c) Albumin addition technique incubating at 37°C.
(d) Indirect anti-human globulin technique incubating at 37°C.
(e) Papain technique incubating at 37°C for selected cases only preferably
      by the one-stage technique (technique No. 8.5a).

The patient's serum is then run into all appropriate tubes and its presence in
them checked.

The patient's red cells and those from each unit are washed three times in
saline, and are then diluted to make 2 per cent suspensions. The usual control for
albumin and anti-human globulin tests of a weak incomplete anti-D with known
D positive and D negative red cells is included. After the red cells have been
added to the tubes, the saline tests are incubated for 2 hours, the albumin tests for
1 to 1½ hours after which one drop of albumin is added to each tube and they are
allowed to stand for a further 30 minutes, and the indirect anti-human globulin
tests for 1 hour. At the end of 1 hour the latter can be completed and read while
the remainder of the tests are undergoing the further incubation. The tubes
containing papain are read after 1 hour's incubation.

Results should be recorded in detail giving strengths of agglutination by means
of the usual symbols. Incompatibility detected between the patient's serum and
the red cells of any of the donors necessitates the identification of the causative
antibody. For this investigation technique No. 22.1 may be required. A positive
reaction between the patient's serum and his own cells due to auto-agglutination
is likely to be reflected in the results obtained against donor red cells also, since
auto-agglutinins are almost invariably pan-agglutinins. A positive reaction
between the patient's serum and his own red cells must be followed up by a direct
anti-human globulin test (technique No. 8.3b) since this is likely to be positive
indicating that the patient's red cells are sensitised by antibody *in vivo*. In such
cases a further investigation must be undertaken (*see* Chapter 27).

Technique No. 23.4. Cross-matching of blood for hypothermia patients

The Whole Blood Test. Whole blood for the patient is made up using equal
volumes of the patient's serum and packed washed cells. Citrated blood in the
proportions of 4 parts of blood to one of ACD as in stored blood of the
appropriate group is used as the donor whole blood.

The patient's whole blood and the donor whole blood are then run into 9×50-
mm tubes in the following proportions:

Patient's whole blood	9	8	7	6	5
Donor whole blood	1	2	3	4	5

A tube containing patient's whole blood and a tube containing donor whole
blood are included in the test as controls.

The blood is left at the appropriate temperature (usually 10°C) for 2 hours. Saline is cooled to the temperature of the test and is used to dilute the whole bloods on a microscope slide before reading microscopically.

This test is used in addition to the normal cross-matching technique (No. 23.3).

CARE OF A HOSPITAL BLOOD BANK

It is not inappropriate as an addendum to this chapter to consider the workings of a hospital blood bank since this is the source of the donor blood that is used for cross-matching.

Keeping of Records

The documentation for such a bank is relatively straightforward. Blood is received weekly or fortnightly from the Transfusion Service and should be booked into a ledger keeping the various groups separate and also the Rh positive and Rh negative supplies within these groups. The fate of the blood should also be recorded here, *i.e.* to whom transfused and the outcome of the transfusion or, if unused, the date of return to the Transfusion Centre.

Refrigeration

The blood must be stored at a temperature of 4°-6°C. It is important that this temperature should not vary by more than plus or minus 2°C so that some kind of temperature recorder, such as the Cambridge recorder, must be employed to keep a running check on the temperature inside the refrigerator. If blood should happen to be over-cooled and thereby partially frozen, it must be discarded as dangerous for transfusion. Care should be taken to ensure that the temperature within the refrigerator is even and that there are no areas in which the blood might become frozen; in particular it must always be protected from coming in contact with the freezing compartment. It is convenient, where possible, particularly in hospitals running a large bank, to have alternative refrigerator accommodation in case one refrigerator breaks down or becomes inefficient.

Ageing of Blood

It is generally agreed that the effective life of a unit of blood is three weeks from the day of bleeding the donor, although blood stored for longer periods can be used with safety but with slightly less good results. Blood should be used in strict date order, the oldest being issued first unless there are special indications for the use of fresh blood.

Cross-matched Blood

A label must be attached to any unit of blood which has been cross-matched giving full details of the patient—name, date of birth, ward, and most important of all, the serial number from the patient's identity disc.* This will have been obtained from the label of the blood sample from the patient used for cross-match. This number, on the label of the cross-matched blood, must be *checked again with the patient's wrist identity disc* before the transfusion is begun.

---

*If the method of having a wrist identity disc is used.

It cannot be emphasised too often that careful and meticulous cross-matching procedure in the laboratory has sometimes been of no avail on account of mistaken identity in the wards.

REFERENCES

Batchelor, E.M., Boorman, K.E., Lincoln, P.J. & Zeitlin, R.A. (1966) Technique for the evaluation of cold antibodies in cases for operation under hypothermia. *J. clin. Path.*, **19**, 348.
Mollison, P.L. (1959) Blood group antibodies and red cell destruction. *Brit. med. J.*, **ii**, 1035 & 1123.
Mollison, P.L. (1972) Blood Transfusion in Clinical Medicine. 5th ed., pp. 474. Oxford: Blackwell.
Mollison, P.L., Polley, M.J. & Crome, P. (1963) Temporary suppression of Lewis blood group antibodies to permit incompatible transfusion. *Lancet*, **i**, 909.

Chapter 24. Emergency Transfusions

An emergency transfusion is a matter for close co-operation between the pathologist and the clinician who has requested and will give the blood. The degree of the emergency has to be weighed against the risks involved if there is insufficient time for the normal cross-match to be performed. There is no emergency so great that some sort of cross-matching cannot be carried out even if it is done while the transfusion apparatus is being set up or while plasma or blood substitutes are being given.

Sometimes a state of emergency is created unnecessarily as when the laboratory is requested at the last minute to provide blood for a patient whose time of operation was booked days beforehand. Once a laboratory allows itself to be persuaded to enact such requirements these will become a habit which may dangerously reduce the efficiency of the cross-matching service.

The wisdom of appointing experienced workers for emergency serological procedures cannot be over-emphasised; particularly is this essential for night emergencies when even a specialist may find the conditions a strain and the inexperienced find themselves without an authority to whom to refer in difficulty.

Materials for Emergency Work

A laboratory which normally undertakes a fair amount of routine serological testing will probably find it unnecessary to make special preparations for emergencies which may occur during the day. They can be dealt with using the materials which are readily available but for night work a special rack of reagents should be set aside. This rack should contain the following:

(1) Anti-A, anti-B, and anti-D anti-sera all well tried for the emergency technique selected.
(2) Positive and negative control cells on these anti-sera.
(3) Anti-human globulin reagent diluted ready for use.
(4) Controls for the anti-human globulin test ready washed for preliminary testing of the reagent and for the direct ahg technique. For the actual cross-match, controls should be set up at the same time as the test itself and receive exactly the same treatment.

Choice of Rapid Typing Techniques for Emergency Work

Choice of method for emergency tests will be influenced by the availability of potent anti-sera. Rapid ABO grouping presents little difficulty providing both

Table 24.1 Rapid Methods for Rh Typing

Type of method	Designation	Principle	Advantages	Disadvantages	Time taken		Reference
					For incubation (min)	Complete test* (min)	
(a) capillary	1. Chown	Angled capillary. Positives show beaded appearance	Sensitive. Economical	Macroscopic only. Occasional false positive which should show up in control	20	35	Technique No. 24.1
	2. Chown with papain	As above	As above. Range of suitable sera increased because of papain	As above	15	30	Technique No. 24.2
(b) Slide	3. Moist chamber	Saline or albumin type anti-D incubated in moist atmosphere	Wide range of anti-sera suitable. Rapid. Microscopic	Fewer false negatives than 3. Easy to prepare	15	25	Technique No. 7.1
	4. Papain slide	Incomplete anti-D + papain + cells on slide	Rapid. Microscopic	Only certain anti-sera suitable. Some false negatives. Papain control essential	15	25	Hekker et al. (1957)
(c) Tube	5. Papain tube	Incomplete anti-D + papain + cells in tube centrifuged	Rapid. Wide range of anti-sera. Microscopic	Papain control essential	10	20	Technique No. 24.3
	6. Centrifuge tube	Saline or albumin type anti-D incubated in tube and centrifuged	Rapid. Microscopic	Only certain anti-sera suitable. May give false positives with albumin anti-sera	15	25	Technique No. 24.4
	7. Polyvinyl-pyrroli-done	Incomplete anti-D + Polyvinylpyrrolidone	Rapid	Macroscopic only. Tendency to false positives if read microscopically	15	25	McNeil et al. (1952)

*Includes time for washing cells.

cells and serum are tested and a control of the patient's cells suspended in saline is examined under the conditions of the method chosen.

There is considerable variation in preferred methods between different laboratories. The following points should be noted when selecting an Rh-typing method for emergency work. Several hundred tests by the chosen technique should be compared with tests done by standard tube method before it is put into general use. Choice should be made in favour of a method which will give false negative rather than false positive results. Rh negative blood can almost always be safely given to an apparently Rh negative recipient who is in fact Rh positive but the reverse procedure may be disastrous. It is an advantage to select a method by which the result may be confirmed microscopically if necessary.

The authors cannot claim detailed knowledge of every rapid Rh typing technique. Table 24.1 gives a representative selection; methods considered most reliable are described at the end of the chapter.

The methods are broadly divided into 3 classes:

(*a*) capillary,
(*b*) slide,
(*c*) tube with use of centrifuge.

Each class has both its advantages and drawbacks. Capillary methods are extremely sensitive and a wide range of anti-sera are suitable. The chosen technique either with or without the addition of papain can become very reliable in experienced hands particularly if a control of patient's red cells put up with AB serum in place of the typing serum, is included. The chief disadvantage is that the results cannot be easily confirmed under a microscope. It is possible to blow gently the contents of a capillary on to a slide but it is not easy to do this without breaking up the fragile clumps of cells.

It is easier to acquire proficiency at slide tests and they are very reliable provided controls are never omitted. In practice it will be found that most saline and many albumin routine Rh typing sera are suitable so that supply of anti-sera for this method is not a problem.

The papain slide test has been used by the originators for an impressively large number of tests. Our impression however was that only certain anti-D sera were suitable; we prefer the papain centrifuge tube test which is very good indeed and does not require the selection of particularly potent anti-sera as does technique No. 24.4.

The tube tests using a centrifuge are very easy to set up and centrifugation after approximately ten minutes' incubation hastens the development of the agglutination. Nevertheless, there is always the possibility with centrifuge methods of obtaining both false positives and false negatives when re-suspending the cell sediment after centrifugation. This tendency is reduced to a minimum when the anti-serum selected gives good macroscopic agglutination after the tube is tapped gently with the finger.

The polyvinylpyrrolidone method is mentioned as being representative of a class of technique employing substances to develop rapidly the agglutination of the incomplete anti-D. There is a high tendency to rouleaux formation which makes the test unreliable unless read only macroscopically. It is not recommended.

In Table 24.2 can be seen the procedures that are recommended for varying lengths of time available for cross-matching. The times quoted do not allow for the collection of the patient's blood or the assembly of the necessary apparatus and reagents. The ABO group and Rh type will often be known (arising from the practice of testing at the ante-natal or outpatients clinics); the procedure when this is so, is given in section (a) while section (b) deals with completely untested cases.

Procedure No. 1 in this table is the full-scale non-emergency technique which is recommended as being the safest procedure and is included for comparison. A reduction in the overall time available, to 2 hours (procedure 2) means a reduction in the incubation period with the attendant hazard of missing agglutination that may not be very strong by saline and albumin techniques. The indirect anti-human globulin technique with its normal incubation period of 1 hour will be unaffected. A modification of the ahg test using cells suspended in a low ionic strength medium (0.03 M NaCl) allows the incubation time of the test to be reduced to 5-10 minutes without loss of sensitivity (Löw and Messeter, 1974). These workers have used this method routinely for more than six years. Preliminary experiments in our laboratory have yielded favourable results. Procedure No. 3 relies upon the moist chamber slide technique (a slight modification of technique No. 2.1) to detect an ABO incompatibility and the rapid indirect anti-human globulin for warm atypical antibodies. In procedure No. 4 the emergency slide test (technique No. 24.6) is by no means infallible but is preferable to no cross-match at all. Procedures No. 5 and 6 recommend moist chamber slide grouping of patient (technique No. 2.1) with a rapid method of determining whether the patient is D positive or D negative (see Table 24.1).

Table 24.2(a) Cross-matching procedure. ABO Group and Rh type of Patient Known

Time	Cross-match techniques	Remarks
(1) 2½-3 hr	Saline, R.T. Saline, albumin, and indirect anti-human globulin at 37°C Papain, trypsin, trypsin anti-human globulin or indirect anti-human globulin + complement where indicated. Maximum incubation time, 2hr.	The procedure for all but emergencies.
(2) 2 hr	As (1), but maximum incubation period reduced to 1 hr	Cell sediments should be handled with extreme care as agglutination may be fragile
(3) ¾ hr	Moist chamber slide technique at R.T. Indirect anti-human globulin at 37°C incubating for 20 min in water bath	Will detect ABO incompatibilities and strong atypical antibodies. May miss antibodies of low titre
(4) ¼ hr or less	Emergency slide test 24.6 followed by procedure (3)	Allow blood to go to ward on result of slide test

Table 24.2(*b*) ABO Group and Rh type of Patient Unknown

Time	Testing of recipient	Cross-match techniques	Remarks
(5) 3 hr	ABO moist chamber Rh moist chamber	As for (1)	The typing of the recipient is checked by standard tube techniques at the same time as the cross-match
(6) 1½ hr	ABO moist chamber Rh moist chamber	As for (3)	
(7) ¾ hr or less	ABO slide	As for (3) or (4)	Cross-match one unit of Rh negative blood of appropriate ABO group. For any further blood required proceed as (6)

Procedure No. 7 allows no time for Rh typing. ABO grouping by slide method is done and Rh negative blood of the appropriate ABO group used pending Rh typing.

TECHNIQUES

Technique No. 24.1. Chown capillary technique (Fig. 24.1)

The apparatus for this technique consists of capillary tubes, internal diameter 0.5 mm (the diameter is important and must be between 0.4 mm and 0.6 mm) and length 10-15 cm, and a rack with notches to hold the tubes at an angle of 45°. For reading purposes the tubes are illuminated from behind and a hand magnifying lens is used.

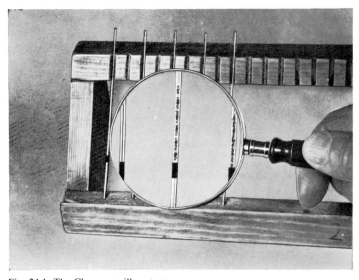

Fig. 24.1. The Chown capillary test.

The anti-serum should be saline agglutinating and of such potency that it can be diluted at least 1 in 4 with saline. It is essential that the red cells should be thrice washed and made up to a 50 per cent suspension in saline. One end of a capillary tube is dipped into the anti-serum and a column of fluid approximately 2 cm in height is permitted to run in. The capillary is next dipped into the washed cells and a column of red cell suspension equal in length to the column of serum is drawn up. Care must be taken to ensure that there is no air bubble between serum and cells. The capillary tube is then inverted so that the red cells are above the serum and the lower end quickly dipped into petroleum jelly to seal. It is then placed in the special rack. Controls of known D positive and D negative red cells are included and also the patient's cells with AB serum.

The tests are incubated for 20 minutes at 37°C and then read against a white illuminated background with, if necessary, the assistance of a hand lens. A beaded appearance of cells formed along the lower side of the capillary indicates a positive reaction wheras a thin smooth line of red cells indicates a negative.

Comment. This method, when performed with suitable sera, washed cells and adequate controls, can, in the hands of the experienced worker, become very reliable. Unfortunately, it is quite often performed with unwashed or insufficiently washed cells, with undiluted sera, without discrimination between saline and albumin anti-sera and even sometimes with serum diluted in albumin. In these circumstances it is a very unreliable technique. The supplies of sera suitable for this technique are not adequate for all the Rh testing that has to be done; moreover it is very risky to assume that Rh sera issued for use by the tube technique will give satisfactory results by the Chown test.

Technique No. 24.2. Chown capillary technique (modified Gilbey) using papain

This is essentially the same as the previous technique. The anti-serum used is incomplete anti-D and need not be of particularly high titre. It is mixed in a tube with an equal part of Löw's papain before being drawn up into the capillary. With the papain present, the reactions develop a little more quickly than in the first Chown method described.

Technique No. 24.3. Papain tube technique

One volume of incomplete anti-D is pipetted into each of the requisite number of precipitin tubes followed by an equal volume of Löw's papain. Then a 2 per cent suspension of once washed red cells from the patient and from Rh positive and Rh negative controls are added to the appropriate tubes. These are then incubated in a water bath at 37°C for 5-10 minutes and then slowly centrifuged.

Reading is effected by tapping each tube gently with the finger; positives give strong macroscopic agglutination. Tests appearing negative are examined under the microscope.

Technique No. 24.4. Centrifuge tube technique

This is essentially the same as the papain tube technique but omitting the use of papain. It is most satisfactory when a potent saline anti-D is used. Incubation is for 15 minutes in a water bath. The tubes are tapped gently but great care must be exercised to avoid the false positives which may be obtained when handling gently to avoid false negatives!

Technique No. 24.5. Emergency cross-match (½ to 1 hr)

When an emergency arises which will not allow time for the full cross-matching technique (technique No. 23.3) we recommend a modification (*see* Table 24.2) which will detect an ABO incompatibility and most atypical antibodies. It consists of two tests only:

(1) Moist chamber slide at R.T.

One drop of the patient's serum is mixed with one drop of 2 per cent suspension of washed red cells on a carefully labelled slide (*see* technique No. 2.1). The tests are allowed to stand in the moist chamber for 10-15 minutes, and the results read, all negative reactions being checked microscopically.

(2) Indirect anti-human globulin at 37°C. As in technique No. 23.3, the tests should be made with the patient's serum against red cells from each proposed donor and his own cells. This control of own cells should never be omitted.

The indirect anti-human globulin test is set up in the usual way except that as the incubation time is cut to a minimum of 20 minutes, it is advisable to warm the tubes, saline, etc., to 37°C before setting up the test. Moreover, a water bath is preferable to a hot air incubator. After 20 minutes' incubation the procedure is as in technique No. 8.3a.

It is possible that this technique may fail to reveal an incompatibility due to a weakly reacting antibody. For this reason the clinician should always be informed that only an "emergency" cross-match has been done.

Technique No. 24.6. Emergency cross-match (¼ hr or less)

It should be emphasised that this method will not detect every incompatibility and it must never be used when the transfusion of blood can be delayed for as much as 30 minutes. In fact its use is restricted to those grave emergencies in which the only alternative would be to transfuse without a cross-match. It will detect most ABO incompatibilities, a few Rh incompatibilities, *e.g.* those caused by potent saline agglutinins, some very potent cold agglutinins but very little else.

The sample from the patient should be taken into heparin or sequestrene and centrifuged. Two drops of the supernatant cell-free plasma are mixed on an opalescent tile with one drop of blood direct from the bottle (*i.e.* whole blood diluted with ACD). The use of recipient plasma rather than serum allows blood from the bottle to be used without washing—serum would cause a clot. The sensitivity of the test is slightly reduced by using unwashed cells but there would be no time available for washing. The tile is gently rocked and read, preferably over a light, after 2 and 5 minutes. If there is any agglutination the blood should not be used. If the blood appears compatible it may be given, the results being confirmed while the transfusion is in progress.

REFERENCES

Hekker, A.C., Klomp-Magnee, W., Krijnen, H.W. & Van Loghem, J.J. (1957) A papain slide test for
    Rh mass typing. *Vox Sang.*, **2**, 128.
Löw, B. & Messeter, L. (1974) Anti-globulin test in low-ionic strength salt solution for rapid antibody
    screening and cross-matching. *Vox Sang.*, **26**, 53.
McNeil, C., Trentelman, E.F., Sullivan, N.P. & Argall, C.I. (1952) A new rapid Rh tube test using
    polyvinylpyrrolidone (PVP). *Amer. J. clin. Path.* **22**, 1216.

Chapter 25. The Investigation of Haemolytic Transfusion Reactions

A haemolytic transfusion reaction may be defined as the occurrence of abnormal destruction of red cells of either the donor or the recipient following a transfusion. Antibodies *per se* do not directly damage red cells possessing the corresponding antigen but because the cell becomes coated with antibody either complement is activated allowing haemolysis to occur or, the antibody-coated cell is engulfed by a phagocyte and removed from the circulation.

After a normal compatible transfusion of fresh blood the donor's red cells are destroyed at a slow rate, a little less than 1 per cent of the total being eliminated per day. When incompatible blood is given the donor's erythrocytes are usually rapidly destroyed, even within a few hours of transfusion, and clinical signs of the rapid red cell destruction may develop. Destruction of some of the recipient's own cells may follow transfusion of blood, if the plasma contains high titre incompatible agglutinins.

Although the clinical diagnosis of incompatible transfusion is outside the province of the serologist, it is useful for him to be able to interpret the findings in a given case because the clinical picture will often influence the serological testing. Where the clinical diagnosis is in doubt the search for an antibody which could have caused the reaction need not be so extensive.

The clinical features any of which may accompany an incompatible transfusion reaction are as follows: rigor, generalised tinglings, bursting headaches, constricting chest pains, feelings of heat and severe lumbar pains. In addition, signs of collapse, cold clammy skin, cyanosis, feeble pulse and hypotension may be noted. Later, jaundice, haemoglobinuria, and oliguria may develop. Alternatively, there may be no clinical symptoms at the time of transfusion. This, of course, constitutes a grave danger since in these circumstances a large amount of blood can be transfused without the incompatibility being suspected.

When it is thought from the clinical findings that a haemolytic transfusion reaction has occurred, the first point to establish is that haemolysis of red cells has taken place. Some of the clinical features mentioned above, particularly severe rigors* can accompany compatible transfusions and, therefore, cannot be used for differential diagnosis. The clinical picture is also affected by whether the destruction is mainly intra-vascular or extra-vascular. In the first case there will

---

* Rigors due to pyrogens are not now common and any severe rigor should be investigated; besides a haemolytic reaction other causes may be due to an allergic reaction, to HLA antibodies, to IgA antibodies etc.

be massive liberation of haemoglobin from cells destroyed in the circulation, while in the second there will only be at most a mild degree of haemoglobinaemia. This is believed to be the result of a small number of incompatible red cells being partially digested by monocytes and forming microspherocytes which subsequently lyse.

INTRAVASCULAR AND EXTRAVASCULAR HAEMOLYSIS

Intravascular haemolysis of transfused incompatible red cells is produced almost exclusively by those antibodies which are readily haemolytic *in vitro e.g.* anti-A and anti-B. Up to 90 per cent of the red cells may be lysed in the plasma when the antibody is powerful, the remainder being phagocytosed. If the haemolysis shown by the antibody *in vitro* is only weak then the elimination of cells may be chiefly extravascular.

Anti-Le^a sometimes haemolyses Le^a positive cells at 37°C *in vitro* but the rate of haemolysis is slow and the destruction of the cells *in vivo* is mainly extravascular.

Antibodies which do not cause haemolysis *in vitro* cause extravascular destruction of the red cells in the liver and spleen. This does not mean, however, that haemoglobin is not sometimes seen in the plasma. Some red cells may become damaged by macrophages or the reticulo-endothelial system may not be able to clear haemoglobin-haptoglobin complexes and so haemoglobin builds up in the plasma.

Influence of antibody properties on red cell destruction

Antibody concentration, IgG class, ability to fix complement, temperature of activity and concentration of antigen are all factors influencing the rate and site of destruction of incompatible red cells.

The antibodies mentioned above as causing intravascular haemolysis are mainly IgM and are capable of activating complement. The most important examples of both IgG and IgM antibodies which do not activate complement are those of the Rh system. Red cells sensitised by IgM Rh antibodies are removed predominantly by the liver while those sensitised by IgG are removed mainly by the spleen.

The relationship between the immunological characteristics of examples of various antibodies and the destruction of red cells by them *in vivo* is given in Table 25.1. Example rates of destruction are also given in this table but these vary considerably according to factors such as the amount of incompatible cells given. As might be expected, antibodies which haemolyse red cells rapidly *in vitro* produce the fastest removal of cells *in vivo*. Also, complement binding IgG antibodies destroy red cells more efficiently than those which are non-complement binding.

The volume of incompatible cells influences their rate of destruction in that larger volumes are eliminated more slowly than smaller amounts. Also the number of antigen sites per red cell appears to play a part. For example there is evidence that A$_1$ cells are eliminated more rapidly than A$_2$ when injected into a

Table 25.1 Relationship between immunological characteristics of antibodies and their effect upon incompatible red cells *in vivo*.

Immunological characteristics	Examples	IgG Class	Destruction *in vivo*	Examples of rate of destruction *in vivo*
Haemolytic				
Rapid	Anti-A, anti-B	IgM or IgG	Mainly intravascular	Rapid *e.g.* 90 per cent in 2 min (small vol. cells) 50 per cent in 2 min (large vol. cells)
Slow	Anti-Le^a, anti-Le^b	IgM	Mainly extravascular	Slow *e.g.* 60 per cent in 4 min (small vol. cells)
Agglutinating				
C-binding	Anti-P$_1$ (if potent)	IgM	Extravascular (mainly in liver)	25 per cent in 20 min (1 ml cells)
Not C-binding	Anti-Rh (D, c etc)	IgM	Extravascular (mainly in liver)	50 per cent in 2-3 min (anti-c)
Incomplete				
C-binding	Anti-Jk^a, some anti-Fy^a and anti-K	IgG	Extravascular (mainly in liver)	50 per cent in 4-6 min (anti-Fy^a, anti-K) 50 per cent in 1 hr (small vol.)
Not C-binding	Anti-Rh (D, c etc)	IgG	Extravascular (mainly in spleen)	50 per cent in 14 hr (large vol.) } anti-D

Data from Mollison P.L. (1972) Blood Transfusion in Clinical Medicine Oxford, Blackwell.

group O recipient and that red cells of individuals homozygous for an antigen are destroyed more quickly than those of the heterozygote *e.g.* $Jk^a Jk^a$ cells are removed more rapidly than $Jk^a Jk^b$ cells.

Evidence for haemolysis

For this at least 10 ml. of blood taken as soon as possible after the incompatible transfusion has occurred together with later samples at intervals are required. It is useful to have available a pre-transfusion specimen of serum from the patient.

A sample of blood removed from the patient by venepuncture within an hour of a haemolytic reaction occurring will usually have plasma stained pink with free haemoglobin. Providing it is certain that this staining cannot be due to mechanical red cell damage during the taking of the sample, this forms good evidence for intra-vascular haemolysis having taken place. Mechanical cell damage can be minimised by taking blood into a syringe rinsed with sterile saline through a wide bore needle, removing the needle and emptying the syringe slowly into a suitable anti-coagulant with gentle mixing. No blood should be allowed to dry on the side of the container as cells lysed by drying will give a false haemoglobin level.

If haemoglobin is present in too small a concentration to be apparent to the naked eye, a spectroscopic examination of the plasma may reveal its presence. Usually haemoglobin is rapidly broken down and haematin is formed which combines with the plasma albumin to form methaemalbumin, which also may be detected spectroscopically.

Having confirmed that haemolysis of red cells has taken place, the next step is to establish the cause. Haemolytic transfusion reactions commonly have a serological basis, but it should be noted that they may also occur when haemolysed donor blood is given. Such haemolysis may be due to: (*a*) overheating; (*b*) freezing; (*c*) overlong storage; (*d*) contamination of the blood by haemolytic bacteria. If the above possibilities have been satisfactorily excluded, a serological investigation should be undertaken.

SEROLOGICAL INVESTIGATIONS

It is proposed here to describe first of all a general routine which should be carried out whenever an incompatible transfusion reaction is suspected, after which incompatibilities due to the various systems will be considered separately. Occasionally the circumstances are such that an inkling of the cause of the reaction is known before a serological investigation is commenced. An example of such is the finding of a clerical or labelling error. In this case the serological tests will be appropriately modified. In all instances the specimens of blood required for a full investigation are the following:

(1) Pre-transfusion sample.
(2) Post-transfusion sample taken as soon as possible after the reaction has taken place.

(3) Samples from each unit, wholly or partly transfused.

(4) A post-transfusion sample taken 5-10 days after the transfusion is also valuable as the results on samples (1) and (2) may occasionally be misleading (see below).

At the outset it is helpful to examine microscopically a 2 per cent red cell suspension in saline from sample (2) as it sometimes contains agglutinates. Except in the case of incompatibility due to donor antibodies, these agglutinates are composed of donor cells which have been agglutinated by an antibody contained in the serum of the recipient. Eventually the agglutinated cells are broken down and removed from the circulation. In fact often their destruction is effected so rapidly that there are no agglutinated cells apparent when a suspension is examined. The absence of agglutinates is therefore no contra-indication to a diagnosis of haemolytic transfusion reaction. An alternative reason for their absence is that no agglutination *in vivo* but merely sensitisation and subsequent destruction of the transfused cells has taken place. Evidence for this can sometimes be obtained if a direct anti-human globulin test (technique No. 8.3b) is performed on sample (2) in cases in which no agglutination is apparent. A "mixed blood" appearance may develop through the agglutination of sensitised donor cells by the anti-human globulin serum which confirms their sensitisation *in vivo*. It is often worthwhile doing the direct anti-human globulin test even when there is some evidence of agglutination without it, since the anti-human globulin often increases the size and number of the clumps.

The next step is the retyping of the red cells of both donor and recipient and the re-cross-matching of blood from each unit transfused using serum from both pre- and post-transfusion specimens (1) and (2) from the patient (technique No. 23.3).

The conduct of the case after this point will vary according to the results of the re-typing and re-cross-matching tests. It is probable that they will reveal which blood group system is involved or at least indicate the most profitable further line for investigation. If a particular blood group system is implicated by the above tests, details for further investigation can be found in the appropriate section of this chapter. When an incompatibility is detected without it being clear to which blood group system the causative antibody belongs an attempt should be made to identify the antibody (technique No. 22.1). Negative results (*i.e.* the blood appearing compatible) probably indicates either that a haemolytic reaction has not taken place or that it has no serological basis. However, such a conclusion must be reached with caution, due consideration being given to the clinical, haematological and biochemical findings. Moreover, there are three circumstances in which the serological findings may be negative in spite of a haemolytic reaction due to blood group antibodies. The first of these is caused by the absence of the causative antibody in both pre- and post-transfusion samples. The absence of the antibody in the pre-transfusion specimen is most unusual but occasionally occurs either because it has become inert as a result of storage or because the antibody causing the reaction only appeared in the bloodstream in response to stimulation by an antigen present in the blood given. In the latter case the transfusion reaction is usually delayed and relatively mild. The absence of the antibody in the post-transfusion sample (2) is unlikely to be due to a badly preserved sample since this will have been tested almost immediately after taking. The most usual reason for not being able to detect an antibody at this stage is that it has been absorbed by the transfused blood. The antibody is usually clearly demonstrable in sample (4) taken several days post-transfusion.

A second reason for negative findings, in spite of a genuine haemolytic reaction having occurred, is that antibodies of high titre in the donor's blood have caused destruction of the recipient's own red cells. This possibility must always be borne in mind if group O blood has been given to patients of groups A, B, or AB.

A third reason for the apparent compatibility of the blood given may be that the techniques employed will not detect the particular antibody which may be present. The cross-match should be repeated using additional methods such as papain, papain anti-human globulin, and anti-human globulin plus complement. All the above reasons for an incompatibility remaining undetected must be considered before concluding that the blood given was compatible.

VARIOUS HAEMOLYTIC TRANSFUSION REACTIONS

Haemolytic Transfusion Reactions Due to ABO Incompatibility

Since anti-A and anti-B are always present and show haemolytic properties *in vitro,* the haemolytic process resulting from an ABO incompatibility is usually rapid and the destruction intra vascular.

Table 25.2 Incompatible transfusion. A to O

	Cell grouping			Serum grouping	
	Anti-A	Anti-B	O serum Anti-A + Anti-B	A cells	B cells
Pre-transfusion sample of patient	−	−	−	C	C
Post-transfusion sample of patient	Mixed blood appearance	−	Mixed blood appearance	+	C
Unit given	C	−	C	−	C

	Repeated cross-match			
	Saline		Albumin	indirect ahg
	R.T.	37°C	37°C	37°C
Pre-transfusion serum	C	++	(+)	Not done*
Post-transfusion serum	+	(+)	w	Not done*

*Anti-human globulin tests not carried out because saline tests were positive.

M

The serological findings in a case of ABO incompatibility wherein the group O patient received a transfusion of 120 ml. of group A blood will be described as being a typical example. (Table 25.2.) The "mixed blood" appearance shown by the post-transfusion sample with anti-A serum is due to the presence of transfused group A cells in the recipient's circulation. Its development is, of course, due to the reaction between the anti-A grouping serum and some of the transfused group A cells which have not yet been destroyed by the recipient's own anti-A. It can be seen that this anti-A has not been completely neutralised, in spite of the presence of circulating transfused group A red cells. This is by no means an uncommon phenomenon. The anti-A and anti-B titres before and at intervals following the transfusion are shown in Fig. 15.5. From the immune response of the anti-A it could have been deduced that group A blood had been given even if a sample from the donor had not been available. Thus in cases where no sample of donor blood has been kept, the immune response is a valuable guide to the group of the blood given.

When selecting blood for transfusion it is not usually necessary to take the sub-groups of A into account. Atypical anti-A_1 antibodies are normally only active at low temperatures. It is only in the rare cases when they are active at body temperature that they will cause destruction of transfused A_1 red cells. Nevertheless in any suspected transfusion reaction where a group A or group AB patient has been given homologous blood, the red cells of patient and donors should be typed with anti-A_1 (technique No. 4.2). The pre- and post-transfusion samples of serum should be tested with known A_1 and A_2 red cells both at room temperature and at 37°C.

Destruction of Recipient's Red Cells by Incompatible ABO Antibodies of High Titre in Donor Plasma

If homologous blood is always used for transfusion this problem will not arise. However, should group O blood with high titre antibodies be given to patients of groups A, B, or AB, a haemolytic transfusion reaction may result. The range of severity of the reaction is wide, occasionally resulting in the death of the patient, sometimes in less severe clinical symptoms, but more often merely in a failure to obtain the expected post-transfusion increase in red cell count and haemoglobin level.

In cases where no incompatibility can be demonstrated between the recipient's serum and the donor erythrocytes but it is known that incompatible agglutinins have been transfused, these should be titrated. At the same time the donor's sera should be titrated for anti-A or anti-B haemolysins (technique No. 25.1), as it is considered that these haemolysins play the major role in such transfusion reactions. Anti-A or anti-B agglutinin titres of less than 1,000 will not cause appreciable destruction of the recipient's blood unless associated with potent haemolysins, except when the recipient is particularly anaemic or several units containing incompatible agglutinins are given.

Typical findings of a case of high titre antibodies in group O blood given to a group A patient are shown in Table 25.3. In the recipient's post-transfusion

Table 25.3 Incompatible transfusion. O to A

| | Cell grouping | | | Serum grouping | | | |
	Anti-A	Anti-B	O serum Anti-A + Anti-B	A cells	B cells	Titre of Anti-A	Titre of Anti-B
Pre-transfusion sample of patient	C	—	C	—	C		
Post-transfusion sample of patient	MB*	—	MB*	(+)	C		
Unit given	—	—	—	C	C	2,000**	256

Repeated cross-match

| | | Saline | | Albumin | Indirect ahg |
		R.T.	37°C	37°C	37°C
Pre-transfusion serum		—	—	—	—
Post-transfusion serum		—	—	—	—

*Mixed blood appearance   ** with some haemolysis

sample we have the anomaly of free anti-A agglutinins in the serum of a group A patient, evidenced by the serum reacting with group A cells. The persistence of free anti-A in the recipient's plasma renders group A blood (*i.e.* blood of the recipient's own group) temporarily incompatible. Therefore, if a further transfusion is contemplated, it is advisable to wait until the anti-A has been eliminated; or if this is not possible, to transfuse washed group O red cells resuspended in group AB plasma to avoid giving the patient more incompatible antibody.

That a haemolytic transfusion reaction is due to transfused antibody is difficult to prove conclusively except by the demonstration of a normal survival of donor cells, by the inagglutinable cell count technique (the Ashby method), technique No. 25.2. If the donor cells are eliminated at the normal rate for compatible blood, then the haemolysed red cells must be the recipient's own.

Haemolytic Transfusion Reactions Due to Rh Antibodies

In the consideration of Rh antibodies as causative factors of transfusion reactions some attention must be given to the fact that they are atypical antibodies which normally only appear in the serum in response to stimulation by the corresponding antigen. If an Rh antibody is present in the patient's serum before the transfusion is given, the sequelae are similar to those already described for haemolytic reactions due to anti-A or anti-B except that the red cell destruction is mainly extravascular. In the sample taken immediately after the transfusion agglutinates are not usually seen but they may develop if a direct anti-human globulin test is carried out. There is a greater possibility of this happening than with ABO incompatibilities because of the common occurrence of incomplete Rh antibodies.

Rh antibodies also show the typical immune response curve such as that shown in Fig. 15.5. A protocol of the findings in a case of a D negative patient whose serum contained anti-D antibodies, transfused with one unit of D positive blood, is shown in Table 25.4.

Table 25.4 Incompatible Transfusion due to Rh antibodies

	Cell grouping					Serum grouping	
	Anti-A	Anti-B	O serum Anti-A + Anti-B	Anti-D	Anti-D	A cells	B cells
Pre-transfusion sample of patient	−	−	−	−	−	C	C
Post-transfusion sample of patient	−	−	−	Mixed blood appearance +	+	C	C
Unit given	−	−	−	V	V	C	C

	Repeated cross-match			
	Saline		Albumin	Indirect ahg
	R.T.	37°C	37°C	37°C
Pre-transfusion serum	−	−	+	+
Post-transfusion serum	−	−	w	+

A patient who has been sensitised either by previous transfusions of Rh positive blood or by an Rh positive foetus *in utero,* but in whom antibodies have not yet developed, may be stimulated to produce them by a transfusion of Rh positive blood. In these cases the elimination of the transfused red cells is comparatively slow and the clinical symptoms are usually confined to the appearance of a fairly transitory jaundice which may easily be overlooked. If the appropriate tests are made the survival time of the transfused cells will be found to be greatly decreased (technique No. 25.2) and when they have all been eliminated from the circulation the atypical antibody will be detectable in the serum. This type of haemolytic transfusion reaction in which the causative antibody is not present in the recipient's serum pre-transfusion but appears in response to the transfused blood is often called a "delayed reaction". The extreme case of a "delayed reaction" is one which shows "intermediate cell survival". The atypical antibody develops so slowly that the donor red cells remain in the circulation for a long time although they do not survive as long as normal compatible red cells.

All the Rh antibodies are potential causes of haemolytic transfusion reactions. At one time anti-D was most commonly implicated but transfusion reactions due to this antibody are becoming more rare. Although the sub-typing of Rh positive patients is not routine practice, the time is soon coming when all recipients will be tested with anti-c and c negatives, women in particular, will receive c negative (phenotype R_1R_1) blood. Two other factors which are sufficiently antigenic and common to merit selection are E and K although because of their lower frequency their antibodies are less likely to be involved as causative agents of transfusion reactions. The possibility of other Rh antibodies being the causative factors, must be borne in mind when investigating haemolytic reactions wherein both patient and donor are D positive. In these cases a full Rh sub-typing of patient (both pre-and post-transfusion samples) and donors may give a clue to the identity of the antibody responsible. For example, if the pre- and post-samples are completely negative with anti-c and one of the donors is c positive this is direct evidence that blood from that donor has been eliminated. If the post transfusion sample gives a mixed blood picture with anti-c then at least some of the transfused blood is surviving.

The general principles of antibody identification already discussed in Chapter 22 should be followed when investigating transfusion reactions due to atypical antibodies whether of the Rh or other blood group systems.

Haemolytic Transfusion Reactions Due to Other Blood Group Systems

Little need be said regarding haemolytic reactions due to other blood group systems, as these follow the same general pattern. Moreover they seldom occur although most of the known blood group antibodies have been incriminated in transfusion reactions from time to time. The antibody responsible can usually be identified if the procedure outlined in Chapter 22 is followed.

Demonstration of Transfused Red Cells *in vivo*

There are three ways of demonstrating the survival of transfused red cells *in vivo*. The basic principle is that there must be some method of distinguishing between the two red cell populations, that of the recipient and that of the donor. Two methods depend upon the fact that if the populations contain different blood group antigens, using an appropriate anti-serum one population can be agglutinated and the other left free. The third method makes use of isotope-labelled red cells, whose presence is, of course, detected by the radioactivity emitted.

The first method is simply a qualitative detection of transfused cells involving the selection of an anti-serum by which they are agglutinated leaving the recipient's own cells free; the finding of a "mixed blood" picture demonstrates that donor cells are still present in the circulation (cf. technique No. 22.1). It is obvious that the sensitivity of the test will depend upon the amount of blood transfused. Cells from a compatible transfusion of 500 ml. of blood can be detected up to about ninety days after transfusion.

The second method, the Ashby inagglutinable cell count technique (technique

No. 25.2) is a quantitative procedure for following the rate of survival of large amounts of transfused red cells. Here it is the recipient's red cells which are agglutinated leaving those of the donor free for counting. The success of this method depends mainly upon the choice of a powerful and avid anti-serum. This high standard of avidity restricts the method in practice to cases where anti-A, anti-B, anti-M or very potent anti-D can be used. It will be found that for fresh compatible blood a sample taken 24 hours later contains more free cells than one taken at the end of the transfusion. This is because the recipient's blood volume is increased by the transfusion but will have returned to normal by this time. Whenever, therefore, the 24 hour count is the greater, it, and not that obtained immediately post-transfusion, is taken as denoting 100 per cent survival. From this point blood will normally be eliminated at the rate of approximately 1 per cent per day. When stored blood is used there may be an initial drop in count but thereafter the rate of elimination will normally be of the same order as for fresh blood. Incompatible blood will be eliminated much faster; in cases where a strong antibody, e.g. anti-A or potent anti-D, is present in the serum at the time of the transfusion all the transfused cells may be eliminated in a few hours. As has already been remarked intermediate survival may occur when an antibody which was absent at the time the transfusion was given is being produced in the recipient in response to an antigen contained in the transfused red cells.

The technique of injecting very small volumes of red cells labelled with radioactive isotopes is an invaluable procedure for studying incompatibility. ^{51}Cr has been found to be a very useful label. In most tests 1-2 ml of labelled cells is a convenient quantity but when it is known that the patient has potent incomplete antibodies the quantity is reduced to 0.5 ml to avoid risk of a febrile reaction. Patients with haemolytic antibodies are not given more than 0.1-0.2 ml of labelled cells. The test is of great value in determining whether an antibody detected in vitro, especially one which appears to have little or no 37°C activity, will in fact destroy transfused red cells in vivo. It thus forms a very sensitive and reliable biological test for compatibility. The tests can also be applied when it is thought that the patient's own cells may have an abnormal life-span, as his tagged red cells can be re-injected and studied in his own circulation.

The method does not usually lend itself to the investigation of a haemolytic transfusion reaction, although the injection of isotope labelled red cells from the same donors or from others having red cells of known antigenic constitution may be of value in certain cases. For an authoritative account of the method and its applications Mollison's Blood Transfusion in Clinical Medicine (1972) should be consulted.

TECHNIQUES

Except for those given below the serological methods have all been described in previous chapters and the technique reference numbers have been included in the text.

Technique No. 25.1. Titration of haemolysins

Serial dilutions of the serum are made by technique No. 3.2 in the serum which is being used as the source of additional complement (*see* below). A convenient range of dilutions is from 1 in 1 to 1 in 32. In order to have adequate fluid in which to view the colouration caused by haemolysis it is advisable to make master dilutions large enough for the use of a unit volume of 0.06 ml. when running out the individual titrations. When estimating the content of anti-A haemolysin in a group B serum, titrations are made in duplicate, using fresh group A cells, similar rows being set up using cells of group B or O as controls. The titration of anti-B haemolysin in a group A serum requires B cells with either A or O cells as controls. Group O serum, is titrated against both group A and group B cells with group O cells as control. After the serial dilutions are made a half volume (0.03 ml.) of packed well-washed cells of the appropriate group is added to each tube. The tests are then incubated at 37°C for 2 hours. Control tubes are set up containing a unit volume of complement serum mixed with each kind of red cell used in the test. At least once during and at the end of the incubation period the tubes are shaken. Then they are centrifuged and the supernatant fluid from each is pipetted into a separate row of clean tubes. Care must be exercised lest red cells are drawn up with the fluid. The degree of haemolysis is read by holding the tubes in a good light, preferably daylight, against a white background. Each dilution of serum should be read by comparison with the corresponding dilution tested with group O cells; thus, any colouration produced may be matched against a negative control. A convenient method of scoring results is as follows:

++++ = complete haemolysis.
+++ = deep red serum.
++ = serum red.
+ = serum less red.
± = traces of haemolysis.
– = colour identical with negative control.

The haemolysin titre is expressed as the reciprocal of the highest dilution showing haemolysis.

If the titration is carried out on a serum which has been drawn within 24 hours it is worth while titrating in saline as its own complement may give better results than complement added from another source in spite of the fact that the complement is being diluted. However, in some cases and indeed in all if the serum is less fresh, complement from another source is necessary so fresh human complement is usually used. When selecting this it must be borne in mind (*see* Chapter 16) that sera of groups A, B or AB will contain, in varying amounts, soluble A or B antigens which may neutralise any anti-A or anti-B haemolysin present in the serum under test. It is better therefore to select as source of complement a serum which is of the same group as the test serum. Even so there is the problem of the antibody content of the serum; one may be adding haemolysin to the system as well as complement. The best source of complement is therefore either serum of the same group as the serum under test or group O serum, both of which must be of low agglutinin titre and giving no haemolysis.

Technique No. 25.2. Quantitative test for the survival of transfused red cells (Ashby technique)

From a well mixed sample of patient's blood, an accurate 1 in 30 dilution in 3 per cent sodium citrate is made. To a convenient volume (0.3 ml) of the diluted blood an equal quantity of the appropriate anti-serum is added. The mixture is left at room temperature for 2 hours (or at 37°C if anti-D is being used) and then centrifuged at 150g for 1 minute. The tube is tapped to break up the agglutinates into small clumps. The process of centrifugation and re-suspension is repeated once or twice more. On the last occasion the largest clumps are then allowed to sink to the bottom of the tube while the upper three-quarters of the suspension is transferred by means of a Pasteur pipette into a second tube which is centrifuged as before. The sediment is then re-suspended by a standard technique consisting of fifty inversions through an angle of 90°–120° at the approximate rate of one inversion per second. A counting chamber is filled from the top of the fluid; this minimises the number of agglutinates withdrawn. Most of the agglutinated cells will appear as tight clumps but any cells that are free but distorted in shape should be regarded as agglutinated and, therefore, not included in the count. Two spreads are made and a total of about a thousand free cells counted.

In calculating the number of transfused cells per cubic millimetre of whole blood, the figure for the inagglutinable cell count must be subtracted. Where no pre-transfusion sample is available an approximation to this figure may be obtained by a count made on blood of the same type as the recipient. It should be remembered that the dilution factor in this method is 1 in 100 whereas for total red cell count as normally performed it is 1 in 200.

When using this technique to follow the survival of transfused red cells, counts are performed at intervals and the results recorded graphically, so that the curve obtained can be compared with that given by fresh, compatible normal blood.

Section 3. Blood groups and Disease.

"The fault, dear Brutus, is not in our stars,
But in our genes. . .

W. Shakespeare, JULIUS CAESAR (ADAPTED)

Chapter 26. Haemolytic Disease of the Foetus

Levine and Stetson (1939) first demonstrated that haemolytic disease of the newborn is caused by antibodies passing from mother to foetus. The causative antibody in the majority of cases is anti-D. In the remainder, other blood group antibodies are implicated, the least uncommon of these being anti-c, anti-E, anti-K and the ABO antibodies. In theory, any antibody which occurs in the IgG class and is active at 37° C is a potential causative antibody and in fact blood group antibodies of almost all specificities when they are of this type, have been implicated in isolated cases.

Modern treatment of haemolytic disease of the newborn is prophylactic rather than therapeutic, at least as far as the disease in the families of Rh negative women is concerned and effort has to be directed towards maintaining supplies of Rh immunoglobulin for injection into Rh negative women giving birth to Rh positive infants.

However some cases of haemolytic disease due both to anti-D and to various other 'warm' antibodies continue to occur and are investigated as described in this chapter.

CLINICAL PICTURE

A detailed account of the clinical features and of the treatment of haemolytic disease of the foetus is beyond the scope of this book. However, laboratory work and the clinical assessment of the case must, of course, go hand in hand. When the clinical picture is typical but no antibodies are detected by the standard routine, a more extensive investigation has to be made.

The most common clinical features of the disease are anaemia and jaundice. Usually they occur together but it is possible for an infant to have a low haemoglobin without any jaundice and occasionally a high degree of jaundice is associated with haemoglobin values of over 110 per cent. The anaemia is usually accompanied by an increase in reticulocytes and nucleated red cells. Infants with severe anaemia may have up to 50-60 per cent of reticulocytes and as many as 200,000 nucleated red cells per cubic millimetre of the peripheral blood. A proportion of infants die in utero, most of them with hydrops and showing some degree of maceration at delivery. It should be noted, however, that cases of hydrops foetalis have been described in which no materno-foetal incompatibility has been demonstrated.

The degree of jaundice in the infant can be measured by performing a bilirubin test on the cord serum. The time of onset of the jaundice in suspected cases of haemolytic disease is important. In most genuine cases the infant is either born jaundiced or the jaundice appears within 24 hours of birth. If an infant becomes jaundiced at a later period of its neonatal life then the jaundice is usually "physiological" and is not due to haemolytic disease of the newborn.

It might be expected that once an infant with haemolytic disease had been born alive it ought to recover as after birth the infant is cut off from any further intake of Rh antibody. However, some infants born alive with the disease die despite treatment. Some die within 24 hours from cardiac failure, some die of cardiac failure during or soon after exchange transfusion; some die of progressive anaemia (this should be prevented by "top-up" transfusions if the haemoglobin level drops significantly 3-14 days after exchange transfusion) and others develop signs of damage to the central nervous system at about the third day and may die later on. Examination of the brain may show a yellow staining of many of the nuclei particularly in the basal ganglia. This condition is known as kernicterus. Modern methods of lessening hyperbilirubinaemia such as treatment with phenobarbitone, phototherapy and where needed exchange transfusion, has virtually eliminated kernicterus.

SEROLOGICAL PICTURE

The serological picture associated with haemolytic disease of the newborn is of an infant having inherited an antigen from the father which is absent in the mother and which has caused her to form the corresponding antibodies. These antibodies traverse the placenta and cause damage to the foetal red cells. In the majority of cases, a positive direct anti-human globulin test on the infant's red cells can be obtained thus demonstrating that they are sensitised by the antibody.

Only IgG immunoglobulin is capable of passing the placental barrier. This means that IgM agglutinins even though produced in response to the stimulus afforded by the foetus *in utero,* play no part in the aetiology of haemolytic disease of the newborn. IgG anti-D has been the causative antibody in the majority of cases and until the method of suppression of Rh immunisation by passively administered antibody was introduced, 1 in 180 of all newborn infants in Caucasian populations suffered in some degree from haemolytic disease.

The knowledge that haemolytic disease of the newborn has an antigen-antibody basis and the introduction of serological tests has greatly facilitated the differential diagnosis of the disease from other causes of stillbirth, neonatal death, neonatal jaundice, etc. It can now be rapidly diagnosed and often prognosed with some degree of accuracy before the baby is born.

When the clinical picture is typical or suggestive of haemolytic disease serological tests should be done as soon as possible, especially when the mother is found to be Rh positive, as the confirmation of the diagnosis, the identification of the causative antibody and the provision of compatible blood may take the laboratory some time.

The result of the serological tests, however, must not be viewed out of perspective. Although positive serological findings may be used as a basis for the diagnosis of haemolytic disease in cases when it is not certain clinically from what disease an infant is suffering, the mere finding of an atypical antibody in the mother which has sensitised the infant's red cells does not necessarily mean that the infant is a clinical case of haemolytic disease and in need of treatment. In some cases where the serological findings are typical of the disease, the infant may be only very lightly affected or even apparently quite normal. Obviously in these instances treatment is undesirable.

An assessment of the value of the serological findings during pregnancy for prognosis is attempted below.

Ideally the first serological steps are taken in early pregnancy, so that when the baby is born it is a matter of only a few simple tests and the treatment can be begun in the first 12 hours of life.

Although antibodies do not often appear in an Rh negative mother during a first pregnancy with an Rh positive foetus (unless a prior transfusion of Rh positive blood has been given) some women may develop antibodies within six months following delivery of a first Rh positive child. This is due to an immune response to foetal red cells entering the maternal circulation at delivery. However many women do not form antibodies to this primary immunisation until some months after becoming pregnant with a second Rh positive child. A more detailed description of the immune response due to pregnancy is to be found in Chapter 15 in which Figure 15.4 should also be consulted.

Surprisingly, in 97 per cent of cases where her Rh positive foetus has stimulated a woman to produce Rh antibodies there is no materno-foetal ABO incompatibility in contrast to normal pregnancies, for which the corresponding figure is 81 per cent. This may be because the foetal cells which are incompatible with the mother's ABO antibodies on coming into her circulation are destroyed before they can act as an antigenic stimulus.

Most antibodies of the Rh and other blood group systems have been the causative factors in haemolytic disease of the newborn. Although anti-D is becoming less common as the causative antibody in HDN, the serological routine still tends to be directed towards the care of the Rh negative woman if only for the fact that, where appropriate, she is the recipient of anti-D immunoglobulin.

ANTE-NATAL AND POST-NATAL SEROLOGICAL TESTING OF MOTHER

It is usual at the present time for all pregnant women to have routine serological tests performed.

It is recommended that all women at their first attendance at a clinic should have ABO grouping, Rh typing with anti-D and an antibody screening test with

R_1R_2 cells by albumin and papain or trypsin techniques. If the papain technique is not included in the routine screening some Rh antibodies will go undetected. Many of these, later in pregnancy, will be detectable by other methods. A few will remain "enzyme type" antibodies throughout the whole of the pregnancy.

Table 26.1 Scheme for Antenatal and postnatal serological investigations

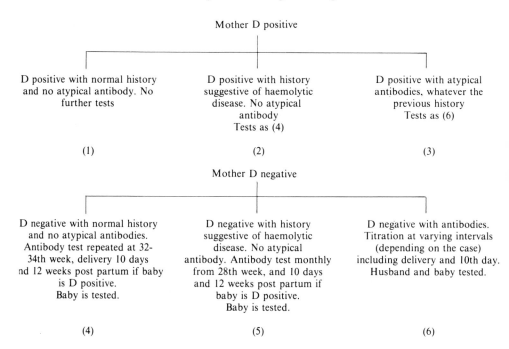

Mother D positive

D positive with normal history and no atypical antibody. No further tests	D positive with history suggestive of haemolytic disease. No atypical antibody Tests as (4)	D positive with atypical antibodies, whatever the previous history Tests as (6)
(1)	(2)	(3)

Mother D negative

D negative with normal history and no atypical antibodies. Antibody test repeated at 32-34th week, delivery 10 days nd 12 weeks post partum if baby is D positive. Baby is tested.	D negative with history suggestive of haemolytic disease. No atypical antibody. Antibody test monthly from 28th week, and 10 days and 12 weeks post partum if baby is D positive. Baby is tested.	D negative with antibodies. Titration at varying intervals (depending on the case) including delivery and 10th day. Husband and baby tested.
(4)	(5)	(6)

The women can be divided into six classes as shown in Table 26.1

When an antibody is found at any time during pregnancy, it must be investigated for specificity and for strength. If the antibody is of the Rh system Chapter 11 will be helpful in determining the exact specificity. An anti-human globulin test with Rh negative K positive and Fy^a positive cells should also be included. In an appreciable proportion of cases where Rh antibodies have been produced and the husband is K+, anti-K antibodies are also formed. If the antibody is not Rh it can usually be identified by technique No. 22.1. If the antibody is so weak that identification is difficult, repeat samples should be requested monthly as the strength may well increase as the result of stimulation.

Once the antibody has been detected and identified no further tests are necessary or indeed helpful until about the 28th week of pregnancy. It is then that the changes in titration values may be of importance in the prognosis for the present pregnancy. Therefore the antibody should be titrated at regular intervals thereafter and a check made with a panel of Rh negative cells for the possible formation of later developing antibodies of which the most likely are anti-K, anti-Fy^a and anti-Jk^a.

SEROLOGICAL TESTING OF FATHER

The father should be tested for ABO group and for Rh sub-type. A knowledge of his ABO blood group (and that of the mother) will enable the laboratory to have suitable blood standing by for the infant. (*See* below.)

The so-called Rh "genotyping" of husbands is, of course, really phenotyping with the available sera. As explained in Chapter 10 laboratory tests cannot in many cases determine an individual's precise genotype; it can only determine the phenotype or as it is often called the probable genotype. This is why most laboratories when asked to perform an Rh genotyping test will report the actual reactions obtained and give the probable genotype.

When a woman has developed antibodies as the result of stimulation by a foetal antigen inherited from the father, the question that needs to be answered is whether this man is homo- or heterozygous for the antigen concerned. When the antigen is, for example, C or E the question can be answered accurately by the use of anti-C and anti-c or anti-E and anti-e sera. In the cases when the antigen in question is D no simple test is possible; it is, however, possible by testing with anti-C, anti-D, anti-E, and anti-c, with the addition in some cases of anti-e, to obtain an idea as to the chance that any given individual is homo- or heterozygous with regard to D. In Table 9.3 the Rh subgroups are arranged in phenotype groupings determined by these sera and there it can be seen that some phenotypes comprise many genotypes and most phenotypes include homozygous DD and heterozygous Dd genotypes. In each phenotype, however, there is always one genotype that is more common than the rest and, with one exception, among these common genotypes d is associated with c.

In Table 26.2 the probable genotype is given for each phenotype followed by the next most probable as well as the percentage occurrence of each of these and whether each one is homo- or heterozygous for D. The figures given for the relative frequencies in each phenotype apply to the general population and are of course applicable to husbands of Rh negative women who have not formed antibodies. The husbands of Rh negative women who have formed Rh antibodies are a selected rather than a general population. This means that there is a higher probability of the husband being homozygous with regard to D than is suggested by the figures given here. In any individual case, however, if the most probable genotype is one heterozygous for D it is quite justifiable to consider that there is the chance of a D negative unaffected child resulting from the present or any subsequent pregnancy. Where the parents are very anxious to have another child but are hesitant because the husband appears to be homozygous for D it may help to test his parents and any surviving children he may have; the finding of a D negative parent or a D negative child would prove that he must be heterozygous for the D antigen.

ESTIMATION OF THE SEVERITY OF THE HAEMOLYTIC PROCESS DURING PREGNANCY

The first question to be answered is whether or not the foetus *in utero* is Rh positive. Several criteria can be applied.

Table 26.2 Interpretation of the Rh D positive phenotypes in terms of DD (homozygous) and Dd (heterozygous)

| Reactions with anti-sera | | | | | Phenotype | Genotypes | | | | Relative frequency of heterozygous: homozygous | Relative frequency of heterozygous: homozygous for whole phenotype |
C	D	E	c	e		Most frequent	per cent of phenotype	Next most frequent	per cent of phenotype		
+	+	−	+		R_1r	$R^1r\ (Dd)$	93.7	$R^1R^0\ (DD)$	6.2	15 : 1	15 : 1
+	+	−	−		R_1R_1	$R^1R^1(DD)$	95.5	$R^1r'(Dd)$	4.5	1 : 21	1 : 21
+	+	+	+		R_1R_2	R^1R^2	88.4	$R^1r''(Dd)$	7.5	1 : 12	1 : 8
−	+	+	+	+	R_2r	$R^2r(Dd)$	93.3	$R^2R^0(DD)$	6.2	15 : 1	15 : 1
−	+	+	+	−	R_2R_2	$R^2R^2(DD)$	85.6	$R^2r''(Dd)$	14.4	1 : 6	1 : 6
−	+	−	+		R_0r	$R^0r(Dd)$	96.8	$R^0R^0(DD)$	3.2	30 : 1	30 : 1
+	+	+	−		R_1R_z	$R^1R^z(DD)$	97.1	$R^zr(Dd)$	2.4	1 : 40	1 : 41

1. If Rh antibodies which were not present early in pregnancy, develop later during pregnancy, it is likely that the foetus is Rh positive.
2. Rh antibodies showing a steady rise in titre during pregnancy are usually but not invariably indicative of an Rh positive foetus.
3. A knowledge of the father's phenotype is important since if he is homozygous for D, the infant is D positive.
4. The presence of Rh antibodies in the amniotic fluid strongly suggests an Rh positive foetus and the degree of severity of the haemolytic process is related to the amount of Rh antibody present.

The situation in which it is most difficult to predict the infant's Rh type is the one where Rh antibodies are present and constant in titre throughout the pregnancy and the husband is almost certainly heterozygous for D.

The value of estimating the concentration of Rh antibodies in the maternal plasma at intervals during pregnancy as a guide to prognosis, is regarded as doubtful by some workers but Tovey and Valaes (1959) found a correlation between anti-globulin titres and disease severity, particularly in the pregnancy in which Rh antibodies were first detected.

A series of 1429 cases analysed by Zeitlin and Boorman (1965) pointed to a relationship between the titre by an anti-globulin spin technique and the clinical condition of the baby. When the titre was below 32, provided there was no history of stillbirth, less than 2 per cent of infants were stillborn or died neonatally and 50 per cent required no treatment. This means that whether or not there has been a previous affected infant (unless stillborn) the pregnancy can be allowed to go to term provided the maternal antibody titre remains below 32. Above this level amniocentesis is of value (see below).

Harrison (1974) investigating the correlation between foetal outcome (using a scoring system to indicate the degree of severity of the haemolytic disease) and anti-human globulin and albumin titres, found a highly significant correlation with both. For anti-human globulin titre (339 cases) $r = 0.549$ ($P < 0.001$) and for albumin titres (492 cases) $r = 0.49$ ($P < 0.001$). He also showed that the correlation was equally good for the first and second affected child of two consecutive affected children.

Tests on amniotic fluid

Collection of amniotic fluid by amniocentesis is indicated when the antiglobulin titre reaches 32 or over by about 28 weeks gestation particularly if the previous obstetric history is one of stillbirths and/or neonatal deaths.

Amniotic fluid from normal infants is almost colourless but that of infants with a severe haemolytic process is bright yellow. A spectroscopic examination is adopted, the basic principle of which is to measure the quantity of bilirubin pigments.

If the height of the spectral absorption curve at 450 nm is measured above a line drawn to the curve from 365 nm and 550 nm this gives a direct measure of bilirubin as this "tangent" corresponds to the absorption expected if no bilirubin were present. This height is known as the optical density deviation. Typical

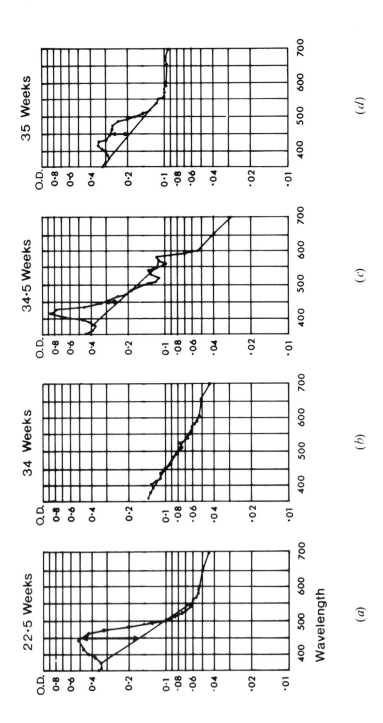

(a)   (b)   (c)   (d)

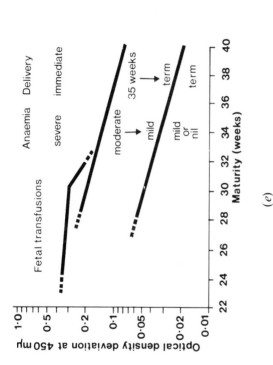

Fig. 26.1 Relation between optical density of amniotic fluid and infant maturity during gestation.
(a) Curve showing optical density deviation of amniotic fluid where the infant was severely affected with haemolytic disease. (b) Normal curve of optical density (infant Rh negative). (c) Curve showing difficulty in finding optical density deviation due to haemoglobin pigments. (d) Curve showing optical density deviation of amniotic fluid where the infant was mildly affected with haemolytic disease (same case as (c)). (e) Significance of optical density deviation at various periods of gestation (after Liley).

curves are shown in Figure 26.1. The pigment peaks shrink with increasing maturity due to a fall in protein and therefore in bilirubin levels. It is important therefore to have an exact knowledge of maturity to assess the significance of any optical density deviation.

Figure 26.1(e) is a diagram (after Liley 1963a) for the interpretation of the significance of optical density deviation in relation to weeks of gestation.

Figure 26.1(a) shows an optical density deviation of 0.32 at 22½ weeks. On Liley's diagram this suggests a severely affected infant. Figure 26.1(b) shows no optical density deviation and was associated with a normal infant. Figures 26.1(c) and (d) are from the same case, in (c) the amniotic fluid was coloured with haemoglobin pigments giving a peak at 400 nm-this makes the "tangential" line difficult to draw and the optical density deviation not so reliable - for what it is worth it suggests a normal or mildly affected infant (deviation 0.035 at 34 weeks), the sample taken one week later was uncontaminated and gave a deviation of 0.08. This plotted onto Liley's diagram prognosed a mildly affected infant, which was in fact the case.

When the deviation prior to 32 weeks is sufficient to bring it into the top section of Figure 26.1(e) it is an indication for intra-uterine transfusion. After 32 weeks, a high deviation suggests the advisability of immediate induction.

Specimens of amniotic fluid should be protected from light because bilirubin is photosensitive. The yellow colour of amniotic fluid results from the presence of closely related bilirubinoid pigments which makes biochemical estimation inferior to spectro-photometric assay. A modification was suggested by Alvey (1964); he measured the absorption at 454 and 574 nm as the extinction co-efficient of oxyhaemoglobin is identical at these wavelengths. The difference in the two readings he called the "Bilirubin Index". Using this method he claims to be able to sub-divide his cases into three categories according to the levels obtained and to prognosticate an unaffected, mildly affected or severely affected infant accordingly.

The tests on the amniotic fluid are particularly informative when the husband is heterozygous. The past history may be bad and the titre high and even rising but if there is no peak at 450 nm and no bilirubin in the amniotic fluid this indicates that the child is Rh negative and not in need of treatment (see Liley, 1963a).

The value of Liley's method for estimating the severity of the disease during pregnancy has recently been improved by estimating the Rh antibody concentra-tion of the amniotic fluid as an additional indication of the haemolytic process (Fraser and Tovey, 1972). These workers found that even if the maternal serum contains a high concentration of Rh antibody it is usually only found free in the amniotic fluid if the infant in utero is Rh positive. (It will be appreciated of course that it always remains a possibility that antibodies found in the maternal serum during a particular pregnancy may be a "hand-over" so to speak from a previous pregnancy.)

Fraser and Tovey found that with antibody protein levels below 0.2 μg per ml in the amniotic fluid the subsequent cord haemoglobin value was over 11.0 g per 100 ml, .but when the antibody protein level was above 0.6 μg per ml, the cord haemoglobin was less than 8.0 g per 100 ml and the infant severely affected with haemolytic disease.

If accidentally a blood stained sample of amniotic fluid is obtained it may be possible to type this for ABO and Rh (D). The result, together with a Kleihauer test may show whether the cells are of foetal or maternal origin. If foetal cells have been withdrawn the opportunity to perform a direct anti-globulin test should not be missed. Even if the amniotic fluid is cell free it is possible to determine the foetal ABO group from testing the fluid by inhibition technique for A, B and H substances. This test can be made sensitive enough to detect even the traces of ABH substances in non-secretor foetuses (Harper *et al.*, 1971).

INTRA-UTERINE TRANSFUSION

After amniocentesis, if the foetus is considered to be severely affected an intra-uterine transfusion is sometimes given. By this technique, red cells introduced into the foetal peritoneal cavity find their way into the foetal circulation. Not all workers are prepared to attempt such transfusions but there is little doubt that this treatment improves the outlook for women with a previous history of hydrops foetalis. The technique of intra-uterine transfusion was evolved by Liley (1963b). There are several modifications, one in fairly general use is that of Holman and Karnicki (1964). A needle is inserted into the foetal abdominal cavity, the position being checked by X-ray.

About 100 ml of fresh blood is transfused. Most workers use group O Rh negative blood for the intra-uterine transfusion, but others use Rh negative blood of the same ABO group as the mother. In either case the blood is cross matched with the maternal serum. Possibly group O Rh negative cells suspended in AB plasma are the ideal as these avoid giving A or B blood to an O baby on the one hand, or anti-A and anti-B to an A or B baby on the other. When a sample of amniotic fluid is available the ABO group of the infant can be determined by inhibition technique on the spun down tissue cells in the fluid and the blood given can be of the same ABO group as the infant.

Intra-uterine transfusion is usually performed not later than the 32nd week of pregnancy. The procedure is often repeated two weeks later. Delivery is usually at about 36th week of pregnancy often by lower segment Caesarean section.

When the cord blood is tested it may well be found to be almost entirely adult blood and type as Rh negative with a negative or only weakly positive direct anti-human globulin reaction. In spite of this the infant may need exchange transfusion, the criteria being falling haemoglobin and/or rising serum bilirubin.

The infant should be tested at about the age of 6 months to determine its true group and Rh phenotype.

ESTIMATION OF THE SEVERITY OF THE DISEASE PROCESS AT DELIVERY

Not all infants suffering from haemolytic disease require treatment. According to Mollison (1972) about 40 per cent of infants born with a positive direct anti-globulin test require no treatment. Nor is the strength of the direct anti-globulin reaction a guide to severity since mildly affected infants may give a strong positive reaction.

The best single indication of severity is the cord haemoglobin level and it is important that the sample tested is, in fact, the cord because a sample taken after birth even at so short a time as 30 minutes is of far less value.

The cord haemoglobin levels used by Fraser and Tovey (1972) (Table 26.3) to assess the disease severity at birth may be taken as a guide.

Table 26.3 Assessment of the severity of haemolytic disease at birth (after Fraser and Tovey, 1972)

Hb level (g per 100 ml)	Degree severity HDN
13.5 or over	Mild
11.0 − 13.5	Mild to moderate
8−11	Moderate to severe
below 8.0	Severe

There is also a correlation between cord bilirubin concentration and severity but it is less close than the cord haemoglobin. During the neonatal period however the serum bilirubin is the parameter which determines whether or not an exchange transfusion is necessary as it should never be allowed to rise above 20 mg per cent.

SEROLOGICAL TESTING OF BABY

The tests on the baby's cord blood include: (a) ABO grouping; (b) Rh typing with anti-D sera; (c) direct anti-human globulin test; (d) full antibody test on cord serum; (e) red cells against maternal serum by saline, albumin and indirect anti-human globulin techniques. Before any tests are attempted, the cells must be carefully washed three times. Difficulty is sometimes experienced if the samples of blood are contaminated with Wharton's jelly which often causes aggregation of the red cells. When this occurs it may be necessary to obtain a fresh sample by heel prick. Contamination with Wharton's jelly can be avoided if the sample is obtained by venepuncture from a placental vein.

ABO Grouping.

Anti-A and anti-B agglutinins do not develop until a few months after birth; any such agglutinins that may be detected in the serum of the cord are of maternal origin having traversed the placenta, and are usually present in low titre only. Thus it is not possible to rely upon serum grouping to confirm the results obtained by testing the infant's red cells with anti-A and anti-B grouping sera. It is, therefore, recommended that the infant's red cells be grouped by two methods.

Rh typing

The red cells of babies present a special problem in Rh typing. Firstly, if the cells are not completely free of Wharton's jelly, any anti-serum used with bovine albumin may give false positive results.

Secondly, positive results obtained with albumin typing antisera may be invalidated because the red cells have been sensitised *in vivo* by maternal antibody. Therefore a control of AB serum and bovine albumin is especially important when testing infant's cells since it is likely to be positive if the cells are sensitised thus indicating that results of the Rh typing, using albumin antisera, are unreliable. In such a situation it is usual to test the infant's cells with anti-D sera containing agglutinins (but not the so called "saline" sera, commercially produced, which have additives which themselves may cause clumping of sensitised cells).

Furthermore, in some instances where the infant's cells are sensitised by maternal antibody (direct ahg test positive and AB serum control positive) typing with saline antisera may result in false negative reactions because the D antigen sites are blocked by the maternal incomplete anti-D. In this situation the elution of anti-D from the cells will confirm that the infant is D positive. Also the cells from which the anti-D has been eluted should in theory give satisfactory results for D typing but in practice it is difficult to elute sufficient antibody from them. It is very rarely that any C or E determinants which the cells may possess will be blocked as well. Typical findings in these cases are negative or indeterminate reactions with anti-D sera associated with strong positive reactions with sera containing anti-C or anti-E. Although unlikely, the possibility that the infant's cells are D negative and the sensitising antibody is other than anti-D must be considered.

Direct anti-human globulin test

It is advisable to test with more than one anti-human globulin reagent or with a single reagent at more than one dilution. Ocassionally a prozone is noted *i.e.* with certain concentrations of antibody coating the red cells, a negative reaction or weak positive is obtained. The use of a different reagent or increasing the dilution of the same reagent will probably give a positive result.

Full antibody test on cord serum

In cases in which the maternal serum contains an atypical antibody, this may or may not be found free in the infant's serum. A high titre of incomplete antibodies in the cord serum is sometimes associated with slow recovery from haemolytic disease. In spite of treatment by exchange transfusion, some remaining antibody carries on the destruction of the infant's own red cells.

Red cells against the maternal serum by saline, albumin and indirect anti-human globulin techniques

Tests against the maternal serum are pertinent since the infant's red cells must contain the antigen responsible for the maternal stimulus and therefore if these tests are negative it is fairly safe to assume that the case is not one of haemolytic disease. When a rare, or "private" antigen, not contained in any of the standard cells is the cause of the immunisation, the infant's and father's red cells will be the only ones capable of revealing the corresponding antibody. Obviously if there is an ABO incompatibility between the maternal serum and the infant's red cells these tests will not provide any information about possible maternal atypical antibodies. In such cases, if the clinical and haematological pictures strongly suggest haemolytic disease, other antibody tests will have to be exhaustive.

PREVENTION OF ALLO-IMMUNISATION BY INJECTION OF ANTI-D

Experiments were carried out using Rh negative male volunteers. They received D positive red cells followed within 72 hours by an injection of anti-D. In this way it was found that immunisation to the D antigen was prevented (Finn *et al.,* 1961; Freda, *et al.,* 1964). The next step was to see whether injection of anti-D prevented antibody formation in Rh negative women following pregnancy with a Rh positive infant.

Clarke (1968) in a review article on the results of several years work showed that a high degree of protection was obtained using concentrated purified IgG anti-D. It is now standard practice to protect Rh negative women in this way. At delivery an estimate is made of the number of foetal cells in the maternal circulation. This is done by an elution technique based on the method devised by Betke and Kleihauer (1958); which is given in technique No. 26.4. If the infant is ABO incompatible with the maternal serum any foetal cells entering the maternal circulation are usually promptly destroyed therefore it is not necessary to give anti-D. It is however advisable to look for foetal cells as if there is a large spill into the maternal circulation it may be a wise precaution to give anti-D immunoglobulin to speed their destruction.

The treatment is almost always initiated within 48 hours after delivery. The recommended dose is 100 μg. This standard dose is sufficient to eliminate 100 foetal cells per 50 low-power fields. It is usual to give a further 100 μg for every 200 foetal cells per 50 low-power fields.

In addition Rh negative mothers who have therapeutic or spontaneous abortions are given 50 μg of anti-D immunoglobulin.

The anti-D used for injection comes from the following sources, (a) from women who have produced it as the result of pregnancies, (b) men who already have a weak Rh antibody which can be stimulated by injection of Rh positive cells and (c) from male volunteers immunised to produce an antibody *de novo*.

The titre in the original serum must be at least 64 by albumin technique. The sera are pooled and the concentrated IgG prepared by a Swiss adaptation of the Cohn fractionation technique.

It seems likely that haemolytic disease due to anti-D will become uncommon. For the next twenty years or so, of course, cases will continue to occur in families where the mother already has Rh antibodies or where no immunoglobulin was given at a previous pregnancy; at present about 5 per cent of negative multiparous women fall into this category. A few cases will also occur where the spillage of foetal cells and the immunisation of the mother has occurred some weeks prior to delivery or where the number of foetal cells in the maternal serum at delivery has been underestimated. Another factor is that immunoglobulin is often not administered in cases of spontaneous abortion occurring at home.

HAEMOLYTIC DISEASE DUE TO BLOOD GROUP ANTIGENS OTHER THAN D

The other antigens of the Rh system

Of the other antigens and antibodies of the Rh system c and anti-c have been most often incriminated as causing haemolytic disease of the newborn, but as all the Rh antibodies are "warm" antibodies active at 37°C they must all, if found, be regarded as likely to cause the disease.

The routine antibody screening, as has been explained in Chapter 11, should detect and identify any of the Rh antibodies, although their specificity will need confirmation, see Table 11.1 and 11.2. If the mother is Rh positive, her Rh sub-type should be determined as well as that of the father. Blood of suitable Rh sub-type can then be selected for the baby. In addition, at least two units of compatible blood should be held in readiness for the mother, since, in the event of an A.P.H. or P.P.H., she will need at short notice blood of known Rh sub-type which is not normally available in the hospital.

If any of the Rh antibodies (*e.g.* anti-c) is detected at the first antibody testing (*i.e.* at about 12-15th week of pregnancy), the mother must be tested at regular intervals as if she were Rh negative with antibodies. If the antibody is only detectable by enzyme techniques throughout pregnancy, the baby will almost certainly be clinically normal. If it becomes detectable by anti-human globulin technique it must be titrated and in the main the prognosis will be related to titre as for anti-D.

Sometimes the antibody is not detectable early in pregnancy, and as the mother is Rh positive she may not be tested again. In any case where the infant is jaundiced and the mother is Rh positive, Rh sub-typing and tests for all Rh antibodies should be an essential part of the investigation especially if the direct anti-human globulin test on the baby's cells is positive.

ABO haemolytic disease

In spite of the regular presence of anti-A and anti-B in the plasma of individuals lacking the corresponding antigen, haemolytic disease, severe enough to warrant transfusion, due to these antibodies is uncommon although about one in five A (or B) infants born to a group O mother show some signs of a mild haemolytic process. In a series report by Voak and Bowley (1969) exchange transfusion was required in 6 out of 5704 infants of group O mothers.

It is of interest that it is almost exclusively the A or B children of group O mothers who are affected. This is likely to be related to the fact that group O people are capable of producing more highly immune sera than people of groups A or B as judged by the proliferation of IgG antibodies and haemolysins. Moreover the immune anti-A or anti-B formed in people of groups A and B is largely IgM immunoglobulin and therefore unable to cross the placenta.

When haemolytic disease due to ABO occurs it is not unusual for the first child in the family to be affected. This is not surprising when it is considered that anti-A and anti-B are always present and therefore readily stimulated. That the disease, in view of the high incidence of hetero-specific pregnancies is not more common is thought to be due to the presence of A and B substances in the foetal tissues and fluids which neutralise the anti-A and anti-B antibodies before they can attack the foetal red cells. Since there is no association of the disease with babies who are non-secretors this is either not the whole explanation or the amount of substance in the tissues and the trace amounts in the fluids of non-secretor babies is a sufficient protection.

Diagnosis

The problem for the serologist is that of proving that a given case is one caused by ABO incompatibility because the mere presence post-natally of anti-A or anti-B in high titre even of the immune type in the maternal serum does not justify their incrimination as the cause of the disease. Such antibodies are often present after the birth of an ABO incompatible but clinically normal baby. Moreover, the direct anti-globulin test may be only weakly positive or even negative although the infant is showing definite symptoms of haemolytic disease. Various workers have used various devices for the improvement of the direct anti-globulin test on the red cells of infants with ABO haemolytic disease. Rosenfield and Ohno (1955) used a spin anti-globulin technique in which equal volumes of antiglobulin and a 2 per cent suspension of four times washed infant's cells were mixed, immediately centrifuged at 2000 r.p.m. for 10 seconds and then examined both macroscopically and microscopically. In 14 per cent of cases in which the infant's cells were incompatible with the mother's serum, there was a positive result and in all these children there were signs of a mild haemolytic process.

Romano and Mollison (1975) have shown that a simple suspension of the infant's cells in plasma on a tile may be the most satisfactory answer to the problem of demonstrating ABO antibodies on the cells of an affected infant. Cells sensitised with ABO IgG antibodies are agglutinated by this technique. It would seem that fibrinogen macro-molecules contribute in some way to the agglutination. A "build up" antiglobulin test (technique 22.7) is also worth trying in a suspected case of HDN due to ABO incompatibility in which the normal direct antiglobulin technique is negative.

The difficulty in demonstrating anti-A or anti-B on the infant's red cells has remained a puzzle. By means of radio-iodine labelled antibody Romano *et al.* (1973) found that the amount of anti-A or anti-B on the red cells of diseased infants ranged from 0.25 μg to 3.5 μg antibody per ml of red cells and only five infants had more than 0.55 μg. These quantities are far smaller than those found in most cases of haemolytic disease due to Rh. Since ABO haemolytic disease, when it occurs may be quite a severe process, it would seem that IgG anti-A and anti-B molecules are more efficient than anti-Rh in causing red cell destruction. This efficiency however would seem not to be due to their haemolytic properties since complement binding by cells coated with IgG anti-A requires at least 14 μg of antibody per ml cells (Romano and Mollison, 1975).

Attempts at eluting antibody from the infant's red cells may be rewarding, as any infant which has a maternal antibody attached to its red cells should probably be considered to be a case of haemolytic disease but may or may not need treatment. However it has to be realised that antibody can be eluted sometimes from the cells of clinically normal infants but Voak (1969) showed that with clinically normal infants the indirect anti-globulin titre of the eluted anti-A was less than 4 while in affected infants the range was 8 or higher.

A further guide is the free antibody demonstrable in the infant's serum. Anti-A (or anti-B) is seldom present in the serum of unaffected babies.

A full investigation of the serum by technique No. 22.1 to eliminate the possibility of there being an atypical antibody which might be causing the disease must be made before assuming the disease is due to anti-A or anti-B. If these results are negative and the maternal serum can be shown to have the typical features of an immune serum it is safe to treat the case as one caused by ABO incompatibility, whether or not the direct anti-human globulin test is positive. This means that the infant if requiring a transfusion should receive washed group O red cells resuspended in AB plasma since it is undesirable to give the baby further anti-A or anti-B antibody incompatible with its own red cells. The cross-matching is performed in the usual manner (technique No. 23.3) using maternal and not infant's serum. Thus, even in the event of the disease not being due to ABO incompatibility but to some other maternal antibody, blood compatible with this and therefore suitable for transfusion to the infant will have been given.

Prognosis of ABO haemolytic disease during pregnancy

The fact that ABO haemolytic disease is not easy to diagnose by testing maternal serum has led some workers to question the value of tests during pregnancy. However Voak (1968) has shown that in cases in which the infant is affected with haemolytic disease, a high maternal titre of IgG anti-A accompanied by haemolysins is a constant feature during pregnancy. As a guide, sera which are seen to be haemolytic when performing serum grouping with A and B cells, are selected for a further test using the maternal serum 1/4 plus if necessary one volume of human complement. At this dilution approximately 1 per cent of maternal sera are found to give haemolysis. These are selected for preparation of the IgG fraction. This is done either by treatment with 2-mercaptoethanol (technique No. 26.6) or by separation on DEAE cellulose, by a modification of the batch technique (technique No. 26.3), Sherwood (1970).

In a series investigated by the authors 0.2 per cent of group O mothers had a titre of IgG anti-A/anti-B of 400 or over by ahg or enzyme technique.

In 81 such cases in which the infant was A or B and the corresponding maternal IgG antibody titre 400 or over, 64.2 per cent of infants showed serological signs of haemolytic disease. Of those cases where a clinical report was obtainable 42.6 per cent of infants showed clinical signs as well.

Other blood group systems

Haemolytic disease caused by the less common antibodies in no way differs in its manifestations and treatment from that caused by Rh. The crux of the investigation is the demonstration and identification of the causative antibody and if treatment is needed, the selection of compatible blood. If there is a significant titre of antibody, amniocentesis and spectroscopic examination of the amniotic fluid is of value, although the critical values differ slightly from those found for infants affected by anti-D.

It is worth remarking—since at times serologists, however experienced, become obsessed with the consideration of one blood group system to the exclusion of others which may be relevant—that infants who are Rh negative must always receive Rh negative blood whatever rare and fascinating antibody the maternal serum may contain.

TREATMENT OF INFANTS SUFFERING FROM HAEMOLYTIC DISEASE

Not all infants suffering from haemolytic disease will require treatment. In any assessment of a given case, clinical, haematological and serological findings must all be considered. The decision to transfuse cannot depend upon positive serological findings alone, since these bear little or no relation to the severity of the disease process. On the other hand, the finding of anaemia (cord haemoglobin below 95 per cent) and/or raised serum bilirubin (above 5 mg/100 ml approximately) are strong indicators for treatment. It must be realised too, that some cases in which no treatment is necessary at birth, may deteriorate during the first few days of life.

Treatment is by transfusion of blood compatible with the maternal antibody causing the disease. This means that where the mother is D negative, the infant D positive and the atypical antibody in the mother is anti-D, D negative blood (*i.e.* Rh negative *cde/cde*) is chosen for the transfusion.

The cross-match should be performed, wherever possible, with the mother's serum. Full details as to the choice of blood and the mode of cross-matching are given below (technique No. 26.2).

After treatment, haemoglobin and serum bilirubin estimations should be made at regular intervals. If these are unsatisfactory a further transfusion may be necessary.

SELECTION AND CROSS-MATCHING OF BLOOD FOR TRANSFUSION OF BABIES AFFECTED WITH HAEMOLYTIC DISEASE

The blood chosen should be of the same ABO blood group as the baby and should not contain the antigen corresponding to the maternal antibody which has caused the disease. Where the disease is due to an ABO incompatibility it is obvious that these two rules are in conflict; the second, being the most important, takes precedence and the blood given is group O which has been washed to prevent the transfusion of anti-A and anti-B.

The blood used should be as fresh as possible and certainly not more than 5 days old as this will give minimal initial destruction and maximal survival in the infant's circulation. If the baby needs a transfusion it is probable that this will be given in the first few hours of life so it is convenient to have suitable blood standing by before the baby is born. If the causative antibody is identified it will be simple to choose blood which is compatible with it. In the majority of cases it will be anti-D and the type of the blood to be transfused will be Rh negative (*cde/cde*). The ABO blood group needed, however, is not quite so easy to prognose. Table 26.4 shows how a knowledge of the ABO blood groups of mother and father will enable a determination of the possible groups of the baby to be made. If a sample of amniotic fluid has been obtained for spectroscopic

Table 26.4 Selection of blood for transfusion of infant

ABO grouping of Rh negative blood to have ready cross-matched for the infant in each of the mother-father ABO combinations.

Blood group of father	Blood group of mother							
	O		A		B		AB	
O	O		O and A		O and B		A and B	
A	O	(A)*	O and A		O and B	(A)* (AB)*	A	(B) (AB)
B	O	(B)*	O and A	(B)* (AB)*	O and B		B	(A) (AB)
AB	A* and B*		A	(B)* (AB)*	B	(A)* (AB)*	A and AB(B)	

( ) Indicates that blood of this group is only rarely needed.
*Indicates that blood of this group cannot be cross-matched against maternal serum.

investigation it can also be tested for the infants ABO group using technique No. 6.4. Bearing in mind that there is rarely an ABO blood group incompatibility between the maternal serum and the infant's erythrocytes in cases of haemolytic disease of the foetus due to Rh incompatibility, it is possible to have Rh negative blood of one, or at most two, blood groups standing by, which will in all but 3 per cent of cases not only be of the suitable ABO blood group but also compatible with the maternal ABO antibodies, if any. This latter point is important as the cross-match wherever possible should be performed with maternal serum.

TECHNIQUES

Technique No. 26.1. Direct anti-human globulin test on infant's red cells

A few drops of the infant's red cells are washed four times in saline. One drop of a 2–5 per cent suspension of washed cells is then mixed with one drop each of two different anti-human globulin reagents (or with two different dilutions of a single reagent) on an opalescent tile. The usual controls necessary for such tests, *i.e.* each reagent with: (a) D positive red cells weakly sensitised with incomplete anti-D, (b) D negative red cells treated with the same anti-D, (c) unsensitised cells of group AB, and (d) the infant's own red cells mixed with saline, are included.

The tests are set out and read as described in technique No. 8.3a.

Technique No. 26.2. Cross-matching of blood for baby

For all but cases of ABO HDN blood of the baby's ABO group is selected, two units for an exchange or a half unit for a simple transfusion.

Immediately after delivery a sample will have been taken from the mother and it is the serum from this sample which is used for the cross-match. The blood is cross-matched against the maternal serum by technique No. 23.3.

As discussed above there will be 3 per cent of cases where it is not possible to cross-match the selected blood against the maternal sample because of an ABO incompatibility. In such cases group O cells suspended in AB plasma cross-matched against the maternal serum can be used for the transfusion.

Technique No. 26.3. A short method for the preparation of a serum fraction containing the IgG antibodies followed by antibody evaluation

The technique is based on the well tried DEAE-cellulose column chromatography technique; DEAE cellulose is equilibrated with the Sorensen's phosphate buffer pH 8.0 and 0.02 M. This is conveniently done in a column by running about 2 litres of buffer down a 2×30 cm column containing 5 gm of DEAE cellulose (Whatman D.E.11). It is made up to 100 ml with buffer, by blowing out into a measuring cylinder and adding buffer up to 100 ml.

0.1 ml of serum is added to 2.2 ml of the 5 per cent (w/v) DEAE cellulose solution (well mixed) in 1×5-cm tubes. The tubes are stoppered and then slowly rotated (on for instance a Matburn rotator) for 20 minutes at room temperature. After centrifugation, the supernatant is removed and made isotonic by the addition of 10 per cent saline (0.1 ml to 1 ml of supernatant).

The serum fraction is titrated by saline and anti-human globulin techniques at R.T. The doubling dilutions start with the neat fraction which represents approximately 1 in 25 dilution of the original serum.

The anti-globulin tests are incubated for two hours at room temperature before the cells are washed and tested with a broad spectrum anti-human globulin reagent at the optimum dilution for detection of IgG antibodies. It is not necessary to use a pure anti-IgG reagent. Titres of 800 and over almost invariably indicate that the infant, if ABO incompatible with the maternal serum, will be affected and suffer from haemolytic disease of the newborn. Occasionally titres of 200 or 400 will be associated with an affected infant.

Technique No. 26.4. The demonstration of foetal cells in the maternal circulation (modified from Nierhause and Betke (1968)).

Reagents

80 per cent ethanol.

Stock solution A:- 0.75 per cent haematoxylin in 96 per cent ethanol.

Stock solution B:- 2.4 g $FeCl_3$ and 2.0 ml of 25 per cent HCl are made up to 100 ml with distilled water.

Elution solution. Two parts of A are mixed with one part of B and one part of 80 per cent ethanol to give a mixture of pH 1.5.

The solution can be used for up to six weeks, but after about 4-5 days it will require filtering as a precipitate of ferric chloride is formed. After filtration it is perfectly satisfactory for use.

Counterstain. Either 0.1 per cent erythrosin or 0.5 per cent aqueous eosin.

Method

Whole blood is diluted with an equal quantity of saline and used for making films. The slides are fixed in 80 per cent ethanol for 5 minutes at room temperature. They are thoroughly dried. They are then placed for 20 seconds in the elution solution, rinsed in distilled water and counter stained for 2 minutes. At least fifty fields are examined using a 1/6 objective. The finding of any foetal cells is an indication for treatment of the mother with anti-D immunoglobulin.

It is the practice now to give immunoglobulin as a safety measure even if no foetal cells are seen. The main use of the technique is in determining the size of dose to be given.

Comment

This method produces good films with the foetal cells easily distinguishable. The white cells, including lymphocytes, stain grey, the adult red cells appear as "ghost" cells while the foetal cells stain bright red.

Technique No. 26.5. Examination of amniotic fluid for bilirubinoid pigments

The sample of amniotic fluid should be protected from light in transit to the laboratory *e.g.* kept in a dark bottle. If kept in the laboratory it should be placed in the refrigerator until it is tested. Usually undiluted fluid can be used but if there is a great deal of bilirubinoid pigments present it may be diluted with an equal part of distilled water. A glass cuvette of 1-cm light path is filled and readings taken between 375 nm and 700 nm at 10 nm intervals. These are plotted on two cycle logarithmic graph paper to give a curve similar to those shown in Figure 26.1 a-d.

A line is drawn to touch the curve at 365 nm and 500 nm, this excludes bilirubin, and the height of the peak at 450 nm above the line is measured. This gives the optical density deviation which is plotted on Liley's diagram (Fig. 26.1e) according to the week of gestation. The position of this point is an indication as to whether an intrauterine transfusion should be given, premature labour induced or the pregnancy allowed to proceed to term.

Technique No. 26.6. Treatment of serum with 2-mercaptoethanol

Mercaptoethanol may be obtained from Koch-Light. A 0.1 M solution is made in isotonic saline buffered to pH 7.4.

Equal volumes of undiluted serum and 0.2 M mercaptoethanol are incubated for ½-1 hour at 37°C. The mixture is then dialysed overnight against buffered saline at 4°C. As a control the same serum is incubated with the buffered saline alone followed by dialysis overnight at 4°C.

Satisfactory results are often obtained without resort to dialysis, using the serum in serological tests directly after the incubation period (Moores and Grobbelar 1969). However Freedman et al 1976 find that by this method satisfactory results are obtained when the treated samples are diluted before being tested but that undiluted treated samples may give false positive results.

REFERENCES

Alvey, J.P. (1964) Obstetrical management of Rh incompatibility based on liquor amnii studies. *Amer. J. Obstet. Gynec.*, **90**, 769.

Betke, K. & Kleihauer, E. (1958) Fetaler und bleibender blutfarbstoff in erythrozyten und erythroblasten von venschlichen feten und neugeborenen. *Blut*, **4**, 241.

Clarke, C.A. (1968) Prevention of Rhesus iso-immunisation. *Lancet*, **2**, 1.

Finn, R., Clarke, C.A., Donohoe, W.T.A., McConnell, R.B., Sheppard, P.M. Lehane, D. & Kulke, W. (1961) Experimental studies on the prevention of Rh haemolytic disease. *Brit. Med. J.*, **i**, 1486.

Fraser, I.D. & Tovey, G.H. (1972) Estimation of antibody protein in amniotic fluid to predict severity in Rhesus haemolytic disease. *J. Obstet. Gynaec. Brit. Cwlth.*, **79**, 981.

Freda, V.J., Gorman, J.G. & Pollack, W. (1964) Successful prevention of experimental Rh sensitisation in man with an anti-Rh gamma$_2$-globulin preparation. *Transfusion (Philad.)*, **4**, 26.

Freedman, J., Masters, C.A., Newlands, M., & Mollison, P.L. (1976). Optimal conditions for the use of sulphydryl compounds in dissociating red cell antibodies. *Vox Sang*, **30**, 231.

Harper, P., Bias, W.B., Hutchinson, J.R. & McKusich, V.A. (1971) ABH secretor status of the Fetus, a genetic marker identifiable by amniocentesis. *J. med. Genetics*, **8**, 438.

Harrison, J. (1974) Personal communication and report to British Soc. Immun.

Holman, C.A. & Karnicki, J. (1964) Intra-Uterine transfusion for haemolytic disease of the newborn. *Brit. Med. J.*, **ii**, 594.

Levine, P., and Stetson, R. E. (1939) An unusual case of intra group agglutination. *J. Amer. Med. Ass.* **113.** 126.

Liley, A.W. (1963a) Errors in the assessment of haemolytic disease from amniotic fluid. *Amer. J. Obstet, Gynec.*, **86**, 485.

Liley, A.W. (1963b) Intra-Uterine transfusion of foetus in haemolytic disease. *Brit. Med. J.*, **ii**, 1107.

Mollison, P.L. (1972) *Blood transfusion in clinical medicine.* p. 630. Oxford: Blackwell.

Moores, P. and Grobbelar, B.G. (1969) A screening test for antibodies using 2-Mercaptoethanol. *J. Forens. Med.*, **16**, 143.

Nierhause, K. & Betke, K. (1968) Eine vereinfachte modifikation der sauren elution fur die cytologische darstellung von fetalem haemaglobin. *Klin. Wschr.*, **46**, 47.

Romano, E.L., Hughes-Jones, N.C. & Mollison, P.L. (1973) Direct anti-globulin reaction in ABO haemolytic disease of the newborn. *Brit. med. J.*, **i**, 524.

Romano, E.L. & Mollison, P.L. (1975) Red cell destruction in vivo by low concentrations of IgG anti-A. *Brit. J. Haemat.*, **29**, 121.

Rosenfield, R.E. & Ohno, G. (1955) A & B haemolytic disease of the newborn. *Rev. Hemat.*, **10**, 231.

Sherwood, F. (1970) Personal communication.

Tovey, G.H. & Valaes, T. (1959) Prevention of stillbirth in Rh haemolytic disease. *Lancet*, **ii**, 521.

Voak, D. (1969) The pathogenesis of ABO haemolytic disease of the newborn. *Vox Sang.*, **17**, 481.

Voak, D. & Bowley, C.C. (1969) A detailed serological study on the prediction and diagnosis of ABO haemolytic disease of the newborn. (ABO HD) *Vox Sang.*, **17**, 321.

Voak, D. (1968) The serological specificity of the sensitising antibodies in ABO heterospecific pregnancy of the group O mother. *Vox Sang.*, **14**, 271.

Zeitlin, R.A. & Boorman, K.E. (1965) Proceedings of 10th Congress International Society of Blood Transfusion Stockholm. 933.

Chapter 27. Auto-immune Haemolytic Anaemias

Auto-immune haemolytic anaemia is brought about through the destruction of red cells by auto-antibodies. This is in contrast to other forms of haemolytic anaemia, including herditary spherocytosis, hereditary eliptocytosis and sickle cell disease which are all due to inherited abnormalities of the red cells and do not involve antibodies.

The auto-immune haemolytic anaemias are a rich source of antibodies, often comprising a mixture of specificities not easily identifiable. The antibodies in these cases are of particular interest because they constitute an exception to the fundamental law of immunity whereby immune antibodies are not formed against any antigen which an individual possesses. The recognition that these auto-immune antibodies had blood group specificity provided striking evidence for the failure of the mechanism which should have recognised such antigens as "self".

The first example of a blood group antibody of this type (Weiner *et al.,* 1953) was an anti-e in a patient of Rh genotype *CDe/CDe*; since then anti-e has been found to be a common auto-antibody in this disease.

Usually there is no known cause for the development of the antibody and the term primary or idiopathic is applied to this type. This is in contrast to the secondary type which occurs in association with some malignant diseases or develops in patients treated with certain drugs (*e.g.* α-methyldopa). Both types appear to show the same serological picture.

The diagnosis of auto-immune haemolytic anaemia depends on the demonstration of auto-antibodies on the patient's red cells and this of course can be demonstrated using the direct anti-globulin test. A positive result in such a test is not in itself diagnostic, but if found in a patient showing signs of haemolytic anaemia, it is good evidence that the haemolytic anaemia is of the auto-antibody type.

The auto-immune antibodies will be either of the "warm antibody type" or the "cold antibody type". The "warm type" have antibodies active at 37°C but no abnormal cold antibodies. In the "cold type" the patient's serum contains high titre cold agglutinins, optimally active at 2°C but with a temperature range which may go as high as 32°C.

A positive direct antiglobulin test will be found in both types; in the "cold type" it is complement which sensitises the cells and gives rise to the positive direct antiglobulin test rather than specifically bound antibody, whereas in the "warm type" it is more usually the attached antibody, although occasionally it may be due to complement.

Information regarding the antibody sensitising the red cells can be obtained using antisera for IgG, IgA, IgM and complement components. Leddy, in 1966 reported three patterns of reactions when he studied the direct antiglobulin tests using four such sera: (1) agglutination with anti-IgG only, (2) with anti-complement only, and (3) agglutination with both anti-IgG and anti-complement. Anti-IgA and anti-IgM were not found to give any positive reactions but since then the occasional positive with anti-IgM has been demonstrated.

Where a positive test is obtained with anti-complement only in the absence of cold agglutinins, this may indicate the presence of an antibody which has failed to be detected. When an eluate is made from such cells no antibody is found and Dacie and Worlledge (1968) have suggested that the complement may become fixed to the cell by an antigen-antibody complex which is removed during the washing. When complement is bound to red cells *in vivo* it is usually only the C3d (α_2D) component of C3 which can be detected on the cells, Englefriet et al (1970), Stratton (1975).

Recently interest has been focused on the subclass of immunoglobulin present on the surface of the red cells and Englefriet has found that IgG1 is the commonest type while IgG2 and IgG3 are much less frequent and IgG4 uncommon.

There appears to be no direct correlation between the intensity of the antiglobulin reaction and the clinical evidence of haemolysis, but in any particular patient clinical improvement is usually associated with a weaker positive antiglobulin reaction. However, Stratton (1975) has obtained positive direct antiglobulin results with anti-C5 in some rare cases and makes the observation that a strong positive result with this antiserum is indicative of more severely damaged red cells.

[The preparation of suitably coated red cells as controls on the various antiglobulin sera used for the detection of complement components is given at the end of this chapter. Further observations on this subject can be found in Freedman and Mollison (1976).]

The auto-antibody is usually but not invariably found free in the patient's serum. The percentage of cases showing free antibody is higher when an enzyme technique rather than the anti-globulin technique is used. This may be due to a continual *in vivo* absorption of antibody on to the red cells in which antibodies of high combining capacity compete successfully against low affinity antibodies detectable only by enzyme, thus leaving such antibodies free in the serum. Alternatively a sufficient concentration of the low affinity antibody may build up to give a positive anti-globulin test.

When the direct anti-globulin test is positive only with anti-IgG the free antibody is likely to be IgG. When the direct test is positive with anti-complement only, the free antibody is likely to be IgM and will haemolyse (and agglutinate) enzyme treated red cells. Sometimes mixtures of antibodies occur.

The warm-type antibodies

The specificity of the antibodies is of considerable interest and may be studied on eluates prepared from the patient's red cells as well as on the plasma. Satisfactory eluates can be prepared usually only when IgG antibodies are sensitising the patients cells. The predominance of Rh specific antibodies is well established, anti-e being a common specificity. Most Rh specificities have been implicated and often can be present as a mixture of antibodies which can be demonstrated using Rh $_{null}$ cells which lack the C, D, E, c and e antigens. However, Mollison (1972) considers that the conclusion that the antibodies are of mixed Rh specificity because they do not react with Rh $_{null}$ cells may have to be modified since such cells have an abnormal red cell membrane and may not agglutinate well because of this.

The nature of the apparent "non-specific" antibodies is particularly interesting because although these antibodies were thought to react with an antigen or antigens present on all red cells, it has now been shown that most such antibodies react only weakly or not at all with En(a–) cells. Thus the specificity of some of these so called "non-specific" antibodies appears to be anti-En[a]. However Goldfinger et al (1975) found an antibody which was not only negative with En (a–) cells but also with Wr (a+b–) cells. Furthermore Issitt et al (1976a) have shown that En (a-) cells are Wr (a–b–) and that the sample of Wr (a+b–) cells was En (a+) therefore the auto-antibody in the case described by Goldfinger et al appeared to have anti-Wr[b] and not anti-En[a] specificity. A detailed paper reporting a high incidence of auto-anti-Wr[b] (39.1%) in auto-immune haemolytic anaemia is presented by Issitt et al (1976b).

The cold-type antibodies

An antibody of the cold variety, can be found associated with both primary (idiopathic) and secondary cases. The syndrome is often referred to as cold haemagglutinin syndrome, and on the whole it is less severe than haemolytic anaemia of the warm type. Idiopathic cases occur among elderly people and may not affect the patient very seriously. Secondary cases occur most often in association with reticulosarcoma and other malignant lymphomas and in atypical pneumonias. The auto-antibodies are essentially similar in both primary and secondary cases.

The antibodies are commonly IgM and can be of very high titre e.g. 20,000 at 2°C. *In vitro* the antibody may be active up to 30-32°C; the temperature in the peripheral blood vessels could be within this range.

The antibodies can bind complement to the red cells as well as cause agglutination. At 37°C agglutination disappears, the antibody and the complement component CI elute off the cells but other complement components, chiefly C3d and C4d, remain attached so that they may be agglutinated by the appropriate anti-complement sera.

The auto-antibodies of this cold type are often anti-I and agglutinate almost all adult red cells. Negative reactions are obtained with the cells of newborn infants whose I antigen is not yet developed and with the few rare examples of adult blood lacking I (ii). A few are anti-i and rarely they do not discriminate between adult and foetal cells *i.e.* not Ii specificity (Marsh and Jenkins, 1968; Moore and Chaplin 1973).

N

At this point it is appropriate to consider paroxysmal cold haemoglobinuria (PCH) because it is associated with cold antibodies. These patients suffer from haemoglobinuria in cold weather, the severity of the disease varying from an isolated attack to repeated attacks over many years.

The antibody concerned is the Donath-Landsteiner (D-L) antibody which is IgG but is complement fixing and capable of haemolysing the cells of the patient or a normal individual. The sensitisation stage takes place in the cold and, if the temperature is subsequently raised to 37°C in the presence of complement, the red cells haemolyse, the optimum pH for the reaction being 7-8. The technique for demonstrating the D-L antibody is given below (technique No. 27.13). In 1963 Levine *et al.* showed that the D-L antibody belonged to the P blood group system. It reacts with all the common P genotypes but fails to react with the rare cells of type pp and P^k and thus has anti-P specificity.

Drug-induced haemolytic anaemia

Certain drugs such as Fuadin (stibophen), quinidine, penicillin and others have been implicated in causing haemolytic anaemia, albeit rarely. In such cases the patients seem to form antibodies against the drug itself and drug—anti-drug complexes are absorbed on to the red cell surface and take complement with them which causes haemolysis. The direct anti-globulin test is positive with anti-complement reagents. The reaction is not a true auto-immune one because the antibody is not primarily directed against antigenic components of the red cell membrane.

However the drug induced haemolytic anaemia which occasionally occurs after a course of α-methyldopa (Aldomet) is an anaemia in which true auto-antibodies, often of blood group specificity, are produced. For example in a series of 202 patients receiving Aldomet, Carstairs *et al.* (1966) found 20 per cent of them developed a positive direct anti-globulin test. The incidence appears to be dose dependent and if the anti-globulin test becomes positive it usually does so 3-6 months after treatment has started. The antibodies are usually of the IgG type. When the drug is stopped the red cell auto-antibodies disappear and the direct anti-globulin test becomes negative although it may take a long time to do so - even up to 2 years. By no means all patients on Aldomet whose red cells give a positive anti-globulin test develop a frank auto-immune haemolytic anaemia. In fact very few patients reach this stage because as mentioned above, when the drug is withdrawn the red cells revert to normal.

Worlledge *et al.* (1966) collected 30 such cases from a wide area over a period of several years. Many of the antibodies possessed by the patients had Rh specificity.

In 1971, Henry *et al.* found that the drug L-dopa was capable of producing serological abnormalities. Out of 80 patients with Parkinson's disease taking part in a drug trial with L-dopa, 5 developed a positive direct anti-globulin test after 8-11 months therapy. Three of these patients had IgG antibody in their cells which appeared to have Rh specificity. Complement only was detected on the cells of the other two patients. All five became anaemic.

Table 27.1 Characteristics of antibodies on red cells in (1) warm-antibody and (2) cold-antibody types of auto-immune haemolytic anaemia

| Antibody type | | Red cells with various ahg reagents | | | | Specificity of eluted antibody |
		Anti-IgG	Anti-IgM	Anti-comp	Anti-IgA	
1. Warm-antibody	(a)	+	−	−	− or rarely +	Usually Rh, rarely anti-LW or anti-U
	(b)	−	−	+	−	No antibodies eluted
	(c)	+	− a few +	+	−	Only IgG antibody eluted. May be anti-En^a or 'non-specific'
2. Cold-antibody		−	−	+	−	No antibody eluted

Serological investigation of a patient suspected of suffering from auto-immune haemolytic anaemia.(AIHA).

The samples required are patient's serum separated at 37°C and patient's red cells taken into ACD (acid-citrate-dextrose) or into EDTA.

1. The first step is to perform a direct anti-human globulin test with a broad spectrum reagent and also with specific anti-IgG anti-IgM and anti-complement reagents (*see* technique No. 27.1). The results should then be interpreted with the help of Table 27.1. A positive reaction with anti-IgG with or without a positive with anti-complement indicates a 'warm type' of AIHA. It can be seen from the Table that a positive reaction with anti-complement only is characteristic both of some warm type antibodies and all cold antibody types. However it should be easy to distinguish the cold type of AIHA on account of its characteristic powerful cold agglutinin. In cold antibody AIHA, although the antibody is IgM, this is not detectable on the red cells with anti-IgM. This is because the antibody readily elutes off the cells but the complement which it binds remains fixed to the red cells and reacts with the anti-complement reagent.

    Occasionally the antibodies appear to be mixtures of the 'cold' and 'warm' types. The direct anti-globulin test usually gives a clue to the type of reaction which may be expected when the patient's serum is tested with enzyme treated cells. For example, when the direct anti-globulin test is positive with anti-IgG only, the free antibody agglutinates but does not usually haemolyse enzyme treated cells, when only anti-complement reagent agglutinates the patient's cells, the free antibody agglutinates and haemolyses enzyme treated cells, and is likely to be IgM (*see* Table 27.2).

2. The second operation if the antibodies are of the warm type is to prepare eluates from the patient's red cells by one of the techniques described. Rubin's technique is to be recommended. The eluates when made are tested in parallel with the serum by technique No. 27.10.

    The specificity of the auto-antibody is easier to identify on antibody eluted from the patient's cells, rather than on the serum since the amount of free auto-antibody in the serum may be small and may also be contaminated with allo-antibodies stimulated by previous transfusions.

ABO grouping and Rh typing in cases of AIHA

These test may present difficulties owing to auto-agglutinins and sensitised red cells.

If the disease is of the 'cold type' and powerful auto-agglutinins are present, the patient's serum against A, B and O cells may not give results consistent with his true ABO group and so the cell grouping may have to be relied upon entirely to give the right answer. If the patient's cells are collected into ACD or EDTA and washed three times at 37°C, there is little likelihood of interference by auto-agglutinins in the ABO grouping of the red cells but the Rh typing results may be falsified by the presence of the incomplete antibodies on the red cells accounting

Table 27.2 Auto-antibody content of serum in (1) warm-antibody and (2) cold-antibody types of auto-immune haemolytic anaemia

Antibody type		Ig Class	Antibody specificity	Reactivity
1. Warm-antibody	(a)	IgG	Usually Rh, rarely anti-LW or anti-U	Optimum papain, may be positive by ahg. No haemolysis
	(b)	IgM	Non-specific	Agglutination and haemolysis with enzyme treated cells
	(c)	IgG and occas. IgM	Often anti-En[a]	Agglutination, occasionally haemolysis with enzyme treated cells
2. Cold-antibody		IgM	Usually anti-I, sometimes anti-i	Agglutination of normal cells in saline. Also haemolysis particularly with enzyme-treated cells or normal cells at acid pH
		IgG(very rare)	Donath-Landsteiner antibody Almost always anti-P	Complement fixing-haemolyses particularly at pH 7-8

for the positive direct anti-human globulin result. This is because strongly sensitised red cells become agglutinated if suspended in a serum albumin mixture or even in serum alone. It is, therefore strictly necessary to include controls of the patient's red cells suspended in AB serum or AB serum/albumin mixture where appropriate when Rh typing or sub-typing. The best approach to the problem is to use high titre agglutinins which will withstand a certain amount of dilution with saline. In cases of extreme difficulty elution of antibody from the surface of the cells may have to be undertaken. Full Rh sub-typing should be done if possible, although for reasons given above it may not be possible to test for anti-c or anti-e because such antibodies seldom occur as agglutinins.

It is as well to test for a full range of blood group systems, particularly Rh subtypes, Ss, Kell, Duffy and Kidd while the patient has no transfused red cells in his circulation. (For the standard techniques for each system see the appropriate chapters.) If the testing has to be done on a "mixed" sample, technique No. 23.1 may be found helpful. In view of the sensitisation of the patient's cells *in vivo* it may not be possible to carry out typing tests which depend upon the indirect anti-human globulin technique. To obtain answers to these it may be necessary either first to elute the auto-antibody from the red cells (technique No. 22.3) or if opportunity arises to type the red cells when they are in a non-sensitised phase (which may occur when the patient is in remission).

Haemolysins

Although *in vivo* haemolysis is a feature of auto-antibody haemolytic anaemia, "warm" haemolysins are difficult to demonstrate. Rapid auto-haemolysis may indeed take place *in vitro* but this is no proof that it is brought about by complement or antibody. Haemolysis may take place for mechanical reasons owing to the presence of spherocytes. This kind of haemolysis can be demonstrated even when complement is inactivated.

However, haemolysins active at 37°C can be demonstrated by using trypsin treated red cells, or red cells from patients suffering from paroxysmal nocturnal haemoglobinuria.

Cold haemolysins are more common and are usually readily demonstrated if the patient has a high titre of cold agglutinins at 2°C. This is particularly true if the pH is adjusted to between 6.5 and 6.8.

Trypsin treated normal cells or PNH cells are readily haemolysed even without the addition of acid but higher haemolysin titres are observed with an adjusted pH. No correlation between titres of haemolysins either "warm" or "cold" and severity of the disease has been noted.

TECHNIQUES

Technique No. 27.1 Direct anti-human globulin test for IgG, IgM and complement

Four reagents are used in this test: (1) a broad spectrum reagent. This will be issued with instructions for use at two different dilutions, the lower chosen to give a good positive with complement components so that complement binding antibodies are detected and the higher, the optimum dilution for the IgG globulin. Both dilutions should be used. (2) anti-IgG reagent. This is specially prepared reagent which reacts with IgG globulins only and should be used at the recommended dilution. (3) anti-complement reagent. Anti-complement can be prepared from a good broad spectrum reagent. To do this the broad spectrum reagent is diluted 1 in 4 and to it is added an equal volume of a 1 per cent solution of pure human IgG globulin. The mixture is allowed to stand for at least 10 minutes before being used in the test. This neutralised reagent will store satisfactorily for 2-3 weeks frozen at –20°C but should be stored in small aliquots as continual freezing and thawing will reduce its efficiency. (4) Anti-IgM.

A ll these special reagents including antisera for complement components, may be obtained commercially.

The patient's red cells are washed four times in a large excess of saline and the direct anti-human globulin test (technique No. 8.3b) is performed using the four reagents, and with saline as a negative control.

Preparation of red cells suitably coated for controls on the various reagents (after Stratton and Rawlinson, 1974 and 1976)

Technique 27.2. Preparation of complement coated cells (EC)

This method makes use of the fact that at low ionic strength complement components become fixed to the red cell surface.

10 ml sucrose-veronal buffer containing 0.25 ml fresh serum is mixed with 0.2 ml washed packed group O cells and incubated at 37°C for 10 minutes after which the cells are washed 4 times in normal saline. These coated cells should be negative with anti-IgM -IgG -IgA but strongly agglutinated by a broad spectrum ahg reagent and anti-complement globulin (anti-C). The cells should also react with various other complement components (*see* Table 15.2).

The low ionic strength buffer with sucrose contains the following ingredients for 1 litre:-

97.22g	sucrose
1.019g	sodium barbitone
0.0167g	calcium chloride
0.017g	magnesium chloride

The pH is adjusted if necessary to 7.4 with HCl (1N).

Technique 27.3. Red cells coated with C3d (α_2D) without C3c or C4d.

To 0.1 ml packed washed group O cells is added 0.25 ml 5% inulin suspension and 5 ml fresh normal serum at 37°C. After 5-10 mins, the mixture is centrifuged and the serum replaced by a further 5 ml of fresh serum. This procedure is repeated 5 or 6 times, the total vol. of serum required being about 30 ml for each 0.1 ml cells. The cells are then separated from the inulin by spinning in a capillary tube for 5 mins on a microhaematocrit centrifuge. The cells are removed by cutting off the bottom of the tube after which they are treated for 4 h. with 10 ml pre-warmed fresh serum at 37°C and subsequently washed 3 times with normal saline. Any activity which may remain with anti-C3c is removed by further treatment of the cells with fresh serum containing a final concentration 0.01 M EDTA.

Technique 27.4. Preparation of cells coated with C3

10 ml of fresh normal serum (about pH 7.8) and 0.5 ml of a 10 per cent concentration of washed group O cells are warmed to 37°C and then mixed together. After 5 minutes 0.3 ml of a 5 per cent suspension of inulin in saline is added and the mixture incubated for a further five minutes at 37°C. The cells are then washed three or four times.

Technique 27.5. Red cells coated with IgM

Anti-Le^a is a suitable IgM antibody for this purpose. Since this antibody normally fixes complement and for a control for anti-IgM, red cells sensitised with IgM without complement are required, EDTA is used to prevent the uptake of complement. The anti-Le^a is mixed wih 0.01 M EDTA in the proportion of 1 volume of EDTA to 10 volumes of anti-Le^a serum (for the preparation of EDTA, *see* technique No. 13.9). For coating the cells 4 vols of a potent anti-Le^a containing EDTA are mixed with 1 volume of 10 per cent washed group O Le (a+) cells. After 30 minutes incubation at 37°C the cells are washed four times in normal saline. These sensitised cells retain their activity for one or two days if stored at 4°C.

With a particular anti-Le^a the optimum proportion of serum to cells may have to be found by trial and error. Too large a proportion of antibody may cause the cells to be agglutinated in saline even after washing but it is necessary to have a potent anti-Le^a in order to obtain a satisfactory positive reaction with anti-IgM.

Technique 27.6. Red cells coated with IgG

Either anti-D or anti-Kell may be used.

Two volumes of suitably diluted anti-serum are mixed with 1 volume of 10 per cent D positive or Kell positive cells and incubated for 20 minutes at 37°C before washing 4 times. If a complement fixing anti-Kell is used 0.01M EDTA must be added.

Red cells coated with IgA

It is difficult to obtain red cells coated with IgA alone and fortunately they are not often required as IgA blood group antibodies are uncommon. Occasional cases of warm type acquired haemolytic anaemia with cells coated with IgA antibody occur and if found it is a good plan to store them frozen for use when the occasion arises.

Technique No. 27.7. Weiner's technique for the elution of antibodies from the red cell surface.

Sensitised red cells from a case of haemolytic anaemia are washed three times with saline, tightly packed and all supernatant fluid removed. They are then placed in the deep freeze at about −20°C until the cells are completely haemolysed. Alternate freezing and thawing will hasten this process. After finally thawing, ten times the original volume of 50 per cent (v/v) ethanol pre-cooled to at least −6°C is added. The tube is rapidly inverted and the alcohol thoroughly mixed with the haemolysed red cells and immediately returned to the deep freeze for 30-60 minutes. The tube is then centrifuged at 3000 r.p.m. for at least 5 minutes. The supernatant is discarded and the tube filled with distilled water. It is then shaken thoroughly to mix and recentrifuged. The supernatant is again removed and a certain quantity of saline depending on the quantity of packed cells used (*e.g.* approximately equal volume) is added to the sediment which is thoroughly mixed with it. The tube is then incubated at 37°C for 30-60 minutes, centrifuged and the supernatant (eluate) collected.

Technique No. 27.8. Rubin's method for elution of antibodies

This is a modification of an adaptation by Rubin (1963) of a method devised by Vos and Kelsall (1956).

The sensitised cells are washed three times in normal saline, packed and then an equal volume of 0.85 per cent saline added to the washed cells. To this mixture is added two volumes of diethyl ether. The container is stoppered and the contents thoroughly mixed. The stopper is loosened and the mixture is incubated at 37°C for 30 minutes. During this time the ether/cell mixture is shaken at regular intervals. The mixture is then centrifuged for 10 minutes at 3000 r.p.m. After centrifugation three clearly defined layers are visible. The upper layer is ether, then comes a layer of denatured stromata and the bottom layer is the eluate. This will be found to be haemoglobin stained. The two top layers are removed and if the eluate is to be stored it is placed in a water bath at 37°C for 15 minutes to remove any traces of ether.

Comment

In spite of the slight disadvantage of producing a haemoglobin-stained eluate this is a most satisfactory method for elution of Rh antibodies, whether these are auto-antibodies as in haemolytic anaemias or from cells sensitised in vitro.

Technique No. 27.9. Elution at acid pH

The patient's sensitised cells are washed four times and frozen at −20°C for 30 minutes after which they are thawed and 20 volumes of ice-cold distilled water added. They are then centrifuged at approximately 10,000 r.p.m. at 0-4°C to separate the stromata, which are then suspended in 5 volumes of bovine albumin (2g/100 ml). The pH of the suspension is then reduced to 3.5 at room temperature, using 0.2N HCl. The suspension is allowed to stand for about 5 minutes, and then centrifuged at 10000 r.p.m.; the supernatant is removed and the pH adjusted to 7.0 approximately, with 0.2N NaOH. The eluate is then dialysed against normal saline overnight.

Technique No. 27.10. Investigation of antibody specificity in "warm" type acquired haemolytic anaemia.

All tests are performed in parallel on patient's serum and on an eluate from the red cells, preferably prepared by Rubin's technique.

Stage one

Initial screening. The serum and eluate are tested by saline, albumin, anti-human globulin and enzyme techniques against OR_1R_1, OR_2R_2, Orr, ORh $_{null}$ and O(-D-/-D-) cells if these are available.

The serum reactions may at this stage be either completely negative and if so no further serum tests need to be done or a specific antibody may be detected, *e.g.* anti-E, anti-e, etc. If so it is important to decide whether this is an allo- or auto antibody. Usually, if it is an allo-antibody the patient's cells will lack the corresponding antigen although if the patient has been transfused a minority population of transfused cells containing the antigen may still be present giving a 'mixed-blood' appearance. If it is an auto-antibody it should also be detectable in the eluate. The usual picture is for both serum and eluate to react with all cells tested except for Rh $_{null}$ cells. If these are not available one is left with a 'pan' reaction. It is likely that there may be a further specific antibody whose reactions are masked by these anti-"complete-Rh-complex" antibodies.

Stage two

The serum and eluate are divided into aliquots and each absorbed with R_1R_1, R_2R_2 and rr cells and tested again as in stage one. This will reveal any underlying Rh specificity *e.g.* anti-e, which can be confirmed with a larger panel of cells in the usual manner. Occasionally the underlying antibody will not be of Rh specificity, but here again the removal of the antibody for the whole Rh complex will probably enable a clear identification to be made.

Technique No. 27.11. Acid lysin technique

The antibodies which are associated with haemolytic anaemias will sometimes haemolyse normal cells in vitro provided that the serum containing them is acidified. A convenient way of ensuring the optimum condition for haemolysis is to make the serial dilutions in fresh acidified normal serum. (The serum should be acidified by the addition of a tenth part by volume of 0.25N HC1.) One volume of a 2 per cent suspension of normal group O red cells is added to each dilution, the tests allowed to stand for 2 hours, at 15°C if the antibody is of the cold type and at 37°C for "warm" antibodies, centrifuged and read for haemolysis as below.

Technique No. 27.12. Haemolysin technique using PNH red cells

The red cells from patients with paroxysmal cold haemoglobinuria are more readily lysed than are normal cells. If an ordinary titration using normal unacidified serum as diluent is tested with group O PNH cells a haemolysin titre is obtained. This titre will often closely parallel the cold agglutinin titre of the serum.

Technique No. 27.13. Qualitative Donath-Landsteiner test

Direct.

A 10-ml sample of venous blood is taken and immediately divided between two dry tubes warmed to 37°C. One is kept at 37°C in a water bath while the other is first placed in crushed ice at 0°C for 30 minutes then, without disturbing the clot, transferred to the water bath at 37°C for an hour. If the test is positive the second tube will show gross haemolysis, the serum will be coloured deep red, while the tube kept at 37°C throughout the test will show no trace of free haemoglobin. This test is diagnostic of paroxysmal cold haemoglobin-uria.

Indirect.

This test must be made on patient's serum which has been separated from the clot without cooling (*i.e.*, at 37°C).

Nine parts of serum are mixed with one part of washed packed normal group O red cells (tube 1). The mixture is allowed to stand in crushed ice at 0°C for 30 minutes and then transferred to the 37°C water bath for 1 hour. A second tube (tube 2) is included using equal parts of the patient's serum and fresh normal serum to act as a source of complement (or guinea-pig complement). The negative controls are provided by keeping a duplicate (tubes 3 and 4) of tubes 1 and 2 at 37°C throughout.

A positive test shows haemolysis in tubes 1 and 2 or in tube 2 alone (if the patient's serum is deficient in complement) with no haemolysis in tubes 3 and 4.

Technique No. 27.14. Quantitative Donath-Landsteiner test

Serial doubling dilutions of (a) the patient's serum (b) control serum, are made in fresh normal serum as a source of complement. An equal volume of a 2-per cent suspension in saline of normal washed group O red cells is added to each tube. The test is immersed in crushed ice at 0°C for 30 minutes and then in a 37°C water bath for an hour. The tubes are centrifuged and the degree of haemolysis read according to the following scale:

4+ = Complete haemolysis
3+ = Deep red supernatant
2+ = Red supernatant
1+ = Pale red supernatant
± = definite but weak haemolysis compared with control

The haemolytic titre is the reciprocal of the highest dilution giving a positive reaction.

The problem of selection of blood for patients with autoimmune haemolytic anaemia

It is rarely possible to select blood for haemolytic anaemias, which is entirely compatible by normal standards. The auto-antibody will usually agglutinate all red cells at least by indirect anti-human globulin and papain techniques if not also by other methods.

Moreover, the problem is intensified when the patient develops blood group antibodies not only to antigens which he lacks and by which he has been immunised by transfusion, but also to antigens which he himself possesses. In such cases it is very difficult to decide whether to transfuse blood of the patient's own sub-type or blood which is compatible with the sensitising antibody but which will inevitably contain antigens which the patient lacks. For example, an R_2r patient who has anti-e auto-antibodies would be given R_2R_2 blood but an rr patient with anti-e would be given rr blood because of the risk of producing anti-D; an R_1r patient with auto anti-e would be given R_2R_2 blood unless he then produced allo- anti-E when R_1r blood (or rr blood) would have to be given.

Usually the best that can be done is to select blood that is compatible with any allo-antibodies that the patient may possess and then compare the reactions that are obtained with this blood against those obtained between the patient's serum and his own cells from which auto-antibody has been eluted. Blood is chosen for transfusion if its reactions are no stronger than the reactions obtained with the patient's serum against his own cells. Often blood can be found which seems more compatible than the patient's own.

"HEMPAS" cells

Certain patients with a particular kind of congenital dyserythropoietic anaemia have defective red cell membranes and their cells are lysed when suspended in T normal, acidified serum. Thus the disorder has been designated Hereditary Erythroblastic Multinuclearity with a Positive Acidified Serum test or HEMPAS for short. (Crookston et al., 1969).

Lysis by normal serum is caused by a naturally occurring antibody, anti-HEMPAS which reacts with an antigen which is expressed only on these cells. In addition the cells are very sensitive to lysis by antibody particulary anti-I. Only small amounts of antibody are required to cause lysis since more than the normal amount of one of the complement components ($C3$) is capable of being fixed by these strange cells.

REFERENCES

Carstairs, K.C., Breckenridge, A., Dollery, C.T. & Worlledge, S.M. (1966) Incidence of a positive direct Coombs test in patients on α-methyldopa. *Lancet,* ii, 133.
Crookston, J.H., Crookston, M.C., Burnie, K.L., Francombe, W.H., Dacre, J.V., Davis, J.A. & Lewis, S.H. (1969) Hereditary erythroblastic multinuclearity associated with a positive acidified serum test; a type of congenital dyserythropoietic anaemia. *Brit. J. Haemat.,* 17, 11.
Dacie, J.V. & Worlledge, S.M. (1968) Auto-allergic blood disease. In *Clinical Aspects of Immunology.* 3rd Ed. P.1149. Oxford: Blackwell.

Englefriet, C.P., Pondman, K.W.,Wolters, G., Borne, A.E.G.V.D.,Beckers, D., Misset-Groenveld G., and Loghem, J.J. van (1970). Auto-immune haemolytic anaemias. III Preparation and examination of specific antisera against complement components and products and their use in serological studies. *Clin. exp. Immunol.* **6**. 721.

Freedman, J. and Mollison, P.L. (1976) Preparation of red cells coated with C4 and C3 subcompo- nents and production of anti-C4d and anti-C3d. *Vox Sang.* **31**, 241.

Goldfinger, D., Zwicker, H., Belkin, G.A. and Issit, P.D. (1975) An auto-antibody with anti-Wr[b] specificity in a patient with warm auto-immune haemolytic anaemia. *Transfusion* **15**, 351.

Henry, R.E., Goldberg, L.S., Sturgeon, P. & Ansel, R.D. (1971) Serologic abnormalities associated with L dopa therapy. *Vox Sang.* **20**, 306.

Issitt, P.D., Pavone B.G., Wagstaff W. and Goldfinger D. (1976a) The phenotypes En(a-), Wr(a-b-) and En(a+), Wr(a+b-), and further studies on the Wright and En blood group systems *Transfusion* (in press).

Issitt, P.D., Pavone, B.G., Goldfinger, D., Zwicker, H., Issitt, C.H., Tessel,. J.A., Kroovand, S.W. and Bell, C.A. (1976b) Anti-Wr[b] and other auto-antibodies responsible for positive direct antiglobulin tests in 150 individuals *Brit. J., Haemat* **34**, 5.

Leddy, J.P. (1966) Immunological aspects of red cell injury in man. *Seminars in Haematology*, **3,** 48.

Levine, P., Celano, M.J., Falkowski, F. (1963) The specificity of the antibody in paroxysmal cold hemoglobinuria (P.C.H.). *Transfusion (Philad.)* **3**, 278.

Marsh, W.L. & Jenkins, W.J. (1968) Anti-Sp.: the recognition of a new cold auto-antibody. *Vox Sang.,* **15**, 177.

Mollison P.L. (1972) Blood Transfusion in Clinical Medicine 5th ed. Oxford: Blackwell. p 374.

Moore, J.A. & Chaplin, H. (1973) Auto-immune hemolytic anemia associated with an IgG cold incomplete antibody. *Vox Sang.,* **24**, 236.

Rubin, H. (1963) Antibody elution from red cells. *J. clin. Path.,* **16**, 70.

Stratton, F., (1975) Recent observations on the antiglobulin test. *Wadley med. Bull.* **5**, 182.

Stratton, F. & Rawlinson, V.I. (1974) Preparation of test cells for the antiglobulin test. *J. clin. Path.,* **27**, 359.

Stratton, F. & Rawlinson, V.I. (1976) Observations on the Antiglobulin tests II. C4 components on Erythrocytes. *Vox Sang,* **31**, (Supp), 44.

Vos, G.H. & Kelsall, G.A. (1956) A new elution technique for the preparation of specific immune anti-Rh serum. *Brit. J. Haemat.,* **2**, 342.

Weiner, W., Battey, D.A., Cleghorn, T.E., Marson, F.G.W. & Meynell, M.J. (1953) Serological findings in a case of haemolytic anaemia, with some general observations on the pathogenesis of this syndrome. *Brit. med. J.,* **ii**, 125.

Worlledge, S.M., Carstairs, K.C. & Dacie, J.V. (1966) Auto immune haemolytic anaemia associated with α-methyldopa therapy. *Lancet,* **ii**, 135.

Further Reading

Dacie, J.V. (1975) Auto immune hemolytic anemia. *Arch. intern. Med.,* **135**, 1293.

Chapter 28. Other Disease Associations and Chimeras

The relationship between blood groups and disease described in the two previous chapters is direct and well authenticated, and blood group antibodies are shown to be the causative agents, for even though viral infection or drugs may be the primary stimulus triggering the onset of auto-immune diseases, blood group antibodies play a major role in the haemolytic process associated with them.

There are however other associations, less-clearly defined where the reasons for the relationship for the most part remain mysterious but where nevertheless certain patterns may be observed.

The possibility of blood groups influencing predisposition to the contraction of diseases has for long been a subject of interest. In this connection the net has been widely cast and ranges from diseases of the alimentary tract to diseases of the mind! The part played by blood groups in such associations has yet to be established. We do not know how directly related they are to the disease or even if, owing perhaps to methods of sampling or failure to take into account all the relevant factors, some of them are indeed associated with blood groups at all!

There are other relationships however which are less vague as will become apparent as we deal briefly with the subject matter under the following headings.

1. Changes in phenotype due to disease.
2. Relationship of the ABO groups to diseases of the gastro-intestinal tract.
3. Blood groups and infectious diseases.
4. The Duffy groups and malaria.
5. Plasma protein associations.
6. Associations between HLA and disease.
7. Chimeras.
8. The implications of blood group and disease associations.

Changes in phenotype due to disease

ABH and leukaemia
The alteration of blood group antigens due to disease notably the effect of leukaemia on the expression of A, B and H antigens has been mentioned in Chapter 16. The first hint of such a possibility is to be found in a paper by Van Loghem *et al.* (1957) in which a weakly expressed A antigen occurred in a patient with myeloblastic leukaemia. A connection between the weak A and the disease was suspected because a year earlier the patient had been grouped as a normal A. Further examples followed, including a case of subacute myeloid leukaemia and

tuberculosis involving the B antigen (Van der Hart *et al.*, 1962). An associated phenomenon in some examples was an apparent "mixed cell" population of group A and group O cells. In one case (Gold *et al.*, 1959) the cells inagglutinable by anti-A, when separated, were capable of absorbing anti-A. On the other hand, Salmon *et al.* (1958) described several cases in which the free cells behaved like group O.

Disturbance of the H antigen as well as A has also been noted. Hoogstraten *et al.* (1961) investigated a group A_1 patient whose red cells, after the onset of leukaemia, became inagglutinable by anti-A but strongly agglutinable by anti-H. The cells reverted to being strongly A and weakly H during a remission of the disease.

Several explanations have been offered for the changes in ABH antigens associated with leukaemia. Salmon has suggested chromosome inactivation. Hoogstraten *et al.* draw attention to the treatment of the disease as a possible reason for the blood group changes observed.

A review of the subject has been made by Salmon (1969).

Acquired B

The best investigated example of a change in ABO phenotype which is bacterial in origin is the acquired B which sufferers from diseases of the gut are particularly prone to develop. A short description of acquired B is to be found in Chapter 16 and its forensic relevance is included in Chapter 29.

The loss of A, B, H substances from cancer cells

Most tissue cells of the body have the appropriate A, B, H substances incorporated in the cell membrane. These antigens are alcohol soluble and occur in both secretors and non-secretors. They have been demonstrated by inhibition, mixed agglutination and immunofluorescence techniques. The work has been extended by Davidsohn and Stejskal (1972) using an adaptation of the mixed cell agglutination technique, called the specific red cell adherence test (SRCA). This test made possible the detection of A, B and H antigens in old stained sections of tissue as well as in fresh material.

Both cancer cells and normal tissue cells were studied and it was found that the cancer cells progressively lost their A, B and H antigens and this may have important implications for prognosis. For example, benign and malignant lesions of the cervix of the uterus were investigated and whereas the appropriate ABH antigens were present in benign lesions, they had disappeared from all cases tested of metastatic carcinomas. Moreover in 32 out of 35 early infiltrating carcinomas without clinical evidence of metastasis these alloantigens had decreased in strength or were absent (Davidsohn *et al.*, 1969; Davidsohn, 1972).

Extension of the work to include carcinoma of the pancreas (Davidsohn *et al.*, 1971) showed a slower loss of blood group activity than in some other carcinomas *e.g.* lungs and cervix. Positive reactions in the SRCA test were often seen simultaneously with negative reactions and sometimes a positive and negative reaction was seen in adjacent cells. An important observation was that the loss of A, B and H in a primary carcinoma seemed to precede the formation of distant metastases.

The secretion of ABH substances in alcoholics

In considering changes in phenotype due to disease it seems relevant to mention a curious connection between the disease of alcoholism and blood groups which affects the secretor phenotype of certain individuals.

In determining the ABO blood group and secretor status of 1,000 alcoholic patients (Camps *et al.,* 1969) and a further 400 patients (Dodd and Lincoln, 1971, unpublished observations), a striking disturbance of the secretor: non-secretor ratio among group A patients was observed. An increase in the frequency of group A non-secretors of the order of 12 per cent was almost exactly balanced by the loss of a similar number of group A secretors so that there was no over-all increase or decrease in patients of group A. Such a balance points to a direct effect of alcohol on the secretor status of an individual and requires that a certain number of genetically constituted group A secretors become non-secretors through the constant imbibition of alcohol. A puzzling feature is the apparent confinement of the observation to patients of group A although there is a hint that group O individuals are not entirely unaffected. The figures obtained do not appear to allow any other explanation than a "change" in status from secretor to non-secretor. So far no individuals have been caught changing in the reverse direction although it would be reasonable to suppose that some would revert to their original type if they remained "dry" for a sufficiently long period. Perhaps they never do!

In spite of the problems yet to be solved in connection with alcohol and the secretion of blood group substances it remains a striking example, perhaps the only one, of blood group changes related to "diet".

The relationship of the ABO groups to disease of the gastro-intestinal tract

The association between ABO groups and diseases of the upper gastro-intestinal tract are too striking to be considered fortuitous although the role of blood groups in these diseases has not yet been elucidated and indeed may be manifold.

The first convincing demonstration of such an association was between group A and carcinoma of the stomach, the A/O ratio being 20 per cent higher in such cancer patients than in normal persons (Aird *et al.,* 1953).

As further investigations have shown a similar association in many parts of Europe and in some non-European populations it seems highly likely that people of group A are for some reason intrinsically more susceptible to carcinoma of the stomach than those of group O.

Further work on cancers of the gastro-intestinal tract show that in general in these diseases there is a raised A/O ratio. This suggests some underlying reason and one that comes to mind is the possibility that some cancer cells irrespective of the ABO group of the patient carry an A-like antigen. If this is true, group A patients might be at a disadvantage since they are tolerant to A and unable to make an antibody against it, whereas the anti-A present in group O and group B individuals might be effective against the A-like antigens of the cancer.

Shortly after drawing attention to the association between the ABO groups and carcinoma of the stomach, the same workers showed that in peptic ulcers there is a very significant excess of group O with an O/A ratio 1.39 times as high as in the general population (Aird et al., 1954). Even more striking is the association between non-secretors of all groups and duodenal ulcers (Clarke et al., 1959). Duodenal ulcers are about 50 per cent more likely to develop in non-secretors than secretors. It has also been demonstrated that group O subjects have an excessive rate of bleeding (Horwich et al., 1966). It is possible that this fact has an important bearing on the apparent association between group O and peptic ulcers since the ulcer cases investigated for blood groups are nearly all hospital cases, many of which are admitted because of their bleeding tendency. This therefore may account for the excess of group O that has been found among patients with duodenal ulcer. A further finding by Clarke et al. (1959) which would tend to support this interpretation of the excess of group O, is the low correlation between blood groups and the occurrence of ulcers among the sibs of patients with ulcers. Moreover, there is now an increasing number of observations which all tend to show that in other diseases in which haemorrhage is likely to occur, patients of group O are more likely to bleed than those of group A.

These observations illustrate well how necessary it is to be cautious about any conclusions drawn from blood group associations. The association which is apparent at first sight, may after all turn out to be fortuitous while the true association may lie elsewhere. It should be pointed out that the strong relationship between duodenal ulcer and non-secretion of ABH substances unlike the association with group O, is reflected in the siblings of ulcer patients. Moreover, there seems to be no association between secretor status and haemorrhage.

It is perhaps not inappropriate in this section to mention the work of Afors et al. (1963) on serum alkaline phosphatase of intestinal origin. Human serum alkaline phosphatases are separable into two major zones by electrophoresis in starch gel. There is a fast moving component present in all sera thought to originate in the liver and probably bone, and a slower component originating in the small intestine. Afors and co-workers found that this slower phosphatase band occurs almost exclusively in sera of groups B and O secretors and is almost always absent from group A secretors or from non-secretors of any ABO group. Later, with more sensitive techniques for demonstrating alkaline phosphatase activity, it was found that small amounts of the enzyme are present in about 15 per cent of group A secretors and somewhat fewer non-secretors. Group AB people are intermediate in the number of positives found and in the amount of phosphatase present in the serum.

The concentration of intestinal phosphatase is lowest in the serum during fasting and rises after the ingestion of fat to a peak after about eight hours. The increase is most apparent in group O and B secretors but is detectable in most people.

The follow up to these findings was the measurement of alkaline phosphatase in the intestinal mucosa. Although Schreffler (1966) found no correlation between alkaline phosphatase measured at this site and ABO groups or secretor type, Langman et al. (1968) observed that group O and group B had the highest mean concentration of alkaline phosphatase, group A the next and non-secretors the lowest amount but the differences were much smaller than those found in serum. Beckman *et al.* (1966) consider that the ABO and secretor genes influence the rate at which the intestinal phosphatase enters the blood or its catabolism, rather than its synthesis in the intestine.

If the relationship which undoubtedly appears to exist between the ABO and secretor genes and intestinal alkaline phosphatase is pointing to the fact that the blood group and secretor genes somehow affect the permeability of the intestinal wall, then this may in some way be related to the tendency to ulceration associated with group O and non-secretors.

Blood groups and infectious diseases

Since blood groups are systems of antigens and antibodies and the agents underlying infectious diseases stimulate the production of antibodies it would not be surprising if ABO groups with their regularly present antibodies exert some influence on the responses of the body to infections. However so far such relationships are less than striking. The best authenticated seems to be the finding by Clarke *et al.* (1968) of a deficiency of group O among patients with rheumatic heart disease which follows haemolytic streptococcal infection. Rheumatic fever believed to be a closely related condition shows but a slight tendency to deficiency of group O while rheumatoid arthritis shows a definite excess of group O. Rheumatic fever is associated with an excess of non-secretors (Glynn and Holborow, 1969).

Vogel *et al.* (1960) put forward an interesting idea based on a relation which they noted between blood group A and susceptibility to smallpox. These workers suggested that the resulting natural selection could be largely responsible for the varying frequencies of group A in different parts of the world. The combined data of all workers investigating this relationship is as yet inconclusive.

There is some evidence that streptococcal infections attack preferentially people of group A with one known exception which is scarlet fever, which although itself caused by a streptococcal infection, is associated with a deficiency of group A!

The Duffy groups and malaria

A refreshingly different approach to the study of blood group and disease associations comes from the work of Miller *et al.* (1975) which began as an attempt to discover why West Africans and approximately 70 per cent of American blacks are restistant to infection by *Plasmodium vivax* although they are susceptible to the other three species of human malaria. From other work there was strong evidence that the resistance factor operated to prevent the merozoite from invading the red cell and so a search was made for red cell receptors for malariae parasites (merozoite stage) by testing the susceptibility of red cells known to lack various antigens to invasion by a simian malaria (*P. knowlesi*). This species also infects man.

Of the red cells tested only those lacking both Fy[a] and Fy[b] antigens were resistant to invasion. Other red cells lacking in common antigens, *i.e.* Rh $_{null}$, Le (a–b–), and Lu (a–b–) were tested but none of these were resistant to invasion. This observation fits remarkably with the distribution of the Fy (a–b–) phenotype in the world and the fact that some African populations have a dramatically higher proportion of Fy (a–b–) individuals than most other ethnic groups. This strongly suggests that Africans developed resistance to *P. vivax* by natural selection of the *Fy* gene.

During the same investigation Miller and his colleagues carried out two further experiments which are of particular interest to serologists: They found that red cells possessing Fy^a and/or Fy^b antigens became resistant to invasion by *P. knowlesi* merozoites after they were enzyme treated, which treatment of course removes the Fy^a and Fy^b receptors. Similarly, coating Fy (a+b–) red cells with anti-Fy^a caused a marked reduction in invasion although a similar experiment coating F (a–b+) cells with anti-Fy^b did not have the expected effect. The authors suggest that the lower titre of the anti-Fy^b, 16 compared to anti-Fy^a 128, may have accounted for the failure of the anti-Fy^a to block invasion of the red cells.

Further work on this association is in progress.

Plasma protein associations

A function has now been assigned to the Gc groups in that Daiger *et al.* (1975) have shown these α_2 lipoproteins to be the carriers of vitamin D in plasma. This fact gave rise to an interesting speculation by Mourant and his colleagues (1976) as to whether there might be a relationship between the Gc polymorphism and the amount of sunshine received by a given population in view of the effect of ultra-violet light in causing the synthesis of vitamin D. From population studies already carried out Mourant *et al.* find that, on the whole, the *Gc^2* allele is commoner in dull than in sunny climates. The inference here, of which there is as yet no direct evidence, is that the *Gc^2* gene product is a better carrier of vitamin D than is *Gc^1*. The same authors suggest that Gc surveys in populations subject to ricketts might be informative.

According to Ritter and Hinkelman (1966), and Kirk *et al.* (1970) the haptoglobin polymorphism is involved in ABO haemolytic disease of the newborn. The findings show that where the father is incompatible with the maternal ABO antibodies, the children show a higher frequency of the *Hp^1* gene than in families drawn from the same population in which the father is ABO compatible with the mother. Kirk (1971) tested 2349 families with 5701 children comprising eight different ethnic populations. Five of these yielded data suitable for studying haptoglobin types in the classes:- (1) father A, B or AB/mother O, and (2) father O/mother A, B or AB. In all five populations the frequency of *Hp^1* was higher in class 1 than class 2. In two of the populations studied the differences were significant ($P = 0.02$, $P = 0.05$). It is known that the *Hp^1* gene product is more efficient than that of *Hp^2* in removing dissolved haemoglobin from the plasma. It is suggested therefore that in cases where children are born suffering from haemolytic disease due to foetal A or B inherited from the father a child who is Hp 1-1 has the best and a child of Hp 2-2 the least chance of survival.

Associations between HLA and disease

Animal studies have revealed in some species the existence of specific immune response genes closely linked to the major histo-compatibility system and also data from mouse experiments show the existence of genes in the H-2 region (mouse HLA) which control susceptibility to virus-induced leukaemias. From these results therefore it would not be surprising to find associations between HLA antigens and disease in humans which come under the general category of immune diseases. Early studies have not shown any associations with Hodgkin's disease but subsequently very definite associations have been found with ankylosing spondylitis, psoriasis, coeliac disease, myasthenia gravis and multiple sclerosis (McDevitt and Bodmer, 1974). The most significant association is between B27 (W27) and ankylosing spondylitis in which 90 per cent of patients with this disease have B27 (W27) whereas the frequency of this antigen in Caucasians is 5-10 per cent. Interestingly, the same association is noticed in African populations where the frequency of B27 (W27) is much lower than in Caucasians as is also the incidence of ankylosing spondylitis. It is believed that the genes responsible for susceptibility to diseases such as these are probably not those of the HLA antigens but rather they are genes closely linked but genetically separable from them (i.e. the D locus; see chapter 19).

Chimeras

We have to find some chapter in which to insert a brief account of chimeras and although they can hardly be said to be associated with disease, they do, neverthless stem from an anatomical abnormality.

A chimera may be defined as an organism whose cells derive from more than one distinct zygote lineage such as the vascular anastomoses which may occur between twins in which, for example, a twin of genetic type O may receive a bone marrow implantation from his twin of group A. Throughout life he will have a major red cell population of group O and a minor population of group A.

Examples began with the work of Owen in 1945 when investigating the vascular anastomoses which commonly occur between dissimilar bovine twin embryos.

Later it was found that, upon rare occasions, the same thing happened in human twin embryos (Dunsford et al., 1953). In this first human example a sample of blood from a healthy blood donor (Mrs McK) was found to be a mixture of two kinds of blood, which was first noticed when a test with anti-A showed agglutinates and many free cells similar to the mixed blood appearance shown in Fig. 23.1. After separating the two populations it was found that 61 per cent of the cells were O, and 39 per cent A_1. There were other differences, the A_1 cells were K+ Jk(a–) while the O cells were K– Jk (a+).

Another example of blood chimerism in twins was studied by Booth et al. (1957) and this paper gives the details of a method of separating the cells which in this case were O and A_1. The principle is to add anti-A to the mixed blood in a Petri dish. The anti-A has to be very avid and capable of forming large agglutinates which are collected and disagglutinated by shaking them in the presence of soluble A substance. The remaining mixture of small agglutinates of A cells with the true O cells are transferred to a long tube and left to settle; the agglutinated A cells sink more quickly than the free O cells which are taken off in the supernatant fluid. If the red cells are A_1, *Dolichos* may be used instead of anti-A. More precise technical details are given in the original paper.

The authors point out that the separation in their particular example could have been made with anti-C, anti-E, anti-s or with anti-Fy^a or anti-Jk^b but the relative weakness of the agglutination of these antisera and their scarcity made the separation with anti-A the obvious choice. Of course in chimeras in whom there is no ABO difference, the antisera of other systems have to be used. In fact in the case of Booth *et al.*, anti-E was used as a cross check and was found satisfactory when Löw's papain was used to enhance the agglutination.

Chimera twins are excellent examples of tolerance to an antigen acquired before birth. If the individual is genetically group O with grafted A cells, anti-A never develops, presumably because the host is exposed to the A antigen during foetal life.

By now about twenty sets of chimeras have been found and all but one were discovered because they involved ABO blood grouping problems showing a mixed cell population and a missing agglutinin. The missing agglutinin seems sometimes to be the first observed clue to the phenomenon. The fact that the known twin chimeras overwhelmingly presented themselves first as ABO discrepancies suggests that there may be others which because each twin has the same ABO group, are missed. A mixed cell population is not so readily seen with antisera that are less avid than anti-A and anti-B. Moreover when other blood group systems are involved there is no opportunity to detect a chimera by means of a missing agglutinin.

The problem with chimeras is to discover the true genotype of each twin. The secretor results on the saliva may give the answer. For example Mrs McK, the original human example had H in her saliva but no A, therefore her true group was O and the A was from her dead twin.

Another method of deducing the true genetic group of a chimera is to look for ABH transferases in the serum, given a difference of ABO group between the pairs. Watkins and Race (cited Race and Sanger, 1975) showed in two sets of twins that the transferases corresponding to the true genetic groups were present in normal amounts whereas the transferase corresponding to the graft had low activity even when the proportion of true genetic cells was small.

A significant point of interest is the finding that a chimera who is a secretor is able to secrete only those ABH antigens which are part of his own genetic constitution. Some observations relevant to this were made by Crookston *et al.* (1970) when investigating a twin chimera pair in which the serum of the female contained anti-A_1 Le^b. This antibody agglutinated the A_1 Le (a–b+) cells of her brother but did not agglutinate those cells originally grafted from her brother, which were present in her own circulation. It would seem therefore that the ability to make the compound antigen A_1 Le^b cannot be grafted but requires A_1 Se, and Le genes to be part of the true genetic make up of the host. Furthermore this shows that the compound antigen is not made in the bone marrow but must be made at some as yet unknown site and secondarily taken up by the red cells.

It has been shown that group O cells grafted into an A chimera twin take up some of the host's A antigen from the serum. However this A antigen appears to be detectable only by selected anti-A+B (group O) sera (Tilley *et al.,* 1975). We think that this is due to the presence in these sera of cross reacting antibody, the combining site area of which may be best suited to the distribution of the acquired A antigen, which is probably sparse. This means that when estimating the relative proportions of O and A cells in a chimera, anti-A and not anti-A+B from group O serum, should be used.

In practice of course, genuine examples of chimerism have to be distinguished from other reasons for the appearance of a mixed cell population. Common causes for mixed cell appearances are transfusions or, in pregnant women, bleeding of the foetus into the maternal circulation. There are also as mentioned in other chapters various antigens which normally give a mixed field type of appearance with appropriate antisera *e.g.* weak A, particularly A_3, Lu^a, Tn and Sd^a.

Some implications of blood group and disease associations

All the major blood group systems are considered to be balanced polymorphisms, but that which has "balanced them", so to speak, is as yet cloaked in mystery. The classical definition of a balanced polymorphism is one in which the heterozygote enjoys some advantage over either homozygote. One of the best examples is to be seen in the relationship between haemoglobin S and malaria in which it has been found that those who have sickle cells due to the effect of the haemoglobin S gene are more resistant to malarial infections than are those with normal adult haemoglobin. So that the situation obtains wherein the homozygote for sickling dies of sickle-cell disease, the homozygote for haemoglobin A tends to die from malaria, while the heterozygote is relatively free from both disadvantages.

No clear example such as this is found in association with blood groups. In fact it would seem that as far as haemolytic disease due to Rh incompatibility is concerned, until recent years, the heterozygote D-d suffered a disadvantage.

The one or two known blood group homozygotes who are known to be at a disadvantage, such as pp which is associated with early abortion and K_O associated with granulomatous disease, are too few to have any appreciable selective power.

Any genuine association between a blood group and a disease whose onset occurs in later life is unlikely to have much effect upon blood group frequencies. Diseases contracted earlier in life either before or during the child bearing period could affect blood group frequencies through natural selection *e.g.* an association between group A and smallpox as mentioned above.

Now it would seem that striking examples of natural selection involving blood groups are coming to light such as the Duffy and *Plasmodium* association if confirmed, which operates in favour of the FyFy phenotype and the relationship between Gc and vitamin D may prove to be another.

Any blood group genes showing marked variation in different parts of the world are worth studying from the point of view of their possible influence on various diseases. Large scale grouping on populations has been carried out already but these have not often been related to the disease patterns within the population studied. We are beginning to acquire good evidence that this aspect of blood groups should prove rewarding in the future.

Readers interested in a detailed treatment of blood group and disease associations are recommended to study Mourant *et al.* (1978).

REFERENCES

Afors, K.E., Beckman, L. & Lundin, L.G. (1963) Genetic variations of human serum phosphatases. *Acta genet.*, **13**, 89.
Aird, J., Bentall, H.H. & Fraser-Roberts, J.A. (1953) A relationship between cancer of stomach and the ABO blood groups. *Brit. med. J.*, **1**, 799.
Aird, J., Bentall, H.H. Mehigan, J.A. & Roberts, J.A.F. (1954) Blood groups in relation to peptic ulceration and carcinoma of colon, rectum, breast and bronchus. *Brit. med. J.*, **2**, 315.
Beckman, L., Björling, E. & Heiken, A. (1966) Human alkaline phosphatases and factors controlling their appearance in serum. *Acta genet*, **16**, 305.
Booth, P.B., Plaut, G., James, J.D., Ikin, E.W., Moores, P., Sanger, R. & Race, R.R. (1957) Blood chimerism in a pair of twins. *Brit. med. J.*, **i**, 1456.
Camps, F.E., Dodd, B.E. & Lincoln, P.J. (1969) Frequencies of secretors and non-secretors of ABH group substances among 1,000 alcoholic patients. *Brit. med. J.*, **4**, 457.
Clarke, C.A., Evans, D.A.P., McConnell, R.B. & Sheppard, P.M. (1959) Secretion of blood group antigens and peptic ulcer. *Brit. med. J.*, **i**, 603.
Clarke, C.A., McConnell, R.B. & Sheppard, P.M. (1960) ABO blood groups and secretor character in rheumatic carditis. *Brit. med. J.*, **i**, 21.
Crookston, M.C., Tilley, C.A., Crookston, J.H. (1970) Human blood group chimera with seeming breakdown of immune tolerance. *Lancet* **ii**, 1110.
Daiger, S.P., Schanfield, M.S. & Cavalli-Sforza, L.L. (1975) Group-specific component (Gc) proteins bind vitamin D and 25-hydroxyvitamin D. *Proc. nat. Acad. Sci. USA*, **72**, 2076.
Davidsohn, I., Kovarik, S. & Ni, L.Y. (1969) Isoantigens A, B and H in benign and malignant lesions of the cervix. *Arch. Path.*, **87**, 306.
Davidsohn, I., Ni, L.Y. & Stejskal, R. (1971) Tissue isoantigens A, B and H in carcinoma of the pancreas. *Cancer Res.*, **31**, 1244.
Davidsohn, I. (1972) Early immunologic diagnosis and prognosis of carcinoma. *Am. J. clin. Path.*, **57**, 715.
Davidsohn, I. & Stejskal, R. (1972) Tissue antigens A, B and H in health and disease. *Haematologia* **6**, 177.
Dunsford, I., Bowley, C.C. Hutchison, A.M., Thompson, J.S., Sanger, R. & Race, R.R. (1953) A human blood group chimera. *Brit. med. J.*, **ii**, 81.
Glynn, L.E. & Holborow, E.J. (1969) Blood groups and their secretion in rheumatic fever. *Rheumatology*, **2**. 113.
Gold, E.R., Tovey, G.H., Benney, W.E. & Lewis, F.J.W. (1959) Changes in the group A antigen in a case of leukaemia. *Nature (Lond.)*, **183**, 892.
Hoogstraten, B., Rosenfield, R.E. & Wasserman, L.R. (1961) Change of ABO blood type in patients with leukaemia. *Transfusion (Philad.)*, **1**, 32.
Horwich, L., Evans, D.A.P., McConnell, R.B. & Donohoe, W.T.A. (1966) ABO blood groups in gastric bleeding. *Gut*, **7**, 680.
Kirk, R.L., Kinns, H. & Morton, N.E. (1970) Interaction between the ABO blood groups and haptoglobin systems. *Am. J. hum. Genet.*, **23**, 384.
Kirk, R.L. (1971) A haptoglobin mating frequency, segregation and ABO blood group interaction: analysis for additional series of families. *Ann. hum. Genet.*, **34**, 329.
Langman, M.J.S., Constantinopoulos, A. & Bouchier, I.A.D. (1968) ABO blood groups, secretor status and intestinal mucosal concentrations of alkaline phosphatase. *Nature (Lond.)*, **217**, 863.
McDevitt, H.O. & Bodmer, W.F. (1974) HL-A immune response genes and disease. *Lancet*, **i**, 269.

Miller, L.H., Mason, S.J., Dvorak, J.A., McGinnis, M.H. & Rothman, I.K. (1975) Erythrocyte receptors for (*Plasmodium knowlesi*) malaria: Duffy blood group determinants. *Science,* **189,** 561.

Mourant, A.E., Tills, D., Domaniewska-Sobczak, K. (1976) Sunshine and the geographical distribution of the alleles of the Gc system of plasma proteins *Hum. Genetics,* **33,** 307.

Mourant, A.E., Kopéc, A.C. & Domaniewska-Sobczak, K. (1978) *Associations Between Polymorphisms and Diseases.* Oxford University Press.

Owen, R.D. (1945) Immunogenetic consequences of vascular anastomoses between bovine twins. *Science,* **102,** 400.

Race, R.R. & Sanger, R. (1975) *Blood groups in Man.* P.521. Oxford: Blackwell.

Ritter, H. & Hinkelman, K. (1966) Zur balance des polymorphismus der haptoglobine. *Humangenetik,* **2,** 21.

Salmon, C., Dreyfus, B. & André, R. (1958) Double population de globules, différent seulement par l'antigéne de groupe ABO, observée chez un malade leucémique. *Rev. Hémat,* **13,** 148.

Salmon, C. (1969) A tentative approach to variations in ABH and associated erythrocyte antigens. *Ser. Haemat.,* **II,** 3.

Shreffler, D.C. (1966) Relationship of alkaline phosphatase levels in intestinal mucosa to ABO and secretor blood groups. *Proc. Soc. exp. Biol. Med.,* **123,** 423.

Tilley, C.A., Crookston, M.C., Brown, B.L. & Wherrett, J.R. (1975) A and B and A₁ Leᵇ substances in glycosphingolipid fractions of human serum. *Vox Sang.,* **28,** 25.

Van der Hart, M., Van der Veer, M. & Van Loghem, J.J. (1962) Changes of blood group B in a case of Leukaemia. *Vox Sang.,* **7,** 449.

Van Loghem, J.J. Dorfmeier, H. & Van der Hart, M. (1957) Two A antigens with abnormal serologic properties. *Vox Sang.,* **2,** 16.

Vogel, F., Pettenkofer, H.J. & Helmbold, W. (1960) Über die populationsgenetik der ABO-blutgruppen 2. Mitteilung. Genhäufigkeit und epidemische erkrankungen. *Acta genet.,* **10,** 267.

Section 4. The Forensic Application of Blood Groups

"When blood is their argument"

Shakespeare, KING HENRY V.

Chapter 29. Blood Groups Applied to Cases of Doubtful Parentage and the Identification of Stains

Forensic science deals often with problems of ientity. Blood groups are excellent aids to these pursuits. They do not however show a positive identity, for example: "This man is the father of this child" or "This blood stain originated from this person" but they do show a definite non-identity, for example: "This man is not the father of this particular child" or "This blood stain cannot have originated from that person". However such an extensive range of polymorphisms is now applied to forensic problems that it is often possible to contribute significant (although not conclusive) evidence towards proving paternity or the origin of a blood stain.

It is not our intention to write exhaustively on the subject of forensic blood grouping and immunology. Many of the techniques used are beyond the scope of this book. However, some of them are merely adaptations of those already described in other chapters and others can be readily mastered by workers who have become familiar with the practical application of blood grouping to clinical and transfusion problems. It must be stressed that although a good theoretical and practical grounding in blood grouping is essential for the forensic serologist, it does not by itself provide the necessary experience for forensic work. This must be gained in the laboratory while studying forensic problems, which are very different from clinical ones.

The chapter is divided into two parts dealing with (a) paternity tests and (b) blood grouping of stains.

BLOOD GROUPING APPLIED TO CASES OF DOUBTFUL PATERNITY

General principles

Since blood group antigens are inherited according to Mendelian laws, they may be of value in problems of identity, for example in cases of doubtful paternity. The two relevant rules of inheritance are as follows:-

(1) A blood group gene cannot appear in a child unless present in one or other (or both) of the parents.

(2) If one or other parent is homozygous for a particular blood group gene, its product must appear in the blood of the child.

A simple example dependent upon (1) would be the situation in which the mother and putative father were both of group O and the child group A. The A gene of the child must be inherited from its father who could not, therefore, be group O. The serological test has thereby excluded him from paternity.

An example dependent upon (2) would be a putative father of Rh type CC who must therefore pass C to all his offspring and who could not be the father of a child of type cc. However the application of the second rule cannot be quite so reliably made since homozygosity for a particular gene cannot be so accurately determined; the possibility of a rare allele being passed to the child which goes undetected must be considered.

Exclusions of paternity based on the first rule of inheritance are termed "first order exclusions" while those based on the second rule which depend upon the assumption that the putative father and child are homozygous for a gene, are termed "second order exclusions". The forensic serologist is reluctant to base an exclusion of paternity on a single second order exclusion and prefers to have at least one other second order exclusion as a back up.

Dosage titrations can be of value in determining in the case of a second order exclusion whether or not the individuals are homozygous for a particular antigen, for, with selected sera, the homozygote will give a 'double dose' reaction and a higher titration score than the heterozygote which will give a 'single dose' reaction (see technique No. 29.1).

Blood group systems used in problems of parentage

These include tests for ABO (including A_1 and A_2), MNSs, Rh (D, C, C^w, E, c and e) and most of the following: Fy^a, K, Lu^a, Jk^a, Gm(1). This brings the chance of proving non-paternity, if such is the case, to about 66 per cent.

As well as the above, haptoglobins, Gc groups and red cell enzymes are routinely included in some laboratories. The combined exclusion rate if all these systems are used is raised to 90 per cent (Table 29.1). This means that, if 100 cases were investigated in which the putative father is not the child's true father, the application of the full range of tests would be expected to exclude 90 of the men from paternity.

Techniques for typing for haptoglobins, Gm and Gc groups all of which are genetically inherited serum groups will be found in Chapter 20. The specialised biochemical procedures for detection of red cell enzymes are beyond the scope of this book, but see Sonneborn 1976.

The suitability of the various blood groups systems for paternity testing

ABO system

The inheritance of ABO has been well worked out and is entirely reliable.

Table 29.1 Probabilities of exclusion of non-fathers

| | Probability of exclusion by:- | |
	Individual systems	Combined systems
Red cell antigens		
MNSs	0.321	
Rh	0.280	
ABO	0.176	
Duffy	0.048	
Kidd	0.045	
Kell	0.033	
Lutheran	0.033	0.657
Serum proteins		
Hp	0.175	
Gc	0.145	
Gm^1	0.065	0.341
Red cell enzymes*		
EAP	0.210	
GPT	0.190	
PGM	0.145	
EsD	0.090	
AK	0.045	
ADA	0.045	
6 PGD	0.025	0.558
Total combined systems		0.901

*EAP, Erythrocyte acid phosphatase; GPT, glutamate-pyruvate transaminase; PGM, phosphoglu-comutase; EsD, esterase D; AK, adenylate kinase; ADA, adenosine deaminase; 6-PGD, 6-phosphogluconate dehydrogenase.

The exceedingly few abnormalities, e.g. one apparent mutation where mother was AB and child O, or a case where a *B* gene was suppressed in one generation (*see* Chapter 16), which have been found are the accumulation of years of work by many serologists and are drawn from many thousands of family studies.

The rarities and anomalies in the system are unlikely to lead to erroneous conclusions about paternity if red cells are routinely tested with group O serum and sera are tested with A_1, A_2, B and O red cells.

For example, O_h ("Bombay" phenotype) is disclosed by the presence of a powerful anti-H in the serum. A_m patterns as a group O with a missing anti-A and A_x is agglutinated by group O serum only (*see* Chapter 16).

The very rare families in which an AB child has one group O parent, are recognisable by the comparative weakness of the B antigen and the presence of a fraction of the anti-B spectrum of antibodies in the serum (*see* Chapter 16).

MNSs system

The MN typing of family material has been studied for over 40 years and the results establish beyond doubt its reliability as a tool for the solution of problems of parentage. Nevertheless, the rare MN alleles (*e.g.* N^2, M^g etc) must be remembered in a medico-legal context (*see* Chapter 18).

In practice, the possible presence of such rare alleles must be considered wherever the putative father is M and the child N or when the putative father is N and the child M *i.e.* in second order exclusions. If, in either of these, the father and the child had, for example, M_g, an entirely opposite interpretation of results would have to be made. The man, far from being excluded from being the father of the child, would be virtually proven to be the father since they both would have this very rare allele. However, M_g has not been found in testing at least 60,000 English blood donors. Moreover, anti-M_g can be obtained fairly readily and should be included in the tests where appropriate. M^k producing no M, N, S or s is of similar rarity to M_g but anti-M^k is not available. "Dosage" titrations may be helpful as confirmatory tests.

The Rh system

This system is one of the most valuable in excluding paternity but there are sometimes difficulties in connection with alternative genotypes. Paternity could appear to be excluded by the probable genotypes of the persons tested but there may be an uncommon genotype on the basis of which there would not be an exclusion. An example taken from an actual paternity problem will help to make this point clear.

Mother	- phenotype R_1R_1 *i.e.* C+ D+ E− c−
probable genotype	*CDe/CDe*
Child	- phenotype R_1r *i.e.* C+ D+ E− c+
probable genotype	*CDe/cde*
Putative father	- phenotype R_1R_2 *i.e.* C+ D+ E+ c+ e+
probable genotype	*CDe/cDE*

Given that the probable genotypes are the actual genotypes in the above case, the putative father could not be the father of the child. But should the putative father be of the alternative genotype *CDE/cde* or even *CDE/cDe* he could be the father of the child. Tests with anti-ce and anti-Ce are invaluable in this situation. The genotypes *CDE/cde* and *CDE/cDe* are positive with anti-ce and negative with anti-Ce whereas for the genotype *CDe/cDE* the reverse is true, the cells are positive with anti-Ce and negative with anti-ce.

Uncommon Rh alleles, C^x, E^w etc must be remembered and if possible sera capable of detecting them used to check any apparent exclusion (*see* Chapter 17). In Rh second order exclusions, −D− has to be considered. A selected incomplete anti-D capable of agglutinating −D−without the addition of albumin, is useful for the detection of−D−in the heterozygote.

The Lutheran system

With good anti-Lu^a sera, a first order exclusion of paternity is accepted. However, in rare instances modifying genes are present and so if an exclusion of paternity is being based solely on the presence of Lu^a in the child and its absence from both mother and putative father, a suppressed Lu^a in one or other of the adults has to be considered. However the suppressor gene has been shown to inhibit both Lu^a and Lu^b so testing the family with anti-Lu^b will indicate whether or not a suppressor gene is present (Tippett, 1971).

The Kell system

Tests with anti-K are suitable for paternity work but the frequency of K is such that only 4 per cent of non-fathers can be excluded by this system.

The Duffy System

The Fy^a antigen is useful for paternity tests providing a reliable pure anti-Fy^a serum is available for testing. Unfortunately, anti-Fy^a often occurs in a mixture of antibodies and care must be exercised that the serum is specific. Anti-Fy^b is also suitable but the possibility of the presence of the alleles which are negative with anti-Fy^a and anti-Fy^b must not be overlooked, particularly in coloured families (*see* Chapter 18).

The Kidd system

Anti-Jk^a and anti-Jk^b sera, if reliable examples are available may be included but the allele which is Jk (a−b−) must not be forgotten.

The Lewis system

This system is unsuitable for cases of doubtful paternity. However if saliva samples have been tested, the Lewis typing of the red cells may be a useful confirmation of the results, particularly when the putative father and mother are non-secretors and the child is a secretor (see below).

Secretion of A, B and H substances

The secretor genes can be applied with confidence to problems of parentage, but only the "mating" *sese* x *sese* shows an exclusion if the child is a secretor. Such a mating occurs in 5 per cent of English families.

P groups

Like secretion, the P system is only helpful in 4-5 per cent of cases in which the mother and alleged father have no trace of P_1, while the child has a strongly developed P_1 antigen.

A rare family in which a P_2 x P_2 mating produced a P_1 child has been described (Contreras and Tippett, 1974). The upset in inheritance was caused by the influence of the Lutheran inhibitor gene on the P locus. In the event of obtaining an apparent exclusion of paternity due to P, tests with both anti-Lu^a and anti-Lu^b would disclose whether or not one of the adults was Lu (a−b−).

Reliability of results in general

Blood grouping in cases of doubtful paternity should not be attempted until a long apprenticeship in the blood grouping field has been served. However in the hands of experienced serologists, aware of possible pitfalls and in the habit of repeating critical tests with other examples of the appropriate antisera and taking fresh samples from the original sample tubes, the application of blood groups to problems of paternity is both reliable and rewarding.

The possibility of mutation occurring and affecting the reliability of results is a question which sometimes arises. Can a blood group gene mutate (*i.e.* change) between one generation and the next? If it can in fact do so, a blood group character might appear in a child which is absent from both parents. No convincing example of a blood group gene mutating between two generations has been found. Moreover the total mutation rate for humans has been estimated at 1 in 1,000,000 gene generations (Stevenson and Kerr, 1967) and for blood group genes alone it would be even lower.

As pointed out above rare variants if undetected may give rise to false conclusions about paternity. Most of the blood group systems listed in Table 29.1 have uncommon or rare alternative genes which may occur from time to time at a particular locus on the chromosome instead of the common gene. Experienced workers are aware of their existence and are able to include tests which will reveal the presence of a number of them. When they do occur in paternity problems they often yield important results, either excluding the alleged father from paternity or because of their low frequency in the general population the finding of one of them in both alleged father and child furnishes highly significant evidence that the two individuals are related.

A single apparent second order exclusion is particularly difficult to interpret when it is obtained in the haptoglobin system or in some of the red cell enzyme polymorphisms, particularly phospho-glucomutase (PGM) and glutamate-pyruvate transaminase (GPT). These systems show evidence for the existence of both 'silent' and very rare alleles Cook *et al*, 1969, Herbidy *et al*, 1970, and Olaisen, 1973. Therefore in the absence of a confirmatory exclusion by a second polymorphic system, some idea of the expected frequency of the appropriate 'silent' allele must be given.

A few rare alleles may remain undetected. However a sensible perspective has to be maintained concerning rarities. In the last analysis it is for the Court to decide after taking into account *all* the evidence in a case, which is the more likely state of affairs, a false result due to a rare abnormality or variant, or the existence of another man who is the true father of the child.

A potential danger exists when individuals connected with a particular case are not all tested in the same laboratory and every effort should be made for a laboratory to receive all the samples relevant to the case. The testing of the putative father in one laboratory and the mother and child in another should be avoided, particularly because the usual routine of repeating critical results cannot be carried out as it will not be known which these are. In addition there is always the possibility that an error may occur when different laboratories using different reagents each handle a part of the same case.

The possibility of proof of paternity from blood groups

Proof of paternity (*i.e.* determining that only one particular man can be the father of a particular child) is at the present time, impossible. However, assistance towards giving a judgement can be obtained by calculating the chance, in a given case, in which an exclusion has not been found, of a putative father who is not the true father being able to pass on the blood group genes necessary for making him a possible father for the child. If this chance is small enough to be statistically significant then the putative father, who besides having the required genes and being known to the mother, is likely to be the true father of the child.

Table 29.2 The result of a blood group analysis in which the putative father Mr W is not excluded from paternity of baby R and the probability of his paternity of baby R is highly significant.

Name	ABO	MNSs	D	C	Cʷ	c	E	Luᵃ	K	Fyᵃ	Gmˡ	PGM	EAP	Hp	Gc	GPT	ADA	AK	EsˡD
MrW	O	NS−	−	+	−	+	−	−	−	+	+	1	BA	2-1	2-1	1	−	−	−
Miss R	O	MS+s−	−	−	−	+	−	−	−	+	−	1	BA	1	1	2-1	−	−	−
Baby R	O	MNS+s+	−	+	−	+	−	−	−	+	−	1	B	2-1	2-1	2-1	−	−	−

If, after completion of a blood group investigation upon putative father, mother and child, no exclusion of paternity is evident, the blood group genes which have been shown to be of paternal origin are noted. The chance the putative father has of passing on these genes all together in one single sperm is compared with the chance of obtaining such a sperm from a man in the general population (for, if the putative father is not the true father, he is an unrelated man selected from the general population).

The combined chance of obtaining the known paternal genes from the putative father is arrived at by multiplying together either 1 or 0.5 according to whether he is known to be homozygous or heterozygous for these genes. If this is unknown, he is arbitrarily taken to be heterozygous thus eliminating any bias towards his paternity.

The figure for the probability of obtaining the genes from an unrelated man is calculated by multiplying together the known frequencies of the genes in the appropriate racial population.

The balance of these probabilities gives the odds in favour of paternity. A whole range of results is obtained. If, in testing a family, only common blood group genes are found, or if only one or two genes are known for certainty to come from the father, the odds in favour of paternity is not significant. We do not consider that much weight should be given to the figure obtained unless the odds in favour of the paternity of the named man are at least 50 to 1 and preferably nearer to 100 to 1.

An alternative method, which is more commonly used is that of making a simple calculation of the expected percentage of men in the general population who, after the same set of tests have been performed, would not be excluded from paternity. A figure of 1-2 per cent or lower is taken as significant.

Members of the legal profession usually find a comparison of men more comprehensible than a comparison of sperm!

However it will be readily appreciated that since the alternative method is based on phenotypes, in situations in which a phenotype includes a number of different genotypes, the whole phenotype will have to be included. For example, if the A_2 gene is known to be of paternal origin, the whole of the group A phenotype and A_2B must be included in the calculation because there are no tests which will disclose which group A_1 individuals are A_1A_2.

The example shown in Table 29.2 is illustrative.

Method 1

Baby R has to receive *Ns, Cde, Hp*^{2} and *Gc*^{2} from her father as the mother lacks them all.

In addition, one each of the genes *O, PGM*^{1}, *EAP*^{B}, *ADA*^{1}, *AK*^{1} and *EsD*^{1}

Table 29.3 Calculation of probability of paternity by method 1.

	O	Ns	Cde	Hp²	Gc²	PGM¹	EAPB	ADA¹	AK¹	EsD¹	Probability
Sperm from Mr W	1	1	0.5	0.5	0.5	1	0.5	1	1	1	0.0625
Sperm from unrelated man	0.68	0.39	0.01	0.58	0.27	0.76	0.60	0.94	0.95	0.88	0.00008

must be of paternal origin, since the child is homozygous for these genes. Mr W's probability of paternity is worked out as shown in table 29.3.

These figures in table 29.3 show a balance of probability in favour of Mr W of 780 to 1.

Method 2

This method merely requires the product of the frequencies of all the appropriate phenotypes to be calculated. As already explained above giving the A_2 gene as an example, large phenotypes may have to be included. In the selected case shown in table 29.2 although the gene complex *Cde* has a frequency of only 0.01, nevertheless this method of calculation requires the whole C positive phenotype to be included which is 67 per cent of the population.

The full calculation for the given example is therefore as follows:

O	Ns	Cde	Hp²	Gc²	PGM¹	EAPB	ADA¹	AK¹	EsD¹	Combined frequency
97	67	67	84	44	93	84	99.3	99.5	99.1	12%

This means 12 per cent of men in the general population, if the same tests were performed, would be expected to have a blood group combination which would not exclude them from possible paternity of baby R.

It is clear therefore that in this example the calculation performed by method 1 is significantly in favour of Mr W being the true father whereas the figure obtained by the second method is not significant.

We consider that, in any given case, the first method is that of choice since it reflects more accurately the probability of the putative father being the true father of the child (*see also* Race and Sanger, 1975; p.505).

Caution is required before drawing too firm a conclusion from the figures obtained for probability of paternity. It is sometimes difficult to obtain accurate knowledge of the most appropriate general population with which to compare the putative father's blood group combination. This is particularly the case when non-European families are involved. Moreover the calculation is completely invalidated if the named man's brother is a second possible father for the child.

In other European countries more sophisticated methods of calculating probability of paternity are often used. These have been well summarised and discussed by Salmon (1974). We do not think they offer the Courts appreciably more guidance than the simple calculations described above.

Doubtful Maternity

There is a case on record (Wiener, 1943) in which a woman who had borrowed a child from an orphan asylum claimed that it was hers by a particular man who thereby had been persuaded to marry her. The results obtained in the MN system were found to exclude her from maternity. Other examples of doubtful maternity are also cited by Wiener (1959).

It is not unusual for the occasional case of doubtful maternity to arise when a mix up of babies on a maternity ward is suspected. These cases of course also

O

involve doubtful paternity and thus increase the capacity of a blood group solution to the problem.

If the accidental exchange of infants is known to have occurred between two particular mothers then blood of all four parents as well as the two infants may be tested.

Doubtful maternity is also involved when blood grouping expertise is sought in cases of kidnapping. Such a case, in which two families accused a third of kidnapping a child from each of them has been reported from the authors' laboratory (Lincoln and Dodd, 1968). It is of interest that the samples from each individual were received from abroad in the form of blood stains on cotton cloth (see below).

Sampling

A few ml of blood from each individual is sufficient. From young babies from whom it may be difficult to obtain blood by venepuncture 1-2 ml samples taken by heel prick are very satisfactory. 2 ml lithium heparin or EDTA containers are excellent for blood sampling since any amount up to 2 ml can be put into them. Surprisingly perhaps, about 1 ml of blood taken by heel prick into these containers is ample for tests for all the red cell antigens and enzymes and the plasma is sufficient for the ABO serum check, Gm^1, Gc and haptoglobin typing.

Provisions under Part III of the Family Law Reform Act 1969

In civil proceedings the Family Law Reform act 1969, Part III, gives the courts power to make a direction for blood grouping tests at the request of one or other party involved in any case of doubtful paternity.

A court direction is not an order so that a person failing to comply with the direction is not in contempt of court. However, under the Act, the court is at liberty to draw whatever conclusion seems appropriate from failure to respond to a direction.

The Act brings greater uniformity into the whole procedure. Only members of a panel of blood grouping specialists approved by the Home Secretary are authorized to undertake Court directed blood group investigations. An Advisory Committee of blood grouping experts scrutinizes the qualifications of those who apply for membership of this panel. Although testers do not all apply exactly the same range of blood group systems, submission of their proposed selection of systems to the Advisory Committee ensures that solicitors and others obtain a comparable service from whichever tester they happen to select. There are some 16 specialists who undertake such blood group investigations, scattered throughout the country but with a higher proportion situated in or near London. However, if the individuals requiring the tests do not live near a testing laboratory, they may be sampled by any willing medical practitioner and the samples sent to the tester by first class mail.

When a court direction is made the Clerk of the Court is responsible for initiating the proceedings and special direction forms with attached photographs of each adult, and child if over 12 months, are sent to the acting solicitor or straight to the doctor who is prepared to take the samples. The photographs are particularly important in ensuring an individual's correct identity and the parties should be encouraged to provide passport photographs even when their case, and there are still many such, has not been brought as a definite court direction. A putative father anxious to ensure a result of non-paternity might be tempted to send a friend to impersonate him. Mutual identification if the parties are willing to attend at the same time for sampling is usually accepted as good evidence of correct identity but circumstances can be envisaged in which prior collusion between the parties to falsify an identity might suit them both.

Presentation of results

Results have to be presented at two levels. First the findings must be given in sufficient detail to satisfy a second blood grouping expert, because occasionally the legal profession will call upon another blood group specialist to do confirmatory tests.

Secondly, the results must be intelligible to solicitors and the courts who, in respect of blood groups, are in the position of laymen.

The report forms introduced at the time of the implementation of Part III of the Family Law Reform Act are designed to satisfy both these points. Part I of the report form states whether or not the putative father is excluded from paternity or if not excluded, a figure indicating a probability of paternity is given. This figure may or may not be significant. Part II of the form allows for a more detailed and technical protocol of the results obtained in each system, and this may be presented in whatever form the serologist wishes.

IDENTIFICATION OF STAINS AND FRAGMENTS FROM INDIVIDUALS

Since the subject of this book is blood group serology we are mainly concerned with the blood group aspect of the identification of stains from body fluids. However, it must be realised that, in any actual forensic problem, the identification of a stain as being, for example, human blood must precede any attempt to ascertain its groups. These preliminary tests make a claim on material which may already be inadequate in quantity and is always irreplaceable. No criminal who accidentally stains his coat with blood will obligingly offer a repeat sample for the convenience of the laboratory! Thus, techniques which have the merit of requiring small amounts of material for their performance are those of choice providing they satisfy the major criterion of reliability.

For the sake of completeness and clarity, a brief summary of the identification of various body fluids follows.

For blood very often a chemical screening test is necessary because stained areas are not always easy to distinguish particularly on dark or dirty clothing.

There are various chemical screening tests but none of them is completely specific for blood since they detect peroxidases which are found, although they are less strongly active, in a number of other biological fluids besides blood. Hitherto the benzidine test has been most often used but owing to the carcinogenic nature of the reagent, it has been replaced by the phenolthalein (Kastle-meyer) test. (Gradwohl's Legal Medicine 1968; *see also* Chapter 20). This is highly sensitive, being capable of detecting blood spots practically invisible to the eye and there is little point in undertaking grouping procedures or species identification on areas when the Kastlemeyer test is negative.

A test for acid phosphatase is the screening test for seminal fluid although it is not entirely specific as vaginal fluid also contains this enzyme. Seminal fluid is identified by the examination of a smear for spermatozoa. Also, contamination by vaginal fluid can be disclosed by taking advantage of the fact the acid phosphatases present in these secretions have different electrophoretic mobilities (Adams and Wraxall, 1974). The detection of semen in cases of aspermia or vasectomised males may depend upon this method.

Saliva reveals itself by the starch test for amylases together with a histological examination for buccal cells. Vaginal fluid shows squamous epithelial cells but is negative for amylase, and is usually found in different situations.

Species identification

The species of origin is determined by using antisera more or less specific for the proteins contained in the serum of the stain. The laboratory must, therefore, possess a collection of reliable antisera capable of making distinctions between various common species e.g. Man, dog, cat, ox, sheep, chicken, etc. In some countries it may be necessary to make the rather difficult distinction between ape and Man, for which carefully absorbed antisera are required. Antisera specific for various animal species can be obtained commercially.

In many cases, however, all that is necessary is the establishment of the blood as human, so an anti-human globulin is used first and, if this test (with suitable controls is positive, the investigation need proceed no further. A negative test may either mean that the blood is other than human or that the proteins in the stain have denatured to the extent of being inactive. At this point tests should be made for other species.

Methods by which species specific anti-globulins may be used

The Ring Test

The classical species identification is by the ring technique in which a drop or two of stain extract (the antigen) is layered carefully above a similar volume of antiserum in a precipitin tube or capillary. In a positive test a ring of white precipitate forms at the interface. This is a sensitive test and requires but small quantities of the reactants. Fairly strong antisera are required and the fluids must be clear.

The anti-globulin consumption test

This test has been used by many workers. It is based on the absorption of a standard anti-globulin reagent by the globulin contained in an extract of the stain to be examined. Any reduction in titre of the anti-globulin caused by its absorption by globulin contained in the stain is shown by means of red cells coated with globulin. For the detection of human globulin red cells sensitised by incomplete anti-D are used. These would normally become agglutinated by the anti-human globulin used in the test but remain unagglutinated or less strongly agglutinated if the anti-human globulin has been taken up already by the stain (*see* technique No. 29.2). The technique is not so readily applicable to the detection of proteins other than human since these require red cells sensitised with protein from the particular animal species for which the test is being made.

Immunoelectro-osmophoresis

When it is necessary to test for the protein of species other than human, an electrophoretic method in agar gel is recommended; this method is also excellent for identifying human globulin in stains. Using the same buffer system as for Gc groups, the movement of the gamma globulins, the antibodies (*e.g.* anti-human globulin) is toward the cathode under the influence of endosmosis while all the other proteins, including those of the stain extract, move towards the anode. Thus it can be arranged that the non-gamma globulins from a stain to be tested for its species of origin, move towards the gamma type antibody in an anti-species specific globulin (anti-human, anti-cow, anti-pig, etc.). At a point between the anodic and cathodic wells, the reactants meet and a line of precipitate is formed (*see* technique No. 29.3) (Culliford, 1964).

The grouping of blood stains

It will be appreciated that direct agglutination tests are not possible for the detection of antigens in blood stains since the red cells have been destroyed and, in the case of stains from other body fluids, the blood group substances are in soluble form.

The inhibition method by which the specific absorption of antibody by the stain is measured has been used both experimentally and in case work. However the method has its limitations. The minimum requirement is that the blood group antigen in the stain must be capable of absorbing, and thus inhibiting the activity of at least three quarters of the antibody content of the serum with which it is tested. Nothing less than this produces a reduction in titre of the original antiserum sufficient to be sure of the presence of the corresponding antigen in the stain. Thus the method is not very sensitive and may require larger areas of stained material per test than are often available. Although it still remains the method of choice for the detection of Gm and Km characters in blood stains, it has largely been abandoned for the detection of red cell antigens in favour of a micro-elution method.

By allowing stained threads or small squares of material to absorb antibody which is subsequently eluted, a high degree of sensitivity is attained, particularly if a low concentration (about 0.1 to 0.05 per cent) of cells is used. Sometimes enzyme treated cells are used as indicator cells for the detection of the eluted antibody. This technique has the further advantage of requiring only small amounts of stained material. Figure 29.1 illustrates this point. The stain on the left of the diagram is 1 x 0.5 cm. A piece of equal size cut from the same stain has been apportioned between tests using the various reagents shown on the right. It

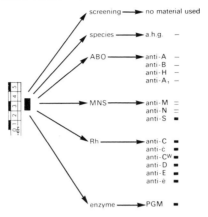

Fig. 29.1 Diagram showing the optimum amounts of blood-stained material required for grouping tests.

will be seen that the amounts required vary from single 3-mm threads for species testing and ABO grouping, to 2-mm squares for each Rh antigen. These amounts are optimal and satisfactory results can often be obtained with even less material. When the elution technique is used to investigate blood staining on hard surfaces, for example on a knife blade, the blood is taken up on to cotton threads made damp with distilled water.

Selection of antisera

Special selection of antisera is of vital importance.

It is highly probable that there is a critical relationship between the required potency of the antiserum and the number of antigenic sites on the red cell for the various antigens. This relationship gains its importance almost certainly because the antigenic sites are not in good shape for the uptake of antibody in blood stains, particularly if these are several weeks or months old.

From a battery of antisera of each specificity only certain examples will be suitable and these have to be selected by trial and error using the elution technique before being used in case work. The combining capacity (K) of the antibody is critical. Antibodies with too high a K value may have to be discarded because they are difficult to recover in the eluate, while those with a low K value are not readily enough absorbed by the stain antigens.

Moreover antisera which are suitable for fresh stains may not be sufficiently potent for older stains and adjustments of the dilution at which they are used may have to be made for the detection of less active antigens. The factors affecting the elution of antibodies from blood stains has been discussed by Lincoln and Dodd (1973).

In the ABO blood grouping of stains, in contrast to the ABO grouping of fresh blood, anti-H (from *Ulex*) is a most important reagent since it provides a valuable positive reaction which is particularly applicable to O stains in situations (which are many) when it is not possible to test for agglutinins in stains. When there is sufficient material and it is not too old, an extract of a stain may show sufficient antibody activity for "cross grouping" to be done.

Sometimes papain treated A and B cells may be used with advantage in such tests.

The blood group markers that are detectable in blood stains

Red cell antigens

The elution technique has been used with success for the detection of the following antigens, A, B, H, M, N, S, s, D, C, c, E, e, C^w, K, Fy^a, Fy^b and Jk^a (Nicholls and Pereira, 1962; Pereira, 1963; Bargagna and Pereira, 1967; Lincoln and Dodd, 1968; Lincoln and Dodd, 1975).

Gm and Km grouping of stains

These are very rewarding antigens to include in the grouping of stains as they are very stable, resistant to heat and detectable after quite long periods of time. Satisfactory results both with experimental stains and in case work using Gm (1), Gm (2) and Km (1) have been reported by Khalap et al. (1976) and there seems no reasons why Gm (4), Gm (5) and other Gm antigens cannot be added to the list provided suitable antisera and the appropriate anti-D for red cell sensitisation can be obtained. Details of the method are described under technique No. 29.7.

Haptoglobins

The usual electrophoretic technique using starch gel is unsuitable for the detection of haptoglobins in stains mainly because of the unavoidable presence in blood stains of excess haemoglobin.

An acrylamide gradient technique has been developed by Culliford (1971). This requires rather more material than for the detection of red cell antigens but the technique is sufficiently successful to be used in routine case work.

Gc types

The detection of Gc allotypes in stains has been described by Nerstrøm and Skafte-Jensen (1963) in whose opinion success depended on the freshness of the stains and only in good stains up to a few days in age could Gc types be reliably distinguished. However, Wraxall (1977) has found that it is possible to distinguish Gc types in stains up to 5 weeks in age, but it appears that the drying conditions of the stains are very crucial.

Red cell enzymes

Much of the pioneer work on the forensic application of red cell enzymes has been carried out by Culliford and his colleagues at the Metropolitan Police Laboratory in London. The results have been such that the following enzymes can be satisfactorily detected in blood stains:–

Phosphoglucomutase (PGM) (Culliford, 1967) adenylate kinase (AK), adenosine deaminase (ADA), 6-phosphogluconate dehydrogenase (6-PGD), glucose-6-phosphate dehydrogenase (G-6-PD) (Culliford, 1971) glutamate-pyruvate transaminase (GPT) by Welch (1972) esterase D by Parkin and Adams (1975), erythrocyte acid phosphatase (EAP) has been added by Wraxall and Emes (1976).

For the detection of these enzymes in stains normally a modified version of starch gel electrophoresis involving a thin layer technique is used. This obviates the necessity of slicing the gel at the end of the electrophoretic procedure and requires on the whole a smaller amount of blood stained material.

The deterioration of blood stains

Blood group antigens and other polymorphic characters associated with the red cell, deteriorate in stains at different rates and there is also a wide variation due to the conditions to which the stain is exposed before testing. Activity may be diminished considerably after a few days or may survive for some years. The antigens of the ABO system seem particularly able to withstand the passage of time. For example one of the authors has found A activity in a blood crust on floor boards fourteen years after the blood was shed.

Usually stains which have dried out quickly retain their activity for longer periods than those which remain wet. Bacteria tend to flourish in wet conditions and their activity may lead to both false positive and false negative results.

M and N antigens are more labile than A and B but good results can often be obtained from stains that are a few months old. Cross reactivity particularly between anti-N and M stains is the main problem with all MN typing of stains.

All the Rh antigens, S, s and K are often detectable after many months and Rh even up to two years in good conditions. However Rh antigens are known to deteriorate rapidly in sunlight.

Red cell enzymes lose their activity in stains more readily than red cell antigens and are, on the whole, inactive after a few weeks. Haptoglobins however retain their activity longer.

Procedure in case work

Although, as will be appreciated from the foregoing paragraphs, there is now an impressive list of genetic markers available for blood stain classification, not all by any means are investigated in every problem!

The procedure in a typical case, for example, a murder, is to type as fully as possible the liquid blood of the victim and if relevant and available, that of the suspect. Any blood stains found on a suspect's clothing and/or weapons etc are investigated for a selection of those markers present in the victim's blood and distinct from the suspect's own, for which it is most profitable to test. This choice is influenced by the amount of blood stain available, by its age and condition, and by the frequencies of the markers in the general population. The least common markers will be the most rewarding although a combination of several relatively common ones can often have a surprisingly low frequency.

An actual case summarised in Table 29.4 illustrates the present scope of tests on blood stains.

A man suffered a severe neck injury caused by an assault against him by means of a broken glass. Blood on a piece of the glass and stains on shirt and trousers of the accused were tested—the range of systems included ABO, MNS, Rh antigens D, C, E and c and the red cell enzyme system, PGM.

It is apparent from Table 29.4 that the stain on the shirt of the accused gave the

Table 29.4 Results of blood grouping in a case of assault

Victim (14/7/72)	A_1	M*N*S$_1$	cC*Dee	PGM 2-1
Victim (19/10/72)	A_1	MS–	ccDee	PGM 2-1
Accused	A_2	MS+	ccDEE	PGM 2-1

Results of stain groupings:

	A	B	M	S	D	C	E	c	PGM	Frequency
Shirt of accused	+	–	+	–	+	–	–	+	2-1	1 in 1000
Glass	+	–	+	–	+	–	–	+	2-1	1 in 1000
Pocket of accused	+	–	+	+	+	–	+	+	2-1	1 in 100

*Tests showed mixed field.

same reactions as the blood found on the glass fragment and this combination of groups differed in two respects from those of the accused himself in that they were both S negative and E negative. In making a comparison with the victim's pattern of blood types difficulty was for a time encountered because the victim had been so severely injured that it was necessary for him to receive an immediate transfusion of three units of blood. Where shown in Table 29.4 the tests gave a mixed field appearance indicating two red cell populations, one, the victim's own and the other originating from the donors. This phenomenon was seen in tests for M, N, S and C. It was therefore not possible to be certain of the victim's blood types until some months later when the donor red cells had been eliminated from the circulation.

It can be seen that there is a significant probability that the blood on both shirt and glass originated from the victim. In this respect it was fortunate that the victim possessed the less common Rh_0 so that his particular blood group combination was expected to occur in only 1 person in 1000 of the appropriate general population.

The finding of a small blood stain area in the accused person's trouser pocket giving a combination of reactions which accorded with his own blood groups led to the speculation that in assaulting the victim with the broken glass the accused might have injured his own hand which might then have been plunged into his pocket. Later the police confirmed that he had indeed sustained such an injury!

The grouping of stains from other body fluids

Secretors usually produce A, B and H blood group substances in high concentrations in seminal fluid, saliva, vaginal secretion and gastric juice. In other body fluids, such as sweat, tears and urine the concentration is fairly low.

Even in non-secretors there are trace amounts of group specific substances and these can be detected by the micro-elution technique discussed above in connection with blood stains.

The most usual stains which present themselves in forensic problems are those of seminal fluid which may or may not be contaminated with vaginal secretion, but occasionally saliva stains are encountered. In case work it is usual to look for blood group substances using the inhibition technique in parallel with elution and results reported only when there is agreement between the two techniques.

There are some hazards. Bacteria tend to flourish in seminal and saliva stains much more often than in blood stains. Particularly, *Escherichia coli* may be the origin of an acquired B and less often A activity (see also grouping of muscle and organ tissue). However the levels of spurious A and B activity are usually lower than those of the authentic group specific substances, and it is often possible to dilute saliva or other body fluids to the point where the spurious activity is no longer detectable while the specific reaction is retained. So when testing, for example, a seminal stain by inhibition technique, several dilutions of an extract of the stain are made and tested for A, B and H substances (*see* technique No. 29.5).

In spite of the soluble nature of the blood group substances in body fluids it is possible to test for their presence in stains by the elution technique even though this technique involves a washing process. Indeed the method is more sensitive than inhibition but it is important to realise that when using this method false negatives may be recorded due to an *excess* of group specific substance some of which dissolves in the antiserum, neutralising a high proportion of the antibody content so that insufficient remains to combine with the antigen which remains attached to the material under test. An alternative explanation of this phenomenon may be that the inactivity of the eluate may be due to the well known fact that it is difficult to obtain free antibody when elution is attempted in a situation of antigen excess. Sometimes a prozone phenomenon can be disclosed by making dilutions from an extract of the stain, dipping cotton threads into the various dilutions *e.g.* 1 in 5, 1 in 10, 1 in 20, allowing them to dry thoroughly after which the elution test is carried out and a prozone effect is seen. In the region of the prozone the strength of the agglutination is inversely proportional to the activity of the antigen in each test and may even be negative in the test in which the corresponding antigen is strongest.

There remains the problem of stains from non-secretors in which substances are not detectable by inhibition and although the small quantities present are detectable by elution, the results may not be reliable because of spurious reactions. Therefore positive reactions detected only by the elution technique must be interpreted with caution. Pereira and Martin (1976) recommend the Lewis typing of stains which are suspected to have come from non-secretors.

A detailed study of PGM types in seminal fluid has been made by Price *et al* (1976).

Recently Km (1) has been demonstrated in both saliva and seminal fluid (Davie and Kipps 1976).

Mixtures of stains

In trying to solve actual problems of crime, the serologist often has to work with mixed stains—*e.g.* blood contaminated with saliva, or more commonly mixtures of vaginal and seminal fluids. False conclusions may be reached if the possibility of a mixture is not realised. For example, a group O secretor man accused of raping a girl who is a group A secretor might be exonerated if the serologist reports in error that seminal fluid of group A has been identified on the girl's clothing. In this situation the A activity may arise from vaginal fluid or even sweat from the girl. A similar problem arises when grouping tests are carried out on seminal fluid from a vaginal swab in the hope of obtaining the ABO group of the man concerned. Such tests are of use only if the group of the woman is known. For example, if she is group O then authentic A and B activity detected on the swab is of male origin. If she is group AB no information about the group of the man can be obtained.

ABH grouping of body fragments

The antigens of the ABO system are distributed throughout most cells of the body. Their detection is often of value in a forensic problem.

This can be achieved by inhibition, elution (as described above) or mixed agglutination. Coombs et al. (1956) devised the mixed agglutination principle for the detection of antigens in cells such as buccal cells, skin cells and platelets none of which is suitable for direct agglutination tests.

The principle of the reaction is illustrated in Figure 29.2 where it can be seen

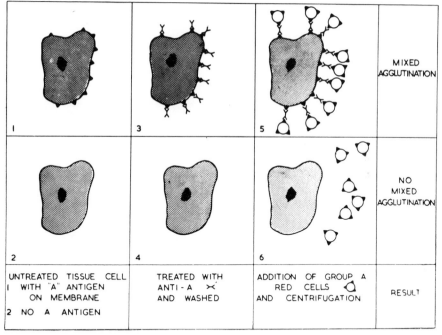

| UNTREATED TISSUE CELL 1 WITH "A" ANTIGEN ON MEMBRANE 2 NO A ANTIGEN | TREATED WITH ANTI - A ⋉ AND WASHED | ADDITION OF GROUP A RED CELLS AND CENTRIFUGATION | RESULT |

Fig. 29.2 Diagram of the mixed agglutination reaction for the demonstration of the A antigen on tissue cells.

that an antigen on a tissue cell may be revealed by a mixed agglutination procedure if the same antigen is available on a suitable indicator red cell so that an antibody reacting both with the tissue cell and the red cell is capable of binding them together in a mixed cell agglutination reaction.

Muscle and organ tissue

Cells from the tissue of organs, or muscle fibres may be grouped by inhibition or elution methods. They may require cleaning up by washing in methyl alcohol followed by ether to remove fat prior to grouping. A knowledge of the ABO group may be useful when assembling the parts of a dismembered body. A hazard is the possibility of bacterial contamination with *Escherichia coli* and related organisms which produce B-like and less commonly A-like substances. Bodies that have been in water are particularly susceptible to this kind of infection. The problem has been investigated by Jenkins *et al.* (1972) and Pereira (1973).

Skin, dander, finger nails and hair

Squamal cells from the surface of the skin and flakes of dander often can be successfully grouped by inhibition elution or mixed agglutination (*see* Technique 29.8). Mixed agglutination has been used by Swinburne, 1962; Poon and Dodd, 1964. Keratinised tissues may require some form of softening up prior to testing with the appropriate antisera and mild alkali or ultrasonic treatment has been used for this purpose. Outteridge (1963) tested a number of finger and toe nails with anti-A, anti-B and anti-H by an elution technique. The absorption phase of the test sometimes required up to 36 hours.

The grouping of hairs has been attempted by a number of workers by various methods such as mixed cell agglutination, elution and a method using ^{125}I-labelled antisera. None of the methods appear to be altogether reliable although some workers claim reliability for their own particular technique. A generally accepted reliable technique for the grouping of hairs would be a useful achievement.

TECHNIQUES

Technique No. 29.1. Titration technique for revealing antigen "dosage"

The technique, given a known dosing antiserum, is designed to find out whether red cells belonging to a particular phenotype are homozygous or heterozygous for a particular blood group gene. This may be particularly useful in blood grouping in cases of doubtful paternity.

For the sake of clarity, the method is described in relation to c and anti-c; other blood group antigens and antibodies can be similarly investigated using other appropriate red cells and antisera.

Serial dilutions of anti-c are made using the master titre technique (No. 3.4) and the required number of titrations run out from this, *e.g.* six. Two examples of rr cells are placed in rows 1 and 2 respectively and two examples of R_1r or other "single dose" c cells are run into rows 3 and 4. Rows 5 and 6 are used for cells under test.

The dosing phenomenon is more usually shown by agglutinins but occasionally the effect is well seen when albumin or anti-human globulin methods are used.

At least a fourfold or preferably an eight-fold difference in titre between "single dose" or "double dose" cells should be found before it can be established that the dosage effect is occurring.

The technique is particularly useful in assessing the true genotype of individuals *e.g.* if red cells behave as "double dose" cells, then they do not possess a rare antigen which has remained undetected in the tests.

Technique No. 29.2. Anti-human globulin consumption test

This test detects human globulin. The basis of the method is that human globulin will inhibit the activity of anti-human globulin serum, the inhibition being demonstrated by the failure of the anti-human globulin to agglutinate red cells sensitised by incomplete antibodies. An anti-human globulin serum, giving a titre of 16-32 against strongly sensitised D positive red cells, is suitable. An extract of the stain under test is made using a few drops of normal saline. If the stain is not fresh it is advisable to extract overnight. This is then mixed with an equal part of the diluted anti-human globulin and the mixture left on the bench for two hours. A control consisting of an extract from an unstained area of the same piece of clothing is also included. The mixtures are then titrated and the contents of each tube set out on a tile in the following manner.

A drop of fluid from each tube of the test row beginning with the most dilute solution, is placed on an opalescent tile. A second row of drops is made from the original titre of the anti-human globulin and a third series from the test made of unstained cloth. A drop of a 2 per cent suspension of D positive red cells, strongly sensitised by incomplete anti-D, is added to each and the mixtures are made uniform with a plastic applicator stick. The tile is rocked gently, for about five minutes and then read in the normal manner for indirect anti-globulin tests. A reduction in titration value of more than two dilutions is indicative of the presence of human globulin in the extract of the stain being tested.

Alternatively the D positive sensitised cells may be added to each tube of the titration and a spin anti-globulin test performed (*see* technique No. 8.3a).

Technique No. 29.3. Identification of blood stains by immuno-electro-osmophoresis in agar

Materials
The buffers and agar used are the same as those given for Gc typing.

Reagents
Anti-human globulin and other anti-globulins specific for various animal species, *e.g.* cow, pig, chicken, sheep. These can be obtained from Wellcome Reagents.

Method
The agar is poured onto microscope slides or a suitable sized glass plate. Glass surfaces must be grease free.

After the gel has set, small wells are punched in the gel in pairs, *see* Fig. 29.3. They should be approximately 1.5 mm. in diameter and 5 mm. apart and should be accurately placed along the line of electrophoretic movement. The

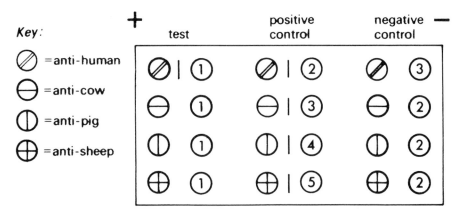

Fig. 29.3 Diagram illustrating species identification by electrophoresis in agar gel. ⊘ Anti-human; ⊖ anti-cow; ⓪ anti-pig; ⊕ anti-sheep.

1. Extract of stain run against 4 anti-species antisera and showing positive result against anti-human serum.
2. Positive control for anti-human serum; extract known human blood stain. Also used as negative control for other 3 antisera.
3. Positive control for anti-cow serum; extract from known bovine stain. Also used as negative control for anti-human serum (4 or 5 equally suitable).
4. Positive control for anti-pig serum; extract from known porcine stain.
5. Positive control for anti-sheep serum; extract from known bovine stain.

stain to be tested is extracted with gel buffer and a drop placed by means of a fine pipette in the cathodic well of a pair. The antiserum is placed in the anodic well. Controls consisting of extracts of known stains of appropriate age and species are included with each batch of tests. Electrophoresis is performed at 5 V/cm for at least 30 minutes.

If the antigen extracted from the stain corresponds to the anti-serum against which it is tested, a line of precipitate forms between two wells where the reactants meet.

Comment

The test is very sensitive and will detect globulin in whole blood diluted to 1 in 20,000 to 1 in 30,000.

The extract of the stain to be tested does not have to be clear or fat free.

The same technique can be used for the identification of seminal fluid or saliva with suitable prepared antisera.

Only the non-gamma globulin in the stain is detected since, in the nature of the test, the gamma globulin is migrating in the same direction as the antibody in the anodic well by endosmosis and therefore cannot meet and react with it.

Technique No. 29.4. A micro-elution technique for the detection of antigens in stains

Absorption

Blood-stained cloth (*e.g.* two 2-mm threads for ABO, 2-mm square for Rh) is placed in 6 x 1 cm plastic tubes. Two volumes (0.06 ml approximately) of suitably diluted antiserum are added to each tube, they are capped and incubated at the appropriate temperature (*e.g.* 4°C for ABO, 37°C for Rh) usually for 16 hours.

After incubation the serum is removed from each tube and the cloth squares or threads are washed five times with ice cold saline. The tubes are left to stand at 4°C during this washing. A final wash is carried out using ice cold 1/100 dilution of 30 per cent bovine albumin in saline. This whole washing process is spread over a period of 2-3 hours.

At each washing care is taken to remove as much liquid as possible.

Elution

One to two unit volumes of the albumin diluent is added to each tube and elution is carried out for 10 minutes in a shaking water bath, the temperature of which is 55–60°C.

Detection of eluted antibody

At the end of this elution process the tubes are removed from the water bath and one volume of the appropriate red cells suspended in 0.3 per cent albumin is added at once to each tube *without removing the cloth.*

Increased sensitivity is gained by using a low concentration of indicator red cells (*e.g.* 0.5 per cent for ABO, 0.05 per cent for Rh and 1 per cent for tests with ahg) and also, in some instances the indicator cells are treated with papain (*e.g.* when testing for the Rh antigens).

After the cells have been added to the tubes the tests are incubated for 1-1½ hours at the appropriate temperature *e.g.* room temperature for ABO, 37°C for Rh. Reading is carried out microscopically and owing to the very thin cell suspension it is often an advantage to remove some of the supernatant fluid before removing the button of cells which is placed on to a microscope slide for reading. Gentle rolling of the slide at this stage aggregates the cells and facilitates reading and in some cases assists agglutination.

Tests for the S, s, K, Fy^a, Fy^b, and Jk^a antigens involve the use of the ahg technique after incubating the cells with the eluted antibody, in which case after the incubation period of 1-1½ hours the supernatant fluid is removed, the tubes filled with saline and the stained material is taken out. The cells are given one further wash and thereafter the procedure follows the normal ahg test.

Technique No. 29.5. Inhibition technique for the detection of A, B and H in seminal and saliva stains

The selected anti-A and anti-B sera are diluted with saline just before use, to give a titre of 16-32. Weak antisera not requiring dilution are usually not so satisfactory. Anti-H (*Ulex*) of about the same titre is also included.

Method 1

Two unit volumes (about 0.06 ml) of each antiserum is added to one of 3 pieces of stained material using about 2 mm square for each test. Controls of unstained material from the same exhibit are treated in the same manner.

The tests are left at 4°C for several hours or preferably overnight. The tubes are then centrifuged and the supernatant fluid in each titrated, after which an equal volume of the appropriate A_2, B or O cells is added to each tube. The tests are read both macroscopically and microscopically for agglutination after 1-2 hours at bench temperature.

The results are compared with those obtained with the unstained cloth controls.

Method 2

An extract of a small portion of stained material (about 6 mm square) and also of a control area is made in a quantity of saline which is no larger than is required for adequate testing afterwards with anti-A, anti-B and anti-H.

The saline is allowed to soak the stain at 4°C for several hours or preferably overnight before being drawn off; this is particularly important if the stain is not very fresh. It is good practice to suck fluid up and down through the stained material with a Pasteur pipette.

The extract is then mixed with an equal volume of antiserum (anti-A, anti-B or anti-H) and from this point, the procedure is the same as for method 1. If the extract is highly active it is an advantage to titrate the extract and to use the dilutions for testing for inhibition with anti-A, anti-B and anti-H (see technique 6.4).

Technique No. 29.6. The detection of A, B and H in seminal and saliva stains by the micro-elution method

The micro-elution technique as designed for blood stains may be used for the detection of A, B and H in body fluids as already mentioned earlier in this chapter.

The technique requires antisera sufficiently potent to overcome the neutralisation effect of the blood group substances in the stain if these are present in high concentration. Washing the stain once in saline before the addition of the antiserum is sometimes effective. Alternatively extracts of various dilutions of stain may be dried on to clean cotton threads. It must also be realised that a high concentration of blood group substance on stained material may also affect the elution stage of the test, by creating a situation of antigen excess in which circumstances it is difficult to obtain a satisfactorily active eluate.

Bearing in mind the above precautions, the directions for elution from blood stains may be followed.

Technique No. 29.7. Gm and Km grouping of stains

Selection of antisera

Serial doubling dilutions of anti-Gm (1), anti-Gm (2) and anti-Km (1) are made in saline and to each tube is added an equal volume of a 2 per cent suspension of the appropriately sensitised red cells. The tests are left at room temperature for 1½ hours after which they are lightly centrifuged and the contents of each tube examined for agglutination both macroscopically and microscopically. The last dilution giving good strong macroscopic agglutination is used as the working dilution in the following inhibition technique.

Inhibition method

For Gm (1) and Km (1) pieces of blood stained thread about 6 mm in length are used and for convenience are cut into 2 mm lengths. It is recommended that double this amount of material is used for Gm (2). [With some materials it may be preferable to make extracts of stains and mix equal amounts of extract with the Gm antisera.]

The pieces are placed in suitable tubes (0.5-mm diameter). One drop of anti-Gm serum at the working dilution is added to each tube and the tests are left to absorb at 4°C overnight. Controls of known blood stains providing a positive and negative control for each anti-serum and unstained cloth controls are set up at the same time.

The following morning the threads are removed with forceps taking care, by squeezing the threads, to retain as much fluid as possible in the tubes. One drop of a 2 per cent suspension of cells sensitised with the appropriate Gm or Km antigens is added to each tube and these are left for 1 hour at room temperature after which they are centrifuged at 1000 r.p.m. for 30 seconds. The cells are examined for agglutination both macroscopically and microscopically.

Technique No. 29.8. The mixed cell agglutination technique

This is a useful technique for the detection of A, B and H antigens on tissue cells other than red cells. The technique is described here for buccal epithelial cells.

Materials

Anti-A and anti-B. These must be monospecific reagents. High titre immune sera are usually particularly satisfactory but standard grouping sera may be suitable. It must be emphasised that the sera have to be specially selected and not all high titre sera are equally good. The sera are heated to 50°C for 30 min and are centrifuged before use.

The optimal dilution has to be found by experiment.

Anti-H. Anti-H, from *Ulex europeus* used either neat or can sometimes be diluted up to 1/5.

Diluents. Diluents and washing fluids are more satisfactory if they contain a little protein and a 1 in 100 dilution of 30 per cent bovine albumin is found satisfactory.

Indicator red cells. Three times washed A_1, B and O red cells made to a 0.5 per cent suspension in the diluent are used.

Buccal epithelial cells. These are collected by scraping the inside of the cheek with a wooden spatula and washing off the cells into about 2 ml of saline.

Large flakes and debris are allowed to settle out then the supernatant is removed and centrifuged and the buccal cells are washed twice in saline, followed by a final wash in diluent. After the final wash a suspension of the buccal cells is made in diluent (ideally there should be approximately 20 epithelial cells per microscope field when using a $\times$ 10 eyepiece and $\times$ 10 objective).

Method

The buccal cell suspension from each sample is tested with anti-A, anti-B and anti-H. Two drops of suitably diluted antiserum are mixed with two drops of buccal cell suspension and the tubes are rotated slowly at room temperature for 1-2 hours or left at 4°C overnight.

After incubation the tubes are centrifuged, the supernatant carefully removed, the cells washed twice in saline and then a final wash in diluent.

Two drops of 0.5 per cent suspension of the appropriate red cells are added to each tube. The tubes are shaken gently to mix the contents and left at room temperature for 30 minutes preferably with gentle rotation. They are then lightly centrifuged and after careful resuspension a generous drop of the contents is transferred to a microscope slide using a wide-bore pipette. Ideally they are viewed after covering under phase contrast microscopy, but mixed agglutination can be examined using ordinary bright field illumination.

Results

A typical positive result is denoted by the coating of the buccal cells by indicator red cells. Sometimes the indicator cells break away from the buccal cells as free agglutinates. The negative appearance is of buccal cells against a background of unagglutinated indicator cells.

When recording the results it is advisable to make two readings with suitable symbols denoting the strength of reaction. Reading (a) is of the mixed agglutination proper *i.e.* the degree to which the indicator cells are bound to the buccal cells. Tapping the coverslip with a pointed instrument sometimes facilitates this reading in that the free and attached cells may be more clearly distinguished.

Reading (b) is the degree of agglutination of the background indicator cells. Providing the control of buccal cells lacking the particular antigen is negative, showing that the washing has been adequate, agglutination of red cells unattached to the buccal cells is indicative of a specific reaction having taken place between an antigen on the buccal cell and the particular antiserum.

Comments

The mixed agglutination test seems to be suitable mainly for the detection of the ABH antigens and even then careful selection of the few antisera which are suitable is essential.

This technique is however useful for the detection of ABH antigens in cells other than red cells and it has the advantage of displaying the distribution of a particular antigen in tissues (see adaption of this technique by Davidsohn and Stejskal, chapter 28).

REFERENCES

Adams, E.G. & Wraxall, B.G. (1974) Phosphatase in body fluids. The differentiation of serum and vaginal secretion. *Forens. Science,* 3, 57.
Bargagna, M. & Pereira, M. (1967) A study of absorption-elution as a method of identification of Rhesus antigens in dried blood stains. *J. forens. Sci. Soc.,* 7, 123.
Contreras, M. & Tippett, P. (1974) The Lu(a–b–) syndrome and an apparent upset of P₁ inheritance. *Vox Sang.,* 27, 369.
Cook, P.L., Gray, J.E., Brack, R.A., Robson, E.B. & Howlett, R.M. (1969) Data on haptoglobin and D group chromosomes *Ann. hum. Genet.,* 33, 125.

Coombs, R.R.A., Bedford, D. & Rouillard, L.M. (1956) A and B blood group antigens on human epidermal cells demonstrated by mixed agglutination. *Lancet*, **i**, 461.

Culliford, B.J. (1971) The examination and typing of blood stains in the crime laboratory. *National Institute of Law Enforcement and Criminal Justice.*

Culliford, B.J. (1964) Precipitin reactions in forensic problems. *Nature (Lond.),* **211**, 872.

Culliford, B.J. (1967) The determination of phospho-gluco-mutase types in blood stains. *J. forens. Sci. Soc.,* **7**, 131.

Davie, M.J., and Kipps, A.E. (1976). Km(1)[Inv(1)] typing of saliva and semen. Vox. Sang. **31**, 363.

Family Law Reform Act 1969. Chapter 46. HMSO.

Gradwhol's Legal Medicine, (1968) Ch. 12. Bristol: Wright.

Herbidy, J., Fisher, R.A., Hopkinson, D.A. (1970). Atypical segregation of human red cell acid phosphatase phenotypes: evidence for a rare 'silent' allele P°. *Ann. hum. Genet.,* **34**, 145.

Jenkins, G.C., Brown, J., Lincoln, P.J. & Dodd, B.E. (1972) The problem of the acquired B in forensic serology. *J. forens. Sci. Soc.,* **12**, 597.

Khalap, S., Pereira, M., and Reid, S. (1976) Gm and Inv grouping of bloodstains. *Medicine Sci. Law,* **16**, 40.

Lincoln, P.J. & Dodd, B.E. (1968) The detection of the Rh antigens C, C^w, c D, E, e and the antigen S of the MNSs system in blood stains. *Medicine, Sci, Law,* **8**, 288.'

Lincoln, P.J. & Dodd, B.E. (1973) An evaluation of factors affecting the elution of antibodies from blood stains. *J. forens. Sci. Soc.,* **13**, 37.

Lincoln, P.J. & Dodd, B.E. (1975) The application of a micro-elution technique using anti-human globulin for the detection of the S, s, K, Fy^a, Fy^b and Jk^a antigens in stains. *Medicine, Sci. Law,* **15**, 94.

Nerstrøm, B. & Skafte-Jensen, J. (1963) Immuno-electrophoretic analysis of blood stains with special reference to Gc grouping. *Acta path. microbiol. Scand.,* **58**, 257.

Nicholls, L.C. & Pereira, M. (1962) A study of modern methods of grouping dried blood stains. *Medicine, Sci, Law,* **2**, 172.

Olaisen, B. (1973) A typical segregation of erythrocyte glutamic-pyruvate transaminase in a Norwegian family. Evidence of a silent allele. *Hum. Hered.,* **23**, 595.

Outteridge, R.A. (1963) Determination of the ABO group from finger nails. *Medicine, Sci, Law,* **3**, 275.

Parkin, B.H. & Adams, E.G. (1975) The typing of Esterase D in human blood stains. *Medicine, Sci, Law,* **15**, 102.

Pereira, M. (1963) The identification of MN groups in dried blood stains. *Medicine, Sci, Law,* **3**, 268.

Pereira, M. (1973) ABO grouping of decomposed tissue. *J. forens Sci. Soc.,* **13**, 33.

Pereira, M., and Martin, P.D (1976) Problems involved in the grouping of saliva, semen and other body fluids. *J. forens. Sci. Soc.* **16**, 151.

Poon, W.L. & Dodd, B.E. (1964) The subdivision of blood stains into A$_1$and A$_2$ and the detection of H on epidermal cells. *Medicine, Sci, Law,* **4**, 258.

Price, C.J., Davis, A., Wraxall, B.G.D., Martin, P.D., Parkin, B.H., Emes, E.G., and Culliford, B.J. (1976) The typing of phosphoglucomutase in vaginal material and semen.*J. forens Sci. Soc.* **16**, 29.

Race, R.R. & Sanger, R. (1975) Blood Groups in Man. P. 505. Oxford: Blackwell.

Salmon, D. (1974) Probabilité de paternité estimée a partin des groupes sanguins et des marqueurs genetiques. *Nouvelle Revue Francaise d'Hematologie,* **14**, 477.

Sonneborn, H.H. (1976) Human erythrocyte iso-enzyme polymorphisms theory and methods. Obtainable from Biotest Serum Institut, Flughafenstrasse 4, D-6000, Frankfurt 73.

Stevenson, A.C. & Kerr, C.B. (1967) On the distribution of mutation to genes determining harmful traits in Man. *Mutation Res.,* **4**, 339.

Swinburne, L.M. (1962) The identification of skin. *Medicine, Sci. Law,* **3**, 3.

Tippett, P. (1971) A case of suppressed Lu^a and Lu^b antigens. *Vox Sang.,* **20**, 378.

Welch, S.G. (1972) Glutamate Pyruvate Transaminase in blood stains. *J. forens. Sci. Soc.,* **12**, 605.

Wiener, A.S. (1943) *Blood Groups and Transfusion.* P.389. Springfield, Ill: Thomas.

Wiener, A.S. (1959) Application of blood grouping tests in cases of disputed maternity. *J. forens. Sci.,* **4**, 321.

Wraxall, B.G.D. (1977) personal communication.

Wraxall, B.G.D. & Emes E.G. (1976) Erythrocyte acid phosphatase in bloodstains. *J. forens. Sci. Soc.* **16**, 127.

Section 5.   The National Blood Transfusion Service

"In letting of blood three circumstances are to be considered, who, how much, when?"

Robert Burton, THE ANATOMY OF MELANCHOLY

Chapter 30. The Functions of the Regional Transfusion Centres

In the next three chapters we deal very briefly with the work of the British National Blood Transfusion Service and in particular the Regional Transfusion Centres, although the work of the Blood Group Reference Laboratory and the Blood Products Laboratory will be mentioned as appropriate. While much of the following applies to all the Transfusion Centres, the detail of the organisation is that of the South London Regional Transfusion Centre.

FUNCTIONS OF REGIONAL CENTRES

The functions of the Regional Centre are as follows:-

1. Recruitment of donors.
2. The holding of sessions at which donors are bled.
3. Testing donor blood for ABO and Rh groups and selected donors for most other blood group systems.
4. Syphilis testing.
5. Screening for Hepatitis B surface antigen (HB_s) (*see* Chapter 31).
6. The supply of blood to hospitals, both routine requirements and rare types where necessary.
7. Fulfilling the role of a regional standards reference centre for hospital blood transfusion laboratories.
8. The preparation of various blood products or the production of pools suitable for processing by the blood products unit (*see* Chapter 32).
9. Acting as a reference centre for hospital ante-natal testing.
10. The training of technologists and pathologists especially those pathologists taking the M.R.C.Path. examinations in Haematology and Blood Transfusion.

1. Recruitment of donors

Blood donors in this country are volunteers. The paid donor system tends to recruit the wrong type of donor in that many are poor and undernourished, and there tends to be a large proportion of alcoholics and drug addicts. Among such donors there is a very high incidence of carriers of hepatitis and even the most modern techniques of detection (*see* Chapter 31) of the HB_s antigen miss a proportion of carriers. In fact commercial drug houses who are almost entirely dependent on paid donors are very concerned about the number of cases of hepatitis in patients receiving, in particular, Factor VIII concentrate where unfortunately the hepatitis virus is concentrated together with the Factor VIII.

The maintaining of an active donor panel is by no means easy as the demand for blood and blood products is continually increasing, and there are many reasons why any individual donor may have to retire. Throughout Great Britain many thousands of new donors are recruited every month, and more are needed.

They are recruited by a number of methods, for example by voluntary organisations, *e.g.* British Red Cross and W.V.S., by donors bringing along their friends and so on—and, in our experience the most effective method, by a local campaign. These campaigns are conducted in the busy shopping areas by means of a loudspeaker van and a team of donor attendants who carry forms for the enrolment of volunteers. The volunteer is called to a blood collection session in his area.

2. The blood donation session

In many ways the ideal blood donation session is held in a permanent clinic belonging to, and preferably either part of the transfusion centre, or near to it. Where such a clinic can be situated in a community sufficiently large to produce at least a hundred donors every day, it is well worth the cost of keeping it open and manned. In actual practice few such communities exist; most areas visited by our mobile teams provide less than five hundred donors every four months!

The usual pattern therefore, is that a mobile team of doctors, nurses, technicians with all the equipment needed sets up a temporary clinic in any suitable large hall in areas in which the donors live.

Another very valuable source of donors is their place of work, whether factory, office, or hospital etc. With the co-operation of the management, often via the welfare officer, a session is arranged actually on work premises, and in working time. This type of session has many advantages. From the donors point of view it is convenient and he can be given a definite appointment time. From the Centre's point of view there are two main advantages; the number of donors attending a session within a few can be regulated for maximum efficiency, and when the session is near to the Centre supplies of blood can be available early in the day for processing. This is especially useful for acquiring good yields of Factor VIII in cryo-precipitate and for the preparation of platelet concentrates.

On attendance at the session a medical history is taken; any donors who have ever had jaundice are rejected. (This is still done as a precaution although all donors are tested at every donation for hepatitis B surface antigen (HB_s) as described in Chapter 31.) This virus can be transmitted by blood transfusion and the resultant jaundice may be very severe, in some cases resulting in liver atrophy and the death of the patient. Malaria is another disease which can be transmitted from donor to recipient. Donors who have had malaria are however accepted as their blood can be used for the preparation of serum. Those among them who happen to have a high allo-agglutinin titre are invaluable for anti-A and anti-B typing. Serum which is not suitable for this purpose is pooled and dried.

The new donor is tested for ABO group by a tile method using whole blood from a finger or ear prick. This method has an appreciable error although it is less than 1 per cent in the hands of an experienced operator, but it enables the blood pack to be given a group label which means that only one donation per hundred will have to be relabelled after the full testing has been done in the laboratory.

It has been agreed that donors shall not be bled if their haemoglobin level is less than 85 per cent. Only a screening test is done, as elaborate and time-consuming tests cannot be performed during a blood-collecting session where about thirty to forty donors are bled per hour. The screening method makes use of the fact that a drop of blood allowed to fall into copper sulphate solution of specific gravity 1.052 will sink to the bottom if the Hb is 85 per cent or over but will float if the Hb is below this figure. Those who fail this rapid screening test and also a confirmation test using a fresh bottle of copper sulphate solution have a 5-ml sample taken from which a more accurate estimation of the haemoglobin level is made in the laboratory. Should it be 85 per cent or over the donor is recalled next time the mobile team is in the area but if not, such donors are not recalled until passed by their own doctor as fit to donate blood.

The donor who has passed the haemoglobin screening test has his name entered on to a serially numbered work-sheet from which this number is copied on to the back of his card; five small labels bearing the same number are issued to him together with a larger, coloured, group label. The label for each group has a different colour: group O, blue, group A, yellow, group B, pink and group AB, white. Individuals who have donated previously are given labels with their appropriate ABO group and Rh type according to their record card.

New donors are given a coloured group label on the result of the tile grouping (see above). All new donors have labels printed Rh positive. Those subsequently found in the laboratory to be Rh negative, have the label changed accordingly.

The donor is bled into a plastic blood pack which may be either single, double or triple depending upon the use to which the donation is to be put (see Chapter 32). At the end of the donation suitable pilot samples are taken for the laboratory each bearing the same number as the bag or bags (the five numbered labels allow for a triple pack, i.e. 1 main bag and two satellite bags, in addition one citrated sample and one clotted sample for the laboratory).The latter samples are collected while the needle is still in the vein after the full main bag has been clamped off.

Immediately the blood is taken it is put into the refrigerator. The pilot tubes are placed in numerical order and transferred to the serological laboratory. Serological tests are normally done on the day following the actual blood-taking.

3. Testing of donor blood

The citrated samples are checked for numerical order and for suitability. For testing on the 15-channel blood grouping AutoAnalyser, the sample must be adequate but not too large so that the double probe will sample cells and plasma separately and there must be no clots in the sample as these will block the probes. To minimise errors all the Transfusion Centres have agreed a standard pattern for ABO and Rh typing on the AutoAnalyser as below.

Channel 1	2	3	4	5	6	7	8	9	10
Anti-A	Anti-B	O serum	AB serum	A_1rr cells	A_2rr cells	Brr cells	Orr cells	Anti-D	Anti-D

Channels 11 to 15 are available for extra tests as each region may decide. In practice channels 11 and 12 are often used for further testing of D negatives using anti-CD and anti-DE or anti-CDE reagents, and 13 and 14 for antibody screening. Channel 15 can be adapted for automated Reiter Test for syphilis and phased to conform with the blood grouping channels. All donors are tested on the AutoAnalyser unless no suitable sample has been obtained, in which case manual testing is done on the clotted sample. It is our practice to test new *i.e.* first time donors manually as an added check.

The clotted samples are also checked for strict numerical order, and serum removed for HB_s antigen testing, for serum check on new donors, and for a manual antibody screen using papain treated cells (technique No. 30.2) which in our hands will detect some antibodies missed by the AutoAnalyser screen.

If antibodies are found either by manual or AutoAnalyser tests they are identified and if sufficiently potent used for typing and subsequent donations are also used for this purpose provided that the titre remains high. Blood with a low titre of Rh antibodies is issued for known Rh negative adults; it is not used for emergency transfusion or for babies.

All r', r" and D^u donors are used for the transfusion of Rh positive recipients as all D negative recipients are transfused with Rh negative (*cde/cde*) blood.

The results of all the above tests are entered on the original work-sheet compiled at the session; where more complicated tests are necessary the results are entered on a "Repeat Sheet" and the conclusions entered back on to the original sheet. The original work-sheet has a perforated section where the group and Rh type of each donation of blood is entered and at the same time the blood is inspected for fitness for use. Then the perforated portion of the work-sheet goes to the blood issue department together with the "passed" donations of blood for issue to the hospital blood banks. In a few cases *e.g.* where the donor's serum contains an atypical agglutinin, it is useful to have a bench work card which is filed under the donor's name and on which results can be entered for each donation.

The donor holds a booklet giving his group and Rh type to which a certificate is added at each donation; in addition special cards are issued to the Rh negative, r' and r" donors for their own protection should they ever need to be transfused. The National Blood Transfusion Service also gives badges to their long-service donors, bronze for 10 donations, silver for 25 donations and silver-gilt for 50 donations.

Donors who have a sufficiently high titre of anti-A and/or anti-B allo-agglutinins are used as donors of grouping sera. These donors are bled into double packs their plasma being collected, recalcified and processed and their concentrated cells used for transfusion. This is also done with donors who have Rh antibodies but here the cells are used for Rh negative adults only and never for transfusion to infants. Some antibodies may not survive recalcification and so are taken into dry bottles e.g. Duffy, Kidd, Lewis.

4. Syphilis Testing

This is often done on a channel of the 15-channel AutoAnalyser or by any of the well recognised tests such as Wasserman, PPR (Price's Precipitin Reaction) or VDRL. We test any donors where the sample for AutoAnalyser was inadequate by the VDRL (technique No. 30.1) and also any samples giving a positive or doubtful reaction by AutoAnalyser testing. Any donor giving a positive reaction is referred for investigation and treatment and removed from the panel.

5. Hepatitis B surface antigen (HB$_s$) testing

This is done on the serum from the clotted sample, if possible, as plasma does not give such a distinct precipitation line on immunoelectro-osmophoresis. (IEOP). Details of the techniques employed and precautions taken are given in Chapter 31. As soon as a positive reaction has been obtained the suspect donation is removed from the storage refrigerator and incinerated. When the confirmation tests are complete the donor is notified and removed from the panel.

6. Maintaining stocks and distribution to hospitals

Except in times of shortage the transfusion centres will supply all the hospital blood banks in their region with group O, group A and group B, Rh negative and Rh positive blood, and AB Rh positive blood. AB Rh negative blood is in great demand for processing and is usually only supplied on request for specific patients.

A proportion of the donor panel is tested for a variety of blood group systems but the transfusion centre rather than the hospital blood bank will hold stocks of these. On application for any specific case R_1R_1, R_2R_2, KK, Fy(a+b−) Fy (a−b+) or Le (a−b−), should be readily available either of group O or group A. Also special stocks are held for any case where an antibody or combination of antibodies makes compatible blood difficult to find. The centre also has access to the National and International rare-donor panels and with the National stock of frozen blood of very rare cell types *e.g.* Lu(a−b−), Fy(a−b−), Vel−, etc.

7. Standards and Reference Centre

Many Regional Centres prepare standard anti-sera and panels of red cells for distribution to the hospital blood bank laboratories of their region. In some cases the anti-sera will have been prepared at the centre itself and the rest will probably have come from the Blood Group Reference Laboratory. In this way many thousands of units of ABO and Rh typing sera are prepared and issued free of charge by the transfusion service every year. Exhaustive testing for specificity means that anomalous results due to unsuspected contaminants are unlikely to occur and if obtained merit further investigation by the issuing laboratory as a very rare antigen or antibody may be involved. As well as the screening for blood group antibodies of unwanted specificity (the most common contaminants are other Rh antibodies in the various Rh sera, anti-K, anti-P_1, anti-Lewis and anti-Wr^a), the sera are tested for Gm antibodies before being used as standard reagents.

Any anti-serum, whether from the Transfusion Service or from commercial sources should be used by the method recommended, as a variation may bring to light an unwanted antibody; (e.g. in anti-C reagents recommended for use by saline technique albumin reactive anti-D is common and would cause C—D+ cells to be typed as C+ if used in a protein medium or by an enzyme technique.) If the method is varied the serum must be re-standardised by the method chosen, a long procedure and entailing the use of rare cells unlikely to be readily available. A distinction must be made between many commercial saline anti-D sera and those issued by the Transfusion Service as the former will be sera containing incomplete antibodies 'fortified' by the addition of various proteins and/or gums and are unsuitable for testing any cells that may be sensitised, while the latter will contain only complete antibodies i.e. agglutinins.

With the coming of storage solutions which enable panels of diluted cells to be stored at 4° C for several weeks, commercial firms are now marketing standard red cells. These are of two kinds: (1) A pool of cells from several donors designed to include as many different antigens as possible; these are intended for antibody screening. They will of course give a mixed cell population appearance (see Fig. 23.1) with some antibodies. (2) A panel of eight to ten different red cell samples each from a single donor. These are issued as aids to the identification of the specificity of antibodies. Some Regional Transfusion Centres also circulate panels of test cells in similar storage media which usually contain inosine or tyrosine; for the reagent used by the South London Transfusion Centre see Technique No. A.II.9.

So called "Quality Control" in the Centre, as in the hospital laboratories, is partly assured by good organisation, the use of standard reagents and appropriate controls with each batch of tests. The introduction of "control" samples into the day's work unknown to the operator can be of value, although it presents some difficulty and can cause confusion. It is perhaps an advantage for the operator to know that a sample is a control, although of course not necessarily the results expected.

"Quality control" exercises are designed by the various Regional Centres for the benefit of the hospitals in their area and the latter participate on a voluntary basis. They are strongly to be recommended as they enable each individual hospital to assess its standard of serological proficiency. Most exercises include the detection of unknown antibodies of varying degrees of potency by the standard techniques recommended for cross-matching. The better planned exercises take care that the tests set are not too easy. Strong and weak antibodies are included both separately and as mixtures of one strong antibody mixed with a weak one of another specificity *e.g.* an anti-D titre approximately 128 with an anti-Fy^a or anti-Jk^a titre 4 to 8. These are interspersed with bland sera and it is a good exercise to duplicate some test sera. A further variation is the inclusion of a serially diluted serum containing a fairly potent antibody but with the dilutions out of order.

Results of such exercises in general show that while most hospital laboratories are proficient at red cell typing and the detection of potent antibodies, the standard of detection of weak antibodies is by no means so high and the errors do not always occur in the same direction. For example with a typical antibody of titre of 8 or less, both false positive and false negative readings tend to occur. Moreover an antibody test by anti-human globulin technique, in which the serum contains both strong and weak antibodies incompatible with the cells used, particularly if read on tiles may result in the tests being discarded after the strong antibody makes its appearance but before the weaker one has a chance to show up (*see also* Chapter 23).

It is a good plan for the results of an exercise to be confirmed by a second specialist laboratory as well as the Regional Centre by which the exercise is set. A copy of the expected protocol and a summary of the errors occurring in the exercise are of great value to the participant hospitals.

Regional Centres act as reference centres for hospitals for identification of antibodies if necessary with the help of the Blood Group Reference Laboratory. They also undertake to supply blood of suitable phenotype and in cases of particular difficulty will also carry out the cross-match.

8. Blood components, preparation and therapy

This subject is dealt with in Chapter 32.

9. The ante-natal service

The Regional Transfusion Centres are willing to perform the full range of blood group, antibody detection and quantification for the ante-natal service (*see* Chapter 26). It will depend on the peripheral laboratory at what level, if any, cases are referred to the Centre. For instance at one end of the scale a general practitioner may send a maternal sample for routine ABO and Rh typing antibody screening and syphilis testing or at the other end the hospital laboratory may do a complete serological investigation of the mother (including antibody titration), father and infant and only refer cases when unable to identify the maternal antibody.

Rh antibody quantification using the AutoAnalyser is usually confined to the Transfusion Centres (Chapter 21). Cases of suspected haemolytic disease due to ABO antibodies are usually referred to the Centres for confirmation and for various specialist tests (*see* Chapter 26).

10. Training

Wherever courses are held for examinations which include blood group serology members of the staffs of the Regional Transfusion Centres are likely to be found among the lecturers and demonstrators and much of the material used is supplied by the centre either directly or indirectly. Many centres also provide supplementary courses on their own premises, some with examinations in mind, others directed to one aspect of importance to the local blood bank such as cross-matching techniques. In our experience attendance at a course arranged at the centre for a number of participants is superior to the alternative whereby a single individual visits the centre for one or two days, as more coherent training can be given and there is also a lively exchange of ideas and information with not only the lecturers but other course members.

TECHNIQUES

Technique No. 30.1. The VDRL reaction

Materials
(1) VDRL antigen (we use "Wellcome" brand).
(2) Buffered saline
    0.093 g Na_2HPO_4 $12H_2O$ ⎫
    0.170 g KH_2PO_4 ⎬ Made up to 1 litre with distilled water
    10.0 g NaCl   ⎪
    0.5 ml formaldehyde.   ⎭
The pH of this solution is 6.0 ± 0.1.
(3) Isotonic saline.

Preparation of antigen emulsion
The antigen is made up by dropping 0.5ml of the antigen into 0.4 ml of buffered saline, rotating the solution while the antigen is being added and for a further 10 seconds to ensure a good mixing. Then 4.1 ml of buffered saline is added, the bottle (a 30-ml bottle is recommended) is stoppered and vigorously shaken for a further 10 seconds. The prepared antigen emulsion is stored in a $4°C$ refrigerator until needed. This emulsion is quite stable but a fresh supply should be made each week. Each batch should be tested with known negative and positive sera; if the results are not clear cut the preparation of the emulsion has not been satisfactory and a fresh batch should be prepared giving special attention to the mixing.

The quantitative slide test
Using the VDRL as a screening test the quantitative slide test is the method of choice.
The sera to be tested are inactivated for 30 minutes at $56°C$. The actual test is satisfactorily performed in welled tiles, and plastic tiles with eight rows each of ten wells are a convenient size.
Each serum is tested by placing 0.05 ml of serum into a well of the slide and adding one drop (1/60th ml) of antigen emulsion. The slides are rotated for 4 minutes on a mechanical rotator (a suitable one is supplied by Luckhams). The tests are read microscopically immediately after rotation at $100\times$ magnification

against a black spot background. The latter is not essential but we find it more satisfactory particularly when large numbers of test have to be read. The positive reaction is a clumping of the emulsified particles. Large and medium clumps are read as a definite positive, an even distribution of small clumps as a weak positive—no clumping as negative. Occasionally irregular clumping or a loose formation of clumps is seen; this is a zonal reaction and the serum should be retested at 1 in 5 and 1 in 25 dilutions in physiological saline.

Comment

This is a simple and reliable technique. A few false positive reactions are obtained but in a screening test this is an acceptable fault.

Technique No. 30.2. Blood group antibody screening using VDRL dilutions

Some time ago we wished to add a second antibody screening test to all our donor samples without greatly increasing the work. A method using the VDRL tests as a source of the donor's serum was devised in our own laboratory. When the VDRL tests have been read one drop of papain treated OR_1R_2K positive red cells are added to each well. The tiles are stacked and the top one covered by an empty tile. They are then incubated for 30 minutes, gently rotated for about 4 seconds and examined for agglutination with the naked eye. Any serum giving a positive reaction is investigated by normal techniques to determine the specificity of the antibodies detected.

Comment

This has proved a very useful additional technique - we have not missed an Rh antibody (anti-D, anti-c, anti-e, etc.) detected by the more conventional techniques, anti-K has been detected, anti-Le[a] and anti-Le[b] and anti-P[1]. Papain type auto antibodies are also detected.

Chapter 31. The detection of Hepatitis B Surface Antigen

The fact that serum hepatitis could be transmitted by the transfusion of blood or blood products had been known for many years but until 1967 the causative agent could not be demonstrated. In that year Blumberg *et al.,* while studying serum proteins in Australian aborigines discovered an antigen which seemed identical to the infective agent responsible for serum hepatitis, hence the name Australia antigen (Au (1)). Other nomenclatures are Hepatitis Associated Antigen (HAA) Hepatitis B antigen (HBA) and Hepatitis B surface antigen (HB$_s$Ag). The latter is in most common usage at the present time.

It is now known that the antigen can be transmitted by contact as well as innoculation and has been found in faeces, urine, bile, saliva and semen.

The Virus

In a typical electron microscope picture of a serum containing Hepatitis B antigen, there are three distinct forms (1) a 20-nm spherical form, (2) a long form 20 nm in diameter and of variable length, (3) the Dane particle which is a 40-nm spherical body with a 27-nm electron dense inner core (Fig. 31.1).

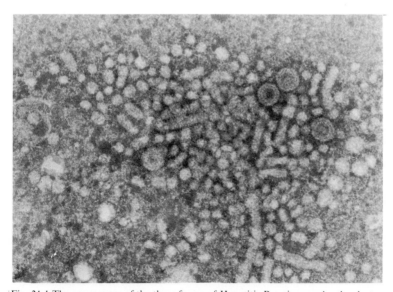

Fig. 31.1 The appearance of the three forms of Hepatitis B antigen under the electron microscope.

The Dane particle is believed to be the complete virion with the Au (1) antigen being on the outer coat (Hepatitis B surface antigen (HB_sAg)) and the inner core being immunologically distinct (Hepatitis B core antigen (HB_cAg).

The Antigen

Little is known of the structure of the antigen but it has an immuno-electrophoretic mobility similar to α_1 macroglobulin and is associated with varying amounts of lipid.

The Heterogeneity of the Hepatitis B_s antigen

There are several antigenic differences in the HB_s antigen; of these "a" is common to all antigens and "d" and "y" are mutually exclusive. Associated with "d" and "y" are "w" and "r" which are also mutually exclusive (Kim and Tilles, 1971; LeBouvier, 1971). The actual function and structure of these antigens has yet to be defined. On immuno-electrophoresis "d" is slower moving than "y" and there is a slight difference between these two on isoelectric focusing. There is also a geographical variation in the frequencies of the various antigens.

HB_c and "e" immune systems

The presence of anti-core antibodies (anti-HB_c) is now believed to be a more sensitive indicator of persistent viraemia than the presence of HB_s Ag, (Hoofnagel et al., 1973). At the moment the materials needed for the detection of anti-core antibody are not easily obtained, so therefore, are not available for routine laboratory screening.

Another immune system connected with the HB virus is the "e" antigen and its corresponding antibody, anti-"e" (Magnius and Epsmark, 1972). The detection of this is also believed to give a truer picture of infectivity. The "e" antigen seems to be associated with Dane particles, (Nielsen J.O. et al., 1974), and is found in those patients with severe liver damage but rarely found in carriers or those recovering normally from acute hepatitis.

Anti-"e" persists in carriers and those patients with chronic inactive liver disease and rarely found in those with chronic active hepatitis, (Eleftheriou et al., 1975).

The Antibody and selection of antibody for screening reagent

The antibody is found in the IgM or IgG fraction of serum. In the selection of anti-sera for routine screening of HB_s antigen, the heterogeneity of the antigen must be taken into account. The anti-sera must be polyspecific and able to detect "ad" and "ay" antigens. Anti-sera can be obtained from the normal blood donor population or from multi-transfused patients such as haemophiliacs.

The Incidence of the HB_s antigen and antibody

In the blood donor population of the South London Regional Blood Transfusion Centre the incidence of the HB_s antigen is 1 in 1200 and of the HB_s antibody 1 in 500. There are sections of the population that have a higher incidence of the antigen *e.g.* drug addicts, patients with Down's syndrome and multi-transfused patients such as haemophiliacs. Also there is considerable variation in the incidence in different parts of the world. In Western Europe and North America the frequency is approximately 0.1 per cent rising as high as 20 per cent in some tropical countries.

Techniques for the detection of HB$_s$ antigen and antibody

The techniques for detection of the HB$_s$ antigen and antibody vary considerably in sensitivity. The least sensitive is the Ouchterlony two dimensional immunodiffusion technique, then in order of increased sensitivity, immunoelectro-osmophoresis (also called counter current electrophoresis or crossover electrophoresis), latex aggregation, complement fixation, haemagglutination and radio immune assay.

TECHNIQUES

Technique No. 31.1. Ouchterlony two dimensional immunodiffusion technique (Prince, 1968).

In our laboratory a modification of the Ouchterlony technique is used for confirmation of positives using concentrated sera. This technique has the advantage of demonstrating identity of antigen and antibody (Fig. 31.2).

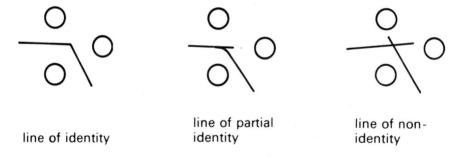

line of identity line of partial identity line of non-identity

Fig. 31.2 Ouchterlony two dimensional immunodiffusion technique.

Principle
The antigen and antibody diffuse through a solid supporting medium *i.e.* agarose and where they meet a line of precipitation forms.

Reagents
   Princes' buffer p H 7.6:
   Sodium chloride   11.6 g
   Tris   2.42 g
   EDTA   0.58 g
   Protamine sulphate   2.0 g
   The volume is made up to 2 litres in distilled water and the pH is adjusted to 7.6.

Agarose: made up to a concentration of 0.9 per cent in Princes' Buffer.

Concentration of Sera

The sera are concentrated × 5 using commercially available acrylamide gel pellets (Lyphogel, Gelman Instruments Co).

Method

2 ml of 0.9 per cent agarose is poured into a 30-mm diameter disposable plastic petri dish (Sterilin) to give a depth of 3 mm. The plate is left to dry at room temperature for 1 hour with the lid off and then overnight with the lid on.

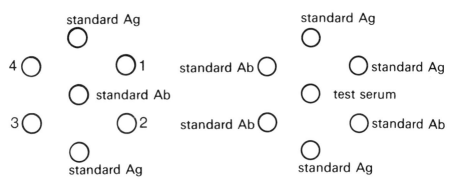

Fig. 31.3(a) Standard pattern for plating-out. (b) Modified pattern for plating-out to give confirmation against three known HB$_s$ antigens and three HB$_s$ antibodies. Ag, antigen; Ab, antibody; 1–4, test samples.

The plates are cut in a seven well pattern (Figs. 31.3 a and b). The wells are 2.5 mm in diameter and the distance centre to centre is 4.5 mm.

The wells are filled with the appropriate reagents and test material (*see* Figs. 31.3a and b) using a pasteur pipette and allowed to diffuse into the gel for 2 hours by which time the wells should be empty. (If they are not empty the plates have not been dried sufficiently.) They are then refilled and the plates are left at room temperature overnight after which they are read for precipitation lines.

Technique No. 31.2. Immunoelectro-osmophoresis (IEOP)

Principle

In a medium of pH 8.6 the gamma-globulin fraction of the serum containing the antibody is electrically neutral while all other serum proteins *e.g.* HB$_s$ antigen are negatively charged. In an electric field these negatively charged proteins will migrate to the positive pole—the anode—and due to positively charged water molecules moving towards the negative pole—the cathode—the gamma-globulin fraction is carried towards the cathode. This movement of water molecules is called electro-endosmosis.

There are two main techniques for IEOP, (a) continuous buffer and (b) discontinuous buffer and many variations within these two. In the continuous buffer system, the buffers in the gel and tank are of the same molarity but in the discontinuous system the molarity of the buffer in the gel differs from that in the tank.

The technique used in our laboratory is a discontinuous buffer method and a modification of Culliford (1964).

Reagents

Buffer. Barbitone acetate buffer for electrophoresis (Oxoid).

This buffer is used at 0.08M concentration in the tank and at 0.02M concentration in the agarose.

Agarose. This is made up at a concentration of 0.65 per cent in 0.02M barbitone acetate buffer.

For this technique the agarose should be selected as suitable for the detection of the Hepatitis B$_s$ antigen. Not all batches are suitable. British Drug Houses have available agarose which has been pre-selected for HB$_s$ antigen testing.

Method

30 ml of gel is poured into a disposable plastic square petri dish $100 \times 100 \times 18$ mm (Sterilin) to give a depth of 3 mm. While the agarose is liquid, wicks 100×100 m of Whatman 3 MM chromatography paper are inserted down two opposite sides of the plate. The plate is allowed to set for 2 hours with the lid off. It can then be stored up to 7 days at 4° C with the lid on. The plate is cut in a 3 well pattern for simultaneous detection of antigen and antibody (Fig. 31.4). The wells

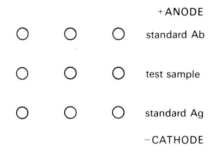

Fig. 31.4 Layout for immunoelectrophoresis. Ag, antigen; Ab, antibody.

are 2 mm in diameter and a distance apart of 7 mm centre to centre. Forty samples can be tested on one plate.

The wells are filled with a fine pipette, the standard HB$_s$ antibody is placed in the anodic well, the standard HB$_s$ antigen in the cathodic well and the test sample in the centre well. The plate is then placed on the electrophoresis tank.

The tank chambers are filled with 0.08 M barbitone acetate buffer and the contact between plate and tank is made by double thickness wicks of 100×100 mm of Whatman 3MM chromatography paper. The wicks are well wetted with tank buffer and one end is overlapped onto the wick already inserted in the plate and the other end is in the buffer in the tank.

The plate is run at a constant current of 3.5 mA per cm *i.e.* 35 mA per plate for 90 min. After which the reading of results is made over an indirect light source and may be assisted by the use of a hand lens.

The test samples should be run both neat and 1 in 20 to overcome any prozone effect.

P

Technique No. 31.3. Haemagglutination method

In this technique purified HB_s antibody is attached to tanned red blood cells. The coated red cells are mixed with the test serum either in test tubes or microtitre plates and read for agglutination.

There are three commercially available haemagglutination kits; Hepanosticon (Organon Scientific Development Group) which uses sheep red cells and sheep HB_s antibody, Wellcome Reagents Ltd. which uses equine HB_s antibody and turkey red cells and Auscell (Abbott Laboratories).

The haemagglutination kit used in our laboratory is Hepatest (Wellcome Reagents).

Method

The test serum is diluted 1:8 in the Diluent Buffer (0.15M phosphate buffered saline). 0.025 ml of HB_s antibody coated turkey cells is added to 0.025 ml of diluted test serum in a rigid styrene disposable 'U'-bottom plate (*e.g.* Cooke Microtiter System plate).

The tests are mixed by shaking and allowed to settle at room temperature.

The results are read after half to one hour. A positive reaction is indicated by a layer of agglutinated cells covering the bottom of the well. A negative reaction is indicated by a tight button of cells in the centre of the well. A positive result is confirmed by titrating the test serum against HB_s antibody coated cells and uncoated cells. A true positive will give a titre at least fourfold greater against HB_s antibody coated cells than uncoated cells.

Other techniques available

Latex Aggregation

Pfizer have a commercially available kit for Latex aggregation.

The reagent is prepared by attaching purified HB_s antibody to latex particles. In the test one drop of the latex reagent is mixed on a slide with one drop of test serum. The presence of HB_s antigen is indicated by aggregation of the latex particles (Leach and Ruck 1971).

Complement Fixation

When an antigen/antibody reaction takes place in the presence of complement, the complement is bound by the antigen/antibody complex. For the detection of the HB_s antigen (or antibody) the test serum is mixed with either a standard HB_s antigen (or antibody), animal complement is added and after incubation, indicator sensitised red cells are added. A positive result is indicated by the absence of haemolysis *i.e.*, the complement has been used in an antigen-/antibody reaction. A negative result is indicated by the lysis of the red cells, *i.e.* the complement is still present, therefore has not been used in an antigen/antibody reaction.

Radioimmuneassay

The commercially available kit for radioimmuneassay is Ausria II - 125

(Abbott Laboratories) which is the sandwich type solid phase radioimmuneassay. This kit uses plastic beads coated with HB_s antibody. The beads are immersed in the test serum or recalcified plasma, in welled trays and are incubated for 2 hours at 45° C (or overnight at room temperature if the samples are plasma). The beads are washed and purified HB_s antibody labelled with ^{125}I is added. After a further incubation at 45° C for 1 hour the beads are washed and counted in a gamma counter. The principle is that the HB_s antigen becomes sandwiched between the HB_s antibody on the beads and the ^{125}I-labelled HB_s antibody.

Abbott Laboratories also have available for the detection of HB_s antibody AusAB which is similar to Ausria II. The beads are coated with HB_s antigen which are incubated with the test serum at room temperature for 18 hours. After washing, the beads are re-incubated with serum containing HB_s antigen labelled with [125]I. After a further incubation at room temperature for 4 hours the beads are washed and counted in a gamma counter.

A GUIDE TO PRECAUTIONS IN THE LABORATORY (see also Safety in Pathology Laboratories, 1972)

1. The area used for HB_s testing should be inaccessible to any but those directly concerned with the work.
2. Samples that are suspected or known to be HB_s antigen positive should be clearly marked "High Risk".
3. The opening of "High Risk" parcels and the plating out of tests should be done in a filter cabinet such as the one made by Hepaire Filtration Ltd.
4. Plastic aprons should be worn to prevent contamination of clothing, plastic gloves to protect hands especially if there are any cuts or abrasions of the skin, and masks in case of aerosol droplet contamination.
5. No paper work should be taken out of the working area.
6. The use of sharp instruments should be discouraged.
7. All samples and any disposable material should be incinerated after soaking in 1 per cent hypochlorite solution.
8. Benches and floors to be washed every day with 1 per cent hypochlorite solution.
9. No smoking or eating should be allowed in the laboratory.
10. All specimens to be treated with respect.

"PRITCHARD" ANTIGEN

While screening blood donors for the HB_s antigen using immunoelectro-osmophoresis we encountered some samples that gave positive results which could not be confirmed as being HB_s antigen positive although the samples did appear to be positive by immune electron microscopy. However on close inspection of the micrographs obtained by immune electronmicroscopy the particles, although similar to the HB_s particles, were in fact morphologically classifiable as a parvo-virus. We named this antigen "Pritchard" after the first donor in whom we clearly recognised it (Cossart *et al.*, 1975; Paver *et al.*, 1975a; Paver *et al.*, 1975b).

Parvo-viruses have only recently been described in Man. They are much more common in the animal kingdom where they are known to produce severe diseases of one sort or another particularly in rodents.

The incidence of the virus in random donors is very low indeed (Cant and Widdows, 1975). We have only found eleven cases in testing over half a million donors. However the antibody is very common. Cossart *et al.* (1975) reported the incidence of antibody to antigen at 30 per cent in a small series. In a larger series we found nearly 40 per cent to possess the antibody.

So far we have no clue of any pathological condition for which this virus may be responsible.

The presence of this contaminating antibody "Anti-Pritchard" in the serum used for routine HB_s antigen screening and in the HB_s serum used in immune electron microscopy allowed this agent to be demonstrated.

REFERENCES

Blumberg, B.S., Gerstley, B.J.S., Hungerford, D.A., London, W.T. & Sutnick, A.I. (1967) A serum antigen (Australia antigen) in Down's syndrome, leukaemia and hepatitis. *Ann. intern. Med.,* **66,** 924.

Cant, B. & Widdows, D. (1975) The incidence of a human serum parvo-virus and its antibody. *Abstracts Int. Congr. Blood Transfusion, Helsinki.* P.75.

Cossart, Y.E., Cant, B., Field, A.M. & Widdows, D. (1975) Parvo-virus like particles in human sera. *Lancet,* **1,** 72.

Culliford, B.J. (1964) Precipitin reactions in forensic problems. *Nature,* **201,** 1092

Eleftheriou, N., Thomas, H.C., Heathcote, J. & Sherlock, S. (1975) Incidence and clinical significance of "e" Antigen and Antibody in acute and chronic liver disease. *Lancet,* **2,** 1171.

Hoofnagel, J.H., Gerety, R.J., Barker, L.F. (1973) Antibody to Hepatitis B virus core in man. *Lancet,* **2,** 869.

Kim, C.Y. & Tilles, J.G. (1971) Immunologic and electrophoretic heterogeneity of hepatitis-associated antigen. *J. Infect. Dis.,* **123,** 618-628.

Leach, J.M. & Ruck, B.J. (1971) Detection of hepatitis associated antigen by the latex agglutination test. *Brit. Med., J.,* **4,** 597.

Le Bouvier, G.L. (1971) The heterogeneity of Australia antigen. *J. Infect. Dis,* **123,** 671-675.

Magnius, L.O. & Epsmark, J.A. (1972) New specifities in Australia antigen positive sera distinct from Le Bouvier determinants. *J. Immunol.,* **109,** 1017.

Nielsen, J.O., Dietrichson, O., Juhl, E., (1974) Incidence and meaning of the "e" determinant among Hepatitis B Antigen positive patients with acute and chronic liver diseases. *Lancet,* **2,** 913.

Paver, W.K., Caul, E.O. & Clarke, S.K.R. (1975a) Parvo-virus like particles in human sera. *Lancet,* **1,** 232.

Paver, W.K., Caul, E.O. & Clarke, S.K.R. (1975b). Parvo-virus like particles in human faeces. *Lancet,* **1,** 691.

Prince, A.M. (1968) Ouchterlony gel diffusion technique. *Proc. Nat. Acad. Sci., USA,* **60, 814.**

Safety in Pathology Laboratories (May 1972). *Department of Health and Social Security and Welsh Office.*

ADDITIONAL READING

The Australian Antigen, Hepatitis Associated Antigen (HAA) and corresponding Antibodies. (Munich, 1970) Symposium on virus hepatitis antigen and antibodies. *Vox Sang.,* **19,** 193-416.

Bulletin of the World Health Organisation (1970) Memorandum. Viral hepatitis and tests for the Australia (hepatitis—associated) antigen and antibody, **42,** 957.

Zuckerman, A.J. (1972) *Hepatitis Associated Antigen and Viruses.* 1st ed. Amsterdam: North-Holland.

Chapter 32. Blood Products

In the early days of Transfusion Services the emphasis was largely on the supply of whole blood. During the 1939-45 War the supply of intravenous fluids to support the injured soldier presented a major problem. The need arose for a product which could be stored for prolonged periods of time without special controlled temperature storage facilities. Freeze-dried plasma, prepared from large pools of plasma harvested from many blood donations, provided an answer. Until the late 1950's the situation remained much the same with the transfusionist's armoury consisting of whole blood, freeze dried plasma - now made from the supernatant plasma of time expired donations, fresh frozen plasma made from pools of plasma harvested within hours of the donation being taken, fibrinogen, small amounts of anti-haemophiliac globulin concentrate and immunoglobulin preparations. There was little progress until the early 1960's partly because there was little demand for other products and also techniques for their preparation on a large scale were not available. In the last ten to fifteen years the situation has been changed completely and there are now enormous demands for anti-haemophiliac globulin, platelets, white cell poor blood, etc.

One of the principle keys to this change has been the introduction of plastic bag systems for blood collection. Using various combinations of multiple bags it is possible to separate a blood donation into two or more components in a completely closed sterile system. Various workers are now developing methods whereby single bags may be joined together in a transfusion unit using sterile "docking" systems (Zuck and Bensinger, 1975). This would allow a range of satellite bags to be added to a single bag containing blood and allow processing to be carried out in a sterile closed system. The preparation of frozen blood, which now is an open procedure, at least in part, might be performed using such a closed system from the time of donation, through freezing and recovery processes right up to the issue of the unit for transfusion.

In examining the available products which may be harvested from a blood donation it is convenient to divide them up into those which are within the capability of the average Regional Transfusion Centre in the United Kingdom and those which require the facilities of a central processing laboratory. A list of these products is given in Table 32.1 and we will consider each of them in turn, starting with those which may be prepared within a Transfusion Centre.

RED CELLS

The tremendous pressure which has built up for the collection of other components such as cryoprecipitate, platelets and semi-purified albumin solutions has led to a reappraisal of the need for red cells to be given as whole blood.

437

Table 32.1 Summary of blood products

	Products preparable in a transfusion centre		
Red-cell orientated	*White-cell orientated*	*Platelet orientated*	*Plasma orientated*
Whole blood	White-cell concentrate	Platelet-rich plasma	Fresh frozen plasma
Fresh blood	White-cell poor red cells	Platelet concentrate	Cryoprecipitate
Concentrated red cells			
Packed cells			
Washed cells			
Frozen blood			
	Products requiring fractionation facilities		
Plasma expanders	*Clotting factors*	*Immunoglobulin*	*Others*
Freeze-dried plasma	Fibrinogen	Non specific	Transfer factor
Plasma-protein fraction	Factor VIII, IX, etc.	Specific:-	
		Anti-D	
		Vaccinia	
		Tetanus	
		Varicella	
		Mumps	
		Herpes simplex	
		Measles	
		Rubella	
		Hepatitis-B antibody	

To meet the demands for anti-haemophiliac globulin and albumin, increasing numbers of donations need to have their fresh plasma partially or completely removed before the red cells are issued. Concentrated red cells must be used when previously this might have been thought desirable but not essential, and ideas are changing about what previously were thought of as absolute indications for the use of whole blood. In order to keep pace with the increasing demand for plasma as a raw material we must aim to use 50 per cent or even more of our donations as concentrated red cells. Perhaps the only absolute indication for the use of whole blood is in the treatment of acute blood loss and J.D. Cash (1976) at the Edinburgh Transfusion Centre has demonstrated that even here a proportion of concentrated red cells may be used.

In outline, the Edinburgh regime for utilisation of concentrated red cells is as follows. All cases not bleeding acutely are given red-cell concentrate only. The first two units of any transfusion for acute bleeding, intraoperative or otherwise, are given as red cell concentrate—any further units over the next twenty-four hours are automatically given as whole blood. Children and burns cases are excepted from the scheme and there is provision for the clinician to overide the rules if he feels it is clinically necessary to do so.

Distinction should be made between the terms concentrated red cells and packed cells. Packed cells are cells from which virtually the whole of the supernatant plasma has been removed. This results in a very viscous fluid which is difficult to transfuse unless it is diluted, and would be an unacceptable product for large scale indiscriminate issue from a Transfusion Centre. In order to both meet the requirement of raw plasma for fractionation and have an acceptable red cell product for distribution it is the practice to remove only a proportion of the supernatant plasma. This proportion varies but if somewhere between 150 and 220 ml of plasma are removed from a unit of 450 ml blood and 75 ml anti coagulant 375 to 300 ml of concentrated red cells remain with a haematocrit of between 56 and 69 per cent and a haemoglobin of between 17 and 21 g per cent. This mixture runs fairly readily through a giving set. Concentrated red cells will probably prove satisfactory for the vast majority of cases where it is necessary to raise the haemoglobin without burdening the circulation with the unwanted volume of the plasma present in a normal bottle of whole blood.

Packed red cells may be required for the treatment of those anaemic patients where it is necessary to raise the patient's haemoglobin though even the added volume of the red cells alone could precipitate cardiac failure. Packed cells can also be of value in the treatment of patients, such as the multi-transfused, who frequently have a mild reaction to some non red cell component of the transfusion. Whilst washing the cells provides the optimum removal of the unwanted component, it is sometimes possible in the milder cases to avoid the reaction by the simple expedient of giving packed cells from which both the supernatant plasma and the buffy coat have been expressed. This is a very simple procedure in a plastic bag collecting system.

Washed cells are prepared simply by centrifuging the unit, removing the supernatant plasma and replacing it with sterile intravenous grade physiologically normal saline. The cells are then re-suspended in the saline, re-centrifuged and the saline supernatant removed. The process of washing can be repeated as required with the red cells finally left for transfusion in a suitable quantity of saline. All steps in this processing must be carried out under fully aseptic conditions and, unless a closed system of processing is used to guarantee sterility, the cells should be transfused within twelve hours of washing. The result of this processing is to remove from the donation all the plasma and a proportion of the white cells and platelets. More efficient removal of the white cells and platelets can be achieved by a dextran sedimentation step at the start of the procedure. There are several variations on this technique. Goldman and Heiss (1971) add 70 ml of 6 per cent Dextran (mol. wt., 70) to a 400-ml donation in 50 ml of ACD. This is allowed to stand at room temperature for 1-2 hours and the supernatant white cell containing plasma is discarded.

Washed or dextran-sedimented red cells are needed for the transfusion of patients with paroxysmal nocturnal haemaglobinuria or who have transfusion reactions due to antibodies to platelets, white cells or protein components. Quite marked reactions can sometimes occur when transfusing patients with antibodies to the Gm system and Pineda and Taswell (1975) have reported very severe reactions as a result of transfusing patients with antibodies to the IgA immunoglobulins.

Fresh blood may be requested occasionally. Mollison (1972a) considers there is no logical case for the use of fresh blood within hours of donation. If specific factors such as platelets, Factor VIII are required then concentrates of these are preferable. There is no evidence to support the concept that there is some magical beneficial ingredient only found in whole blood brought hot foot from the donor to the patient though there are occasions when red cells with maximum survival are needed. Red cells deteriorate on storage such that after twenty-one days storage in ACD 15-30 per cent are non viable and will be removed from the circulation within twenty-four hours of transfusion. This is undesirable for instance in exchange transfusion for HDN, in the treatment of chronic hypoplastic anaemia and for open heart surgery. For this sort of case red cells are needed which will survive virtually as well as fresh cells. The anticoagulent used is important here since red cell 2, 3 Diphosphoglycerate (2, 3-DPG) is better preserved in blood taken into CPD (Citrate-phosphate-dextrose) anticoagulent than into ACD. It is generally regarded that red cells stored up to four days in ACD or seven days in CPD have, for practical purposes, a survival and function as good as fresh blood.

Frozen red cells have been increasingly demanded in recent years. It is not proposed to go into the technical details of their preparation in a book of this size. Readers should refer to the vast amount of published literature on this topic. There are two main methods in current use at the present time. One method uses relatively high concentrations of glycerol as a cryoprotective and the cells are stored at $-80°$C (Merryman and Hornblower, 1972). The other method uses a considerably lower concentration of glycerol and the cells are then stored at $-196°$C (Krijnen et al., 1965; Rowe et al., 1967). The first method has the advantage that the storage temperature can be achieved by a mechanical refrigerator which is relatively cheap to buy and run. But for the recovery of the cells it is almost obligatory to use some form of continuous flow washing device which is usually quite costly to run. The second method has the disadvantage that expensive liquid nitrogen refrigerators are needed and these have to be continually topped up with liquid nitrogen. To offset this, the cells can be recovered by an inexpensive manual batch washing system though automatic continuous flow equipment does make recovery much less tedious. Other cryoprotective agents tried include dimethylsulphoxide and hydroxyethyl starch. Red cells frozen at $-80°$C can be preserved satisfactorily for up to two years whilst it is estimated that red cells stored in liquid nitrogen could be satisfactorily recovered after nearly fifty years storage.

The stimulus to freeze blood was provided initially by the problems of finding compatible blood for patients with antibodies to common antigens such as Kp[b], Vell, etc. It also provided a means of storing blood for auto-transfusion both for those who had these antibodies and for people such as Jehovah's Witnesses who had religious objections to being transfused with blood from other people. Later frozen blood was used in the transfusion of patients with chronic renal failure on dialysis who were candidates for renal transplantation since blood which has been frozen appears to be much less liable to stimulate immunisation to the transplantation antigens than other red cell preparations. Frozen blood has also found a use in the management of non red cell transfusion reactions in the multi-transfused, such as thalassaemics, when the incidence of transfusion reactions after frozen blood is markedly diminished. Lastly, frozen blood has been used as a buffer store in large blood banks, particularly in America, to tide over periods of blood shortage. It is an arguable point as to whether the expense incurred in using frozen blood in this way would not produce a better return spent on recruiting more donors to prevent such shortages.

WHITE CELLS

White cells may be significant in transfusion in two ways, either as white cell concentrate for the treatment of patients with low white cell counts or as white cell poor blood to avoid sensitisation to transplantation antigens. McCredie *et al.* (1974) have shown that white cell transfusion may be beneficial in some cases of leucopaenia. However, it must be remembered that over 90 per cent of the body's granulocytes are normally extravascular and it is not sufficient to calculate the body's requirement purely on a basis of the circulating white cell count. Also, the life span of transfused granulocytes is only a matter of hours and therefore successful treatment depends on frequent administration of vast quantities of white cells. It is almost impossible to get this from normal donations, the white cells from 20 or 30 units of blood would be required once or twice a day to treat a single patient. Efforts have therefore been concentrated on the continuous plasmapheresis, using a continuous flow cell separator, of either members of the patient's family or well motivated donors or, better still, a chronic myeloid leukaemic undergoing leucopheresis as part of treatment. Crowley and Valeri (1974) have shown that functional white cells survive effectively in a blood donation for twenty-four hours and the administration of the buffy coats from some twenty units of blood has produced an effective clinical response. Other efforts to obtain leucocyte concentrate have involved filtration of donor blood through cotton wool filters with the subsequent elution of the adherent white cells. In the treatment of aplastic anaemia it is desirable to irradiate the white cell concentrate with gamma rays before transfusion to kill any stem cells present and prevent them becoming engrafted and setting up a graft versus host reaction.

White cell poor blood has been provided by a variety of methods. These methods have included dextran sedimentation of the red cells, filtration through columns filled with various fibres and frozen red cells. The objective is to be able to transfuse red cells to a patient who is a candidate for a transplant, such as a kidney, without sensitising him to transplantation antigens. Since both white cells and platelets carry these antigens it may be necessary to remove both of them from the unit of blood. Many of the methods devised have been effective in removing one or other but not many of them have been effective in removing both. At least 95 per cent of the white cells must be removed to have any chance of avoiding sensitisation to HLA antigens. Few of the filtration methods currently available reduce the white cell content in a unit of blood to this level though Diepenhorst and Engelfriet (1975) report encouraging results. Frozen blood may be better than any of the other methods but it has not been proved that it itself is completely devoid of the risk of sensitising the patient to a subsequent graft and both Telischi *et al.* (1975) and Crowley *et al.* (1974) have demonstrated the survival of immunocompetent cells in frozen washed blood after storage at −80°C.

The whole foundation of the case for transfusing prospective organ transplant recipients with white cell free blood was turned upside down by the observation in 1974 (Opelz *et al.)* that kidney grafts survived better in patients who had been previously transfused with whole blood than in those transfused with white cell poor blood. This paper has met with some criticism from Perkins (1975) though he reported that grafts in patients who had been transfused fared better than in patients who had not, a finding that was confirmed by Festenstein *et al.* (1976). It is not clear what role HLA and transplantation antigens play in the effect, if any, but Storb (1973) has shown, admittedly in dogs given a bone marrow graft, that the transfusion, prior to grafting, of blood with 99.8 per cent of the white cells removed seriously prejudices graft survival. It may be that the search for blood free from transplantation antigenicity will prove to be an unattainable and even in the case of renal grafting, an undesirable goal.

PLATELETS

A need for platelets has existed for a long time for the treatment of acute thrombocytopaenia. The modern intensive treatments for leukaemia frequently induce profound thrombocytopaenia as a side-effect. Platelet transfusions are vital to support the patient during treatment and a vast amount of effort has been put into developing methods for preparing them. There is considerable argument about the best temperature for preparation and storage. Maintaining the platelets at room temperature (22-23°C) yields platelets which have a reasonable life-span in the circulation of the recipient but do not recover their best haemostatic activity until twenty-four hours after infusion. Preparation at 4°C yields a platelet with good coagulant activity but a relatively short life-span within the circulation. The choice of product used should be governed by the clinical requirements of the patient. An acute thrombocytopaenic haemorrhage will be better controlled with platelets prepared at 4°C and platelets stored at 23°C are better for prophylactic therapy (Kattlove, 1974). Platelets prepared at 22°C can be detected in the patient's circulation for up to eight days after transfusion (Valeri *et al.*, 1974) whereas platelets prepared at 4°C are removed from the circulation within thirty-six hours (Becker and Aster, 1972). Platelets are prepared from single donations in a plastic bag with one or two satellites. The unit is centrifuged at 1000g for nine minutes which spins down the red cells and leaves platelet rich plasma on the top. The platelet-rich plasma (PRP) is then expressed into one of the satellite bags and re-spun at 2000g for thirty minutes. The supernatant plasma can then be returned to the red cells and the sedimented platelets re-suspended in a minimal volume of residual plasma to give platelet concentrate. The two preparation stages can be reversed so that the first spin is a hard one to sediment the platelets down on to the red cells as a buffy coat. The supernatant plasma can then be expressed into one satellite, from which cryoprecipitate can be made, and the residual plasma and buffy coat expressed into a second satellite. The second Satellite, containing the buffy coat, is removed and 3-5 similar buffy coats are pooled in a transfer pack and centrifuged slowly to yield platelet concentrate. This modification of the method has the advantage that both cryoprecipitate and platelets can be recovered from the same donation with relative ease.

Earlier methods have involved acidifying the platelet rich plasma by additional ACD. The affect of this is to reduce the aggregation of platelets which occurs when they are cooled at 4°C but at the same time it reduces the post-transfusion survival of platelets. There is no advantage in adding extra ACD to platelets which are to be prepared at room temperature and, in fact, these platelets should not be allowed to fall below pH 6.5. Platelets have also been prepared by attaching the donor to a continuous flow cell separator. Much work has been done on prostaglandin E_1 which, while extremely potent in preventing platelet aggregation, does not seem to produce improved survival of transfused platelets in the circulation (Becker et al., 1976). Some success has also been achieved in freezing platelets using dimethylsulphoxide (DMSO).

A great deal of work has also been done on the sterility of platelet products. There is no doubt that there is potential danger of infection in any blood product which is prepared by an open process. The work on this is conflicting and it appears from results of some workers that there may be an infection risk, presumably from the original venepuncture, even in platelets made in a totally enclosed system (Buchholz et al., 1973). Other workers have failed to confirm this and have produced evidence to suggest that even an open, but aseptic, process can yield platelet concentrate with a very low level of infection (Mallin et al., 1973). There is also evidence that the survival of HLA incompatible platelets is occasionally diminished in patients with HLA antibodies (Yankee, 1971). Since platelet transfusions themselves can stimulate the formation of these antibodies it has been suggested that consideration should be given to the provision of platelets of the same HLA type as the patient. The evidence that this is necessary in more than a very few cases is lacking and to provide such a service on a large scale would be virtually impossible using random donors and could only be obtained by repeated plateletpheresis several times a week from a single donor. It is unreasonable to expect such dedication from any but relatives and friends of the patient concerned. In addition the workload of building up and organising a panel of HLA typed donors willing to undertake this work has to be taken into consideration.

The decision to transfuse platelets should be based on clinical grounds. Once platelet therapy is started there is a high chance that in about ten days a patient with normal immunological functions will develop antibodies to platelets and become resistant to further treatment. Whilst this may not prevent the use of platelets to terminate an episode of acute bleeding it could make effective prophylactic therapy impossible. It is important therefore not to start treatment too early. In the absence of clinical evidence of platelet deficiency such as bleeding, purpura, etc., platelet transfusion should not be given until the platelet count has fallen to between 10 and 20 $\times 10^9/l$.

PLASMA

Fresh Frozen Plasma (FFP)

FFP is prepared from plasma separated from blood within a matter of hours of donation and is stored below $-20°C$ until needed. The plasma may be prepared in individual units, which should be given to patients whose red cells are ABO compatible with the plasma being transfused, or aliquoted out from pools of about eight units in a selected mix of ABO groups to both dilute and neutralise the ABO antibodies present.

FFP should contain all the non-cellular coagulation factors. As such it can be used to replace any of them but it must be remembered that the volume which a patient can receive without being overloaded is limited and this determines the amount by which a particular factor can be raised in a patient's circulation. This is particularly true of Factor VIII, which has a short *in vivo* half-life, where the patient's Factor VIII level cannot be maintained by the use of FFP at more than 15-30 per cent of normal for longer than a day or two (Biggs, 1972).

Cryoprecipitate

The discovery, in 1965, by Pool and Shannon that a very high degree of concentration of Factor VIII from fresh raw plasma could be obtained in a closed bag system by any Blood Bank, by the simple expedient of freezing and thawing and harvesting the cryoprecipitate, revolutionised the treatment of haemophilia. In outline, the donation is taken into a double bag, centrifuged and the plasma is squeezed over into the satellite bag which is then frozen, still attached to the donation bag by the transfer line, in an alcohol/cardice bath to −40 to −60°C. The plasma is then thawed either overnight in air at 4°C or more quickly in a water bath maintained at 8°C. When thawed the plasma contains a cotton wool like cryoprecipitate, rich in Factor VIII and fibrinogen, which is much slower to dissolve at 0-4°C than are the other plasma proteins and may be centrifuged to the bottom of the satellite. The supernatant plasma is then squeezed back onto the red cells until only a few ml. remain and the satellite is then separated from the parent bag and stored below −20°C in which form it will keep for several months. In expert hands over 80 per cent of the original factor VIII can be recovered in the cryoprecipitate (Burka *et al.,* 1975) and, being a closed system, the sterility of both the red cells and the cryoprecipitate is assured. However, there is at least one European Transfusion Centre that has prepared cryoprecipitate from plasma aspirated from bottled blood using a rigid aseptic technique. The resulting packed cells have been stored at 4°C and given a normal 21 day shelf life. The process has operated without incident for several years but the key to success is the care taken in the "open" separation stage.

The cryoprecipitate is thawed immediately before use and the contents of several units are aspirated into a syringe and given to the patient intravenously. Since the volume of fluid in each bag is small it is very easy to leave a considerable proportion of the activity in the bag unless the bag is flushed out with saline or citrate and care is taken to aspirate as much as possible from the bag. Cryoprecipitate is a very efficient source of Factor VIII but the activity in any individual bag is unpredictable and it is impossible to be certain how much activity the patient is getting. In a large Transfusion Centre it is not easy to ensure that the percentage recovery is identical in every bag and, even if it were so, the activity in the starting plasma varies from donor to donor. This, together with the inconvenience of having to pool many bags of cryoprecipitate to make up a single dose, is one of the chief reasons why Factor VIII concentrate is preferable.

FRACTIONATED PRODUCTS

Under this heading are included those products which require the facilities of a fractionation and freeze drying production unit. In some countries these are provided centrally and separate from the Transfusion Centre. However, in other countries the Transfusion Centre and fractionation plant are all housed under the one roof.

Freeze-Dried Plasma (FDP)

Freeze-dried plasma was originally made from vast pools of plasma which were then aliquoted out and freeze dried. With the recognition that blood donation could carry the risk of transmission of hepatitis and that one infective donation could disseminate the disease through a whole pool of plasma the risk was minimised by restricting plasma pools to no more than the plasma from ten donations of blood. These ten donations were composed of a selected mix of all the ABO groups to both dilute and neutralise the A and B alloagglutinins of each donation. Each pool was then aliquoted out into 400-ml amounts which were freeze dried. Virtually all the plasma used for this purpose came from time expired blood where the plasma had been in contact with the red cells for at least twenty-one days. In consequence, the final FDP is deficient of virtually all non-cellular clotting factors, with the exception of fibrinogen, and can contain quite large amounts of potassium which has diffused from the red cells during their storage period. In a bottle of reconstituted FDP the potassium levels can be as high as 17 mmol/l. Consideration of FDP as a product is now largely historical however. In the United Kingdom it has virtually been replaced by plasmaprotein fraction, though some FDP is preferred by certain specialised units who use it as a replacement solution when plasmapheresing patients with macroglobulinaemia.

Plasma protein fraction (PPF)

Plasma Protein Fraction is a liquid preparation containing about 45 grammes of protein per litre. By itself this would be a hypotonic solution so 130 - 160 mmol of sodium chloride is added per litre. The protein in solution is Cohn fraction V precipitate and consists of 90 per cent or more albumin with not more than 10 per cent α- and β-globulin and is stablised with sodium caprylate. Albumin in this low concentration can be heated to 60°C for ten hours without causing undue aggregation of the protein. This step inactivates hepatitis B virus and hence the final product is non-icterogenic. This was one of the major reasons for introducing PPF but since this decision was made the risk of transmitting hepatitis with freeze dried plasma itself has been dramatically reduced as a result of modern methods of testing donations for the presence of the hepatitis B antigen.

Albumin

This is produced by re-precipitation of the PPF containing fraction. The final product, containing not less than 95 per cent albumin and virtually no sodium, is stabilised with sodium caprylate and freeze dried. Before freeze drying it is heated to 60° C for ten hours to inactivate the hepatitis B virus. The freeze dried product contains not more than 16.3 mmol of Na and 1.3 mmol of K per bottle and is often referred to as "salt free albumin". Albumin is made up for use by dissolving it in the appropriate volume of sterile water for injection. If the final concentration of albumin in solution is intended to be less than 15 g per cent then saline or dextrose saline should be used to avoid administering a hypotonic solution of albumin to the patient. However, if a dilute protein solution is required then PPF rather than albumin is the material of choice.

There is considerable controversy regarding the clinical usefulness of albumin. There is a small, but definite, requirement for treating haemolytic disease of the newborn where the added albumin increases the intravascular binding of bilirubin. Its most common use is in treating the chronic hypoalbuminaemic states that arise in liver or renal disease. Mollison (1972b) states that it is universally agreed that albumin has no place in the treatment of these conditions but Davison (1972) has suggested that in chronic renal disease albumin can play a very important role in the control of oedema in those cases that fail to respond to diuretics.

Fibrinogen

Fibrinogen is prepared as a freeze-dried product from plasma by Cohn fractionation and is mainly used to treat disseminated intravascular coagulation, as occurs as a complication of labour for example. The manufacturing process cannot free it from the risk of hepatitis transmission. Like albumin, it is re-dissolved in the appropriate volume of sterile water for injection. Dissolving both fibrinogen and albumin is sometimes a tedious process which can be simplified considerably by using water pre-heated to 37° C followed by centrifugation. Bottles of sterile water can be kept in a 37° C incubator until required and then added to the freeze dried protein. The protein is mixed with the water, if necessary by moderate shaking, until all the protein is free from the sides of the bottles and floating on the water. The protein is then forced into solution by centrifuging the bottle for 15—20 minutes at as high a speed as the container can safely stand. It is possible to get quite concentrated solutions of fibrinogen (or albumin) by this technique when it would be difficult to dissolve the protein by gentle aggitation in the small volume of solvent.

Factor VIII

Freeze dried concentrates of Factor VIII, and indeed other clotting factors such as Factor IX, VII, etc., can be produced. They are prepared as freeze dried products of high potency and have the enormous advantage that very large doses of the active factor can be easily administered to the patient. Factor VIII concentrate is made from pools of a thousand or more donations. The activity of each batch is assayed and the amount of activity in each vial of the material is indicated. In the case of Factor VIII this is a tremendous advantage over cryoprecipitate which is of largely unpredictable potency. The manufacturing process does not free Factor VIII from the risk of transmitting hepatitis. It is yet to be seen how far modern methods of testing each donor for Australia antigen will reduce the incidence of hepatitis transmitted by these concentrates.

Immunoglobulins

These are usually prepared as liquid preparations for intramuscular injection. Given intravenously, they sometimes cause severe reactions due to the presence of aggregated immunoglobulin molecules. However, some manufacturing units use processes which produce a preparation which is safe for intravenous use. The preparative process renders the material non-icterogenic. Immunoglobulin preparations can be divided into non-specific and specific preparations. Non-specific immunoglobulin, prepared from large plasma pools from random donors contains a mix of immunoglobulins of various specificities. This preparation is invaluable in the maintenance of patients with hypogammaglobulinaemia and has also been used with some success in conferring passive immunity against hepatitis A.

Specific immunoglobulins are prepared from donors with high titres of antibodies to particular antigens. The most celebrated is anti-D immunoglobulin which has had a dramatic effect in reducing the incidence of immunisation of Rhesus-negative mothers by their Rhesus-positive babies.

Most anti-D immunoglobulin is obtained from Rhesus negative donors who have been previously immunised with Rhesus positive red cells as a result of pregnancy or transfusion. A small number of Rhesus negative volunteers, men or post menopausal women, have been deliberately immunised. If a donor's antibody level is too low it can be boosted by the intravenous injection of a small volume of Rhesus positive red cells. These cells must come from a selected donor who, apart from being fit and Hb Ag negative, must have a history of several previous donations which can be shown not to have caused post transfusion jaundice in the patients who received them. Due to the small number of donors available and the large number of women needing protection frequent plasmapheresis of the donors rather than straight donation is needed to obtain enough plasma for fractionation.

Other specific immunoglobulins include those for mumps, measles *varicella* (*herpes zoster*) and *vaccinia* which are used to protect people who have been exposed to infection such as the very young, the elderly and the chronic sick whose lives would be at risk were they to develop the disease. They are also of value for the protection of patients receiving immunosuppressive drugs after an organ transplant.

Human tetanus immunoglobulin can be used in place of immunoglobulin prepared in horses and avoids the risk of anaphalactic reactions and, like horse immunoglobulin, is effective in the treatment of tetanus infection and for producing passive immunisation.

Immunoglobulin to hepatitis B can be prepared from donors found to have the antibody during the course of screening for Australia antigen and antibody. Evidence is accumulating that, if given in large enough doses, it is effective in preventing the development of the disease in those who had inadvertently become contaminated with material thought to be infective.

Rubella immunoglobulin was used extensively for some years in an attempt to prevent pregnant women who had been in contact with the disease from developing the disease during the first three months of pregnancy, the time when the threat to the foetus of deformities induced by the disease was at its greatest. In recent years it has been shown that this immunoglobulin is ineffective in preventing the disease and it is no longer used.

Maintaining sufficient supplies of these materials depends on finding people who have recently had the disease or been vaccinated and who are prepared to come forward as donors. Work by Entwistle (1975) and Eldrige and Entwistle (1975) has shown that it is possible to screen random donors to find those whose plasma contains suitable levels of *vaccinia* or *tetanus* antibody to prepare specific immunoglobulin. *Tetanus* immunoglobulin levels of 5 iu/ml or more were found in 4.4 per cent of random donors but only 1.2 per cent of donors had high enough levels of *vaccinia* antibody from which to make immunoglobulin.

Transfer factor

Transfer factor is the name given to a group of polypeptides of m.wt. between 700 and 5000 which may be extracted from lymphocytes. It appears to have the property of transferring cell mediated immunity from the cells of a patient who has been immunised to the cells of a patient who has not. It has found application in a variety of conditions such as chronic mucocutaneous candiasis, Wiskott-Aldrich syndrome and other conditions (Basten *et al.*, 1975). Recently it has been tried in the treatment of malignant disease (Oettgen *et al.*, 1974). As yet its preparation is difficult and its effects uncertain but should further research demonstrate a clear cut valuable role for transfer factor in the treatment of cancer then the demands for raw material for processing will be enormous.

This has, necessarily, been an incomplete survey of the available products. No mention has been made of some of the other clotting factor concentrates such as Factor IX or prothrombol. It is very likely that the range of products will be yet further extended as new therapeutic materials are found which may be recovered from a blood donation.

REFERENCES

Basten, A., Croft, S., Kenny, D.F. & Nelson, D.S. (1975) Uses of transfer factor *Vox Sang.*, **28**, 257.
Becker, G.A. & Aster, R.H. (1972) Short term platelet preservation at 22°C and 4°C. *Blood*, **40**, 593.
Becker, G.A., Kunicki, T., Aster, R.H. (1974) Effect of prostaglanolin E_1 on harvesting of platelets from refrigerated whole blood. *J. Lab. Clin. Med.*, **83**, 304.
Biggs, R., (1972) *Human Blood Coagulation, Haemostasis and Thrombosis.* Blackwell. P. 338.
Bucholz, D.H., Young, V.M., Friedman, N.R., Reilly, J.A. & Mardiney, M.R.Jr. (1973) Detection and quantitation of bacteria in platelets stored at ambient temperature. *Transfusion*, **13**, 268.
Burka, E.R., Puffer, T. & Martinez, J. (1975) The influence of donor characteristics and preparation methods on the potency of human cryoprecipitate *Transfusion*, **15**, 323.

Cash, J.D., (1976) Personal communication.

Crowley, J.P., Skrabut, E.M. & Valeri, C.R., (1974) Immunocompetent lymphocytes in previously frozen washed red cells. *Vox Sang.*, **26**, 513.

Crowley, J.P. & Valeri, C.R. (1974) Recovery and function of granulocytes stored in plasma at 4°C for one week. *Transfusion*, **14**, 574.

Davison, A.M. (1972) Clinical uses of albumin. *Proc. R. Soc. Edin. (B)*, **71**, Suppl. 9, 83.

Diepenhorst, P. & Engelfriet, C.P. (1975) Removal of leukocytes from whole blood and erythrocyte suspensions by filtration through cotton wool. V. Results after transfusion of 1820 units of filtered erythrocytes. *Vox Sang.*, **29**, 15.

Eldridge, P.L. & Entwistle, C.C. (1975) Routine Screening of donor plasma suitable for the preparation of anti-tetanus immunoglobulin. *Vox Sang.*, **28**, 62.

Entwistle, C.C. (1975) Antibody to Vaccinia. II Prevalence in blood donors. *Vox Sang.*, **28**, 77.

Festenstein, H., Sachs, J.A., Paris, A.M.I., Pegrum, G.D. & Moorhead, J.F. (1976) The influence of HL-A matching and blood transfusion on outcome of 502 London Transplant Group renal-graft recipients. *Lancet*, **i**, 157.

Goldman, S.F. & Heiss, F., (1971) A method for preparing buffy coat poor blood for transfusion—a modification. *Vox Sang.*, **21**, 540.

Kattlove, H.E. (1974) Platelet preservation—what temperature? A rationale for strategy. *Transfusion*, **14**, 328.

Krijnen, H.W., de Wit, Fr.M.J.J., Kuivenhoven, A.C.J. & Reyden, C.V.D., (1965) Freezing of red cells with liquid nitrogen: results with glycerol as an intracellular substance. *Bibl. Haemat.*, **23**, 683.

McCredie, K.B., Freireich, E.J., Hester, J.P. & Vallejos, C. (1974) Increased granulocyte collection with the blood cell separator and the addition of etiocholanolone and hydroxyethyl starch. *Transfusion*, **14**, 357.

Mallin, W.S., Reuss, D.T., Bracke, J.W., Roberts, S.C. & Moore, G.L. (1973) Bacteriological study of platelet concentrates stored at 22°C and 4°C. *Transfusion*, **13**, 439.

Merryman, H.T. & Hornblower, M. (1972) A method for freezing and washing red blood cells using a high glycerol concentration. *Transfusion*, **12**, 145.

Mollison, P.L. (1972a) *Blood Transfusion in Clinical Medicine.* 5th Ed. P. 94. Blackwell.

Mollison, P.L. (1972b) *Blood Transfusion in Clinical Medicine* 5th Ed. P.87. Blackwell.

Oettgen, A.F., Old, L.J., Farrow, J.H., Valentine, F.T., Lawrence, H.S. & Thomas, L. (1974) Effects of dialysable transfer factor in patients with breast cancer. *Proc. Nat. Acad. Sci. USA*, **71**, 2319.

Opelz, G., Mickey, M.R. & Terasaki, P.I. (1974) HL-A and kidney transplants: re-examination. *Transplantation*, **17**, 371.

Perkins, H.A. (1975) Immunologic hazards of blood transfusion. *Transfusion and Immunology 1975*, Plenary session lectures of the XIV Congress of the International Society of Blood Transfusion, Helsinki, 1975. P.107.

Pineda, A.A. & Taswell, H.F. (1975) Transfusion reactions associated with anti-IgA antibodies: report of four cases and review of the literature. *Transfusion*, **15**, 10.

Pool, J.G. & Shannon, A.E. (1965) Production of high potency concentrates of antihaemophiliac globulin in a closed bag system. Assay *in vitro* and *in vivo*. New Engl. J. Med., **273**, 1443.

Rowe, A.W., Eyster, E. & Kellner, A. (1967) Survival of human blood frozen by the low glycerol-liquid nitrogen rapid freeze technique. *Cryobiology*, **3**, 379.

Storb, R., Kolb, H.J., Graham, T.C., Erickson, V. & Thomas, E.D. (1973) The effect of buffy coat poor blood transfusion on subsequent hemopoietic grafts. *Transplantation*, **15**, 129.

Telischi, M., Krmpotic, E. & Moss, G. (1975) Viable lymphocytes in frozen washed blood. *Transfusion*, **15**, 481.

Valeri, C.R., Feingold, H., Marchionni, L.D., (1974) The relation between response to hypotonic stress and the ^{51}Cr recovery in vivo of preserved platelets. *Transfusion*, **14**, 331.

Yankee, R.A. (1971) Importance of histocompatibility in platelet therapy. *Vox Sang.*, **20**, 419.

Zuck, T.F. & Bensinger, T.A. (1975) Implications of sterile docking devices. *Transfusion*, **15**, 339.

Appendix I. A practical guide to laboratory procedure

"I never knew you played the banjo. . ." "Not exactly", replied George, "but it is very easy, they tell me—and I've got the instruction book."

Jerome K. Jerome, THREE MEN IN A BOAT

The subject of human blood groups is a large one and there are many, some would say a bewildering number, of techniques. In spite of the variety it is true, however, that the chief manipulation in a blood grouping laboratory is the mixing together of extremely small quantities of red cells and serum and afterwards observing whether or not the red cells have been agglutinated or sensitised by an antibody in the serum. The mixing is effected most accurately and conveniently by delivering small volumes with a graduated Pasteur pipette into precipitin tubes, or in some circumstances on to slides or opalescent tiles.

Alternatively, blood grouping may be performed in a continuous flow system such as the multichannel AutoAnalyser (*see* Chapter 21).

SEROLOGICAL APPARATUS

Tubes

These can be hard glass and in two main sizes.

(1) *The 50 mm (length)* ×11 *mm (internal diameter) cell suspension tube.* This will be found to be of convenient size for:

(*a*) Red cell suspensions.
(*b*) Anti-human globulin (Coombs) tests—there is room for an adequate volume of saline at the washing stage.
(*c*) Storage of typing serum of various kinds.
(*d*) The serial dilutions of "master" titres, dilutions of saliva, etc.

(2) *The 50 mm (length)* × 5.5 *mm (internal diameter) precipitin tube.* This tube is used for almost all serological tests with the exception of the anti-human globulin technique. In a busy laboratory it is, therefore, required in large numbers.

Alternatively plastic tubes can be used. The most usual sizes are 60 mm × 8 mm (internal diameter) and 35 mm × 5 mm (internal diameter) to take the place of glass tubes (1) and (2) respectively. A disadvantage of plastic tubes is that it is more difficult to deliver a volume of liquid to the bottom of the tube.

Cleansing of Tubes

The adequate cleaning of tubes presents a considerable problem. The least trace of particulate dirt, of previously used potent anti-serum, or of alkali or acid, may be fatal to the subsequent tests. Dirty tubes should be covered with cold water, as soon as possible after the tests are read, and left to soak.

There are a variety of ways of cleaning the tubes. A machine which sprays jets of fluid into the tubes can be used, a satisfactory sequence is tap water, detergent, two rinses with tap water and then steam under pressure. If a machine fitted with jets is not available the tubes must be held under a fast-running tap, thoroughly shaken, boiled in detergent, rinsed in hot and then cold tap water and finally with distilled water. For the rinsing process the tubes are held upright in handfuls so that each tube is filled completely with the rinsing fluid. After each rinse they are vigorously shaken. They are dried quickly in a hot air oven.

The importance of an efficient cleaning process for tubes cannot be over-emphasised; without it first-class work may be ruined.

Racks for Holding Tubes

Small wooden blocks as shown in Figures AI. 2a and b, AI. 3a and b. have now been almost entirely superseded by 50-holed aluminium racks of approximately the same size. A small 50.holed plastic rack to fit the serological centrifuge (*see below*) is most useful for spinning techniques.

Pasteur or Capillary Pipettes

These are the serologist's chief tool.

In Fig. AI.1 eight different Pasteur pipettes are depicted each designed for a different purpose. The first of these (A), is a general purpose pipette graduated to deliver two unit volumes 0.03 ml each; the graduation marks both come well within the straight part of the stem. This is essential for accuracy. If the size of the bore and the required unit volume are such that it is necessary to make a graduation where the stem is starting to widen, the pipette is unsuitable as any slight inaccuracy that may occur in measuring a volume results in a larger error than when the volume is confined to the straight part of the stem. If the bore is such that the unit volume marking is less than 1″ from the tip, the pipette is less accurate. The overall length of the pipette, excluding the rubber teat is 5½-6 in. This is a comfortable length for the average hand but there will naturally be slight variations (of not more than ½ in) according to personal preference. The graduation must be a fine line (not a grease pencilled blob!) which can be made with a mapping pen using either Gurr's glass ink or Chinese lacquer.

The second pipette, (B) in Fig. AI.1, requires little additional comment. It is essentially similar except that it is graduated to deliver three unit volumes instead of two. It is included to emphasise the point that even if further unit volume markings are needed they must all remain within the confines of the narrow part of the stem.

The third pipette shown (C) is designed solely for titration and should be reserved for this purpose. It bears a single graduation situated approximately 1 to 1½ in from its tip.

The fourth pipette (D) is for the delivery of micro-volumes (0.01 ml or less).

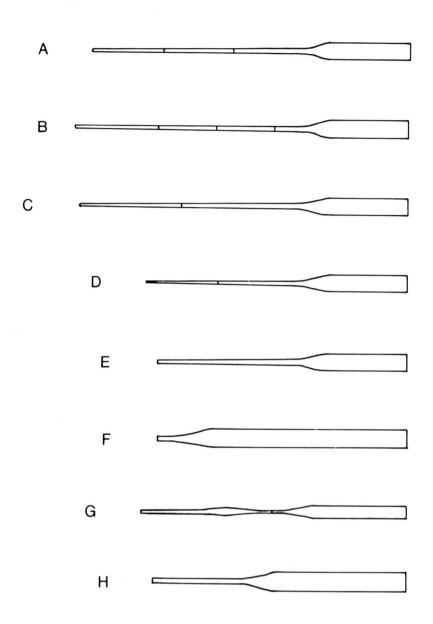

Fig. AI.1. The Pasteur pipettes used for blood group serology.

A. General purpose.   *E.* Reading.
B. Three unit volume.   *F.* Transfer.
C. Titration.   *G.* Master dilution.
D. Micro-volume.   *H.* Dropping pipette.

The bore of this pipette has to be very fine to allow the small unit volume to occupy a reasonable length of the stem (*i.e.* approximately 1 in). It is not advisable to mark such pipettes to deliver more than one unit volume.

The fifth pipette (E) is not graduated since it is used solely for the preparation of smears. It can with advantage be of slightly wider bore than the general purpose pipette.

The sixth pipette (F) shown is designed for the transfer of larger quantities, *i.e.* several millilitres of any liquid, such as serum, from one container to another. Thus, the wide end of the pipette is increased to 5 in and the narrow end reduced to ½ in.

The seventh pipette (G) is for the making of "master" dilutions. The bulge in the stem allows for a large unit volume (up to 0.3 ml to 0.5 ml) while maintaining both the fine point which reduces carry-over to a minimum and a graduation mark made in a narrow region of the stem so that accuracy in actual measurement of the volume is comparable with that of the other pipettes described.

The eighth pipette (H) is designed for use by the dropping technique. The aperture of a dropping pipette must be of standard bore and a gauge is used to ensure that the pipette delivers a drop of the correct size.

Handling of Pasteur Pipettes

For blood grouping techniques Pasteur pipettes are used in a specialised way; the handling of them in other kinds of laboratory does not give the worker experience of their use for serological manipulations.

The measurement and delivery into precipitin tubes of small volumes of fluid requires a delicate touch and much practice, but an amazing degree of accuracy coupled with speed can be attained by the practised worker. The pipettes should be held at an angle, the glass stem just below the teat being gripped between the third and fourth fingers while the thumb and first finger rest gently on the rubber teat (cf. Figs. AI.2a and b). The weight of the pipette is supported by the third and fourth fingers, while the thumb and first finger are used entirely for controlling the measurement of the required volume. The next step is to exert very slight pressure on the teat with the thumb and first finger. The exact amount of pressure required must be learnt by experience but let it be said that it is far less than is usually imagined by the novice! The tip of the pipette is dipped just under the surface of the fluid which is to be measured and the pressure gradually released until the fluid is drawn up exactly to the mark. This is a simple procedure providing the preliminary pressure on the teat has been gauged correctly. The optimum pressure is such that the fluid within the stem just manages to reach the mark with little or no suction left over to raise it any further. If too great a pressure is exerted it will be found that the column of fluid fluctuates wildly, is difficult to control and will not come to rest at the desired level.

Having obtained an accurately measured volume it is next delivered into a small precipitin tube; this also requires knack. The tip of the pipette is placed just overlapping the edge of the tube and pressure is again exerted with the thumb and forefinger, this time fairly sharply. It is released when the whole volume has been delivered. This method of delivery is slightly modified for micro-volumes since these are placed on the bottom of the tube which is taken out of the rack and

Fig. A1.2(a) Typical bench layout; setting-up tests.

Comments

1. Note that the general layout is convenient, everything needed being within arm's reach, also that the beakers and jar are close to the worker's hand.

2. Note the strict alignment of the racks, a precaution against placing volumes of red cell suspension or serum from the unknown samples into the wrong tubes.

3. The blood sample and the corresponding cell suspension tube are both held in the left hand throughout the whole running out process and then exchanged simultaneously for the next tubes in the row, the right hand being used to exchange the cell suspension tube while the left is exchanging the blood sample tube.

4. The serial number or name on the first tube of the row is written on to the label immediately after the tube has been taken from its position on the large rack. Before the last tube is replaced, the number or name on this is also written on the label. This labelling is adequate if, and only if, the procedure described above (3) is adopted.

5. Note the handling of the pipette, especially the way it is supported by the second and third fingers, and there is no great pressure being exerted on the teat.

Fig. A1.2(b) Key to Fig. A1.2(a)

A = Large rack containing 37 unknown samples and A, B and O controls in positions 38, 39 and 40. B = rack for serum-grouping with standard A and B red cells. C = rack for cell-grouping with anti-A and anti-B sera. D = rack for testing with O serum (αβ). E = Beaker containing clean saline. F = Beaker containing saline used for rinsing pipette. G = Discard. H = Bottles containing anti-sera. I = Pipette rack. J = racks for the samples 1-40. K = Label. L = Sample tube. M = Cell suspension tube. N = Pipette. O = Teat of pipette.

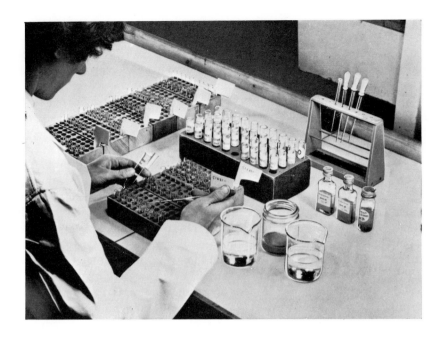

AI.2a

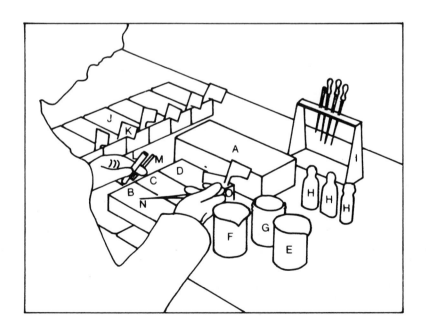

AI.2b

held in the left hand. With practice this method of delivering measured volumes can be carried out very rapidly.

The technique of handling the dropping pipette is entirely different. The teat is squeezed and released sufficiently to allow liquid to enter to about two-thirds of the way up the stem. The pipette is then held vertically and one drop of fluid allowed to fall into each precipitin tube. This procedure is slightly faster than delivering unit volumes of fluid and slightly more inaccurate as the size of the drop is not only dependent on the aperture of the pipette but also on the viscosity of the fluid used, so that drops of, e.g. saline, serum and bovine albumin will not all be exactly equal. For many purposes this is immaterial and provided the pipette is held upright and the fluid allowed to drop (not squirted) into the tube, a dropping technique is adequate for most typing techniques, except when very small quantities of fluid are to be delivered. In our opinion, however, a measuring technique as described above is to be preferred both for its additional accuracy and because the manipulator gains dexterity which stands him in good stead for techniques where it is essential that a measured volume is used.

Alternatively there are several automatic devices on the market. These can save time when large numbers of tests are set up at one time. For example, in one laboratory where we need anti-A, andi-B and group O sera for some 700-1000 tests daily, these sera are run out by means of an automatic syringe graduated to deliver 0.02 ml into each tube.

When using the pipette for preparing smears, it must be remembered that most cell sediments require gentle handling while they are being removed from a tube and spread on a microscope slide. The teat of the smearing pipette, therefore, must be squeezed before dipping the end into the liquid. If the pressure is not applied till after the end of the pipette is under the surface of the fluid, air will be blown on to the sediment and fragile agglutinates may be dispersed.

The cells are drawn gently into the pipette, care being taken that they do not rise as high as the wide portion. They are then pipetted on to a microscope slide and spread. Spreading is accomplished by first holding the pipette in a horizontal position, just touching the right-hand end of the drop of fluid on the slide; the fluid adheres to the pipette by surface tension and can be spread by moving the pipette to the right. If further spreading is required, it can be effected by gentle tilting of the slide. It should never be done by rubbing the pipette backwards and forwards over the surface.

When handling any of the described pipettes, fluid should not enter the teat. Indeed for most manipulations it is entirely unnecessary to allow fluid to reach the wide part of the stem at all. In making serial dilutions the fluid must not be allowed to rise above the graduation as this could introduce a large error. Even when making 2 per cent red cell suspensions from samples of whole blood the fluid need not rise beyond the shoulder. If, inadvertently, it is allowed to get inside the teat, the pipette must be rinsed throughout its entire length, and the teat discarded.

Pipettes are fragile and their tips are easily chipped which makes them unfit for use. They should, therefore, be kept either in special racks or in boxes lined with cotton wool.

Microscope Slides

These are used in large quantities since it is recommended that not more than two smears are made on any one slide. Although in serological work slides are used only for wet preparations which are discarded in a very short time they should be of good quality and should always be of the same thickness so that continual refocusing of the microscope is reduced to a minimum. This may seem at first sight an unimportant detail but for those who read many smears in a normal working day, the use of slides of all makes and thicknesses may become a major trial. As soon as the reactions are recorded the dirty slides are placed in a dish containing enough water to cover them. They should be washed in warm soapy water (detergent can be used if preferred), rinsed in cold water and in hot distilled water. Ideally they are then polished with a clean dry cloth, and care is taken not to finger the polished slides. Some kind of slide holder set at an angle of about 45° to the bench is an asset (*see* Figs. AI.3a and b).

Moist Chamber

This is a box where slides can be kept in a moist atmosphere to prevent drying up of the test during incubation. It can be entirely of glass or perspex but in any case should have a transparent lid so that the tests can be viewed with the lid in position. When results have been recorded the slides are removed from the box and the negative reactions checked microscopically.

Opalescent Glass Tiles and Viewing Box

Squares and strips of white opalescent glass are used for anti-human globulin (Coombs) tests and for any grouping test such as MN that may be done on tiles rather than in tubes. They should be thin enough to allow light to pass through when they are held over a lamp. Alternatively, it is useful to be able to use them in conjunction with a viewing box particularly for anti-human globulin tests. The tiles are placed on top of a box with an opalescent glass lid. Inside the box is a white fluorescent strip light which gives good luminosity with little heat.

It is advisable to keep tiles used for anti-human globulin separate from those used for any other purpose. In this way no human serum should ever come into contact with these tiles.

Incubators and Water Baths

(*a*) 56°C. This is required for the inactivation of complement and for the preparation of eluates.

In laboratories where a large number of Price Precipitation or VDRL tests are carried out, a 56°C water bath which will carry at least 250 samples at one time is convenient.

(*b*) 37°C. For this temperature either a water bath, an air incubator or hot room is needed. With a water bath the required temperature is reached more quickly than with an air incubator but for large-scale work water baths are not practicable because of the space required. Most serological laboratories use air

Fig. AI.3(a) Typical bench layout; reading tests.

Comments

Note convenient arrangement of bench to facilitate the reading of many tests. The worker is at the final stage of preparing a smear. The liquid has been drawn along the slide from left to right behind the Pasteur pipette to which it adheres by surface tension. Note the position of the small precipitin tube A, the content of which has been placed on the slide; the tube is held in the left hand throughout the reading and discarding of the slide and is then exchanged for the next tube to be read. This is a way of marking position in a row of tubes.

Fig. AI.3(b) Key to Fig. AI.3(a)

A = Tube containing test to be examined. B = Microscope slide. C = rack containing tests to be read. D = Special rack for microscope slides. E = Smearing pipette (*see* Fig. AI.1 E). F = Beaker of saline. G = Container for used slides.

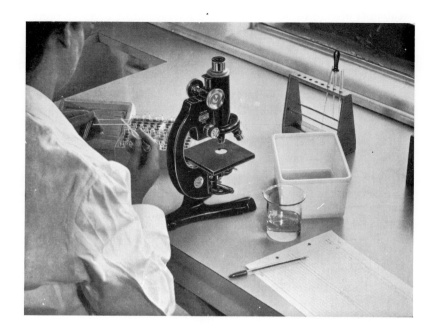

AI.3a

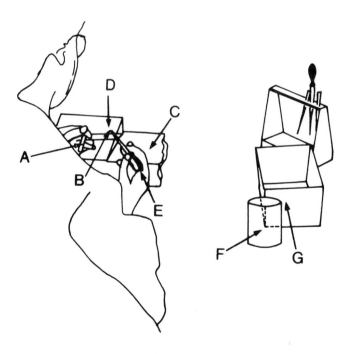

AI.3b

incubators of various sizes to give them a temperature of 37°C. For large scale work an actual room, the temperature of which can be controlled at 37°C, is ideal. This hot room has the added advantage of usually being large enough to accommodate a bench with microscope and centrifuge so that manipulations and readings can actually be carried out at 37°C if desired.

(c) 10°-18°C. These are useful for various reactions, particularly for antibodies that are sensitive to temperature differences and for cross-matching for operations under hypothermia.

Refrigerators

The optimum storage temperature for red cells is 4°C. A large blood bank will require at least one. cold room at this temperature, but for small-scale work a domestic refrigerator is satisfactory. A precautionary measure if this is used, is the checking of the temperature in the various parts of the interior. An unevenness of temperature may sometimes be observed and if this leads to overcooling haemolysis may occur.

Typing sera of all kinds including anti-human globulin serum are best stored at −20°C, therefore, some kind of deep freeze capable of maintaining this temperature is essential.

A cabinet containing carbon dioxide snow can be used but its limitations should be realised. The temperature inside the container will vary widely according to proximity to the snow. In addition the atmosphere within becomes saturated with carbon dioxide which may have serious effects on the contents unless strictly air-tight containers are used throughout.

Any laboratory which stores rare cells may well find it best to keep them in liquid nitrogen. This entails special precautions and will be dealt with in connection with red cell storage (Appendix II).

Centrifuges

The blood grouping laboratory requires a number of centrifuges of varying capacities. In a large laboratory, it is useful to have a centrifuge to hold a large number of test tubes or universal containers at a time.

A useful centrifuge is one which will spin 50 holed plastic racks. This is useful in those techniques where it is wished to speed or improve agglutination by centrifugation. It is also valuable where large numbers of anti-human globulin tests are performed.

Another aid found useful by some workers when washing large numbers of tests is a multi-nozzle vaccuum pump.

Also, there are now available machines for automating the whole washing procedure of anti-globulin tests.

Refrigerated centrifuges, e.g. the MSE Mistral, capable of spinning 6 or 8 blood bottles or packs are needed for the preparation of blood components.

GENERAL ROUTINE PROCEDURE FOR ALL SEROLOGICAL INVESTIGATIONS

A pre-determined bench "lay-out" and pattern for each kind of serological procedure is a great time-saver and encourages a higher degree of accuracy in testing.

The first step is to assemble all apparatus needed, including racks filled with tubes in the pattern required for each test. Fig. AI.2 shows a convenient bench arrangement for the ABO grouping of 37 unknown samples. It is, however, of equal if not greater importance to adhere to a standard procedure even when only one or two samples are to be tested. After putting out the required rows of tubes the racks are clearly labelled with the name of the test. Flag labels, as shown in the photograph are convenient. Then all diluent fluids and standard anti-sera are run into the appropriate rows, rinsing the pipette very carefully 3 or 4 times between each fluid. It is essential to have a rule about which position a particular serum occupies. In the set-up shown, anti-A serum is always run into the front row of a rack and anti-B into the second. Similarly, for serum-grouping A cells go into the front row and B cells into the second. This routine is never varied.

Next, the unknown sera are pipetted into all serum-grouping, and/or antibody detection tests; the pipette must, of course, be rinsed carefully between the delivery of each unknown serum. Before the appropriate red cells are added, the tubes are checked for their serum content. This is an extremely important step in the general procedure, which, if omitted, might have serious consequences. If perspex or metal racks are used a glance will show whether all the tubes have their proper serum content, but with wooden blocks the tubes will have to be picked up.

Red cell suspensions, which are usually required to be 2-5 per cent in saline (as judged by eye), are made from the first unknown sample and without rinsing the pipette they are measured into the appropriate tubes. Note the strict alignment of the racks, a precaution against placing volumes of red cells or serum into the wrong tubes. The sample to be tested and the corresponding cell suspension tubes are both held in the left hand throughout the whole procedure and then exchanged simultaneously for the next tubes in the row, the right hand being used to exchange the cell suspension tube, while the left is exchanging the blood sample tube. The serial number or name on the first tube of the row is written on the label immediately after the tube has been taken from its position on the large rack. Before the last tube is replaced, the number or name on this is also written on the flag label. Standard cells are then run into the appropriate tests and into the controls of the cell typing tests. A known positive and known negative control is included for each anti-serum used and the controls are repeated for each batch of tests set up. The tubes are tapped (except where a layering technique is being used) to ensure good mixing of the contents, then incubated for the required time at the appropriate temperature, after which the controls are read first and then the actual tests. Smears are made as described above. Results are entered as they are obtained although it is permissible to memorise consecutive identical results.

If this basic procedure is followed, each reagent or unknown serum or red cell suspension is handled only once in the whole manipulation, thereby reducing to a minimum the time taken and the risk of errors.

Appendix II Reagents

Technique No. AII.1. Preparation of isotonic saline

A 0.85 per cent solution of sodium chloride in distilled water is isotonic, *i.e.* of the same osmotic pressure as the contents of the human red cell, *e.g.* 8.5 g dissolved in 1 litre of distilled water will probably be a convenient quantity. Saline should be freshly made but need not be sterilised. Alternatively, commercially produced tablets of NaCl of various weights are available.

Technique No. AII.2. Preparation of isotonic trisodium citrate

The isotonic solution of trisodium citrate is 3.8 per cent (*i.e.* 38 g in 1 litre of distilled water).

Technique No. AII.3. Preparation of AB serum

This is obtained from group AB donors and must be completely free from all antibodies. Tests are, therefore, carried out at 37°C, R.T. and 4°C by saline, albumin, papain and indirect anti-human globulin techniques against A_1, A_2, B, and O cells. Not infrequently an identifiable atypical antibody, *e.g.* anti-A_1, is discovered which can then be removed by suitable absorption. The indirect anti-human globulin test at 4°C will detect the "cold incomplete" antibodies which are practically always present, and which can be removed by absorption with an equal volume of pooled group O red cells overnight at 4°C. However if the AB serum is to be used in an enzyme technique it should be absorbed for 1 hour with a fifth of its volume of papain-treated group O cells.

Bovine serum albumin (BSA)

Bovine albumin is supplied by various manufacturers, (*e.g.* Armour Laboratories, Ortho Diagnostics, Biotest Folex) as a 30 per cent solution specially prepared for blood grouping. It usually contains sodium azide as a preservative and should not be frozen but stored at 4°C. For most purposes it is advisable to reduce it to 20 per cent by the addition of one part of AB serum (or normal saline) to two parts of the 30 per cent albumin. This minimises any tendency to cause rouleaux although for the detection of weak atypical antibodies, particularly Rh, reactions are often somewhat stronger if the albumin is used at the 30 per cent concentration at which it is supplied.

462

When changing from one batch of albumin to another in the laboratory it is essential to standardise the new batch by using it in parallel with the former batch, for the titration of several IgG anti-D sera.

The efficiency of bovine albumin as a medium for the activation of incomplete Rh antibodies has been found to be related to the polymer content of the albumin (Jones *et al.*, 1969; Goldsmith *et al.*, 1971; Goldsmith, 1974 see also report by working party 1976). It would seem that those batches of bovine serum albumin which react optimally in agglutinating red cells sensitised with Rh antibodies contain 85 per cent of the albumin in the monomer form with the remainder in dimer or polymer forms. Excess of polymerised material leads to false positive agglutination of unsensitised cells.

There is the occasional problem of an albumin autoagglutinating factor, an antibody found in the serum of some normal individuals which agglutinates unsensitised cells in the presence of most but not all batches of bovine albumin. This has been found to be due to caprylate which is added to bovine albumin in the course of its preparation to ensure that over-polymerisation does not occur. It is thought that the so called "autoagglutination" is due to a non-specific adsorption of an antigen-antibody complex on to red cells. The antibody is a gammaglobulin directed at albumin which has been altered by the caprylate (Golde *et al.*, 1969).

More recently the presence of an agglutination inhibitor in 3 out of 28 commercial preparations of bovine albumin has been found (Gunson and Phillips, 1975). The phenomenon was first noted when a batch of BSA used for the first time, caused a reduction in sensitivity of a standard assay technique on the AutoAnalyser. The inhibiting effect was also apparent using manual methods. The inhibition was not related to the degree of polymerisation of the albumin and in spite of intensive investigation the reason for this inhibiting effect has not yet become clear.

This phenomenon offers yet another reason for the careful standardisation of batches of BSA before they are put into circulation for routine use.

The possibility of bacterial contamination has to be considered. It is perhaps not always appreciated that although BSA is sterile when it leaves the hands of the producers, it is not necessarily maintained in a sterile condition throughout the course of its production and it may therefore contain bacterial metabolites which could have adverse effects upon agglutination tests.

Technique No. AII.4. Preparation of bromelin solution

The exact concentration of the bromelin solution is less critical than for trypsin or papain. A satisfactory bromelin solution can be prepared by making a 0.5 per cent solution by weight (in normal saline) of bromelin.

The solution will store satisfactorily for a week at 4° C, but is best used on the day of preparation. For convenience, therefore, it is as well to weigh out aliquots of 0.05 g of bromelin into a number of screw-capped bottles to one of which 1 ml of saline can be added each day.

Technique No. AII.5. Preparation of trypsin solution

A trypsin solution can be prepared by dissolving 0.1 g of crystalline trypsin in 10 ml. of 0.05M HCl. (Armour Laboratories manufacture a suitable trypsin preparation). If kept at 4°C this stock solution will remain active for some months. As required, it is diluted with 0.1 M phosphate buffer, 1 in 10 v/v. This buffer, of pH 7.7, is prepared by mixing one part of 0.1M KH_2PO_4 (13.6 g/l) with nine parts of 0.1M Na_2HPO_4 (14.2g/l). Eight grams of sodium chloride are added to each litre.

The buffered trypsin solution prepared by either method is then used for preparation of enzyme treated red cells as described in technique No. 8.4.

Technique No. AII.6. Löw's technique for the preparation of papain solution

Reagents. Purified, powdered papain (Merck, Savory & Moore, B.D.H., and Evans all supply suitable products).

0.1M phosphate buffer (Sörensen) pH 5.4
1M cysteine hydrochloride
1M sodium hydroxide

The phosphate buffer consists of a mixture of $M/15$ solutions of Na_2HPO_4 and KH_2PO_4. According to Sörensen's table they should be mixed in the proportions of 0.4 ml of the sodium salt to 9.6 ml of the potassium salt. For each batch of reagent the pH should be checked and any small adjustment of the proportions made to give the required pH. Eight grams of sodium chloride are added to each litre of buffer.

Two grams of powdered papain are ground in a mortar with buffered saline (pH 5.4) and the suspension made up to 100 ml and filtered. It is important that the solution should be clear; this is probably best effected by using a Seitz filter with a clarifying pad, alternatively filtration through fine grade filter paper using celite analytical filter-aid (John-Manville) is very satisfactory. Five ml of the molar solution of cysteine hydrochloride are neutralised with 5 ml of the molar solution of sodium hydroxide. That the solutions have (as they should) exactly neutralised each other can be checked with a pH meter or with litmus paper; if not neutral the proportions are slightly adjusted until neutralisation is achieved. Ten ml of the neutralised solution are added to the 100 ml of filtered papain solution, the whole made up to 200 ml with buffered saline and incubated at 37°C for 1 hour. The solution is stored frozen solid at −20°C in convenient quantities.

$M/15$ solution of $Na_2HPO_4.2H_2O$ contains 11.93 g per litre.
$M/15$ solution of KH_2PO_4 contains 9.07 g per litre.
M solution of cysteine hydrochloride contains 157 g per litre.
M solution of sodium hydroxide contains 40 g per litre.

Technique No. AII.7. Preparation of ficin

Crude ficin is weighed out in 250 mg amounts. The powder is stable indefinitely so it can be kept dry until needed. It must be handled with care and always weighed into stoppered containers as in sensitive individuals it is capable of causing sloughing of the mucous membranes. It is therefore recommended that mask and goggles are worn when handling the powder.

When needed, each 250 mg is dissolved in 25 ml of Hendry's buffer (pH 7.4). This is the stock solution. The buffer is designed to be isotonic with human red cells and is prepared by adding 19 ml of a solution containing 2.34 g $NaH_2PO_42H_2O$ per 100 ml to 81 ml of a solution containing 1.63 g Na_2HPO_4 per 100 ml.

ANTI-COAGULANT SOLUTIONS FOR THE PRESERVATION OF STORED BLOOD

There are two important functions of the solution into which blood is taken for storage, first it must be an efficient anti-coagulant and secondly red cells stored in it for three to four weeks must survive well in the recipient's circulation.

The present solution, ACD, combines reasonably good storage with a good degree of anti-coagulant activity and a low caramelisation.

Technique No. AII.8. Preparation of ACD (acid-citrate-dextrose)

Each MRC bottle for the collection of 430 ml of blood contains 120 ml of ACD containing 2 g of disodium citrate and 3 g of dextrose. A convenient quantity of this solution can be prepared by adding 800 ml of a 15 per cent solution of anhydrous dextrose to 4 litres of a 2 per cent solution of disodium citrate $(Na_2H(C_6H_5O_7). H_2O$; molecular weight 254).

The solution is filtered through filter paper—Whatman No. 1—and then through a medium grade (3 or 4) cintered glass filter. It is then put into the bottles, using a simple mechanical apparatus to deliver exactly 120 ml into each bottle; the cap is loosely screwed on and the bottle is ready for the autoclave. Since plastic bags are now in common use it is more usual to take about 450 ml of blood into a plastic bag containing 60-75 ml of the following citrate solution:-

Trisodium citrate (dihydrate)	2.2 g
Citric acid (monohydrate)	0.8 g
Dextrose	2.5 g
water	to 100 ml.

Storage of standard cells

Careful selection of standard cells is of utmost importance. They must be chosen with a view to their sensitivity, specificity and availability.

Fresh standard cells are usually to be preferred to stored cells and are used wherever suitable donors are readily available. Red cells are taken from an ear or finger prick into 3.8 per cent trisodium citrate. The tube is inverted frequently to prevent the blood from clotting. The cells are washed and can then be used for making saline or albumin suspensions or for enzyme treatment.

Q

Alternatively plastic containers designed for up to 2 ml of blood and containing either sequestrine or sodium (or lithium) heparin are very convenient for the collection of small samples. Moreover, the quantity of blood collected in these containers is not critical; any amount up to 2 ml is permissable. Such samples, if stored at 4°C are fresh enough for most purposes up to one week from bleeding.

Red cells stored under their own unadulterated serum in a sterile clotted sample will keep in good condition for even longer than a week but may of course become sensitised by cold incomplete auto antibodies.

Another good storage medium is Alsever's solution.

The composition of this is as follows:-

Trisodium citrate (dihydrate)	8.0 g
Dextrose	19.0 g
Sodium chloride	4.2 g
Citric acid (monohydrate)	0.5 g

One volume of this solution is added to one volume of blood.

Storage solutions which enable cells to be stored at 4°C for 4-5 weeks are also useful. Such a preservation fluid used in our own laboratory is essentially that described by Burgess and Vos (1971) and is given below (technique AII.10).

Even in the preservative solutions just described red cells have only a limited life. If it is desired to keep them for several months or even years they can be frozen in glycerol at −20°C or in liquid nitrogen.

Technique No. AII.9. Fluid for preserving cells for 4-5 weeks at 4°C

Glucose	10.00 g
Trisodium citrate ($Na_3C_6H_5O_7 2H_2O$)	5.88 g
Di-sodium phosphate ($Na_2HPO_4.2H_2O$)	3.56 g
Citric acid ($H_3C_6H_5O_7H_2O$)	0.55 g
Adenine	0.08 g
Inosine	0.35 g
Calcium chloride ($CaCl_2.6H_2O$)	0.06 g
Chloramphenicol	0.33 g
Neomycin sulphate	0.1 g
30 per cent lipid free bovine albumin	13 ml

The mixture is made up to 1 litre with distilled water and the pH adjusted to 7.3 using 1N NaOH.

Cells for preservation are packed by centrifugation and then washed twice in the preservation fluid. Immediately after washing a 5 per cent cell suspension is prepared in the fluid. Universal containers or bijoux are used for storage but they are only half filled with cell suspension to allow air space in the container above the cells. Storage is then at 4°C and the cells do not need to be washed before use.

Technique No. AII.10. Storage of standard red cells in glycerol

The concentration of glycerol in the red cell-glycerol mixture should be about

30 per cent w/v for efficient storage. This is achieved by adding an equal quantity of 40 per cent v/v glycerol in buffered tripotassium citrate to packed cells. The packed cells are obtained from blood which has been taken into ACD, centrifuged and the supernatant plasma removed; they are thus suspended in a minimal quantity of their own plasma plus ACD. Red cells stored in this way can be recovered into saline.

(a) Preparation of the Standard Solutions

Buffered Tripotassium Citrate. This is a mixture of tripotassium citrate and phosphate buffer. It contains 3.25 per cent tripotassium citrate $(K_3C_6H_5O_7.H_2O)$, 0.47 per cent potassium dihydrogen phosphate (KH_2PO_4) and 0.6 per cent dipotassium hydrogen phosphate (K_2HPO_4). In practice it is probably convenient to make up a litre of this stock solution which would, therefore, contain 32.5 g citrate, 4.7 g potassium dihydrogen phosphate and 6 g of dipotassium hydrogen phosphate.

The "Laying-down" Solution. This is a 50 per cent w/v (approx.) or 40 per cent v/v which will give about a 30 per cent concentration of glycerol when mixed with an equal quantity of packed cells. 40 ml of glycerol well mixed with 60 ml of the buffered citrate is probably a convenient quantity.

The Recovery Solutions. These are 16, 8, 4, and 2 per cent w/v glycerol to buffered citrate.

Owing to the high viscosity of the glycerol it will be found best to make up the 16 per cent solution and then prepare the others by doubling dilution. 200 ml of the 16 per cent can be prepared by adding 25.6 ml of glycerol to 174.4 ml of buffered tripotassium citrate. Care must be taken to ensure that the buffered citrate and glycerol are well mixed.

(b) "Laying-down" Process.

Ideally the blood to be stored is taken into ACD in the usual proportions (*i.e.* four parts of blood to one part of ACD) but blood from other sources can be used. The sample is centrifuged and the supernatant removed. An equal quantity of the 40 per cent v/v laying-down solution is added gradually to the packed cells mixing well so that none of the cells are subjected to excessive concentration of glycerol. The mixture is then frozen at −20°C. If small quantities of the cells will be needed on several occasions the mixture can be divided into 1 ml. quantities before being frozen.

(c) Recovery.

To recover the red cells the mixture is allowed to thaw at room temperature, as much as is needed removed and the rest re-frozen. The sample is centrifuged, the supernatant fluid removed and the cells washed with each of the recovery solutions in turn (beginning with the 16 per cent and ending with the 2 per cent) followed by buffered tripotassium citrate and then twice with saline.

Alternatively a convenient method for the recovery of small quantities of red cells is to place them in a length of dialysis tubing, and dialyse against either saline or the buffered tripotassium citrate for 1 hour. The cells are then washed three times in saline. They can then be used in exactly the same ways as freshly bled cells.

A continuous flow system using buffered saline to remove glycerol which is dialysed out through Visking tubing is described by Moghaddam (1976).

Technique No. AII.11. Storage of red cells in liquid nitrogen

The blood to be stored is taken into either EDTA ll mg/ml)or into ACD in the normal proportions.

The blood should be frozen as quickly as possible and should not be more than two days' old if antigens are to store well. Immediately before storage in liquid nitrogen, the blood is mixed with half its volume of 40 per cent sucrose. The sucrose is added gradually with mixing.

A siliconed 50 ml syringe is fitted with 2-in plastic tubing and a needle from a transfusion "taking" set. It is then suspended over a 2 litre beaker which is lined with cotton-wool on sides and bottom. The beaker is filled with liquid nitrogen and the syringe fitted with the blood prepared as described above. The drop from the needle is controlled by a clip so that the blood forms discrete drops on entering the nitrogen which do not coalesce (a rate of 1-2 ml per minute approximately).

The method can be modified for small or large quantities of blood, *e.g.* for large quantities a fenwal pack is convenient; its tubing fits into the socket of an Iver needle or over an olive mount needle.

Care should be taken to inspect the level of nitrogen in the beaker and the blood may require mixing a little to prevent sedimentation of cells.

The pellets of frozen blood are transferred with a cooled spoon to small containers (pill boxes may be useful) filled with liquid nitrogen before putting down in the liquid nitrogen container.

For recovery the pellets are removed and placed in 1 per cent NaCl at 45°C. They quickly melt and thereafter the blood is washed in isotonic saline until the supernatant fluid shows no haemolysis.

Another method for storing cells for blood grouping tests and one which produces the minimum of haemolysis on recovery is as follows:-

Glycerolised cells are prepared as described above and are then aspirated into special PVC straws 135 mm in length and 4 mm in diameter holding 1.5 ml cells. The secret of successful storage, with little haemolysis on recovery, is to cool them slowly, ideally by placing in a Union Carbide 3-2- biological freezer or if this freezer is not available the cooling rate can be slowed own by placing the straws on styrofoam floating on liquid nitrogen.

Thawing is achieved by shaking the straws manually in a water bath at 37°C; the glycerol is removed by dialysis as described above.

Choice of Standard Red Cells

Sensitivity of red cells will vary with different antigen content. It is best to use the most sensitive cells when testing unknown sera for antibodies and to use weakly reacting cells for the positive controls on standard sera.

ABO.

For ABO testing the required standard cells are A_1, A_2, B and O. The A_1 and

A_2 cells must have been tested with at least two and preferably three anti-A_1 sera, and results must be clear cut, negative for A_2 and positive for A_1. Having selected cells on the basis of their reactions with anti-A_1 sera, their strength is found by titration with a known anti-A serum in parallel with known A_1 and A_2 cells. This may show that the A which was negative with anti-A_1 is really an A_3 or weaker subgroup of A and not A_2 and is, therefore, not suitable for use. The sensitivity of B cells can be found in the same way by titration with anti-B serum, but this is not normally done since the variation is slight. It is not usually considered necessary to test the sensitivity of the group O cells. Both in selecting test cells and in interpreting results it must be remembered that any red cell has many blood group antigens, and anomalous results may arise because the serum contains an antibody belonging to another blood group system. Atypical Rh antibodies are among the most likely to be encountered and it is as well to select ABO standard red cells that are Rh negative; this is especially important when samples from pregnant women are being tested.

Rh.

For Rh antibody screening a panel of four group O cells are required R_1R_1, $R_2(R_2R_2$ or $R_2r)$, R_1R_2, and rr. These must all be established by sub-typing with at least two anti-C, anti-D, anti-E and anti-c sera, and, as in ABO testing, results must be unequivocal.

For positive controls on anti-Rh sera, cells which have only a single dose of antigen should be used. These controls have been discussed in some detail in the Rh chapters especially with regard to using sera containing more than one specific antibody.

Other Blood Group Systems.

Cells for other blood group systems must be chosen on the same principles and with as much care. The method used to select the cells must be the same as that by which they are to be used.

In all cases it is essential to confirm the specificity of standard cells with more than one anti-serum. It is preferable to have the full typing for all known blood group systems of any standard cells used. For antibody detection a strong positive is needed.

The positive control for a typing serum as far as possible should be equivalent to the weakest positive expected to occur in the tests.

SPECIFIC ANTI-SERA

These are dealt with in some detail in Chapters 3 and 13 for ABO and Rh and in the appropriate chapters for the other blood group systems.

Technique No. AII.12. Preparation of anti-human globulin serum (Coombs reagent)

The rabbit is the animal most commonly used for the production of anti-human globulin sera, although it is possible to immunise other species e.g. goats.

Not all strains of rabbit are equally good antibody producers. Hybrid species or brown rabbits if obtainable are often the most suitable.

Human group O serum pooled from several donors is used as a source of antigen. Groups A, B or AB, should be avoided, as it is undesirable to risk stimulating the animals to produce unwanted anti-A or anti-B antibodies. For a broad spectrum anti-globulin reagent* the gamma globulins are precipitated with a saturated solution of ammonium sulphate. A proportion of two parts serum to one of ammonium sulphate should be satisfactory. The resulting precipitate is carefully washed twice in 40 per cent ammonium sulphate, dissolved in a small quantity of Na_2HPO_4 and dialysed at $4°C$ against normal saline.

The separated globulin then has to be mixed with Freund's adjuvant. The material required can be obtained from Difco (Agents Baird and Tatlock) in complete and incomplete (without Mycobacteria) forms.

It may also be made up as follows:

Bayol F (Esso Ltd.)	17 parts
Arlacel A (Honeywill and Stein Ltd.)	3 parts
Dried Microbacterium butyricum (Difco)	0.5 to 1.0 mg per ml

Equal volumes of adjuvant and 1 g/100 ml antigen solution are emulsified together. This process is greatly facilitated by using a homogeniser, as the final product should be of the consistency of stiff toothpaste and should be completely emulsified. A drop placed in water should not spread. There is great variation possible in the schedule of injections, and they should be subjected to trial and error.

The first injection is usually 1-2 ml emulsion intramuscularly into each leg (4 injections). After two weeks or later, a second similar injection into each shoulder. About one week after this there can be a short intravenous course of 1 ml of 1 per cent aqueous solution of antigen without adjuvant. These injections can be given every two days for about ten days. The animals must be carefully watched for signs of anaphylaxis as indicated by respiratory distress. If this occurs the injections must be stopped. Small test bleeds are made before a larger quantity, 60-80 ml by ear, is taken. After 2-6 months' rest a further intravenous course without adjuvent may be tried.

Absorption of Unwanted Antibodies

The serum is freed of antibodies for human red cell antigens by absorbing with group O and group AB red cells. It is first heated at $56°C$ for 30 minutes to prevent possible haemolysis of the red cells used for absorption. The cells used for the absorption must be very carefully washed in a large excess of saline, approximately one part of cells to ten parts of saline. At least six washings are necessary to free the cells completely of serum globulin. The supernatant saline from the last wash of the cells should be tested with sulphosalacylic acid to ensure it is protein free. The absorptions are carried out at $4°C$ using equal parts of

---

*There are several methods for the preparation of more specific antisera. See Mollison (1972), Stratton & Rawlinson (1976) and Freedman & Mollison (1976).

serum and cells and allowing the mixture to stand for 2 hours. A second or even a third absorption may be needed.

Technique No. AII.13. Standardisation of anti-human globulin (Coombs reagent)

The absorbed reagent is tested for residual "anti-Man" agglutinins. This is done by making serial dilutions of the serum and testing them with washed group A, B and also group O cells by the actual technique by which the standardised reagent will be ultimately used.

Once the rabbit serum has been successfully absorbed it is then titrated for its ability to react with sensitised red cells. Rabbits differ in the type of anti-human globulin that they produce, nearly all of them produce antibodies against the IgG, IgM and complement components of the globulin but the proportion of each of the antibodies will vary from serum to serum and often from immunisation to immunisation of the same rabbit. The routine laboratory will in the main require a broad spectrum reagent which will detect both IgG and complement binding antibodies at one dilution so it should contain anti-C3c (β_1A) to detect complement bound *in vitro* where incubation time is short and anti-C3d (α_2D) to detect complement where incubation has been prolonged and, more important, to detect the coat on red cells from cold auto-immune acquired haemolytic anaemia.

It is not always possible to produce a reagent fulfilling all these criteria in one animal, so it may be necessary to pool antibodies from different animals but of the same species. This pooling is done after the serum has been absorbed for heteroagglutinins. In order to ensure that the pool may be satisfactory, it is a good precaution to prepare an initial trial pool containing small quantities of the sera before the final large-scale product is prepared. An average dilution would be 1 in 40 for a broad spectrum reagent although a pure anti-complement may only need diluting 1 in 10 and a pure anti-IgG may possibly require a much higher dilution.

Tests for potency of anti-IgG

The potency of anti-IgG in a reagent is usually determined by a checker-board titration with group O (D+) cells sensitised with a high titre incomplete anti-D and group O (D+) cells sensitised with a weak incomplete anti-D. The weak anti-D must not be a high titre anti-D diluted but a "weak response" antibody.

Both anti-D's are diluted by doubling dilutions in saline from 1 to 16. Suitable volumes of D-positive cells are incubated with each of these dilutions of antibody. Meanwhile, serial dilutions of the anti-globulin serum from 10 to 5120 are prepared in saline. Using the technique by which the anti-globulin reagent is to be used, each dilution of the anti-globulin reagent is tested against the Rh-positive cells sensitised with the various concentrations of anti-D. These results will indicate the optimal dilution of the reagent particularly for the weak response antibodies.

Alternatively a procedure using group O Rh positive cells (1) strongly, (2) moderately, (3) weakly sensitised with Rh antibodies as shown in Table AII.1 can

Table AII.1 The standardisation of an anti-human globulin rabbit serum

Type of serum		Dilutions of anti-human globulin serum										
	Neat	1/10	1/20	1/40	1/60	1/80	1/100	1/200	1/300	1/400	1/500	Time (min)
(1) O D positive cells strongly sensitised	±	2+	2+	4+	5+	5+	5+	5+	4+	4+	3+	2-5
(2) O D positive cells moderately sensitised	3+	4+	4+	5+	5+	5+	5+	4+	3+	3+	2+	2-5
(3) O D positive cells weakly sensitised	3+	4+	4+	4+	4+	4+	4+	3+	2+	–	–	2-5
(4) O D positive cells unsensitised	+	±	–	–	–	–	–	–	–	–	–	15
(5) O D negative cells	+	+	–	–	–	–	–	–	–	–	–	15
(6) A_1B D negative cells	3+	+	–	–	–	–	–	–	–	–	–	15
(7) O cells sensitised with complement	5+	5+	5+	4+	4+	2+	–	–	–	–	–	5

Table AII.2 Serum preparation chart

		Dilutions of anti-human globulin serum									
	Neat*	1/10	1/20	1/40	1/60	1/80	1/100	1/200	1/300	1/400	1/500
ml of serum		0.2									
" " 1/10			0.5	0.25	0.15	0.1	0.2				
" " 1/100								0.5	0.3	0.25	0.2
Saline		1.8	0.5	0.75	0.75	0.7	1.8	0.5	0.6	0.75	0.8
Total (ml)		2.0	1.0	1.00	0.90	0.8	2.0	1.0	0.9	1.00	1.0

*Often omitted as rather wasteful of the reagent.

be adopted. An additional row of cells coated with complement (for preparation *see* Chapter 27) is also included. Table AII.2 is a chart for the preparation of suitable dilutions of a serum.

Specimen results are shown in Table AII.1. (Note the prozone with the strongly sensitised Rh positive cells). On the basis of these results the serum could be used at 1/60, at which dilution it will detect both complement and IgG and 1/200 for detecting IgG only. At this last dilution it would be very useful for testing cells for the presence of D^u with incomplete anti-D as it will not detect any sensitisation with "cold" antibody—in particular the incomplete "cold" auto-antibody which would otherwise give a false positive reaction.

Tests for potency of anti-complement components can be made using cells coated as described in Chapter 27.

Finally, if the anti-globulin is found satisfactory it should be possible to recommend it at one dilution *e.g.* 1 in 40 for the detection of complement components and at a higher dilution *e.g.* 1 in 100 or even 1 in 200 for the detection of IgG.

Once the optimal dilution of the anti-globulin reagent has been determined it should be tested at that dilution against a panel of cells of various phenotypes sensitised with a wide range of "incomplete" blood group antibodies including "weak response" and complement binding antibodies.

REFERENCES

Burgess, B.J. & Vos, G.H. (1971) The preservation of laboratory panel cells. *Vox Sang.,* **21,** 109.
Freedman, J. & Mollison, P.L. (1976) Preparation of red cells coated with C4 and C3 subcomponents and production of anti-C4d and anti-C3d. *Vox. Sang.,* **31,** 241.
Golde, D.W., McGinnis, M.H. & Holland, P.V. (1969) Mechanism of the albumin agglutination phenomenon. *Vox Sang.,* **16,** 465.
Goldsmith, K.L.G., Jones, J.M. & Kekwick, R.A. (1971) The effects of polymers on the efficiency of bovine serum albumin used as a diluent in the detection of incomplete Rh antibodies. *Proc 12th Congr. Int. Soc. Blood Transf.* Moscow (1969) *Bibl. haemat.* No. 38 part 1, p.138. Basel: Karger.
Goldsmith, K.L.G. (1974) The effect of bovine serum albumin on red cell agglutination. In *Enhancement of Serological Reactions.* Proceedings of Symposium published by Biotest Folex Ltd.
Gunson, H.H. & Phillips, P.K. (1975) An inhibitor to erythrocyte agglutination in bovine albumin preparation. *Vox Sang.,* **28,** 207.
Jones, J.M., Kekwick, R.A. & Goldsmith, K.L.G. (1969) Influence of polymers on the efficacy of serum albumin as a potentiator of "incomplete" Rh agglutinins. *Nature,* **224,** 510.
Moghaddam, M. (1976) An improved method for the reconstitution of frozen red blood cells. *Vox Sang.,* **30,** 317.
Mollison, P.L. (1972) *Blood Transfusion in Clinical Medicine.* 5th edition. P.409 *et seq.* Blackwell.
Stratton, F. & Rawlinson V.I. (1976) Observations on the antiglobulin tests. C4 components on erythrocytes *Vox. Sang.,* **31,** 44.
A study performed on batches of serum albumin used as diluents in Rh testing (1976).
A report to the International Society of Blood Transfusion/International Committee for Standardisation in Haematology by their albumin working party. *Brit. J. Haemat,* **32,** 215.

Appendix III—Glossary

Absorption. Removal of antibodies from a serum by adsorption on to red cells. Hence, absorbed serum—a serum from which antibodies have been so removed.

Acquired antigen. Antigen not genetically determined and sometimes transient.

Adsorption. The attachment of one substance to the surface of another, in particular the attachment of antibody to specific determinants on the red cell surface.

Agglutinates. Clumps of agglutinated cells.

Agglutination. The clumping of red cells by antibodies.

Agglutinin. An antibody which causes agglutination of red cells in a saline medium by virtue of reacting with the specific antigen.

Auto-agglutinin. An agglutinin which reacts with the red cells of the individual in whose serum it is found; it usually agglutinates the red cells of most other individuals also.

Atypical agglutinin. One which is occasionally present in the serum of some individuals whose red cells lack the corresponding antigen.

Cold agglutinin. An agglutinin whose optimum temperature of reactivity is in the cold, whose potency decreases rapidly with increase of temperature, and whose reaction at 37°C is negative (except in rare circumstances).

Hetero-agglutinin. An agglutinin directed against antigens found in another species, cf. allo-agglutinin.

Iso-agglutinin. (now called allo-agglutinin) An agglutinin directed against antigens found in the same species, cf. hetero-agglutinin.

Normal or typical agglutinin. An agglutinin which is regularly present in the serum of all individuals whose cells lack the corresponding antigen.

Pan-agglutinin. An agglutinin which agglutinates the red cells of all individuals, irrespective of blood group.

Agglutinogen. Old-fashioned term for red-cell antigen.

Albumin. *See* Bovine Albumin.

Allele, allelomorph, or allelic gene. One of two or more genes which determine alternative characters which are located at the same locus on homologous chromosomes.

Allotypes. Genetically determined polymorphic variants. The term was first introduced to describe the different antigenic forms of rabbit gamma globulins. It was then extended to include polymorphic variants of plasma proteins in general (*e.g.* haptoglobins, Gc groups) but now includes red cell and white cell polymorphisms.

Amino acid. Any one of a class of organic compounds containing the amino (NH_2) group and the carboxyl ($COOH$) group. Amino acids form the chief structure of proteins.

Amorph. A gene which apparently has no end product *e.g.* a specific antigenic determinant. Sometimes called a 'silent' gene.

Anaemia. A condition in which the blood is deficient either in quantity or in quality.

Anamnestic response. The redevelopment of antibodies on the introduction of an antigen different in specificity from the one which provided the initial stimulus.

Antibody. An antibody is a substance which appears in the plasma or body fluids as a result of stimulation by an antigen and which will react specifically with that antigen in some observable way.

Anticoagulant. A substance which prevents coagulation or clotting of the blood.

Antigen. Any substance which, when introduced parenterally into an individual who himself lacks the substance, stimulates the production of an antibody, and which when mixed with the antibody, reacts with it in some observable way.

Antigenic determinant. The particular site on an antigen molecule which combines with the corresponding antibody.

Antigenicity. Potency as an antigen.

Anti-human globulin. (Coombs reagent.) An antibody produced in an animal (often a rabbit) in response to the injection of human globulin.

Atypical antibody. An antibody which occurs as an irregular feature of the serum, *e.g.* anti-D.

Australia (Au) antigen. Synonyms, Hepatitis-associated antigen or HAA Hepatitis B antigen (HBA), Hepatitis B surface antigen (HB$_s$ Ag). See chapter 31.

Auto-antibody. An antibody which reacts with the red cells of the individual in whose serum it is found; usually reacts upon the red cells of most other individuals also. *See* Auto-agglutinin.

Autosome. Any chromosome other than a sex chromosome.

Avidity of an antiserum. A measure of the ability and speed with which the antiserum agglutinates red cells. Is a property of the combining constant (K).

Bilirubin. A red pigment found in the bile and present in the serum.

Blocking. The coating of a red cell determinant by an incomplete antibody in such a way as to render it partially or completely inagglutinable by agglutinins of the same specificity—hence, blocking antibody.

Blood group substance. *See* Group specific substance.

Buffer. Any substance or substances in solution which resist changes in pH.

Chimera. An organism whose cells derive from two or more distinct zygote lineages *e.g.* the vascular anastomoses which may occur between twins (a twin of genetic type O may have a bone marrow implantation from his twin of group A. Throughout life therefore he has a major red cell population of group O and a minor population of red cells of group A).

Chromosome. One of a number of more or less rod-shaped, dark staining bodies situated in the nucleus of a cell. It is only distinguishable at the time of cell division. It is made up of a series of genes in linear arrangement.

Cis position. Being on the same chromosome and within the same cistron.

Cistron. A collection of genes situated so close together that they can have conjoint expression effects when in the cis position.

Clone. A group of cells which are homogeneous because they are descendants of a common precursor cell.

Closely-linked genes. Genes in close proximity on a chromosome so that they are inherited together, usually without cross-overs occurring.

Co-dominant genes. Two or more allelic genes, each capable of expressing itself in single dose.

Cold agglutinin. *See* Agglutinin.

Compatible blood. Blood, the red cells of which are not sensitised or agglutinated by the recipient's serum.

Complement. A complex of substances present in normal serum which cause lysis of red cells sensitised by haemolysins. Heating the serum at 56°C for ½ hour destroys the thermolabile components which are necessary for haemolysis.

Complete antibody. Agglutinin.

Conglutination. The clumping of sensitised red cells by a substance conglutinin, present in normal bovine sera, in the presence of complement. It is sometimes erroneously applied to the clumping effect of human serum or bovine albumin on cells sensitised by incomplete Rh antibodies, which is independent of complement.

Crossing-over. The process by which genetic material is exchanged between homologous chromosomes. It can occur at mitosis or meiosis.

Cryo-globulin. Globulin which precipitates from serum at 0-4°C.

Deletion. Loss of genetic material from a chromosome.

Dominant gene. One which gives rise to its corresponding character, whether present in "double dose" (in the homozygote) or in "single dose" (in the heterozygote).

Dosage. A quantitative difference in the strength of the antigen between the homozygote and the heterozygote.

Electrophoresis (of serum). The separation of serum proteins according to their rate of travel when an electric current is passed through a buffer solution. The supporting medium can be a Whatman paper, or starch or agar gels.

Eluate. In serology, denotes an antibody solution made by recovery into a fluid medium of antibodies that have been taken up by red cells. Saline is usually the fluid selected and the recovery of antibodies from the red cells is effected by, for example, raising the temperature of the sensitised cells to 56°C.

Elution. The process of making an eluate.

Enzyme. *See* Proteolytic enzyme.

Equilibrium or **combining constant (K).** The measure of the goodness of fit of the antibody to the corresponding antigen. When the equilibrium constant is high the bond between antigen and antibody is less readily broken. An antibody with a high equilibrium constant is more avid than one with a low K (*see also* avidity).

Erythrocyte. Red cell.

Experimental error. The maximum variation in results obtained by any technique in the hands of an expert.

Fertilisation. The fusion of the male and female sex cells to form the zygote.

Gamete. A sex cell.

Gene. One of a number of portions of chromosomal DNA in linear arrangement along a chromosome and coding for the synthesis of a single inherited character.

Genotype. A group of individuals having the same genetic make-up with regard to particular alleles, *e.g.* AO.

Globulin. A class of proteins to which antibodies belong. They can be separated by electrophoresis into α, ß and γ fractions (*see also* Immunoglobulins).

Group specific substance. A term applied to an antigen or hapten which possesses blood group specificity.

Haemoglobin. The oxygen-carrying red pigment of the red blood cells.

Haemolysin. An antibody which causes haemolysis of red cells, in the presence of complement.

Haemolysis. The breaking-down of the red cell envelope with the liberation of haemoglobin.

Haemolytic. Causing haemolysis.

Haemolytic anaemia. Anaemia caused by excessive destruction of red cells.

Haemolytic disease of the newborn. The modern name for erythroblastosis foetalis. A disease of the foetus or newborn which is caused by a maternal antibody attacking the foetal red cells.

Haemolytic transfusion reaction. A reaction due to an increased rate of destruction of red cells *in vivo* following transfusion.

Haploid. Having half the number of chromosomes present in the body (somatic) cells. Is the characteristic state of gametes.

Hapten. A substance which will combine specifically with the corresponding antibody but will not stimulate the formation of antibodies *in vivo*. Haptens are often polysaccharides, *e.g.* group specific substances A and B as isolated from saliva and pseudomucinous ovarian cysts.

Heparin. An anti-coagulant.

Hetero-agglutinin. *See* Agglutinin.

Heterospecific pregnancy. A pregnancy in which the maternal serum contains an anti-A or anti-B antibody incompatible with the foetal red cells, *e.g.* O mother, A foetus.

Heterozygous. Having unlike alleles on the corresponding loci of a pair of chromosomes.

Homologous chromosome. One of a pair of identical chromosomes.

Homologous blood. Blood of the same group. Is usually restricted to mean of the same ABO group.

Homozygous. Having like alleles on the corresponding loci of a pair of chromosomes.

Hydrops foetalis. One form of haemolytic disease of the foetus (or newborn) in which the foetal tissues retain abnormal quantities of fluid.

Hyper immunisation. Immunisation to an unusually high degree—hence hyper immunity, hyper immune antibody, etc.

Hypertonic solution. A solution of greater osmotic pressure than blood.

Hypotonic solution. A solution of less osmotic pressure than blood.

Icterus. Jaundice.

Icterus gravis neonatorum. Severe jaundice of the newborn—one of the manifestations of haemolytic disease of the newborn.

Immunisation. The process by which antibodies are produced in response to antigenic stimulus—hence immune antibody and immune response.

Immuno-electrophoresis. The identification of proteins separated by agar gel electrophoresis by means of lines of precipitation formed against specific antisera diffusing through the agar.

Immunoglobulin (Ig). Antibody containing globulins but also includes those proteins without apparent antibody activity which have the same antigenic specificity and are produced by similar cells.

The following classes of immunoglobulins are recognised:

IgG   (γG)Contains most incomplete antibodies and some agglutinins. Can be divided into subclasses IgG1-4.

IgA   (γA)Blood group antibodies in saliva and milk are characteristically of this type.

IgM   (γM)These are macro-globulins, this group contains most agglutinins and a few incomplete usually 'enzyme type' antibodies.

IgD   (γD)Is not usually antibody active but some anti-nuclear antibodies are IgD.

IgE   (γE)Contains antibodies to allergens.

Inactivation of serum. The heating of serum at 56°C for 30 minutes to destroy the heat labile fractions of complement.

Incomplete antibody. Any antibody which sensitises red cells suspended in saline but fails to agglutinate them.

Inhibition. The prevention of the normal reaction between an antigen and its corresponding antibody, usually because an antigen of the same specificity but from another source is present in the system—hence to inhibit.

Inhibition technique. A test which can be either qualitative or quantitative, devised for the detection of group specific substances by means of their inhibiting effect on the corresponding antibody.

Irregular. Atypical.

Iso-agglutinin (now allo-agglutinin). *see* Agglutinin.

Isotonic solution. A solution having the same osmotic pressure as blood.

Karyotype. An individual's set of chromosomes.

Kernicterus. Damage and pigmentation of the brain nuclei, particularly of the basal ganglia, associated with severe neonatal jaundice.

Linked genes. Genes which are carried on the same chromosome and are within measurable distance of each other *c.f.* syntenic genes.

Locus. The position on a chromosome occupied by a gene.

Lysis. The breakdown of cells.

Meiosis. The cell division which produces mature sex cells with half the number of chromosomes possessed by the original cells.

Mitosis. Cell division which produces daughter cells with the same number of chromosomes as the original cells. All cell division, with the exception of that which produces mature sex cells, is mitotic.

Modifying gene. A gene which modifies the expression of another gene.

Mosaic. A mixture of characters produced by a cross-over occurring within the confines of a gene.

Mutation. A change in a gene resulting in the formation of another allele. Allelomorphs are thought to have arisen as the result of mutations. Mutation is very rare in man.

Naturally-occurring antibodies. *See* Agglutinin (typical).

Non-secretor. An individual who does not secrete the appropriate A, B, or H group specific substances in his body fluids.

Normal saline. Isotonic saline.

Ovum. The female gamete or sex cell.

Pan-agglutinable cells. Red cells which are agglutinated by all human sera irrespective of blood group.

Panel of cells. A set of standard red cells specially selected to detect and identify blood group antibodies.

Pan-agglutinin. *see* Agglutinin.

Phenotype. A group of individuals who when tested with a particular set of antisera are found to belong to the same type or sub-type, but who may not necessarily all be of the same genotype, *e.g.* Group A, which includes the genotypes *AO* and *AA*.

Plasma. The fluid portion of unclotted blood.

Poly-agglutinable red cells. Cells that are agglutinated by most but not all human sera regardless of blood group.

Polypeptide. A long chain of amino-acids linked by peptide bonds.

Polysaccharide. One of a group of complex carbohydrates of large molecular size.

Position effect. The effect which blood group antigens have upon each other by virtue of the relative position of their genes on the chromosome pair, *e.g.* the different effect of E upon D in the genotypes R^2r (*cDE/cde*) and R^0r'' (*cDe/cdE*).

Potency. Strength, particularly strength of antiserum.

Precipitin. An antibody which reacts with its corresponding antigen to form a precipitate.

Propositus. Member of family through which the family came to be investigated.

Proteolytic enzyme. An organic compound which specifically effects the digestion of protein, *e.g.* trypsin.

Protocol. The original record made of the results of a test.

Prozone phenomenon. In an antigen-antibody system, a negative reaction obtained with low dilutions of the antibody, although a positive reaction is obtained with higher dilutions of the same antibody.

Pseudo-agglutination. Clumping of red cells by other agents than antibodies. The cells are not distorted or damaged.

Pseudomucinous ovarian cyst fluid. A fluid from certain ovarian cysts which is rich in blood group substances.

Putative. Reputed, supposed—hence putative father, the reputed father of a particular child.

Pyrogen. A substance capable of causing rise of temperature when injected into an animal. Distilled water pyrogens are filtrable, thermostable products probably of bacterial origin, and tend to cause a severe rigor if injected intravenously.

Recessive gene. A gene which only gives rise to its corresponding character when present in "double dose" (in the homozygote).

Recombination. The re-arrangement of genes at gametogenesis so that offspring have new combinations which differ from those of either parent.

Rouleaux formation. A form of pseudo-agglutination in which the red cells give the appearance of piles of coins.

Screening. Preliminary testing.

Secretor An individual who secretes the appropriate A, B, and H substances in the body fluids.

Sensitisation of red cells. Red cells are said to be sensitised when they have antibody specifically attached to their receptors but are not agglutinated.

Sensitisation of individuals. Stimulation of an individual by an antigen which renders him liable to form antibodies.

Serum. The fluid portion of clotted blood.

Siblings. Children of the same parents.

Somatic cells. Body cells as opposed to sex cells.

Specificity. The special affinity between an antigen and its corresponding antibody.

Sperm. The male gamete or sex cell.

Suppressor gene. A modifying gene which will completely or partially suppress the expression of another gene.

Syntenic genes. Genes known to be on the same chromosome whether or not linkage can be directly measured between them.

Thermal amplitude. The temperature range within which an antibody reacts.

Titrate. To make a series of dilutions. To determine the strength of an antigen or antibody by making a series of dilutions and testing their strength against the corresponding antibody or antigen—hence titration.

Titre or titration value. A numerical evaluation of the strength of an anti-serum, usually expressed as the reciprocal of the highest dilution at which it reacts with the corresponding antigen by a given technique.

Trans position. Being on opposite chromosomes and may or may not be within the same cistron.

Variant. Different type, usually applied to the rarer forms.

Warm antibody. An antibody reacting better at 37°C than at lower temperatures.

Zygote. A fertilised egg cell.

Appendix IV - Numerical Index of Techniques

"One, two, buckle my shoe;
Three, four, shut the door;..."

NURSERY RHYME

Appendices

Index